OUTPATIENT MEDICINE

OUTPATIENT MEDICINE

STEPHAN D. FIHN, M.D., M.P.H.

Associate Professor of Medicine and Adjunct
    Associate Professor of Health Services,
University of Washington;
Chief, Section of General Internal Medicine,
Seattle Veteran Affairs Medical Center,
Seattle, Washington

STEVEN R. McGEE, M.D.

Assistant Professor of Medicine,
University of Washington;
Director, The Medical Follow-up Clinic,
Seattle Veteran Affairs Medical Center,
Seattle, Washington

W. B. SAUNDERS COMPANY

Harcourt Brace Jovanovich, Inc.

Philadelphia, London, Toronto, Montreal, Sydney, Tokyo

W. B. SAUNDERS COMPANY
Harcourt Brace Jovanovich, Inc.

The Curtis Center
Independence Square West
Philadelphia, PA 19106

Library of Congress Cataloging-in-Publication Data

Outpatient medicine / [edited by] Stephan D. Fihn, Steven R. McGee.
   p.   cm.
  ISBN 0-7216-3480-X
  1. Ambulatory medical care—Handbooks, manuals, etc. I. Fihn,
Stephan D. II. McGee, Steven R.
  [DNLM: 1. Ambulatory Care. 2. Preventive Medicine.   WX 205 0942]
RC55.088 1992
616—dc20
DNLM/DLC
for Library of Congress

91-46870
CIP

To Rosalie and Judy without whose help,
hard work, support, and forbearance
this book would have never come to be.

Material in the chapters listed below is in public domain:

CONTRIBUTORS

MOHAMED ABDEL-AZIN, M.D.
Research Fellow in Urology, West Roxbury Veterans Affairs Medical Center, West Roxbury, Massachusetts.
Urinary Incontinence

JESSIE H. AHRONI, A.R.N.P.
Research Assistant, General Internal Medicine Clinic, Seattle Veterans Affairs Medical Center, Seattle, Washington.
Diabetic Foot Care Education; Local Care of Diabetic Foot Lesions

DENNIS ANDRESS, M.D.
Assistant Professor of Medicine, University of Washington School of Medicine, Seattle, Washington. Attending Physician, Seattle Veterans Affairs Medical Center, Seattle, Washington.
Paget's Disease; Osteoporosis

MANUEL J. ARBO, M.D., M.P.H.
Fellow, Infectious Disease Program, New England Medical Center, Boston, Massachusetts.
Ambulatory Cardiac Monitoring

ANTHONY L. BACK, M.D.
Acting Instructor, Division of Oncology, Department of Medicine, University of Washington School of Medicine, Seattle, Washington.
Changes in Mentation in the Patient with Cancer; Management of Pain in the Patient with Cancer; Dyspnea in the Cancer Patient

HOWARD BARNEBEY, M.D.
Assistant Clinical Professor, Department of Ophthalmology, University of Washington School of Medicine, Seattle, Washington.
Screening for Glaucoma; Glaucoma

WILLIAM S. BECKETT, M.D., M.P.H.
Associate Professor of Medicine, Departments of Internal Medicine and Epidemiology and Public Health, Yale University School of Medicine, New Haven, Connecticut. Attending Physician, Department of Internal Medicine, Yale–New Haven Hospital, New Haven, Connecticut.
Screening for Occupational Lung Disease

DONALD W. BELCHER, M.D.
Associate Professor of Medicine, University of Washington School of Medicine, Seattle, Washington. Attending Physician, Seattle Veterans Affairs Medical Center, Seattle, Washington.
Periodic Health Assessment

RICHARD E. BERGER, M.D.
Associate Professor of Urology, University of Washington School of Medicine. University of Washington Affiliated Hospitals, Seattle, Washington.
Male Infertility; Impotence

JUDYANN BIGBY, M.D.
Associate Professor of Medicine, Harvard Medical School, Boston, Massachusetts. Associate Physician, Brigham and Women's Hospital, Boston, Massachusetts.
Diagnosis and Management of Drug Abuse; Diagnosis and Management of Alcoholism

THOMAS D. BIRD, M.D.
Professor of Medicine, University of Washington School of Medicine, Seattle, Washington. Chief, Section of Neurology, Seattle Veterans Affairs Medical Center, Seattle, Washington.
Tremor

EDWARD J. BOYKO, M.D., M.P.H.
Associate Professor of Medicine and Epidemiology, University of Washington School of Medicine, Seattle, Washington. Attending Physician, Seattle Veterans Affairs Medical Center, Seattle, Washington.
Inflammatory Bowel Disease

MICHAEL K. BRAWER, M.D.
Associate Professor, Department of Urology, University of Washington School of Medicine, Seattle, Washington. Attending Physician, University Hospital, Seattle, Washington. Chief, Section of Urology, Seattle Veterans Affairs Medical Center, Seattle, Washington.
Cancer of the Genitourinary System; Prostate Cancer

JOHN D. BRUNZELL, M.D.
Professor of Medicine, University of Washington School of Medicine, Seattle, Washington.
Hyperlipidemia

DIANA D. CARDENAS, M.D.
Associate Professor, Department of Rehabilitation Medicine, University of Washington School of Medicine, Seattle, Washington. Director, Rehabilitation Medicine Clinic, University of Washington Medical Center, Seattle, Washington.
Chronic Pain Syndrome

ROBERT M. CENTOR, M.D.
Associate Professor of Internal Medicine and Chair, Division of General Internal Medicine, Medical College of Virginia, Richmond, Virginia. Attending Physician, Medical College of Virginia Hospital, Richmond, Virginia.
Pharyngitis

MANUEL D. CERQUEIRA, M.D.
Associate Professor of Radiology and Internal Medicine, University of Washington School of Medicine, Seattle, Washington. Director, Nuclear Cardiology, University of Washington Medical Center and Seattle Veterans Affairs Medical Center, Seattle, Washington.
Radionuclide Assessment of Cardiac Function

JAMES J. COATSWORTH, M.D.
Clinical Associate Professor of Medicine (Neurology), University of Washington School of Medicine, Seattle, Washington. Attending Neurologist, Virginia Mason Hospital, Seattle, Washington.
Seizures; Electroencephalography

THOMAS G. COONEY, M.D.
Professor of Medicine and Residency Program Director, Oregon Health Sciences University, Portland, Oregon. Attending Physician, Portland Veterans Affairs Medical Center, Portland, Oregon.
AIDS

MICHELE G. CYR, M.D.
Assistant Professor of Medicine, Brown University School of Medicine, Providence, Rhode Island. Program Director, General Internal Medicine Residency, Rhode Island Hospital, Providence, Rhode Island.
Menopausal Symptoms

DAVID C. DALE, M.D.
Professor of Medicine, University of Washington School of Medicine, Seattle, Washington. Attending Physician, University of Washington Medical Center, Seattle, Washington.
Lymphadenopathy

RICHARD A. DEYO, M.D., M.P.H.
Professor of Medicine, University of Washington School of Medicine, Seattle, Washington. Director, Health Services Research and Development, Seattle Veterans Affairs Medical Center, Seattle, Washington.
Low Back Pain

ANDREW K. DIEHL, M.D., M.S.
Professor of Medicine, University of Texas School of Medicine, San Antonio, Texas. Chief, Division of General Medicine, University of Texas Health Science Center at San Antonio, San Antonio, Texas.
Biliary Tract Disease

DOUGLAS EINSTADTER, M.D.
Assistant Professor of Medicine, Case Western Reserve University, Cleveland, Ohio. Attending Physician, Cleveland Metropolitan Hospital, Cleveland, Ohio.
Cholesterol Screening

DIANE L. ELLIOT, M.D.
Associate Professor of Medicine, Division of General Medicine, Oregon Health Sciences University, Portland, Oregon.
Diagnosis of Pregnancy; Asthma in Pregnancy; Thyroid Disorders in Pregnancy; Diabetes Mellitus in Pregnancy; Gestational Diabetes Mellitus; Pregnancy and Hypertension

STEPHAN D. FIHN, M.D., M.P.H.
Associate Professor of Medicine, Adjunct Professor of Health Sciences, University of Washington School of Medicine, Seattle, Washington. Chief, General Internal Medicine, Seattle Veterans Affairs Medical Center, Seattle, Washington.
Role of the Ambulatory Provider; Redness of the Eye; Colorectal Cancer Screening; Shoulder Pain; Injection of the Shoulder; Dysuria; Nephrolithiasis; Urinary Tract Infections in Women; Back Pain in the Cancer Patient; Bacteriuria in Pregnancy

DAVID G. FRYER, M.D.
Associate Clinical Professor of Medicine, University of Washington School of Medicine, Seattle, Washington. Neurologist, Virginia Mason Clinic, Seattle, Washington.
Dementia

VICTOR Y. FUJIMOTO, M.D.
Fellow, Reproductive Endocrinology Center, University of California, San Francisco, California.
Female Infertility

GREGORY L. GARDNER, M.D.
Assistant Professor of Medicine, Division of Rheumatology, University of Washington School of Medicine, Seattle, Washington. Adjunct Assistant Professor of Orthopedics, University of Washington School of Medicine. Attending Physician, University of Washington Medical Center, Seattle, Washington.
Hip Pain; Wrist and Hand Pain; Knee Pain; Ankle and Foot Pain; Polymyalgia Rheumatica and Temporal Arteritis; Osteoarthritis

MARY ELLEN GILLES, M.D.
Attending Physician, Medical Service, Tucson Veterans Affairs Medical Center, Tucson, Arizona.
Obesity

MICHAEL G. GLENN, M.D.
Assistant Professor, Department of Otolaryngology and Head and Neck Surgery, University of Washington School of Medicine, Seattle, Washington. Attending Physician, University of Washington Medical Center, Veteran Affairs Medical Center, Harborview Medical Center, and Providence Hospital, Seattle, Washington.
Epistaxis

ERIKA GOLDSTEIN, M.D., M.P.H.
Assistant Professor of Medicine, University of Washington School of Medicine, Seattle, Washington. Attending Physician, Harborview Medical Center, Seattle, Washington.
Determinants of Patient Satisfaction; Hyperventilation Syndrome

GEOFFREY H. GORDON, M.D.
Associate Professor of Medicine and Psychiatry, Oregon Health Sciences University, Portland, Oregon. Attending Physician, Portland Veterans Affairs Medical Center and Oregon Health Sciences University, Portland, Oregon.
Somatization

ROBERT J. GRIEP, M.D.
Associate Professor of Medicine and Radiology, University of Washington School of Medicine, Seattle, Washington. Associate Staff Consultant, Providence Medical Center, University of Washington Medical Center, Harborview Medical Center, and Seattle Veterans Affairs Medical Center, Seattle, Washington.
Screening for Thyroid Disease; Common Thyroid Disorders

JOHN S. HALSEY, M.D.
Chief, Endoscopy Services, Skagit Valley Hospital, Mount Vernon, Washington.
Diarrhea; Jaundice; Cirrhosis and Chronic Liver Failure; Viral Hepatitis

KENNETH E. HAMRICK, O.D.
Adjunct Assistant Clinical Professor, Pacific University College of Optometry, Forest Grove, Oregon. Director, Ophthalmology-Optometry Clinic, Seattle Veterans Affairs Medical Center, Seattle, Washington.
Visual Impairment

JODIE K. HASELKORN, M.D., M.P.H.
Assistant Professor (Acting), Rehabilitation Medicine, University of Washington School of Medicine, Seattle, Washington. Attending Physician, Seattle Veterans Affairs Medical Center, Seattle, Washington. Consulting Medical Staff, University of Washington and Harborview Medical Center, Seattle, Washington.
Chronic Pain Syndrome

JAY W. HEINECKE, M.D.
Assistant Professor, Department of Medicine, Washington University School of Medicine, St. Louis, Missouri. Attending Physician, Lipid Research Clinic, Washington University School of Medicine, St. Louis, Missouri.
Hyperlipidemia

DAVID H. HICKAM, M.D.
Associate Professor of Medicine, Oregon Health Sciences University, Portland, Oregon. Coordinator, Health Services Research and Development, Portland Veteran Affairs Medical Center, Portland, Oregon.
Chest Pain; Angina

ALLEN D. HILLEL, M.D.
Associate Professor, Department of Otolaryngology and Head and Neck Surgery, University of Washington School of Medicine, Seattle, Washington. Chief, Otolaryngology Section, Seattle Veterans Affairs Medical Center, Seattle, Washington. Attending Physician, University of Washington Medical Center, Seattle, Washington.
Detection and Initial Management of Oral Cancer

JAN V. HIRSCHMANN, M.D.
Professor of Medicine, University of Washington School of Medicine, Seattle, Washington, Assistant Chief, Medical Service, Seattle Veterans Affairs Medical Center, Seattle, Washington.
Principles of Dermatologic Diagnosis and Therapy; Pruritis; Corns and Calluses; Warts; Superficial Fungal Infections; Scabies and Lice; Eczema; Sebhorrheic Dermatitis; Herpes Zoster; Acne; Psoriasis; Malignant Melanoma; Urticaria

RICHARD M. HOFFMAN, M.D.
Acting Instructor in Medicine, University of Washington School of Medicine, Seattle, Washington. Ambulatory Care Fellow, Seattle Veterans Affairs Medical Center, Seattle, Washington.
Sleep Apnea Syndromes; Assessment of Physical Activity

ROBERT G. HOLMAN, M.D.
Assistant Professor of Surgery, University of Washington School of Medicine, Seattle, Washington. Staff Surgeon, Seattle Veterans Affairs Medical Center, Seattle, Washington. Attending Surgeon, Harborview Medical Center and University of Washington Medical Center, Seattle, Washington.
Diverticulitis

THOMAS M. HOOTON, M.D.
Associate Professor of Medicine, University of Washington School of Medicine, Seattle, Washington. Medical Director, Madison Clinic, Harborview Medical Center, Seattle, Washington.
Sexually Transmitted Diseases

DAVID H. INGBAR, M.D.
Associate Professor of Medicine, Pulmonary Medical and Critical Care, University of Minnesota School of Medicine, Minneapolis, Minnesota. Codirector, Medical Intensive Care Unit, University of Minnesota Hospital and Clinic, Minneapolis, Minnesota.
Pleuritic Chest Pain; Hemoptysis; Pleural Effusion

ANDREW F. INGLIS, Jr., M.D.
Assistant Professor of Otolarygology, University of Washington School of Medicine, Seattle, Washington. Attending Physician, Childrens Hospital and University of Washington Medical Center, Seattle, Washington.
Otitis Media and Externa

KAJ JOHANSEN, M.D.
Professor of Surgery, University of Washington School of Medicine, University of Washington, Seattle, Washington. Acting Chief of Surgery, Harborview Medical Center, Seattle, Washington.
Peripheral Arterial Disease; Doppler Measurement of Ankle Pressures

WISHWA N. KAPOOR, M.D., M.P.H.
Professor of Medicine, University of Pittsburgh School of Medicine. Attending Physician, Presbyterian University Hospital, Montifiore University Hospital, and Pennsylvania Veterans Affairs Medical Center, Pittsburgh, Pennsylvania.
Syncope; Palpitations; Ambulatory Cardiac Monitoring

DANIEL L. KENT, M.D.
Associate Professor of Medicine, University of Washington School of Medicine, Seattle, Washington. Director, Problem Evaluation Center, and Staff Physician, Seattle Veterans Affairs Medical Center, Seattle, Washington.
Screening for Dementia

MICHAEL B. KIMMEY, M.D.
Assistant Professor of Medicine, University of Washington School of Medicine, Seattle, Washington. Director of GI Endoscopy, University of Washington Medical Center, Seattle, Washington.
Peptic Ulcer Disease

SHOBA KRISHNAMURTHY, M.D.
Clinical Associate Professor, University of Washington School of Medicine, Seattle, Washington. Attending Physician, Providence Medical Center, Seattle, Washington.
Constipation

WENDY LEVINSON, M.D.
Associate Professor of Medicine, Oregon Health Sciences University, Portland, Oregon. Assistant Chief, Department of Medicine, and Associate Director, Internal Medicine Training Program, Good Samaritan Hospital, Portland, Oregon.
Effective Communication in the Ambulatory Care Setting

THOMAS D. LINDQUIST, M.D., Ph.D.
Associate Professor, Department of Ophthalmology, University of Washington School of Medicine, Seattle, Washington. Attending Physician, Seattle Veterans Affairs Medical Center, University of Washington Medical Center, Harborview Medical Center, and Childrens Hospital, Seattle, Washington.
Dry Eyes and Excessive Tearing; Cataracts; Foreign Bodies and Corneal Abrasions; Conjunctivitis; Foreign Body Removal

BENJAMIN A. LIPSKY, M.D.
Associate Professor of Medicine, University of Washington School of Medicine, Seattle, Washington. Director, General Internal Medicine Clinic, Seattle Veterans Affairs Medical Center, Seattle, Washington.
Adult Immunizations; Fever; Urinary Tract Infections in Men; Bacteriuria in the Elderly

TIMOTHY E. LITTLE, M.D.
Assistant Professor of Medicine, University of Washington School of Medicine, Seattle, Washington. Attending Physician, Seattle Veterans Affairs Medical Center, Seattle, Washington.
Abdominal Pain; Sigmoidoscopy and Colonoscopy; Upper Gastrointestinal Endoscopy

JAMES B. MACLEAN, M.D.
Associate Clinical Professor of Medicine, University of Washington School of Medicine, Seattle, Washington. Section Head of Neurology, Virginia Mason Clinic, Seattle, Washington.
Multiple Sclerosis

KATHLEEN H. MAKIELSKI, M.D.
Assistant Professor, Department of Otolaryngology and Head and Neck Surgery, University of Washington School of Medicine, Seattle, Washington. Chief, Otolaryngology and Head and Neck Surgery, Pacific Medical Center, Seattle, Washington.
Hiccough (Singultus); Hoarseness

MEREDITH MATTHEWS, M.D., M.P.H.
Associate Professor of Medicine, University of Washington School of Medicine, Seattle, Washington. Attending Physician, Providence Medical Center, Swedish Medical Center, Seattle, Washington.
Chronic Renal Failure; Hematuria; Proteinuria; Electrolyte Abnormalities

THOMAS H. MATSKO, M.D., Ph.D.
Attending Physician, Montana Deaconess Medical Center, Columbus Medical Center, Great Falls, Montana.
Diabetic Retinopathy

STEVEN R. McGEE, M.D.

Assistant Professor of Medicine, University of Washington School of Medicine, Seattle, Washington. Attending Physician, Seattle Veterans Affairs Medical Center, Seattle, Washington.

Weight Loss; Anorexia; Dyspnea; Dizziness; Fatigue; Cerumen Removal; Edema; Congestive Heart Failure; Exercise Tolerance Testing; Dyspepsia; Dysphagia and Heartburn; Hemorrhoids and Anal Fissures; Restless Legs Syndrome; Muscle Cramps; Painful and Swollen Calf; Raynaud's Syndrome; Leg Ulcers; Alcohol Withdrawal; Idiopathic Facial Palsy (Bell's Palsy); Scrotal Pain; Scrotal Mass

ROGER E. MOE, M.D.

Associate Professor, Department of Surgery, University of Washington School of Medicine, Seattle, Washington. Attending Physician, University of Washington Medical Center, Seattle, Washington.

Breast Masses and Breast Pain

DONALD E. MOORE, M.D.

Associate Professor, Department of Obstetrics and Gynecology, University of Washington School of Medicine, Seattle, Washington. Attending Physician, University of Washington Medical Center, Seattle, Washington.

Abnormal Uterine Bleeding

ANNE W. MOULTON, M.D.

Assistant Professor of Medicine, Division of General Internal Medicine, Brown University School of Medicine, Providence, Rhode Island. Attending Physician, Rhode Island Hospital, Providence, Rhode Island.

Cervical Cancer

CYNTHIA MULROW, M.D.

Associate Professor, University of Texas Health Science Center at San Antonio, San Antonio, Texas. Attending Physician, Audrie Murphy Veterans Affairs Medical Center, San Antonio, Texas.

Screening for Hearing Impairment

ALVIN I. MUSHLIN, M.D., SC.M.

Associate Professor of Community and Preventative Medicine and Medicine, University of Rochester School of Medicine and Dentistry, Rochester, New York. Attending Physician, University of Rochester School of Medicine, Strong Memorial Hospital, Rochester, New York.

Breast Cancer Screening; Mammography

KAREN L. NIGUT, M.D.
Fellow in General Internal Medicine, Division of General Internal Medicine, Rhode Island Hospital, Providence, Rhode Island.
Menopausal Symptoms

JAMES C. ORCUTT, M.D., Ph.D.
Associate Professor of Ophthalmology, University of Washington School of Medicine, Seattle, Washington. Adjunct Associate Professor of Otolaryngology and Head and Neck Surgery, University of Washington School of Medicine. Chief, Ophthalmology Section, Seattle Veterans Affairs Medical Center, Seattle, Washington. Attending Physician, University of Washington Medical Center, Seattle, Washington.
Eye Pain

CATHERINE M. OTTO, M.D.
Assistant Professor of Medicine, Division of Cardiology, University of Washington School of Medicine, Seattle, Washington. Attending Physician, University of Washington Medical Center, Seattle, Washington.
Aortic Stenosis; Other Valvular Disease; Echocardiography

DOUGLAS S. PAAUW, M.D.
Assistant Professor, Division of General Internal Medicine, Department of Medicine, University of Washington School of Medicine, Seattle, Washington. Attending Physician, University of Washington Medical Center, Harborview Medical Center, Seattle, Washington.
Gout/Hyperuricemia; Gynecomastia

CAROLYNN PATTEN, M.S., P.T.
Physical Therapist, Motor Control Laboratory, Department of Physical Therapy, Sargent College of Allied Health Professions, Boston University, Boston, Massachusetts.
Principles of Physical Therapy

LAIRD G. PATTERSON, M.D.
Associate Clinical Professor, Department of Medicine, Section of Neurology, University of Washington School of Medicine, Seattle, Washington. Attending Physician, Virginia Mason Hospital, Seattle, Washington.
Entrapment Neuropathies; Parkinsonism

ROGER E. PECORARO, M.D.*

Associate Professor of Medicine, Division of General Internal Medicine, University of Washington School of Medicine, Seattle, Washington. Attending Physician, Seattle Veterans Affairs Medical Center, Seattle, Washington.

Diabetes Mellitus

STEVEN H. PETERSDORF, M.D.

Assistant Professor, Medical Oncology, Department of Medicine, University of Washington School of Medicine, Seattle, Washington. Attending Physician, University of Washington Medical Center, Harborview Medical Center, Seattle, Washington.

Thrombocytopenia; Polycythemia; Anemia; Sickle Cell Disease

JEANNE POOLE, M.D.

Assistant Professor of Medicine, University of Washington School of Medicine, Seattle, Washington. Attending Physician, Harborview Medical Center, Seattle, Washington.

Chronic Ventricular Arrhythmias; Supraventricular Arrhythmias

HUBERT N. RADKE, M.D.

Associate Professor of Surgery, University of Washington School of Medicine, Seattle, Washington. Chief, Surgical Service, Seattle Veterans Affairs Medical Center, Seattle, Washington.

Diverticulitis

PAUL G. RAMSEY, M.D.

Professor and Chairman, Department of Medicine, University of Washington School of Medicine, Seattle, Washington. Attending Physician, University of Washington Medical Center, Seattle, Washington.

Sinusitis

JOHN RAVITS, M.D.

Assistant Clinical Professor of Medicine, University of Washington School of Medicine, Seattle, Washington. Attending Physician, Section of Neurology, Virginia Mason Medical Center, Seattle, Washington.

Muscular Weakness; Electromyography and Nerve Conduction Studies

---

*Deceased.

NANCY RISSER, M.N., R.N., C., A.N.P.
Clinical Instructor, University of Washington School of Nursing, Seattle, Washington. Clinical Instructor, Seattle University, Seattle, Washington. Respiratory Clinical Nurse Specialist and Adult Nurse Practitioner, Seattle Veterans Affairs Medical Center, Seattle, Washington.
Smoking Cessation

NANCY J. ROBEN, A.R.N.P., B.S.N.
Adult Nurse Practitioner, Seattle Veterans Affairs Medical Center, Seattle, Washington.
Chronic Anticoagulation

GERALD J. ROTH, M.D.
Professor of Medicine, University of Washington School of Medicine, Seattle, Washington. Chief, Hematology Section, Seattle Veterans Affairs Medical Center, Seattle, Washington.
Bleeding; Transfusion Therapy

ELAINE SACHTER, M.D.
Physician, Virginia Mason Clinic, Seattle, Washington.
Mitral Valve Prolapse

MARK M. SCHUBERT, M.D., D.D.S., M.S.D.
Associate Professor, Oral Medicine, School of Dentistry, University of Washington, Seattle, Washington. Adjunct Assistant Professor, Otolaryngology and Head and Neck Surgery, University of Washington School of Medicine, Seattle, Washington. Attending Physician, University of Washington Medical Center, Fred Hutchinson Cancer Center, Swedish Hospital, Seattle, Washington.
Dental Disease

JANE SCHWEBKE, M.D.
Assistant Professor of Medicine, Northwestern University, Chicago, Illinois. Medical Director, STD/HIV Clinic, Chicago Department of Health, University of Chicago, Chicago, Illinois.
Vaginitis

KIRK K. SHY, M.D., M.P.H.
Associate Professor of Obstetrics and Gynecology, University of Washington School of Medicine, Seattle, Washington. Attending Physician, University of Washington Medical Center, Seattle, Washington.
Contraception

KATHLEEN C.Y. SIE, M.D.
Clinical Fellow, Childrens Hospital, Boston, Massachusetts. Clinical Fellow, Department of Otolaryngology, Harvard Medical School, Boston, Massachusetts.
Tinnitus

DAVID L. SIMEL, M.D.
Assistant Professor of Medicine, Duke University, Durham, North Carolina. Associate Chief of Staff, Ambulatory Care, Durham Veterans Affairs Medical Center, Durham, North Carolina.
Principles of Screening

GREGORY E. SIMON, M.D.
Acting Instructor, Psychiatry and Behavioral Sciences, University of Washington School of Medicine, Seattle, Washington. Staff Psychiatrist, Group Health Cooperative of Puget Sound, Seattle, Washington.
Screening for Depression; Generalized Anxiety; Management of Depression; Psychosis; Panic Disorder; The Difficult Patient

SHAWN J. SKERRETT, M.D.
Assistant Professor of Medicine, Pulmonary and Critical Care Medicine, University of Washington School of Medicine, Seattle, Washington. Attending Physician, Seattle Veterans Affairs Medical Center, Seattle, Washington.
Cough and Sputum; Upper Respiratory Infection; Lower Respiratory Infection; Asthma and Chronic Obstructive Pulmonary Disease; Pulmonary Function Testing; Thoracentesis; Arterial Blood Gas

C. SCOTT SMITH, M.D.
Acting Assistant Professor of Medicine, University of Washington School of Medicine, Seattle, Washington. Attending Physician, Boise Veterans Affairs Medical Center, Boise, Idaho.
Hypertension Screening; General Principles of Consultation; Preoperative Cardiovascular Problems; Preoperative Infectious Disease Problems; Preoperative Endocrine Problems; Preoperative Hematologic Problems; Preoperative Pulmonary Problems

DAVID L. SMITH, M.D.
Associate Professor of Medicine, Oregon Health Sciences University, Portland, Oregon. Attending Physician, Veterans Affairs Medical Center, Portland, Oregon.
Prepatellar and Olecranon Bursitis

JOHN F. STEEGE, M.D.
Associate Clinical Professor, Department of Obstetrics and Gynecology, Duke University School of Medicine. Attending Physician, Duke University Medical Center, Durham, North Carolina.
Pelvic Pain in Women

SUSAN STEINDORF, M.S., P.T.
Physical Therapist, Children's Orthopedic Hospital, Seattle, Washington.
Principles of Physical Therapy

JOHN F. STEINER, M.D., M.P.H.
Assistant Professor of Medicine, University of Colorado Health Sciences Center, Denver, Colorado. Attending Physician, University Hospital, Denver Veterans Affairs Medical Center, Denver, Colorado.
Compliance; Essential Hypertension

JOHN B. STIMSON, M.D.
Clinical Assistant Professor of Medicine, University of Washington School of Medicine, Seattle, Washington.
Abnormal Taste and Smell; Fibromyalgia; Myofascial Pain Syndromes; Trigger Point Injection; Benign Prostatic Hyperplasia

LYNNE P. TAYLOR, M.D.
Clinical Instructor, University of Washington School of Medicine, Seattle, Washington. Neurologist, Virginia Mason Hospital, Fred Hutchinson Cancer Center, and Swedish Hospital, Seattle, Washington.
Cerebrovascular Disease

WILLIAM M. TIERNEY, M.D.
Professor of Medicine, Indiana University School of Medicine, Indianapolis, Indiana. Attending Physician, Wishard Memorial Hospital, University Hospital, Indianapolis, Indiana.
Determining Disability: The Primary Physician's Role

SUSAN W. TOLLE, M.D.
Associate Professor of Medicine, Division of General Internal Medicine, Director, Center for Ethics in Health Care, Oregon Health Sciences University, Portland, Oregon. Attending Physician, Oregon Health Sciences University Hospital and Clinics, Portland, Oregon.
Death of Clinic Patients

BARBARA WEBER, M.D.
Fellow in General Medicine, University of Pittsburgh School of Medicine, Pittsburgh, Pennsylvania.
Palpitations

CRAIG G. WELLS, M.D.
Assistant Professor, Department of Ophthalmology, University of Washington School of Medicine, Seattle, Washington. Attending Physician, University of Washington Medical Center, Harborview Hospital, and Childrens Hospital. Staff Surgeon, Seattle Veterans Affairs Medical Center, Seattle, Washington.
Ophthalmoscopy

RICHARD H. WHITE, M.D.
Professor of Clinical Medicine, University of California at Davis. Attending Physician, University of California Davis Medical Center, Sacramento, California.
General Approach to Arthritic Symptoms; Interpretation of Serologic Tests; Injection of the Trochanteric Bursa; Aspiration/Injection of the Knee

SUE ANNE WIEDENFELD, Ph.D.
Clinical Assistant Professor, Department of Psychiatry and Behavioral Science, University of Washington School of Medicine, Seattle, Washington.
Insomnia; Psychological Assessment

JOYCE E. WIPF, M.D.
Assistant Professor of Medicine, University of Washington School of Medicine, Seattle, Washington. Attending Physician, Seattle Veterans Affairs Medical Center, Seattle, Washington.
Tuberculosis Screening; Atrial Fibrillation; Headache; Peripheral Neuropathy

PÅL WÖLNER-HANSSEN, D.M.S.
Department of Obstetrics and Gynecology, University of Lund, Lund, Sweden.
Pelvic Inflammatory Disease

SUBBARAO V. YALLA, M.D.
Associate Professor of Surgery (Urology), Harvard Medical School, Boston, Massachusetts. Chief, Urology Section, Veterans Affairs Medical Center, West Roxbury, Massachusetts.
Urinary Incontinence

ACKNOWLEDGMENTS

Much of the credit for this project goes to our many contributors, who were able to condense extensive amounts of clinical literature into readable and practical reviews. We are grateful to Gregory J. Raugi, Charles E. Pope II, Wayne Levy, and Donald Sherrard, who reviewed many of the chapters. We also want to thank Maureen Morrison, Rosalie O'Leary, and Myrna Dumo, who typed and retyped much of the manuscript. BiLan Chiong and Pauline Haley also assisted in this task. John Fitzpatrick at Editorial Services of New England diligently shepherded the manuscript through production. Finally, our sincerest thanks to our editor from Saunders, John Dyson, who through innumerable difficulties, has been a source of constant encouragement, enthusiasm, and counsel.

NOTICE

Medicine is an ever-changing field. Standard safety precautions must be followed, but as new research and clinical experience broaden our knowledge, changes in treatment and drug therapy become necessary or appropriate. The editors of this work have carefully checked the generic and trade drug names and verified drug dosages to ensure that the dosage information in this work is accurate and in accord with the standards accepted at the time of publication. Readers are advised, however, to check the product information currently provided by the manufacturer of each drug to be administered to be certain that changes have not been made in the recommended dose or in the contraindications for administration. This is of particular importance in regard to new or infrequently used drugs. It is the responsibility of the treating physician, relying on experience and knowledge of the patient, to determine dosages and the best treatment for their patient. The editors cannot be responsible for misuse or misapplication of the material in this work.

FOREWORD

Having had the privilege of browsing through this book in manuscript form, my impression is that the editors and contributors have assembled a novel, helpful collection of concise articles that will be of assistance to all physicians who deal with ambulatory adult patients. The intended readership includes not only general internists and family practitioners, but also physicians whose principal interests lie in other fields: the medical subspecialties, obstetrics, and various branches of surgery. Thus its subjects include some minor, early manifestations which tend to be categorized as belonging within the provinces of organized specialties but which actually do not require specialized skills and technologies.

The work recognizes the realities of a new era, in which medical practice has shifted from a preponderance of acute infectious processes afflicting younger patients to today's medicine, in which we deal largely with an older patient population, presenting chronic problems related to more than one disease and more than one organ system.

The authors and editors also recognize the obligation of today's health care providers to limit costs, avoid expensive hospital care, and enable patients to continue their regular activities in normal life settings. Thus we frequently find the statement that a certain diagnostic or therapeutic procedure is *not* warranted. Also there is information about relative costs of medicines which could be prescribed for the same complaint.

I am acquainted with the editors, as well as many of the contributors, and I know their dedication to ambulatory medical care. It has been gratifying to observe their success in teaching this branch of medicine, and to see how warmly it is esteemed by medical students and house officers.

PAUL B. BEESON

PREFACE

The delivery of medical care in the United States has changed radically in the past decade. These changes have included a myriad of new technologies for diagnosis and treatment, a striking transformation in the way medical care is funded, and new demands for physician accountability and patient autonomy. While the process of medical care has become increasingly complex, there has been a paradoxical shift in the primary site where care is delivered from the highly controlled environment of the hospital to the much less structured milieu of the clinic. When they first arrive in the clinic, experienced house officers quickly realize that acumen acquired on the inpatient service is of only limited value in this arena. A whole new set of skills and knowledge are required to practice effectively in the outpatient setting. Unfortunately, the typical busy clinic routine does not allow for the leisurely rounds and lectures that form the core of teaching on the wards. Unlike captives confined to hospital beds, outpatients have schedules to keep just like their physicians. All too often, the clinic attending has no special training for this role and finds his or her outpatient teaching repertoire lacking. Moreover, the attending may also be expected to see his or her own patients along with the residents.

To cope with this demanding set of circumstances we have, for the past decade, held weekly primary care rounds at the Seattle Veteran's Affairs Medical Center, in which the approach to common outpatient problems is discussed in a critical and practical fashion. *Outpatient Medicine* was inspired by these rounds and by the experience of teaching outpatient medicine to house officers. The primary care rounds frequently generate in-depth reviews with fresh insights into common ambulatory problems; many of the presentations are condensed into chapters here. The teaching of residents produced the need for outpatient medicine "mini-lectures," comprehensive enough to be helpful but brief enough to be practical during a busy clinic. We include in the *Outpatient Medicine* these concise reviews that address the most common clinical questions encountered in an adult medicine clinic. We do not intend this book to substitute for a comprehensive ambulatory medicine textbook.

After introductory chapters which survey general aspects of ambulatory care and preventive medicine, the book is divided by organ systems. Within each organ system chapter there are four types of sections: (1) screening for disease, (2) approach to common symptoms, (3) approach to specific problems and syndromes, and (4) procedures. Much of the information is condensed into tables and, if appropriate, diagnostic or therapeutic algorithms. To avoid unnecessary repetition of information, the chapters are extensively cross-referenced. Each chapter concludes with several key references, annotated to guide further reading.

We hope the busy student, house officer, and practicing generalist will carry this book to clinic and refer to it when direction is needed during their encounters with patients. We encourage your comments and criticisms.

STEPHAN D. FIHN
STEVEN R. McGEE

CONTENTS

CHAPTER III

CONSTITUTIONAL SYMPTOMS

CHAPTER IV

DISORDERS OF THE SKIN

CHAPTER V

DISORDERS OF THE EYE

CHAPTER VI

DISORDERS OF THE EARS, NOSE, MOUTH, AND THROAT

CHAPTER VII

RESPIRATORY DISORDERS

CHAPTER VIII

CARDIOVASCULAR DISORDERS

CHAPTER IX
GASTROINTESTINAL DISORDERS

CHAPTER X
MUSCULOSKELETAL DISORDERS

CHAPTER XIII
ENDOCRINE DISORDERS

CHAPTER XIV
WOMEN'S HEALTH

CHAPTER XV

GENITOURINARY AND RENAL DISORDERS

CHAPTER XVIII

THE PATIENT WITH KNOWN CANCER

CHAPTER XIX

THE PREGNANT PATIENT

CHAPTER XX

THE PREOPERATIVE PATIENT

GENERAL ASPECTS OF AMBULATORY CARE

1 ROLE OF THE AMBULATORY PROVIDER

STEPHAN D. FIHN

Life is short, and the Art long; the occasion fleeting; experience fallacious and judgment difficult. The physician must not only be prepared to do what is right himself, but also to make the patient, the attendants, and externals cooperate.

Hippocrates, from the *Aphorisms*

For the past 50 years, the primary setting of adult medical care and of medical education has been the hospital ward. The bulk of expenditures for medical care traditionally has been consumed in the inpatient setting. Medical students and internal medicine residents have spent the overwhelming majority of their clinical rotations addressing the needs of hospitalized patients.

Today, for a variety of reasons, medical care is being delivered more often in the office or clinic than in the hospital. The enormous expense of hospitalization has compelled both payers and patients to seek alternatives, especially outpatient treatment. As a result, inpatient days decreased nationwide between 1984 and 1989, while outpatient visits rose 32%, to over 300 million, in the same period.[1] Many problems that a few years ago would have mandated hospital admission are now routinely treated in the clinic. This trend has been hastened by the development of sophisticated diagnostic and therapeutic interventions that can be safely and effectively used in the outpatient setting. Patients usually prefer the lower cost and morbidity associated with outpatient treatment. Those patients who need hospitalization are now being discharged sooner, in part because of reimbursement schedules that pay a fixed amount for a given diagnosis, irrespective of length of stay. Early outpatient follow-up is typically an integral part of the discharge plan.

The transfer of care to the outpatient setting has made the hospital ward a less attractive site for training students and house staff. Most hospital admissions are now for previously diagnosed conditions or complications occurring

1

in severely compromised hosts. Many types of clinical disorders, such as endocrinologic, rheumatologic, and dermatologic diseases, are seldom encountered in the hospital. There is little opportunity to observe the evolution of disease or understand its effect on the patient's daily life. Trainees develop a narrow perspective of medical care and fail to appreciate the complexity and importance of continuity of care in the outpatient setting. Pressure to reduce the length of hospital stays, an emphasis on technical procedures, and the use of predetermined therapeutic protocols limit opportunities for teaching and independent thought. In response to these concerns, many training programs are steadily increasing the amount of time trainees devote to ambulatory care.

In this rapidly changing environment, the evolving role of the ambulatory care provider is a demanding one. Coincident with the escalating complexity and specialization of medical care, there has been a paradoxically increasing demand for primary care physicians who can deliver comprehensive longitudinal care. Patients look to their primary care provider to take a broad perspective on their medical condition, rather than focusing exclusively on a single organ system. Patients with complex problems also want their primary physician to serve as an advocate and advisor and to coordinate the care delivered by a multitude of specialists. Health care purchasers such as insurers, large corporations, governmental agencies, and health maintenance organizations also look to the primary care physician to plan and coordinate care and, in the process, to control costs. As the coordinator of care, the ambulatory care provider is expected to address the full spectrum of problems that arise, not only medical but social and emotional problems as well. In addition to dealing with diagnostic and therapeutic issues, the practitioner is often asked to assist patients with financial and living arrangements.

Some may view this array of responsibilities as too demanding or as extending unnecessarily beyond the bounds of traditional medical practice. This view is particularly common among trainees who have grown accustomed to the inpatient environment, where most attention is typically directed toward reversing acute problems and correcting physiologic derangements. The goals of outpatient treatment, however, are often substantially different from those of inpatient treatment and mandate a broader view of the provider's role. Many patients may be elderly and suffering from a number of different disorders. Established chronic diseases often cannot be eradicated or reversed, and the primary aims of therapy are to lessen symptoms and improve function as well as to prevent further deterioration. To achieve these ends, it is essential to understand the patient's activities, resources, and support systems. In the process, the provider often develops an intimate bond with the patient and the patient's family—one of the uniquely satisfying experiences of providing continuous care.

Inured as most are to the inpatient setting, trainees frequently find their introduction to ambulatory care unsettling. Unlike inpatients, who are often highly dependent medically and under almost continuous observation, outpatients are independent people with their own agendas and responsibilities. Busy clinic schedules may not allow time to address all issues in complete depth, requiring that problems be prioritized and dealt with selectively. Orders cannot simply be written with the assurance that the patient will actually take a medication or undergo a procedure. Patients may be unable or unwilling to make frequent follow-up visits. They want to be involved in decisions about their care, making negotiation between the patient and provider a common occurrence.

In recent years, several large-scale clinical trials have addressed issues in the management of common outpatient problems. Nonetheless, well-controlled trials dealing with a number of common outpatient topics are lacking, and much of practice remains based largely on experience and opinion. Recognizing this fact, the practitioner should remain flexible and be willing to seek imaginative solutions to thorny problems. For a variety of reasons, it is often impossible to adhere to textbook recommendations. Taking a confrontational approach with a patient is usually ill-advised. It is far better to seek a compromise solution. Partial solutions, though less satisfying, are usually preferable to impractical solutions and many times achieve a successful clinical outcome.

The experienced ambulatory practitioner becomes adept at operating effectively and efficiently in this complicated environment. One important aspect is to involve the patient fully in the process of care. Patients are usually cognizant of time pressures and are eager to forge a successful working partnership with the provider. They appreciate the provider's attempts to tailor diagnostic and treatment plans to meet their special individual needs. They endorse efforts to educate them about the nature of their condition and about beneficial measures they can take. Patients often avidly accept responsibility for aspects of their own care, such as monitoring parameters and adjusting therapy. Well-timed feedback reinforces these positive behaviors.

The deft outpatient clinician also learns to use time effectively as an important diagnostic and therapeutic agent. Simply observing a patient to glean more data before making a decision to intervene is often more informative than any laboratory or imaging test. The therapeutic qualities of "tincture of time" are hackneyed but nonetheless genuine. Most patients are grateful for efforts to limit the time and expense required by numerous clinic visits and extensive diagnostic evaluations. Astute clinicians develop a sense for the tempo of a patient's illness and plan follow-up intervals accordingly. Longer intervals between visits are often possible by scheduling interim telephone contact.

Because imaging tests are often inconvenient and must be scheduled in the future, the outpatient provider must rely heavily on the physical examination. Routine, complete physicals are rarely warranted, whereas the careful, directed exam is essential.

One of the more time-consuming tasks is maintaining medical records. Because of the frequent complexity of outpatient management and involvement of multiple providers, the record of care must be clear and adequately detailed.

Yet, to keep pace, the practitioner must also make notes concise. A modified SOAP (Subjective/Objective Assessment and Plan) format is often a useful way to organize data. An entry for each category of each problem is not necessary at every visit. The advantage of this approach is that it helps to maintain an active problem list, which is essential for tracking patients with complicated problems over time. The use of flow sheets greatly aids in the care of outpatients and saves time. At a minimum, the clinician should use the flow sheet to record preventive services provided and to track important clinical data such as blood pressure, weight, blood glucose levels in diabetics, and the like. Used in this manner, a flow sheet can be a valuable reminder to perform indicated procedures and can save the time otherwise spent reviewing a thick record to determine when a given procedure was last performed. Flow sheets can also be used to update medication profiles, obviating the need to list them anew after each visit.

The clinician must judiciously manage not only time but other resources as well. Many current insurance plans provide only limited outpatient coverage, sometimes resulting in substantial out-of-pocket expenses for patients. Frequent office visits and multiple prescriptions are a financial burden for many families. Providing high-quality care requires sensitivity to the cost of care and making every effort to balance expense against expected benefit. All too often patients are asked to undertake difficult or costly treatment programs for which evidence of effectiveness is absent or marginal. Even some treatments of known efficacy may be of dubious value if other, more serious illnesses are present. Therapies that seem trivial to the provider may be quite vexing to patients. Each time the patient is seen, it is worthwhile reexamining the therapeutic regimen and reconsidering the risks and cost-benefit ratio.

A sensible approach to providing preventive care is also important. A number of screening tests and interventions have been conclusively shown to reduce morbidity and improve survival. The outpatient provider should aggressively implement these procedures whenever indicated. As was recently reviewed in a comprehensive report, many commonly performed procedures, even some vigorously advocated by professional organizations, lack convincing evidence of efficacy.[2] The clinician should apply interventions with the same thoughtfulness that all other types of care are given.

In the hectic clinic atmosphere, clinicians occasionally forget the important role they play in their patients' lives. Even though patients may recognize the inability of medical care to halt or completely palliate an irreversible decline in their health, many derive consolation and comfort from visits with their regular practitioner. The salutary effects of simply listening and caring should never be dismissed.

As society comes to recognize the limits of technology, there is a resurgence of respect and enthusiasm for the central role of the primary care provider. It is an exacting role that is intellectually challenging and emotionally rewarding. The next decade will witness a reorganization of medical delivery centering on outpatient facilities, with the emergence of new tests and treatments for use in this setting.

The astute clinician will master these advances but will continue to recognize that effective practice requires applying this knowledge in an individualized manner guided by a meaningful, personal relationship with the patient.

REFERENCES

1. Eubanks P. Outpatient care: a nationwide revolution. Hospitals 1990;64:28.

2. U.S. Preventive Services Task Force. Guide to Clinical Preventive Services: An assessment of the effectiveness of 169 interventions. Report of the U.S. Preventive Services Task Force. Baltimore, Williams & Wilkins, 1989.

2 DETERMINANTS OF PATIENT SATISFACTION

ERIKA GOLDSTEIN

Despite considerable research, the determinants of patient satisfaction remain poorly understood. General aspects of the provider-patient encounter that may influence patient satisfaction relate to the patient's sociodemographic background, the cost of and access to health care, the organizational and physical aspects of the health care setting, and the provider's behavior.

Patient satisfaction correlates with the provider's humanistic and communicative skills and with the patient's perceptions of the provider's technical competence. Although patients may be poor judges of the technical skills of physicians, their perceptions are paramount in assessing humanistic qualities.

In a study sponsored by the American Board of Internal Medicine, twenty-four aspects of physician behavior were found to influence patients' assessments of a physician's humanistic skills (Table 2–1). The nine aspects rated as most important by patients were (1) courtesy, (2) preparation by the doctor, (3) taking the patients' complaints seriously, (4) maintaining a relaxed atmosphere, (5) listening to and understanding what patients have to say, (6) explaining the examination, (7) providing clear and complete explanations, (8) knowing his or her limitations, and (9) involving the patient in treatment decisions.

These categories translate into specific actions the provider can take to enhance patients' satisfaction. For example, the courteous physician always greets patients and family members by name. To be prepared, the provider should always review the medical record before entering the examining room. A phone call to the patient at home conveys support and interest. Such small but important efforts improve patient satisfaction and, in turn, the quality of

TABLE 2–1.   CHARACTERISTICS OF THE HUMANISTIC PHYSICIAN

Getting the Visit Off to a Good Start
1. Professionalism: neat appearance
2. Professionalism: does not "carry over" from previous patients
3. Respect for patients: punctuality
4. Respect for patients: treats patient as an equal
5. Supportive of patients: courtesy*
6. Supportive of patients: relaxed atmosphere*

Finding Out What the Problem Is
7. Professionalism: preparation by doctor*
8. Professionalism: limits interruptions
9. Respect for patients: listens and understands patients*
10. Respect for patients: explains examination*
11. Supportive of patients: takes patients' complaints seriously*
12. Supportive of patients: concerned about patient's life

Talking About the Problem and What To Do About It
13. Professionalism: clear and complete explanations*
14. Professionalism: knows limitations*
15. Respect for patients: involves patients in treatment*
16. Respect for patients: honesty
17. Supportive of patients: takes time to talk to patient
18. Supportive of patients: encourages patients to ask questions

Following-up on the Problem and Treatment
19. Professionalism: provides access and coverage
20. Professionalism: follows through
21. Respect for patients: involves patient in managing the problem
22. Respect for patients: conscious of patient's financial situation
23. Supportive of patients: checking on patients at home
24. Supportive of patients: follows up on what patient should be doing

Source: Carter WB, Inui TS, UW-ABIM Study Group. How patients judge the humanistic skills of their physicians. [Presented at American Public Health Meetings and available from Dr. Carter, Department of Health Services (SC-37), University of Washington, Seattle, WA, 98195.]
*Rated most important by patients.

care. Carefully eliciting and addressing the patient's concerns is central to patient satisfaction with care. Sound medical knowledge and procedural skills by themselves do not constitute high-quality medical care. Good communication skills, respect, and empathy are as important to patients.

Cross-references: Effective Communication in the Ambulatory Setting (Section 3), The Difficult Patient (Section 195).

REFERENCES

1. Subcommittee on Evaluation of Humanistic Qualities of the Internist, American Board of Internal Medicine. Evaluation of humanistic qualities in the internist. Ann Intern Med 1983;99:720–724.
   Position paper reviewing the charge to the subcommittee and its findings.

2. Carter WB, Inui TS, UW-ABIM Study Group. How patients judge the humanistic skills of their physicians. (Presented at American Public Health Meetings and available from Dr.

Carter, Department of Health Services (SC-37), University of Washington, Seattle, WA, 98195).
Review of an ABIM sponsored study to develop a patient satisfaction questionnaire.

3. Cleary PD, McNeil BJ. Patient satisfaction as an indicator of quality care. Inquiry 1988;25:25–36.
Interesting review of the relationship between satisfaction and quality.

4. Hall JA, Roter DL, Katz NR. Meta-analysis of correlates of provider behavior in medical encounters. Med Care 1988;26:657–675.
This study, one of several meta-analyses of patient satisfaction literature, focuses on provider behavior.

5. Ware JE, Snyder MK. Dimensions of patient attitudes regarding doctors and medical care services. Med Care 1975;13:669–682.
Attempts to define dimensions of patient attitudes towards their health care.

3 EFFECTIVE COMMUNICATION IN THE AMBULATORY CARE SETTING

WENDY LEVINSON

RATIONALE.   During the medical interview, the clinician must efficiently accomplish three tasks: (1) gather necessary medical information, (2) develop rapport and trust, and (3) educate and instruct the patient.[2,3] Specific communication skills can make the interview more effective and efficient. A successful interview promotes diagnostic accuracy, patient compliance, patient satisfaction, and clinician satisfaction. Throughout the interview, the clinician must actively listen to the patient's concerns and express attentiveness.

INFORMATION GATHERING.   The clinician needs information to formulate diagnostic hypotheses, test them, and reformulate new ones. Patients need to inform the doctor about symptoms, the experience of being ill, and how the problem is affecting their life. Helpful techniques to collect data effectively are listed below.

1.   *Use open-ended questions.* Use of open-ended questions early in the interview provides the interviewer with a broad view of what the patient considers to be important. Clinicians should follow open-ended inquiries with more specific questions to gather missing details. Not only does this approach give a more comprehensive picture of the patient's problem, it is also a more efficient strategy than the traditional use of multiple focused questions.

2.   *Permit the patient to speak without interruption.* On average, physicians first interrupt patients 18 seconds into their opening statement about the purpose of the visit.[1] Early interruptions can disrupt the development of trust and

flow of the interview. The efficient interviewer gathers information in the sequence and organization provided by the patient, rather than forcing the patient to conform to a framework.

3. *Survey the breadth of problems early in the interview.* A problem recognized by all clinicians occurs when the patient mentions a new problem as the interview seems to be concluding. This often occurs when the patient has not expressed his or her real agenda early in the interview. To avoid this the clinician should ask the patient "What else?" after the statement of the initial problem, and should continue asking "What else?" until all the problems that the patient wants to discuss have been set forth. Although it may not be possible to cover all the topics during one visit, the provider and patient can negotiate what will be covered that day.

4. *Facilitate the patient's story.* To help patients tell the story of their illness, clinicians may use statements like "Go on," "Tell me more," and indicate nonverbally to the patient that more detail is desirable. This is particularly useful during the initial part of the history when using open-ended questions.

5. *Summarize and check.* Summarizing or repeating parts of the history provides opportunities to correct inaccurate data and allows patients to know that the clinician listens attentively. This can be done briefly following natural breaks in the interview, before moving to a different line of inquiry.

RAPPORT BUILDING AND ADDRESSING PATIENTS' FEELINGS. Each patient comes to an appointment with real concerns about a problem that interferes with his or her life. The patient has usually thought about the appointment for several days and has often formulated ideas about the cause of the problem and possible treatments. Frequently the problem affects the patient's work, relationships, or sense of well-being. Patients frequently are anxious or distressed when they arrive at the office. Addressing the patient's feelings helps build an alliance between the patient and the clinician and makes the interaction more satisfying for both. Often clinicians feel they are "opening a can of worms" by asking about patients' feelings and are worried that this will take too much time in the interview. In fact, addressing the patient's feelings improves the quality of diagnostic information, the therapeutic alliance, and makes the interview more efficient. Communication skills to build rapport and deal with patient feelings include the following.

1. *Express empathy.* The practitioner should name the feeling that the patient is experiencing. Examples of statements that recognize the patient's emotional experience are "It sounds as though you are really frustrated," or "You seem sad." Such comments indicate concern for the patient's emotional experience.

2. *Express understanding or reassurance about the feeling.* Clinicians should indicate that they genuinely believe the patient's feelings are legitimate. For example, the clinician may say, "Many patients feel anxious when they come to the doctor. That's normal." While clinicians may not always agree that the

emotional reaction is appropriate, they can still understand that it is a real feeling for the patient.

3. *Demonstrate respect.* There are many ways, verbal and nonverbal, to demonstrate respect for the patient. Specific strategies include interviewing the patient when he or she is dressed, especially in an initial interview; providing privacy and expressing concern for the patient's comfort; and asking the patient's opinion about the cause of the problem and ideas about treatment. Understanding patient beliefs about the nature of the illness or treatment options is essential to patient compliance.

4. *Prepare for the interview.* Most patients recognize the clinician's busy schedule and wish to use time to maximum advantage. They also want to feel that the clinician has a special interest in and understanding of their concerns. This concern can be readily conveyed by spending a few minutes reviewing the medical record *before* the visit. Even if the physician is behind schedule, it is worth taking time to review the record after notifying the patient that appointments are running late.

EDUCATION AND MOTIVATION.   To realize the benefit of a therapeutic plan, the clinician and patient need to agree on what the problem is and what to do about it. Negotiation is particularly important when helping patients with lifestyle changes (e.g., smoking or dietary change). The key to motivating patients is actively involving them in the development of treatment plans rather than prescribing a treatment regimen. The clinician can use simple questions to actively involve the patient and promote compliance.

1. *What do you know about . . . ?* This question allows the clinician to explore the patient's knowledge and beliefs about the illness or treatment. For example, a clinician might ask, "What do you know about diets to manage diabetes mellitus?" During this discussion information can be corrected or added about the treatment.

2. *How do you feel about . . . ?* This allows the clinician to understand the patient's emotional reaction to a particular illness or treatment option. For example, the patient might say that she feels overwhelmed by having to make the dietary changes necessary. The clinician can then express empathy and understanding about the patient's feelings and incorporate this information into modifications of the treatment plan.

3. *What are you willing to do?* Once the patient has the appropriate information about treatment options, it is essential to find out what part of the proposed treatment the patient is willing to implement. Again, this asks the patient to be an active decision-maker instead of blindly following the clinician's plan.

4. *What help might you need?* This asks the patient to anticipate the type of assistance that might be necessary to carry out the plan. For example, the patient with diabetes might need the help of the spouse with the dietary changes; an appointment for both with a nutritionist might be appropriate.

5. *What problems might arise?* It is helpful to ask the patient to anticipate potential barriers to implementing the therapy and allow an opportunity to plan strategies to address these difficulties. If unmentioned, these barriers might lead to noncompliance.

6. *Now what is your plan?* With this question the clinician asks the patient to reiterate in detail the treatment plan. The clinician can check what the patient has heard and probe any discrepancies between the patient's and clinician's understanding of the plan. The review also reinforces the patient's responsibility for implementing the treatment plan.

Cross-references: Determinants of Patient Satisfaction (Section 2), Compliance (Section 4).

REFERENCES

1. Beckman HB and Frankel RM. The effect of physician behavior on the collection of data. Ann Int Med 1984;101:692–696.

    The average patient has three reasons for a visit and gets interrupted within an average of 18 seconds of starting to tell his or her story. Few patients are allowed to tell their story fully. How these interviewing errors interfere with collection of adequate data and alter the doctor patient relationship is discussed.

2. Bird J, Cohen-Cole SA, Mance R. The three function model of the medical interview. In: Lipkin M, Putnam S, Lazare A, eds. The Medical Interview. New York: Springer Verlag, 1991.

    Describes three functions of the clinical interview: data gathering, emotion handling, and behavior management. A set of basic interviewing skills is described.

3. Lipkin M. The medical interview and related skills. In: Branch WT, ed. The Office Practice of Medicine. Philadelphia: W.B. Saunders Co.; 1987:1287–1306.

    Provides stepwise guidance and insight into the opening of the interview; practical advice about the physical environment, preparing oneself to listen, and how to structure the opening.

4 COMPLIANCE

JOHN F. STEINER

Compliance with therapy is defined as the extent to which a patient's behavior (in keeping appointments, modifying life-style, taking medications, and so forth) conforms to medical advice.[2] Compliance is a crucial link between the *process* of medical care (the interaction between doctor and patient) and the *outcomes* of care (the physiologic and functional consequences of treatment). Clinicians often distinguish patients who are "compliant" with treatment from those who are "noncompliant." In fact, many patients take their medications intermittently; these patients are better viewed as partially compliant rather than as absolutely noncompliant with therapy. For most chronic diseases, rates of partial compliance with medications range from 30% to 50%; lack of adherence to recommended behavioral changes is even more common.[2] Partial compliance has long been identified as a barrier to successful treatment; over 30 years ago, patients with a history of rheumatic fever who failed to take sufficient antibiotic prophylaxis were found to have higher rates of recurrent streptococcal infections. More recent work has confirmed the link between partial compliance and poor therapeutic outcomes. For example, reduced compliance is the most common reason for inadequate blood pressure control in hypertensive patients, a common reason for rehospitalization in hypertensives and patients with congestive heart failure, and a predictor of poor seizure control in epileptics.

Physicians often regard partial compliance simplistically, as the patient's defiance of the doctor's orders. Recent research in the social sciences suggests that variations in compliance are better understood as a component of the patient's attempt to control or regulate the illness,[5] based on his or her understanding of the disease and its treatment. A clinician who understands the reasons for such medication "experiments" can better assist the patient toward their common goal of treating the disease.

DIAGNOSIS OF PARTIAL COMPLIANCE WITH MEDICATIONS.   Identification of partially compliant patients is difficult. Using intuition alone, physicians cannot predict accurately which patients are taking their medications as prescribed. Moreover, attainment of a therapeutic goal, such as a controlled blood pressure, is not an accurate measure of compliance, because many factors other than drug therapy, such as regression to the mean, concurrent nonpharmacologic treatment, or the natural history of the disease, also influence treatment outcomes. Serum drug levels or physiologic effects of drugs (resting pulse in patients on beta-adrenergic blockers, prothrombin times in patients receiving warfarin) are also imperfect compliance measures because of pharmacokinetic and pharmacodynamic variability between individuals. Compliance measures used in clinical trials, such as pill counts and electronic medication monitors, are too cumbersome or expensive for routine use. Measures of medication refill rates from centralized pharmacies in managed health care systems may be helpful in assessing pill acquisition, the first stage in compliance. The best screening test for reduced compliance in clinical care is to ask the patient, directly but nonjudgmentally: "Most people have trouble taking their medicine. Do you ever have trouble taking yours?" In response to this question, about 50% of patients who are partially compliant will acknowledge the fact (that is, the sensitivity of self-report is about 50%), and reports of reduced compliance are generally accurate (positive predictive value of 80% to 90%).[3] However, even those who acknowledge partial compliance will generally report being more compliant than they actually are.

IMPROVEMENT OF COMPLIANCE.   Having recognized partial compliance, the physician should next consider whether the patient would benefit from improved adherence. In their efforts at self-regulation, some patients may have correctly discovered that their medications were unnecessary or were prescribed in excessive doses. If the patient has attained the desired outcome despite partial compliance, it may be possible to stop the drug or reduce the medication dose.

To improve compliance, the clinician should begin by exploring the patient's view of the illness and its treatment. Although attempts to educate the patient about the disease and its consequences are useful, such efforts alone rarely suffice to improve compliance. Simple treatment regimens lead to better compliance; patients are most likely to comply with once-a-day drugs.[1] Strategies for behavior modification can also enhance compliance, in several ways: (1) The individual can learn to monitor the illness through techniques such as home blood pressure measurement or glucose testing. (2) The patient can link medication taking to other routine activities. For example, the patient can store pills next to the coffeepot or hairbrush, where they will be seen every morning. (3) Family members or home health care workers can be enlisted to monitor the disease or assist the patient in taking pills. (4) The clinician can establish contracts with the patient to provide rewards for adherence, such as credit toward the purchase of a blood pressure cuff for home use. (5) Finally, the physician can identify and reschedule patients who drop out of care. Combinations of these behavioral strategies work best, and require continuous reinforcement.[4]

REFERENCES

1. Cramer JA, Mattson RH, Prevey ML, Scheyer RD, Ouellette VL. How often is medication taken as prescribed? A novel assessment technique. JAMA 1989;261:3273–3277.
   This study demonstrates the insights which electronic medication monitors can offer in compliance research, proves the clinical adage that adherence improves with simpler medication regimens, and links compliance to outcomes (seizure control) in a group of epileptic patients.

2. Haynes RB, Taylor DW, Sackett DL, Eds. Compliance in Health Care. Johns Hopkins University Press, Baltimore, 1979.
   The standard textbook in the field; describes the epidemiology, measurement, and implications of compliance for medical practice and clinical research.

3. Haynes RB, Taylor DW, Sackett DL, Gibson ES, et al. Can simple clinical measures detect noncompliance? Hypertension 1980;2:757–764.
   The best evaluation of clinically practical means of compliance assessment; self-report had a sensitivity of 50% and a specificity of 96% for detecting reduced compliance as measured by pill counts.

4. Haynes RB, Wang E, Gomes MD. A critical review of interventions to improve compliance with prescribed medications. Patient Educ Counseling 1987;10:155–166.
   A recent literature synthesis. Emphasizes the need for practitioners to learn and employ techniques of behavior modification to improve adherence.

5. Leventhal H, Cameron L. Behavioral therapies and the problem of compliance. Patient Educ Counseling 1987;10:117–138.
   A view of compliance from the perspective of the social sciences. Summarizes the most common theories of compliance behavior.

5 DETERMINING DISABILITY: THE PRIMARY PHYSICIAN'S ROLE

WILLIAM M. TIERNEY

The traditional problem-oriented approach to diagnosis and treatment often ignores assessments of the patient's function, comfort, and sense of well-being. A more complete description of illness requires the physician to consider a more global framework that encompasses measures of both physical and social function and their effects on quality of life. The integration of medical and social considerations is essential to competent assessment of disability.

In Western society, a person's concept of self and self-worth are inextricably intertwined with occupation and the ability to work. People often introduce themselves by the work they perform: "I am _____ and I do _____." Moreover, income from employment is necessary for most interactions with society.

Disability insurance protects patients from the financial and social consequences of the inability to work. The largest provider of disability insurance benefits is the Social Security Administration, whose Disability Insurance Benefit and Supplemental Security income programs make payments to more than 4 million Americans.[3] Most disability programs deem a person disabled according to rigorous preestablished criteria, based on objective medical information obtained from the physical examination and diagnostic tests. Unfortunately, the disease orientation of modern medical education fails to prepare most clinicians for determining disability. Yet the primary care physician is often asked by the patient, the patient's representative, or the insuring agency to make disability assessments and to supply relevant information or counsel patients.

DEFINING DISABILITY. Disability is an administrative concept defined by explicit criteria outlined in individual policies, and these criteria may differ greatly between policies. For the Social Security Administration's disability program, these criteria are contained in the Listings of Impairments, recorded in the Handbook for Physicians,[2] which can be obtained from state disability determination agencies or any local Office of Hearings and Appeals of the Social Security Administration. These criteria, organized by organ system, list the objective findings that either must have been present for at least a year or are likely to be fatal for a claimant to be deemed disabled.

A claimant may become officially disabled in three ways. First, he may meet all the objective requirements. For example, the claimant may satisfy the Social Security listing for coronary artery disease by having chest pain compatible with angina pectoris and a positive treadmill exercise electrocardiogram (with positive results explicitly defined). Second, when criteria are not exactly met, disability boards may declare other combination of findings equivalent to the impairment criteria. For example, the exercise electrocardiogram may show only nonspecific changes but a thallium scan may reveal an exercise defect. Third, some disability insurance programs judge a patient disabled despite failure to meet all criteria when significant objective evidence of disease exists that reduces the patient's ability to work below some specified level. Each insuring agency strictly defines these levels of functioning, and judgments concerning the applicant's ability to perform past work may also take into consideration nonmedical factors such as age and education. Some insurance policies will pay if a person cannot perform relevant past work, others require that a person be unable to perform any work. The Social Security Administration's disability program does consider past work experience, age, and education.

Each person eligible for disability insurance payments has paid premiums. This includes the Social Security disability program, where the premium is part of the Social Security taxes. Although the merits of any program are debatable, the patient should collect if a particular policy provides payments for a condition and the condition exists. The physician should supply information and not judge the merits of any insurance program.

APPLYING FOR DISABILITY. To file for disability, the patient supplies a detailed medical and work history and identifies physicians likely to have relevant clinical information. The agency sends disability forms for physicians to complete, and these data are forwarded to a person or outside agency who judges whether the claimant's condition meets the objective criteria. The Social Security Administration has contracts with disability determination agencies in each state. If there is a favorable ruling, the patient is awarded disability benefits and the process ends, although the agency usually has the right to reevaluate a claimant at a later date if the condition is one that may improve with time. If the judgment is unfavorable, the patient may appeal through an explicit process that varies among insuring agencies. For the Social Security Administration, the initial appeal is made to the state disability determination agency. If the ruling is again unfavorable, the patient may appeal for a hearing before an administrative law judge who will examine the evidence, question the patient, possibly call on expert witnesses (medical or vocational), and render an independent decision. Many patients secure the services of an attorney to represent them at disability hearings. Social Security regulations require that these lawyers work on a contingency basis, with payment not to exceed 25% of any potential benefits accrued during the period preceding a favorable judgment. If the judge's decision is favorable to the patient, the ruling is automatically appealed to the Appeals Council of Social Security. If the ruling is unfavorable, the patient may also appeal to the council, which can require a new hearing if there is evidence of procedural error or inattention to important details. Finally, if the Appeals Council denies the claim, the patient can appeal to the federal district court. Care and associates list the likelihood of a ruling favorable to the patient at each step of this process for Social Security disability applications.[1]

REQUESTS FOR CLINICAL INFORMATION. In addition to requests from the insuring agency, patients or their representatives (usually attorneys) may ask physicians to supply information. The primary care physician should always comply with these requests when the information is available. For the patient, who often has no other income, attention to these requests may be more important than the attention paid to their clinical problems.

Physicians should supply only the relevant facts whenever possible. It helps greatly to know the specific criteria to which the patient's information will be compared. For Social Security disability, the listings are available,[2] but criteria for other disability insurance programs usually are not readily available. Regardless, the physician's primary role is to supply objective information. For example, if the patient suffers from chronic obstructive lung disease, relevant information would include spirometric measurements, arterial blood gas studies, results of chest radiography, and evidence of acute exacerbations. For arthritis, relevant information includes the range of motion of affected joints, evidence of motor dysfunction, joint deformity and atrophy, and radiographs. For a malignancy, the data should include cell type, location, evidence of local and distant metastases, and response to therapy.

Physicians' opinions about the patient's disability either carry little weight or may adversely influence the determination of disability. If a physician summarily states that a patient is "totally and permanently disabled" without supplying supporting information, this opinion will do little to improve a patient's chances of receiving disability compensation. Conversely, if a patient's data meet an insurance policy's criteria and the physician states that the patient is not disabled, the objective information will often be ignored and the patient may be told that he is not disabled because of the physician's denial. The sensible course is to record all relevant objective information and assiduously avoid making judgments. A prudent physician will not overstate a patient's case or supply misleading information or opinions, even if pressured to do so by a patient, a lawyer, or an insurance company. Such statements rarely aid a patient's application, may give the patient false hope of a favorable decision, and may cast doubt on other information that the physician has supplied.

The one area where the primary care physician's opinion and judgment are important and useful is in estimating the patient's capacity to perform work. Physical labor is usually defined as heavy, medium, light, or sedentary, terms that are specifically defined.[2] Although not expert in vocational matters, the physician may use the Social Security Administration's Listings of Impairments to aid in judging functional ability. For example, if the objective information almost matches the criteria in the listings, the physician may conclude the patient's residual functional capacity is at the lowest level (sedentary). If the evidence shows less severe disease, yet it is more than slight, then many patients will often be limited to light work. These opinions do carry some weight in disability decisions, but they are still contingent upon, and only as helpful as, good objective data.

THE PHYSICIAN'S ROLE.   Supplying information when requested is an important clinical activity. Indeed, the outcome of disability claims may have major effects on a patient's clinical condition, since disability compensation may supply the funds and health insurance necessary to obtain adequate medical care. The physician may also be asked to supply information in person by testifying at a patient's hearing. Although time-consuming, the appearance of the treating physician often carries much weight.

Physicians may be asked to perform consultative examinations of their own or another physician's patient or as in independent examiner. These examinations are extremely helpful, especially if the examination targets the organ(s) whose dysfunction is the basis for the claim and if the report addresses the objective criteria that must be met. The consultative examiner's opinion as to functional capacity also carries weight in disability deliberations.

Finally, the physician often serves as an advisor to patients. Patients may ask whether they are eligible for disability and whether the physician will write a letter supporting an application. Knowing the relevant criteria will allow the physician to estimate with some accuracy whether the patient is likely to be successful. When agreeing to write a letter, the physician should tell the patient that the letter will contain all relevant facts, but the disability agency will determine whether the patient is disabled. This allows the disability determination process to proceed smoothly, efficiently, and with minimum effect on the doctor-patient relationship.

REFERENCES

1. Carey TS, Hadler NM. The role of the primary physician in disability determination for Social Security insurance and workers' compensation. Ann Intern Med 1986;104:706–710.
    Although somewhat out-of-date, this offers the best description of the process of evaluation of disability claims, the success rate for obtaining disability at each step, and where the primary care physician should be involved.

2. Disability Evaluation Under Social Security. Publication N.05-10089; Washington, D.C.: United States Department of Health and Human Services, 1986.
    Comprehensive listing of the clinical findings necessary for a person to be eligible for disability benefits. It also explains the Social Security's disability evaluation process and defines terms such as "residual functional capacity." It is a handbook that should be in every primary care physician's office.

3. McCoy JL, Weems K. Disabled-worker beneficiaries and disabled SSI recipients: a profile of demographic and program characteristics. Soc Secur Bull, 1989;52:16–28.
    Comprehensive description of the recipients of Social Security disability benefits.

6 DEATH OF CLINIC PATIENTS

SUSAN W. TOLLE

ADVANCE DIRECTIVES. Because approximately 80% of patients die in hospitals or long-term care facilities, it is important that families and physicians have previously discussed and understood the patient's preferences regarding life-sustaining treatment. Ideally, these discussions should occur in the clinic, long before the terminal hospital admission. Such conversations benefit the patient, who still has enough good health and time to make thoughtful decisions, and the family and the physician, who become confident that they know the patient's preferences. In one study of surviving spouses a year after a loved one's death,[6] those spouses who made decisions about withholding or withdrawing life-sustaining treatment without the benefit of a prior directive from the patient had many continuing anxieties. They continued to wonder whether or not they had made the right decision, whereas spouses who clearly understood their loved one's wishes were more often at peace with their decisions. Communication both respects the patient's values and facilitates the adjustment of survivors.

Even though most patients wish their doctors would talk with them about advance planning for serious illness, initiating these conversations can be uncomfortable for the physician and the patient.[2] Patients' anxieties often increase when they fear their doctor is encouraging advanced planning for medical reasons (e.g., "I must have cancer or he wouldn't be bringing this up"). Patients find it reassuring to know that the physician talks with all of his or her patients about these issues, and that the patient has not been specifically selected for this discussion because the physician has serious concerns about the patient's health. A helpful approach is to open the conversation with: "I like to talk with all of my patients about advance planning for serious illness. I do not expect any sudden change in your health in the near future but an accident could happen to any of us at any time. There have been some recent changes in the law which clarify a patient's rights to set limits on their health care. Many of my patients want to talk about these laws and share their values and goals. I am open to talking with you about these issues."

Two types of advance directives that patients may complete are commonly available: the living will, which is more prevalent and allows patients the right to refuse life-sustaining treatment when their death is imminent; and the newer and more flexible document, the power of attorney for health care, which allows patients to appoint someone to act as their health care representative should they be unable to speak for themselves. Although advance directives are often completed in the outpatient setting, recent federal legislation (the Patient's Self-determination Act, effective December 1, 1991), requires that all adult patients admitted to hospitals, nursing homes, or hospice programs be informed of their right to refuse life-sustaining treatment and offered the opportunity to sign an advance directive.

NOTIFICATION OF A PATIENT'S DEATH.   Following a patient's death, the needs of the survivors are influenced by the duration of the patient's illness, whether the death was expected, the patient's age, the amount of advanced planning and guidance the patient has provided, whether family members were present at the time of death, and the strength of the physician-family relationship. When desired by the patient after a long terminal illness, death may be a relief for the family and physician. Conversely, sudden and unexpected death in a healthy person can be catastrophic for survivors.

Expected Death.   Most patient deaths, whether they occur at home, in long-term care facilities, or in acute care hospitals, are anticipated. It is important to discuss several issues with the patient and family before the patient's death. (1) Tell patients specifically what to expect regarding their illness. (2) Reassure patients that you will not desert them and that you will help keep them comfortable. (3) Help patients share the diagnosis with friends or family so they can provide support and help with advance planning and legal issues. (4) Discuss advance directives. (5) Encourage conversations about organ donation and autopsy. Family members take particular comfort in knowing they have followed the patient's wishes.

When the patient dies, families appreciate timely notification and privacy (i.e., a room where they can grieve together without interruption), the opportunity to return to the patient's bedside, and the extra time physicians may spend with them. Predictable questions may arise: Did the patient suffer? What was the immediate cause of death? Was the patient aware of the family members' presence? Was there anything the family could have done to prevent the patient's death? What does the family do next? Religious preferences should be considered, and if appropriate, specific denominational representatives should be summoned.

The physician should understand the hospital's administrative procedures regarding completion of forms, return of personal effects, autopsy, and organ donation. Federal legislation requires that family members be offered the opportunity to consent to an anatomical gift if the patient is medically eligible as a donor. Before these discussions take place, however, the physician should determine the patient's eligibility to avoid offering the opportunity to donate only to realize later that the organs or tissues cannot be used. Consent for organ donation and autopsy is the exclusive prerogative of the next of kin or legal guardian; the physician can only advise, explaining potential benefits to the family while respecting their right to accept or refuse.

The physician's support of the family does not end with the patient's death. For close family members, the bereavement period is characterized by depressive symptoms and somatic complaints and, for some, increased rates of hospitalization and even death. Table 6–1 lists different avenues of subsequent contact between survivors and primary physicians; these options provide knowledge and comfort, and tend to reduce the survivor's anxiety.

TABLE 6–1.   OPTIONS IN PROVIDING BEREAVEMENT SUPPORT

Send a sympathy card.
Call the family.
Attend the funeral.
Mail bereavement information*: pamphlets on grief and a community support list.
Provide a lay explanation of the autopsy findings.
Schedule a family conference.
Cultivate a network to facilitate your own support.

*Contact your hospital social worker, chaplain, rabbi, priest, or minister.

Unexpected Death.   The unexpected death of a clinic patient creates special needs both for the family, who have little opportunity for advanced planning, and for physicians, who often experience concern about personal inadequacy. Families are often the first to learn of a patient's death when it occurs outside of the hospital; the physician, once notified, should telephone the family to provide emotional support and, if possible, clarify the cause of death.

When an unexpected death occurs in the hospital, physicians are frequently apprehensive about conveying the news to the family. In general, revealing an unexpected death by telephone should be avoided. Most families prefer to be called and asked to come to the hospital, where they can be notified of the death in person. Some consider this practice deceptive and prefer to be told during the initial phone conversation. It is usually easy to separate these two groups. A few survivors, when asked to come to the hospital, will ask the physician directly if the patient has died. They should be told the truth. Most do not ask, however, and they should be invited to come to the hospital and be informed in person. Most survivors prefer to be at the hospital when they are told because it allows direct contact with the physician, offers the opportunity for family members and close friends to be notified together for mutual support, and allows family members an opportunity to see the deceased. Actually visiting the body confirms the reality of death and helps family members overcome denial and begin the grieving process.

Maintaining open communication with the patient's loved ones is especially critical, though often more difficult, when the death was unexpected (Table 6–1). These survivors are likely to benefit from written information about what to expect in the normal grieving process. The optimal timing for bereavement information varies; although some prefer to receive this information after the memorial service, most find it most helpful 2 weeks to 3 months after an unexpected death. After an unexpected death, families often need longer to adjust and are more likely to benefit from a bereavement support group, although many are unable to attend support groups for at least 3 months following the death. Support is even more valuable for families with a limited social support system and for survivors of patients who have committed suicide.

THE PHYSICIAN'S EMOTIONAL NEEDS.   Physicians commonly believe that their own outward expression of grief over a patient's death somehow falls short of personal, professional, or societal expectations. Surviving family members, however, do not find it offensive when physicians express emotion following a patient's death. Physicians cannot help having feelings about the death of a long-standing clinic patient. These feelings may include sadness, fear of inadequacy, a sense of loss, and even a sense of relief. To ignore these feelings or to allow them to go unaddressed is unhealthy. Physicians also benefit from sharing their fears of inadequacy and feelings of loss with a colleague or a support group. Attending a patient's funeral may not only help physicians express and resolve their own feelings, but shows respect for the patient and family.[3]

REFERENCES

1. Creek LV. How to tell the family that the patient has died. Postgrad Med 1980;68(4):207–209.
    Identifies key considerations in notifying survivors of a loved ones death.

2. Gordon GH, Tolle SW. Discussing life-sustaining treatment: a teaching program for residents. Arch of Intern Med 1991;151:567–570.
    Outlines an educational program for residents to practice their skills in discussing advance directives.

3. Irvine P. The attending at the funeral. New Engl J Med 1985;312:1704–1705.
    Argues that physicians often benefit from attending their patient's funerals.

4. Moseley JR, Logan SJ, Tolle SW, et al. Developing a bereavement program in a university hospital setting. Oncol Nurs Forum 1988;15:151–155.
    Describes the development and implementation of a hospital based bereavement program.

5. Seravalli EP. The dying patient, the physician, and the fear of death. N Engl J Med 1988;319:1728–1730.
    Explores the potential adverse impact of our fears in caring for dying patients.

6. Tolle SW, Bascom PB, Hickam DH, et al. Communication between physicians and surviving spouses following patient deaths. J Gen Intern Med 1986;1:309–314.
    Provides data about unmet needs from interviews with 105 surviving spouses.

PREVENTIVE SERVICES

7 PERIODIC HEALTH ASSESSMENT

DONALD W. BELCHER

PREVENTIVE SERVICES. In selecting general preventive services for adult patients, it is important to distinguish between a test's usefulness for diagnostic versus screening purposes. Many tests of proven value in the diagnosis of symptomatic adults (e.g., glucose and hemoglobin determinations, thyroid studies, chest radiography) perform poorly as screening measures in asymptomatic adults. This discussion is largely based on an authoritative review, the *Guide to Clinical Preventive Services,* by the U.S. Preventive Services Task Force,[6] which uses explicit criteria of efficacy and effectiveness to evaluate preventive activities (see Section 12, Principles of Screening) and compares its recommendations with those published by other authorities.

Because the prevalence of a target condition or related risk factors determines a screening test's predictive value, general preventive services are most effective when directed at subgroups with certain age, sex, or behavioral factors (Table 7–1). Patients at higher risk because of a family medical history, environmental hazards, or other risk factors need special preventive services (Table 7–2). Health maintenance flow sheets that list recommended prevention activities, attributes of target groups, and frequency of testing are helpful aids for practitioners. Over 75% of Americans see a physician each year—far more than are likely to volunteer for separate screening programs. Patient visits for management of chronic or episodic illnesses should serve as opportunities to provide preventive services. Rapport and familiarity with an individual patient's health status assist in the appropriate delivery of prevention services.

Certain preventable behaviors lead to disease. Special attention should be given to smoking cessation strategies (see Section 11, Smoking Cessation) and how to identify and manage alcohol and substance abuse (see Section 8, Diagnosis and Management of Drug Abuse, and Section 9, Diagnosis and Management of Alcoholism), areas where physicians express difficulty in intervening. To avoid overlooking adult immunizations, practitioners need to understand the rationale for immunizing general and high-risk patients (see Section 10, Adult Immunizations). Despite incomplete evidence and conflicting recommendations, physicians must make prevention decisions for individual

TABLE 7–1.   PREVENTION RECOMMENDATIONS FOR GENERAL ADULT POPULATION

Procedure	Target Condition	Target Group	Recommendation
Smoking cessation	Cardiovascular and pulmonary disease, some cancers	Smokers	Annual counseling
Alcohol moderation	Medical conditions; accidents, violence	General	Annual counseling
Diet change	Obesity; medical	General	Periodic assessment
Exercise schedule	Coronary heart disease; various	General	Individualize to needs
Blood pressure measurement	Hypertension	General	At 1–2-yr intervals
Breast examination	Breast cancer	Women 40+ yr	Annual
Papanicolaou smear	Cervical cancer	Women 20–65 yr	3 yr or less intervals
Influenza vaccine	Influenza	Elderly; patients with chronic disease	Annual vaccination
Pneumococcal vaccine	Pneumonia	Elderly; patients with chronic disease	Vaccinate once
Tetanus/diphtheria toxoid	Infections	General	10-yr intervals
Cholesterol (total; HDL)	Coronary heart disease	Men and women 20–60 yr	5-yr intervals
Mammography	Breast cancer	Women 50–74 yr	At 2–3 yr intervals
Fecal occult blood test	Colorectal cancer	Men and women 50–74 yr	Optional; 1–2 yrs intervals

patients and should update these recommendations as additional information becomes available.

THE PERIODIC HEALTH ASSESSMENT.   The periodic health assessment is a set of recommended prevention activities to be conducted at specified intervals for various age groups. Periodic health assessment involves more than an examination. It includes risk factor assessment, immunization, disease screening

TABLE 7–2.   PREVENTION RECOMMENDATIONS FOR HIGH-RISK INDIVIDUALS

Procedure	Target Condition	Target Group	Recommendation
Estrogen counseling	Osteoporosis	Women, perimenopausal, smokers	At menopause
Aspirin counseling	Coronary heart disease	Men aged 50+ with cardiovascular risk factors	Periodically
Skin review	Skin cancer	Family history; history of excess sun, cancer precursors[1]	Special surveillance, annual examination
Oral cavity examination	Oropharyngeal cancer	Smokers, drinkers	Annual
Thyroid examination	Thyroid cancer	History of upper body irradiation	2–3-yr intervals
Papanicolaou smear	Cervical cancer	Women aged 65+ with irregular screening history	Annual × 2 negatives
Testes examination	Testicular cancer	Men <40 years; history of cryptorchidism	Periodic
Vaccination (flu, pneumonia)	Pneumonia	Resident of nursing home or extended-care facility	Annual influenza; pneumococcal once
HIV, hepatitis B	AIDS, hepatitis	Possible HIV exposure	Individualize testing; safe sex counseling
VDRL	Syphilis	Multiple sexual partners	Individualize testing
Mammography	Breast cancer	Family history of premenopausal breast cancer	Start at age 35
Colonoscopy	Colorectal cancer	Family history	Persons aged 50+: every 3–5 yr

[1]Dysplastic nevi, some congenital nevi.

(physical examination, laboratory tests, or other procedures), and patient health education (the acronym RISE). It is more selective and individualized than a routine medical checkup and has a higher yield and a lower cost. The purpose of the periodic health assessment is to prevent certain target diseases altogether (primary prevention) or to detect disease at an early stage and improve outcome (secondary prevention).

A consensus on the content or frequency of the adult periodic health assessment is elusive, with authorities often differing in their interpretation of published evidence or recommendations. There may be insufficient information about a disease's natural course (e.g., prostate cancer), the estimated cost-benefit ratio for different screening intervals (mammography), or the appropriateness of applying trial results to age groups other than those studied (cholesterol screening). Much remains to be learned about prevention in adults over age 65, the group at highest risk for many diseases, including coronary heart disease, most cancers, and strokes. Screening activities for vision, hearing, falls, foot problems, and osteoporosis—important concerns for the elderly—are generally not listed among recommendations because test effectiveness is unknown.

RECOMMENDATIONS.   Table 7–1 lists recommended adult preventive care activities, the target group, and the frequency of testing.

PREVENTIVE CARDIOLOGY.   Because cardiovascular disease dominates disease patterns in the United States and because effective early detection techniques are lacking, primary prevention is an important goal. Epidemiologic studies, such as the Framingham study, link smoking, hypertension, and elevated cholesterol levels to the development of coronary heart disease, stroke, and peripheral vascular disease. Half of coronary heart disease has been attributed to these three risk factors, including the 30% of cases due to cigarette smoking alone.

Smoking Cessation.   The relative impact on coronary heart disease of quitting smoking or controlling hypertension, compared to the impact of reducing elevated cholesterol levels, has been estimated as 3 or 4 to 1. Smoking cessation also reduces lung disease and deaths from cancer, and improves pregnancy outcome. Widespread public acceptance that smoking cessation is beneficial, an increasing awareness of risk from passive exposure, and smoke-free policies in hospitals, domestic airlines, and many job sites help motivate smokers to change. Strategies to individualize smoking interventions are discussed in Section 11 (Smoking Cessation).

Hypertension.   Treatment of moderate to severe hypertension (diastolic blood pressure of 105 mm Hg or higher) clearly reduces the rates of stroke, congestive heart failure, and hypertensive renal failure. Although most trials have involved only men less than 60 years old, comparable results in women and older persons seem likely. The benefits of treating mild hypertension are less clear.

Because about 60% of hypertensives are overweight—twice the rate as in the general population—it is prudent to include advice about weight control, sodium restriction, and adequate exercise. Recent studies indicate that minority groups experience more complications from hypertension, in part because of lower compliance with medication and a belief in nonmedical models to explain hypertension. These are important topics for physician education. The treatment of systolic hypertension remains difficult and controversial (see Section 86, Essential Hypertension).

Elevated Cholesterol Levels.   In the United States, cholesterol levels tend to rise with age. The evidence for an epidemiologic association of cholesterol levels with coronary heart disease is clear, but the exact benefits of intervention trials are debated. Cholesterol reduction appears to offer greatest benefit for younger adults with high levels. Most physicians tell patients with high cholesterol levels to reduce their fat intake, lose weight, and exercise more. In the trials usually cited, diet was not tested alone but in combination with other interventions, such as smoking cessation (Multiple Risk Factor Intervention Trial [MRFIT], Oslo trial), the treatment of hypertension (MRFIT), or the administration of cholestyramine (Lipid Research Clinic). Persons who consistently comply with dietary advice may lower their cholesterol levels about 5%, but responses vary considerably, and relapse is common. Consequently, a decision to intervene usually involves the prescription of a lipid-lowering medication and regular testing (see Section 155, Hyperlipidemia). Many physicians do not have the time, nutritional information, or behavior modification skills necessary to counsel patients regarding diet; these physicians are encouraged to involve dietitians and to refer patients to selected community nutrition education programs.

The total cholesterol level, measured without fasting, was the value used in epidemiologic studies and all primary prevention trials and remains the starting point for assessing an individual's risk. Recent food intake does not affect values. The National Cholesterol Education Program (NCEP) recommends that all adults be tested at 5-year intervals. High-risk persons, defined as those having a total cholesterol level of 240 mg/dl or higher, should also undergo lipoprotein analysis to determine high-density and low-density lipoprotein values before diet modification or lipid-lowering medications are prescribed. Persons with borderline cholesterol levels (200–239 mg/dl) and two or more risk factors (including male sex) or known coronary heart disease are managed as high-risk individuals.

Although the NCEP guidelines are valuable as a structured screening approach, there is concern that they may overstate the potential benefit of cholesterol reduction for women and older persons or for men with only modest cholesterol elevations. All trial subjects were men less than 60 years old for whom interventions were made at higher cholesterol cutoff points. Until future trials in men and women of all ages demonstrate the feasibility and benefits of lowering cholesterol levels, it seems prudent to direct screening efforts toward high-risk groups, including persons with known coronary heart disease, those with a relevant family history (i.e., of hyperlipidemia, heart attack, or sudden death before age 55), or patients who smoke, are hypertensive, or have diabetes mellitus. An optional group to screen might be other adults under age 60, with their age-based 90th percentile ($\geq$265 mg/dl) taken as the level for intervention.

CANCER RISK REDUCTION AND SCREENING. Cancer, the second leading cause of death in the United States, was the focus of the earliest risk reduction and screening studies. Few cancers are amenable to early detection and treatment. Screening trials for lung cancer in male smokers, for example, have been uniformly unsuccessful, which emphasizes the need to dissuade new smokers and to encourage smokers to quit. Research in the causative and protective roles of dietary factors in cancer development is expanding. Available information is retrospective (case-control), with diet trials now underway. The Surgeon General has published diet recommendations consistent with good nutritional practices and aimed at reducing the risk of developing certain cancers. These recommendations include reducing fat intake to 30% of total diet calories; including fruit (especially citrus), vegetables (carotene-rich and cruciferous—e.g., broccoli, cauliflower), and adequate fiber (e.g., whole wheat) in the diet; and minimal consumption of salt-cured, smoked, or nitrite-containing foods.

Several cancers with long presymptomatic stages that are amenable to early detection and intervention have shown improved outcomes with screening; these are described below.

Breast Cancer.   The three modalities used to screen women for breast cancer are physical examination, breast self-examination (BSE), and mammography. As generally practiced, breast examination by physicians fails to detect early-stage breast cancer (without node involvement) in about half of women later diagnosed to have breast cancer. Although physician performance might be improved with better training and monitoring compliance, supplementary tactics are needed. Annual clinical breast examination is recommended for all women aged 40 and older.

The effectiveness of BSE is also being reassessed. In the U.S. Preventive Services Task Force review of BSE studies, BSE was not shown to reduce cancer-associated mortality. Efficacy is hindered by incompetency and irregular compliance. There appears to be decreased BSE sensitivity with increasing patient age, when breast cancer has its highest incidence. A current Canadian trial of BSE should provide additional screening information.

Mammography is the only screening technique proven to lower breast cancer deaths. It demonstrates small, nonpalpable tumors with little risk of radiation side effects. The cost of screening mammography (currently about $100) is a major deterrent to its wider use, although increasing coverage by health insurance should help women for whom cost is an obstacle. Authorities disagree about the age at which a baseline mammogram should be obtained and the intervals for repeat screening in low-risk women. Mammography is recommended starting at age 50 and repeated every 1 to 2 years until about age 75. For high-risk women with a family history of premenopausal breast cancer in first-degree relatives, clinical breast examination and mammography should be started at age 35 (see Section 161, Breast Cancer Screening).

Cervical Cancer.   The marked fall in cervical cancer deaths in the past two decades is attributed to the widespread use of the Papanicolaou smear, a long presymptomatic period, and effective treatment. Based on a large population data base and assumptions about test performance, Papanicolaou smears are recommended for women from about age 20 to age 65, at intervals of 3 years or less.[2] Some individuals have high-risk behavior or inadequate long-term testing. Sexually active teenagers and women with multiple sexual partners warrant earlier and perhaps more frequent testing. Elderly women who have not had regular or recent Papanicolaou tests should have two annual consecutive tests (with negative results) before discontinuation (see Section 160, Cervical Cancer).

Colorectal Cancer. Indirect evidence based on the natural history of colorectal cancer and preliminary results from studies suggest that screening may reduce the mortality from colorectal cancer. Several screening methods have been proposed to detect asymptomatic colorectal cancer when it is potentially curable. These methods include endoscopy, which may be used to identify and remove adenomatous polyps before they progress to cancer. Rectal digital examination is relatively cheap and easy to do. As a screening procedure it assesses only the last 4 inches of the large bowel and has not reduced cancer rates. Because bowel lesions bleed intermittently, the fecal occult blood test has limited sensitivity. Two test samples taken on three different days, for a total of six samples, are recommended. Various fecal occult blood tests, including the Hemoccult II, are available, but all have low specificity for cancer and low predictive power because other gastrointestinal causes of bleeding might exist.

Sigmoidoscopy is more sensitive than the fecal occult blood test but is unacceptable to many patients. The flexible 65-cm sigmoidoscope is more comfortable and detects two to three times the number of cancers identified with the rigid 25-cm instrument. However, flexible sigmoidoscopy requires patient preparation before endoscopy, an experienced operator, and costs $100 or more. Consequently, endoscopy is used chiefly as a diagnostic procedure in persons with a positive fecal occult blood test. Until available evidence strongly supports the use of fecal occult blood testing as a screening measure, its use is optional. A reasonable screening approach for an average-risk patient between the age of 50 and 75 years might be a fecal occult blood test every 1 to 2 years. The addition of flexible sigmoidoscopy (performed with a 65-cm scope) every 3 to 5 years would improve screening sensitivity. If a first-degree relative had colorectal cancer (see Table 7–2), a barium enema examination to assess the entire colon can be substituted for sigmoidoscopy every 3 to 5 years.

Other Cancers. Few of the common cancers are amenable to early detection and treatment. Available tests are too insensitive (e.g., for prostate and bladder cancer), or the cancer develops rapidly (e.g., ovarian cancer), or treatment is ineffective (e.g., lung cancer). If the cancer is slow-growing and usually localized at diagnosis, as is true for 75% of endometrial cancers, patient education (e.g., to report unusual vaginal bleeding) is more beneficial than screening.

OTHER PREVENTION ACTIVITIES. *Alcohol Abuse.* Alcohol abuse, although highly prevalent in a patient population, is generally unrecognized at early stages and even after symptoms develop. Physicians do not screen for alcohol abuse for several reasons. In a society with a high consumption of alcohol, definitions are unclear. Practitioners may feel uncomfortable with the topic, ineffectual in counseling, pessimistic about patient compliance with advice, or may believe that referral services are inaccessible. Patients frequently deny that their problems may be related to alcohol consumption. Increased public awareness of alcohol-related hazards (vehicle accidents, risk during pregnancy, medication effects) may make asking questions about alcohol use more acceptable.

Two questions are recommended to screen for possible alcohol abuse: "Are you currently drinking?" and "Are you or is anyone else concerned about your drinking?" Additionally, a positive response to any of the CAGE questions ("Have you tried to cut down? Are you annoyed when questioned about drinking? Do you ever feel guilty about your drinking? Do you have an eye opener early in the day?") suggests a problem with alcohol. Once a potential candidate for referral is identified, the physician's interpersonal skills, rapport, and persistence will be valuable assets to motivate the patient to accept further diagnostic evaluation at an alcohol rehabilitation program (see Section 9, Diagnosis and Management of Alcoholism).

Infectious Disease.   Adult infection screening and immunization practice received little attention until the recent epidemics of sexually transmitted diseases and AIDS occurred and the aging U.S. population's susceptibility to respiratory infection was recognized. Immunization recommendations are described in detail in Section 10.

High-Risk Categories.   Certain behavioral or exposure factors or a family history place an individual at higher risk of becoming ill than those without such risk factors. Table 7–2 lists prevention activities for persons with predisposing risk factors for skin, oropharyngeal, testicular, or thyroid cancer. Aspirin chemoprophylaxis can be prescribed for men aged 50 years and older who have cardiovascular risk factors such as hypertension, smoking, diabetes, or elevated cholesterol levels. A discussion of estrogen replacement therapy with perimenopausal women at greater risk of developing osteoporosis (e.g., smokers) is recommended (see Section 164, Menopausal Symptoms). For persons whose residence or behavior constitutes additional health hazards, immunization or certain tests should be provided. A more comprehensive set is described in the Guide for Clinical Preventive Services.[6]

REFERENCES

1. Eddy DM. Screening for breast cancer. Ann Intern Med 1989;111:389–399.

2. Eddy DM. Screening for cervical cancer. Ann Intern Med 1990;113:214–226.

3. Eddy DM. Screening for colorectal cancer. Ann Intern Med 1990;113:373–384.
   These three articles review current information about risk factors, evidence of screening effectiveness, and how patient age and the frequency of screening may reduce the probability of developing cancer.

4. Frontiers in disease prevention. J Gen Intern Med (suppl 5) 1990;5.
   Recent Johns Hopkins symposium on issues and strategies in implementing breast cancer screening tests.

5. Lawrence RS, Mickalide AD. Report of the US Preventive Services Task Force. JAMA 1990;263:436–437.
   Concise description of procedures used to select prevention activities, and key findings.

6. U.S. Preventive Services Task Force. Guide to Clinical Preventive Services: An Assessment of the Effectiveness of 169 Interventions. Williams & Wilkins, Baltimore, 1989.
   Outstanding overview of current prevention information, including a comparison of recommendations by USPSTF with those of other authorities.

8 DIAGNOSIS AND MANAGEMENT OF DRUG ABUSE

JUDYANN BIGBY

EPIDEMIOLOGY.   Approximately 1 to 3 million Americans are regular users of cocaine, 500,000 are addicted to heroin, 2 million use heroin occasionally, and over 10 million smoke marijuana regularly. Among primary care patients with substance abuse, about 45% abuse alcohol, 25% abuse drugs other than alcohol, and 30% abuse both alcohol and other drugs.

SYMPTOMS AND SIGNS.   The signs and symptoms of drug abuse depend on the substances abused. Cocaine has been associated with seizures, arrhythmias, myocardial infarction, and sudden death due to cerebral hemorrhage. Regular intranasal administration causes chronic sinus disease, while inhaling or smoking free-base cocaine causes chronic diffusion abnormalities, pulmonary edema, and spontaneous pneumomediastinum. Cocaine dependence produces behavioral abnormalities such as diminished motivation, psychomotor retardation, irregular sleep patterns, sexual dysfunction, and symptoms of depression. Intravenous heroin use is associated with infections such as AIDS, hepatitis, bacterial endocarditis, skin infection, and pulmonary emboli. Marijuana use has been associated with automobile and workplace accidents, depression, and diminished motivation. Patients who abuse prescription drugs, such as opiates and benzodiazepines, frequently suffer from depression, chronic pain, personality disorders, and drug-seeking behavior.

CLINICAL APPROACH.   The physician should ask explicit questions to determine the patient's use of all drugs, legal or not. Routes of administration include intravenous (shooting), subcutaneous (skin popping), inhalational, and oral. Any history of drug treatment should be documented. Routine evaluation of the intravenous drug user should include tuberculin skin testing and testing for syphilis and other sexually transmitted diseases.

MANAGEMENT. Patients with drug abuse may be referred to treatment centers and to self-help groups such as Narcotics or Cocaine Anonymous. Most departments of public health provide information on available inpatient and outpatient treatment resources.

Patients with cocaine addiction are at particularly high risk for relapse after treatment. Antidepressants and dopamine agonists (e.g., amantadine, bromocriptine) are being investigated for their efficacy to suppress the cocaine craving and anhedonia accompanying withdrawal. Patients with heroin addiction can be referred to methadone treatment centers for detoxification over 2 to 3 weeks or for methadone maintenance. Methadone maintenance programs not only improve an individual's social functioning but may also reduce the rate of human immunodeficiency virus (HIV) seroconversion.

It is the physician's responsibility to counsel intravenous cocaine and heroin users about the risk of HIV infection. HIV seroprevalence rates range from 61% of addicts in New York City, to 20% in Hartford and Boston, to 5% in Seattle. The physician should discuss the danger of needle sharing, the benefits of using bleach to clean needles and other paraphernalia, and the risks of sexual and perinatal transmission of HIV.

FOLLOW-UP. The physician should monitor patients for relapse and for complications of drug use. The primary care physician can help prevent the substitution of one substance of abuse for another by limiting the prescription of psychoactive drugs except when they are clearly indicated. To minimize the potential for abuse when prescribing controlled substances, the physician should (1) know the abuse potential of all drugs, (2) monitor prescriptions (store pads in locked areas, do not preprint DEA numbers, spell out the quantity prescribed to prevent changes by patients), (3) document the treatment indications and goals, (4) maintain a record of each prescription for controlled substances given to individual patients, (5) be alert for fraud—if it does not "feel right" to prescribe a drug, there is probably reason for concern, and (6) identify a single physician to prescribe controlled substances if many physicians are involved in the patient's care.

Cross-reference: Periodic Health Assessment (Section 7), Principles of Screening (Section 12).

REFERENCES

1. Cooper JR. Methadone treatment and acquired immunodeficiency syndrome. JAMA 1989;262:1664–1668.
   Methadone treatment delivered in quality centers decreases the HIV seroconversion rate in intravenous drug users.

2. Coulehan JL, Zettler SM, Block M, McClelland M, Schulberg HC. Recognition of alcoholism and substance abuse in primary care patients. Arch Intern Med 1987;147:349–352.
   Epidemiology of substance abuse in primary care patients; 14% of patients are affected.

3. Curtis JL, Crummey C, Baker SN, Foster RE, Khanyile CS, Wilkins R. HIV screening and counseling for intravenous drug abuse patients. JAMA 1989;261:258–262.

    Patients in treatment for intravenous substance abuse reported reductions in the number of sex partners and in personal needle sharing after counseling.

4. Gawin FH, Ellinwood EH. Cocaine and other stimulants. N Engl J Med 1988;318:1173–1182.

    An excellent review of the effects of cocaine, signs of abuse, and treatment dilemmas.

5. Newman RG. Methadone treatment: Defining and evaluating success. N Engl J Med 1987;317:447–450.

    A review of methadone treatment and why it works.

9 DIAGNOSIS AND MANAGEMENT OF ALCOHOLISM

JUDYANN BIGBY

EPIDEMIOLOGY.   Approximately 10% of the general American population have alcoholism. Twenty-five percent of all American families are affected by a member with alcoholism. An estimated 10% to 20% of patients in a typical ambulatory practice have alcoholism or are problem drinkers.

SYMPTOMS AND SIGNS.   The earliest signs of alcoholism reflect the disruptive behaviors of drinkers that occur in families, society, and at work. Medical complications such as chronic liver disease, pancreatitis, cognitive impairment, or severe withdrawal occur in late-stage alcoholism, and are absent in most alcoholics presenting in the primary care setting. Clues to the diagnosis of alcoholism include poor job performance, absenteeism, industrial accidents and recurring minor trauma, poor relationships with a spouse or other family members, and legal problems related to behavior while under the influence of alcohol.

Complaints of poor memory, insomnia, anxiety, depression, sexual dysfunction, and nonspecific gastrointestinal complaints are common in persons with early or mid-stage alcoholism. Reports of blackouts (amnestic episodes occurring during periods of drinking) are diagnostic of alcoholism. Hypertension is a common physical finding among patients with problem drinking. Laboratory abnormalities such as an elevated MCV and abnormal liver function tests are helpful when they are present, but they are not always abnormal.

CLINICAL APPROACH.   The role of the primary care physician is to screen for the disease, establish a diagnosis when alcoholism is suspected, present the diagnosis to the patient, and help the patient identify treatment resources. The diagnosis of alcoholism relies on the identification of complications from drinking (e.g., marital problems, absenteeism), loss of control of drinking (e.g., repeated attempts to cut down), tolerance or addiction to alcohol (e.g., drinking in the morning to steady the nerves), and the quantity and frequency of use.

All patients in the ambulatory setting should be screened. Questions about the quantity and frequency of alcohol use are not sensitive enough to identify problem drinking. The CAGE questionnaire (Table 9–1) has a sensitivity of 75% to 90% and a specificity of 85% to 95% for the diagnosis of alcoholism when two or more questions are answered affirmatively. All affirmative answers should be pursued with explicit questions about the relationship of drinking to the problem.

MANAGEMENT. Physicians should share their concerns with patients: "I am concerned that drinking is a major problem for you. Your stomach complaints, high blood pressure, and your recent emergency room visit after you fell off the ladder all point to alcohol as your major difficulty." The physician can offer counseling and education to family members, make a referral for treatment, and suggest self-help groups such as Alcoholics Anonymous (AA) and Alanon. AA meetings appropriate for the patient can be identified by calling the central chapter of AA, listed in the local telephone directory. Patients with adequate social supports can be referred for outpatient treatment. Patients from unstable social settings or facing impending crises (threatened job loss, divorce) may require inpatient treatment. Most state departments of public health have up-to-date information about treatment centers.

Disulfiram may be used as an adjunct to treatment but is contraindicated in patients with liver disease, cardiac disease, and kidney disease. It decreases the likelihood that a person will drink impulsively, particularly well-motivated patients who have stable social situations and no history of a disulfiram-alcohol interaction. Patients should be willing to take the drug and should be aware of the consequences of drinking. The characteristic disulfiram-alcohol interaction occurs 15 to 20 minutes after drinking and consists of flushing, nausea and vomiting, headache, chest pain, and difficulty breathing. Patients should have abstained from alcohol for 72 hours prior to beginning disulfiram and cannot

TABLE 9–1.   THE CAGE QUESTIONNAIRE

Have you ever tried to cut down on your drinking?

    Why? Was it difficult? Why did you start drinking again?

Have you ever been annoyed by criticism of your drinking?

    Who criticized you and why? Did you attempt to change your drinking?

Have you ever felt guilty about your drinking?

    What caused the guilt? Did you try to change your drinking?

Have you ever had a morning eye-opener?

    Do you feel shaky in the morning? Do you need a drink to get you through the day?

drink until 5 to 7 days after the last dose. The usual dose is 250 to 500 mg once a day for the first week, and then 250 mg three times a week.

FOLLOW-UP.   If the patient refuses to accept the diagnosis, the physician can follow the patient, emphasizing alcoholism as the major problem.

Patients who accept treatment and referral need to be followed up in the early stages of recovery and monitored for signs of relapse. The physician can also reinforce the need not to drink, and how treatment will help accomplish this. Some symptoms of withdrawal (anxiety, insomnia, depression) may last 6 to 12 months. Patients need to be reassured that these will improve.

Patients relapse because they are unable to control their drinking. Physicians should not criticize patients but instead should congratulate them for the period of sobriety achieved. After reevaluation of the patient's previous treatment, the clinician should suggest ways to achieve longer periods of sobriety (e.g., the patient could attend more AA meetings, acquire a sponsor, or follow up with an alcoholism counselor).

Cross-references: Periodic Health Assessment (Section 7), Principles of Screening (Section 12).

REFERENCES

1. Babor TF, Ritson EB, Hodgson RJ. Alcohol-related problems in the primary health care setting: A review of early intervention strategies. Br J Addict 1986;81:23–46.
    The results of several investigations suggest that drinking behavior can be changed and adverse effects from drinking decreased in individuals who are counseled about the consequences of abnormal drinking. Interventions included education, advice, self-help groups, and periodic monitoring.

2. Barnes HN, Aronson MD, Delbanco TL, Eds. Alcoholism: A Guide for the Primary Care Physician. Springer-Verlag, New York, 1987.
    A practical approach to the diagnosis and management of alcoholism, with an emphasis on office treatment.

3. Cleary PD, Miller M, Bush BT, Warburg M, Delbanco TL, Aronson MD. Prevalence and recognition of alcohol abuse in a primary care population. Am J Med 1988;85:466–470.
    Five percent of patients in a hospital-based ambulatory practice had evidence of alcoholism; 20% had a history of alcohol abuse or problem drinking. Men were three times more likely than women to have problem drinking or alcohol abuse.

4. Hays JT, Spickard VA. Alcoholism: Early diagnosis and intervention. J Gen Intern Med 1987;2:420–427.
    An excellent review of the signs and symptoms of alcoholism and strategies for treatment.

10 ADULT IMMUNIZATIONS

BENJAMIN A. LIPSKY

EPIDEMIOLOGY. Vaccines are among the most cost-effective means to improved health care. Nevertheless, immunization in adults is often neglected because it lacks established tradition or broad legal requirements. The three major target groups for inoculation against vaccine-preventable diseases are healthy individuals who are susceptible because they lack previous immunization or infection; persons who are at risk of these diseases because of their occupation or life-style, and patients whose age or medical conditions increase the risk of morbidity or mortality from these diseases. Interest in immunizations for adults has increased in recent years with the recognition that some vaccine-preventable diseases now occur primarily in persons 20 years old or older, yet the majority of adults at risk are not protected against most of these diseases (Table 10–1).

CLINICAL APPROACH. Table 10–2 summarizes the current recommendations for vaccinations of adults in various groups. Contraindications to adult immunization are commonly misunderstood. The following are *not* contraindications to vaccination:

1. A previous vaccination produced local tenderness, redness and/or swelling, or fever less than 40.5°C.
2. Mild acute upper respiratory or gastrointestinal illness accompanied by fever less than 38°C.

TABLE 10–1. VACCINE-PREVENTABLE DISEASES IN ADULTS—UNITED STATES, 1985–1989

Disease	Cases		Population Studied (Age, yr)	% Immune
	Total No.	% in Adults		
Diphtheria	11	63.6	≥60	34–51[1]
Hepatitis B	125,237	87.4	NA[2]	2–90[3]
Measles	34,348	14.9	18–29	85–95[1]
Mumps	34,198	10.6	NA	NA
Rubella	2,108	45.3	15–44	80–90[1]
Tetanus	301	92.4	≥60	16–59[1]
Influenza	*	—	≥20[4]	17[5]
Pneumococcal	*	—	≥20[4]	9[5]

*Influenza and pneumococcal disease are not included in the national system of notifiable disease reporting.
[1]Estimated immunity level derived from serosurveys (actual vaccine coverages unknown).
[2]Not available.
[3]Based on immunization surveys and estimates in selected population.
[4]Includes all persons aged 65 years and high-risk persons aged 20–64 years.
[5]Based on national immunization surveys.

3.   Current antimicrobial therapy, convalescence from a recent illness, or exposure to an infectious disease.

4.   Pregnancy in another household member.

5.   Breast-feeding.

TABLE 10–2.   VACCINE RECOMMENDATIONS FOR SELECTED POPULATIONS IN THE UNITED STATES*

Patients	Vaccines†					
	Td	*MMR*	*Polio*	*Flu*	*Pneu.*	*Hep. B*
General use						
18–64 yr old	V, B	(V)	S			
≥65 yr old	V, B		S	V	V	
Special groups						
Pregnancy[1]		X				S
Occupational						
College students		(V)				
Health care workers		(V)		V		S
Day care personnel		(V)	(V)	V		
Life-styles						
Homosexual men and heterosexuals with multiple partners						V
Parenteral drug abusers	(V)					V
Environmental situations						
Prison inmates						V
Mentally retarded (institutionalized)						V
Nursing home residents				V	S	
Compromised hosts[2]						
Chronic organ system or system disease				V	V	
Immunosuppressed		X		±	±	±

*Special considerations may apply for travelers. There is good evidence from at least one properly randomized controlled trial to support all of these recommendations (except for pneumococcal vaccine).

†TD = tetanus-diphtheria toxoid, MMR = mumps-measles-rubella, Flu = influenza, Pneu. = pneumococcal, Hep. B = hepatitis B, V = routine administration, (V) = administer if not previously infected or vaccinated, B = boosters every 10 years, S = selected high-risk individuals, X = contraindicated, ± = variable immunogenicity.

[1]Pregnant patients:

1.   Live virus vaccines (measles, mumps, rubella, rubeola) should generally be avoided because of theoretical risks to the fetus, although there are no clinical data to support this possibility.

2.   Hepatitis B, pneumococcal, and influenza vaccines are neither specifically indicated nor contraindicated.

3.   Diphtheria-tetanus vaccine should be administered to those not previously immunized.

4.   Polio immunization is not indicated unless traveling to highly endemic areas, in which case inactivated vaccine (IPV) should be given.

[2]HIV-infected patients:

1.   May receive all appropriate vaccines during asymptomatic stages but should not take live virus vaccines (e.g., OPV) when in more advanced stages.

2.   Efficacy of vaccines is best when vaccination is given as early in the course of the HIV infection as possible.

TABLE 10–3. KEY INFORMATION ON RECOMMENDED VACCINES

Disease	Vaccine	Dose/Route	Indications	Precautions	Frequency	Special Considerations	Approximate Cost*
Measles	Measles live virus[1] (Attenuvax)	0.5 ml SQ	All children and adults born after 1956 without previous live virus vaccination or evidence of previous infection	Pregnancy; immunosuppression; egg or neomycin allergy	Once; second dose 10 yr later for young adults entering college, health professions or traveling abroad	Persons vaccinated in 1963–67 may need revaccination	$16
Mumps	Mumps live virus[2] (Mumpsvax II)	0.5 ml SQ	All children and susceptible adults (particularly men)	(Same as measles)	Once; no booster	Measles-mumps-rubella (MMR) is vaccine of choice if all 3 needed	$33 (MMR) $18 (Mumpsvax)
Rubella	Rubella live virus[2] (Meruvax II)	0.5 ml SQ	All children and susceptible adults (particularly women of child-bearing age and those working in congregate situations)	(Same as measles)	Once; no booster	Pregnancy within 3 mo of vaccination may damage fetus; vaccine may cause arthralgias, paresthesias	$17 $33 (MR)
Tetanus/ diphtheria	Adsorbed tetanus and diphtheria toxins (Td)	0.5 ml SQ	All children and adults	History of allergy or neurologic reaction from previous dose	2 doses 1–2 mo apart; 3rd dose 6–12 mo later; booster every 10 yr	See reference 1; boosters at ≤ 10-yr intervals may increase adverse reactions	$1
Pneumococcal	Polyvalent pneumococcal polysaccharide (Pneumovax 23; Pnu-immune 23)	0.5 ml SQ or IM	Children and adults at increased risk, especially those with asplenia, ≥65 y.o., chronic cardiac, pulmonary, and perhaps, other disorders	Previous (recent) pneumococcal vaccination; local soreness may occur	Once; repeat vaccination recommended only for those at highest risk who received 14-valent vaccine or were vaccinated > 6 yr ago	Efficacy is poor in immunocompromised hosts; data to support use in high-risk US populations are limited	$10 (Medicare Part B coverage)

	Type	Dose/Route	Indications	Contraindications	Schedule	Comments	Cost*
Influenza	Inactivated virus (Fluogen: influenza virus vaccine)	0.5 ml SQ	Persons ≥65 yr, or with high-risk conditions or residing in chronic care facilities; also, essential public and health care workers	Egg allergy; local soreness, fever, mylagias may occur	Annually (before December)	Vaccine changes annually; efficacy in high-risk U.S. population is reasonably well established	$4 (free to Medicare beneficiaries)
Polio	Live oral polio virus	OPV: 0.5 ml PO IPV: 1 ml SQ	All children; routine vaccination for adults is unnecessary; vaccinate those at high risk because of travel or occupation, preferably with IPV	OPV: Pregnancy, immunosuppression IPV: streptomycin or neomycin allergy	OPV: 3 doses ≥ 6 wk apart; 4th dose ≥ 6 mo later; IPV: 4 doses, per package, insert	Rare instances of paralysis in recipients of OPV and their close contacts	$12/dose (OPV) $11/dose (IPV)
Hepatitis B	Recombinant HBsAg vaccine (Recombivax-HB, Engerix-B)	1 ml IM (in deltoid)	Multiple sex partners; IV drug abuse; hemophiliacs; health care workers; staff and patients in mental institutions	None	2 doses 4 wk apart; 3rd dose 5 mo later	Effectiveness decreased with increased age, obesity, or injection in buttock	$150 (for 3 doses; Medicare coverage in renal failure)

*Wholesale cost to pharmacist (*Drug Topics Red Book*, 1990).

[1] Also available in: measles-rubella live virus (M-R-VAX II) and measles-mumps-rubella live virus (M-M-R II).

[2] Also available in rubella-mumps live-virus (Biavax II).

- Vaccinations should not be given to persons with a febrile illness (>38°C).
- Do not give live virus vaccines to immunocompromised patients.
- Measles, mumps, rubella, DPT, and OPV can all be given simultaneously.

6.   Personal history of "allergies," excluding anaphylactic reactions to neomycin (for combined measles, mumps, and rubella vaccine) or streptomycin (for oral polio vaccine).

7.   Family history of "allergies," adverse reactions to vaccination, or seizures.

Key information on selected vaccines is listed in Table 10–3.

Cross-reference: Periodic Health Assessment (Section 7).

REFERENCES

1.   Advisory Committee on Immunization Practices: General recommendations on immunization. MMWR 1989;38:205–227.
     Thorough and up-to-date overview of recommendations for all aspects of immunization.

2.   American College of Physicians Task Force on Adult Immunization and Infectious Diseases Society of America: Guide for Adult Immunization, 2nd ed. American College of Physicians, Philadelphia, 1990.
     Recent revision of the most thorough guidelines in this field.

3.   Centers for Disease Control. Public health burden of vaccine-preventable diseases among adults: Standards for adult immunization practice. MMWR 1990;39:725–729.
     As stated in the title.

4.   LaForce FM. Adult immunizations: Are they worth the trouble? J Gen Intern Med 1990; 5(suppl):s57–61.
     Thoughtful review of the data supporting immunization in adults.

5.   Poland GA, Love KR, Hughes CE. Routine immunization of the HIV-positive asymptomatic patient. J Gen Intern Med 1990;5:147–152.
     A review of the risk of vaccine-preventable diseases and the safety and efficacy of vaccination in HIV-infected patients.

11 SMOKING CESSATION

NANCY RISSER

EPIDEMIOLOGY.   Cigarette smoking remains the chief preventable cause of death and illness in the United States, responsible for one-sixth of all deaths. Although the prevalence of smoking decreased from 40% in 1965 to 29% by 1987, 50 million Americans continue to smoke.

RATIONALE.   All patients, including the elderly, receive substantial and immediate health benefits from stopping smoking. Smoking cessation reduces the risk for lung, esophageal, head and neck, bladder, and other cancers, coronary heart disease, stroke, and chronic lung disease. Women who stop smoking before pregnancy or during the first trimester reduce their risk of having a low birth weight infant to that of women who have never smoked. Even with brief interactions, clinicians can influence their patients to stop smoking. Because 70% of adults in the United States see a physician at least annually, even a small increase in the percentage of smokers who quit justifies this effort.

CLINICAL APPROACH. As a minimum, the clinician should (1) ask every patient about smoking habits during each visit; (2) advise each smoker to quit, with a clear, firm, unequivocal message; (3) try to obtain an agreement from the patient to quit smoking; and (4) monitor progress at follow-up visits.

To further increase quit rates, the physician should:

1. Assure the patient that he or she can quit.

2. Discuss the smoker's reasons for quitting and previous attempts. Portray quitting as an evolving process. Successful quitting usually occurs only after several unsuccessful attempts.

3. Motivate cessation by linking abnormalities such as wheezes, cough, abnormal spirometry, or other personal symptoms to smoking. Emphasize the health benefits of quitting. Convince the patient that smoking may injure others (e.g., family).

TABLE 11–1. NICOTINE REPLACEMENT THERAPY

Administration	Directions for Use	Cost
Nicotine Polacrilex Gum		
2 mg (one piece) q20–30 min PRN urges; max 30/24 hours; use enough gum (avg, 1 gum/2 cigs); use for 3–6 + mos.	Do not smoke and use gum. Chew slowly so absorbed through buccal mucosa and not swallowed. When gum is in mouth, use no liquids (to maintain a pH that releases nicotine). Incorrect usage increases side effects such as gastrointestinal symptoms, hiccups, or oral ulceration.	$25—30/box of 96 gums
Nicotine transdermal system		
Begin with one 21 mg patch qd × 4–8 weeks (begin with 14mg qd if cardiovascular disease, weight < 100 lbs, or smokes < ½ pack cigs daily). Taper to 14 mg qd × 2–4 wks. End with 7 mg qd × 2–4 weeks.	Do not smoke and use patch. Apply new patch qd to different, nonhairy, dry intact skin on upper body or upper outer arm; may bathe and exercise during use. Almost 50% experience local irritation.	$50–$60/box of 12 $100–$120/box of 30

4. Secure a commitment to a specific quit date within 3 weeks. Record it on a signed prescription or a written contract and in the chart.

5. Provide self-help materials, such as the American Lung Association's "Freedom from Smoking" manuals.

6. Provide a list of local stop smoking resources for referral and encourage the smoker to select one.

7. Offer nicotine polacrilex gum (Nicorette) or the nicotine transdermal system (Nicoderm) *as an adjunct to counseling* to smokers who demonstrate symptoms of nicotine addiction (smoke their first cigarette within half an hour of awakening, smoke more than a pack of cigarettes daily, or report withdrawal symptoms during previous quit attempts) (Table 11–1). Remind smokers that the gum costs little more than the cigarettes it replaces. Although clonidine may reduce initial nicotine withdrawal symptoms, its benefit in long-term smoking cessation remains unproven.

FOLLOW-UP. A follow-up appointment or telephone contact should occur 1 to 2 weeks after the quit date. The clinician should continue to repeat a clear, consistent, personalized nonsmoking message. A relapse is not a failure; most smokers need more than one attempt at quitting to learn what is necessary for their ultimate success. For smokers who have quit, the clinician should continue to provide positive reinforcement and emphasize the benefits of quitting.

Cross-reference: Periodic Health Assessment (Section 7).

REFERENCES

1. Benowitz NL. Pharmacologic aspects of cigarette smoking and nicotine addiction. N Engl J Med 1988;319:1318–1330.

   Reviews nicotine action, pharmacokinetics, relationship to human disease, interactions with other drugs, and nicotine substitution therapy.

2. Greene HL, Goldberg RJ, Ockene JK. Cigarette smoking: The physician's role in cessation and maintenance. J Gen Intern Med 1988;3:75–87.

   Practical review with 122 references.

3. Kottke TE, Battista RN, DeFriese GH, Brekke ML. Attributes of successful smoking cessation interventions in medical practice: A meta-analysis of 39 controlled trials. JAMA 1988;259:2883–2889.

   Effective interventions used multiple modalities to motivate and assist behavioral change, involved both physicians and nonphysicians in individualized face-to-face efforts, and provided the messages on multiple occasions over the longest possible time period.

4. Lam W, Sacks HS, Sze PC, Chalmers TC. Meta-analysis of randomized controlled trials of nicotine chewing gum. Lancet 1987;2:27–30.

   Twelve-month success in specialized clinics was 23%, compared to 13% with placebo. In general practice settings, 9% quit with the gum, 5% with placebo.

12 PRINCIPLES OF SCREENING

DAVID L. SIMEL

DEFINITION. Screening is the process of detecting disease early, before it causes symptoms. Several factors must be present for effective screening programs:

1. The target disease is an important clinical problem.
2. The screening test is accurate, widely available, and acceptable to patients and doctors.
3. The natural history of the target disease is understood and there is a presymptomatic stage.
4. Treatment for the target condition is available, acceptable, and efficacious.

PRINCIPLE 1. The target disease is an important clinical problem. To be "important," the disease must be common enough that many patients benefit from early detection. In addition, the disease should be associated with significant morbidity or mortality. Examples of common important diseases include hypertension, breast carcinoma, or gestational diabetes.

Prevalence describes the proportion of patients who have disease in a given population (Figure 12–1): Prevalence = $(A + C)/(A + B + C + D)$. Prevalence describes the prior odds that a disease is present before a screening test is performed. Thus,

$$\text{Prior odds} = \frac{\text{Prevalence}}{1 - \text{Prevalence}}$$

For example, if the prevalence of disease is 5%, the prior odds = $(0.05)/(0.95)$ = 0.053.

When reading medical literature, the physician must understand the population used to describe test performance. Because the prevalence of disease may depend on geography and on the sex and age of the patient, the physician's patient population may differ from published study populations.

PRINCIPLE 2. The screening test is accurate, widely available, and acceptable. Screening tests must be acceptable and available (e.g., reasonable cost and little discomfort for patients; easy to perform or order for the doctor).

		Disease	
		Present	Absent
Test Result	Positive	A	B
	Negative	C	D

FIGURE 12–1. 2 × 2 Table (see text).

However, to decide whether a screening test works the clinician uses the operating characteristics of a test, **sensitivity** and **specificity,** together with the prior odds.

$$\text{Sensitivity} = \frac{\text{No. of diseased patients with a positive screening test}}{\text{No. of all patients with the disease}}$$

$$= (A)/(A + C).$$

$$\text{Specificity} = \frac{\text{No. of normal patients with a negative screening test}}{\text{No. of all normal patients}}$$

$$= (D)/(B + D).$$

These values define the odds favoring disease if the test result is positive (also called the positive likelihood ratio, LR+):

$$\text{LR}+ = \frac{\text{Sensitivity}}{1 - \text{Specificity}}$$

or the odds favoring disease if the test result is negative (also called the negative likelihood ratio, LR−):

$$\text{LR}- = \frac{1 - \text{Sensitivity}}{\text{Specificity}}$$

For example, a test with sensitivity of 80% and specificity of 80% has an LR+ of 4.0 and an LR− of 0.25.

The prior odds are multiplied by the appropriate likelihood ratio to yield the odds of disease after performing the test:

$$\text{Posterior odds} = \text{Prior odds} \times \text{LR}.$$

The likelihood ratio is represented by LR+ for a positive screening test result and LR− for a negative screening test. Thus, the posterior odds depends on the prevalence of disease in the population under study and on the operating characteristics of the test. If a test with a sensitivity of 80% and a specificity of 80% yields positive results in a patient from the population described in Principle 1, the odds that disease is actually present increases from the prior odds of 0.053 to the posterior odds 0.053 × 4.0 = 0.212.

Because it is sometimes easier to think of the probability of an event than the odds of an event, the odds ratio can be converted back to probability estimates by the equation:

$$\text{Probability} = \text{Odds}/(1 + \text{odds}).$$

Therefore a positive test result increases the prior probability of disease (prevalence) from 5% to the posterior probability of 17.5% for our example [0.212/(1 + 0.212)].

To assess the likelihood of disease when a test result is negative, multiply the prior odds by LR− to get the posterior odds (e.g., 0.053 × 0.25). In our example, a negative test result decreases the probability of disease from 5% to 1.3%.

Some clinicians prefer to use predictive values rather than likelihood ratios to describe the diagnostic impact of test results. The positive predictive value is figured as the proportion of patients with positive screening tests who actually have disease; the negative predictive value is figured as the proportion of patients with negative tests who actually do not have disease. Predictive values have limited diagnostic utility unless the population prevalence is well described.

PRINCIPLE 3.   The natural history of the target disease is understood and there is a presymptomatic stage. This simple statement is extremely important. If there is no presymptomatic stage of a disease, the disease cannot be detected before it causes symptoms. Thus, for such disease (e.g., impotence, appendicitis, or pneumonia) there will be no effective screening test.

PRINCIPLE 4.   Treatment for the target condition is acceptable, available, and efficacious. This final principle suggests we should only screen for diseases that can be affected positively by treatment. Although this may seem obvious, determining whether treatment is acceptable, available, and efficacious may be difficult. This decision requires a clear understanding of the individual patient's medical, psychological, and socioeconomic conditions and requires the physician to know the best available medical information. For many diseases for which evidence of treatment efficacy from randomized clinical trials is lacking, decision analysis may suggest appropriate strategies that can be considered for individual patients. Screening for cervical carcinoma is a strategy that meets these requirements. Screening for lung carcinoma does not meet these requirements because current evidence suggests that screening has no impact on outcomes.

REFERENCES

1. Feussner JR, Simel DL, Matchar DB. Quantitative approaches to clinical diagnosis of cancer in elderly patients. Clin Geriatr Med 1987;3:447–461.
    Discusses a common problem in ambulatory medicine and integrates sensitivity and specificity issues with decision analysis.

2. Sackett DL, Haynes RB, Tugwell P. Clinical Epidemiology: A Basic Science for Clinical Medicine. Little, Brown, Boston, 1985.
    The single best reference to learn methods for critically appraising evidence of efficacy from the medical literature.

3. Sox HC, Blatt MA, Higgins MC, Marton KI. Medical Decision Making. Butterworth, Boston, 1988.
    Excellent introductory text regarding the tools of decision and cost-effectiveness analysis. The appendix lists likelihood ratios for commonly performed tests.

4. U.S. Preventive Services Task Force. Guide to Clinical Preventive Services. Williams & Wilkins, Baltimore, 1989.
    A recent and well-annotated source that evaluates screening strategies for 169 different diseases.

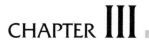
CONSTITUTIONAL SYNDROMES

13 CHRONIC PAIN SYNDROME

Problem

JODIE K. HASELKORN
DIANA D. CARDENAS

EPIDEMIOLOGY. The perception of pain is highly personal and is dependent on the stimulus, the individual, and the individual's environment. An identical painful stimulus may be perceived differently by a single individual at different times and by different individuals at the same time.

Because many factors contribute to pain, the definition of chronic pain syndrome is elusive. Patients with chronic pain syndrome cannot be characterized by the severity or location of the pain. Pain may occur in any region of the body, but it tends to involve the lower back, neck, head, abdomen, and soft tissue.

Chronic pain syndrome generally refers to pain that persists beyond the period when healing or cessation of inflammation should have occurred. The normal time of healing varies from individual to individual and with different clinical conditions, but pain persisting more than 3 months beyond the time expected for healing can be used as a benchmark to differentiate acute and chronic pain.[4]

One important risk factor for chronic pain syndrome is inadequate treatment of an acute injury. Other potential risk factors include stress, dissatisfaction with employment or employer, disability income that equals or exceeds employment income, pending litigation, and family problems.

Because chronic pain syndrome is difficult to define, its epidemiology has not been well described. Roughly one-third of the American population, however, may experience chronic pain, with one-half of this group experiencing temporary or permanent disability. In 1986, the cost of this problem was about $79 billion.[1]

SIGNS AND SYMPTOMS.   In contrast to acute pain, which signals potential harm and promotes rest and healing after injury, chronic pain serves no such useful purpose.

Patients with chronic pain syndrome tend to exhibit accompanying behaviors such as depression, drug dependence, "doctor shopping," an inordinate limitation of activity, and suffering out of proportion to what seems reasonable. Typical symptoms are a depressed affect, appetite and sleep disturbances, and decreased pain tolerance. Patients feel hopeless and helpless, adopt a "sick" role, and often feel that there is no predictable end to their experience. These suffering behaviors, which tend to reinforce the pain experience, are learned, goal-directed, and frequently reinforced by family, friends, and the medical/vocational system. The chronic pain syndrome, therefore, differs from the chronic pain that may occur without these accompanying behaviors (e.g., pain in some patients with cancer). Unlike acute pain, which is characterized by a heightened sympathetic response, patients with chronic pain syndrome typically lack hypertension, tachycardia, diaphoresis, and dilated pupils.

CLINICAL APPROACH.   Chronic pain syndrome usually can be diagnosed with confidence if the risk factors cited above are present and either (1) a physiologic source of chronic pain is not evident after a thorough evaluation or (2) a source is identified, but the patient's suffering behaviors are well out of proportion to those usually seen. Clues to the recognition of chronic pain syndrome include the absence of recovery beyond a predicted recovery date, nonphysiologic physical examination findings, missed follow-up appointments, frequent medical visits to multiple providers, drug-seeking behaviors, and a history of lost medications.

Once the initial evaluation has been completed, there is little to be gained from additional diagnostic efforts. In fact, additional workup is likely to be detrimental because it reinforces the patient's pain perception and suffering behavior. Instead, the clinician should review with the patient all prior diagnoses and the results of previous studies. Clinicians should also emphasize that they understand that the patient is hurting and not malingering, but that the patient's perceptions of the problem exceed actual tissue damage. It is useful to explain that the severity of pain does not represent actual harm but instead reflects learned patterns, and that the problem is common and can be successfully treated.

The patient interview should identify how much the patient's activities are limited and the degree of associated drug use, depression, and suffering. The clinician should obtain a full inventory of all medications, including prescriptions, over-the-counter remedies, alcohol, and illicit drugs. The patient should describe both the negative environmental factors that serve to maintain the patient's suffering behaviors (e.g., the patient receives more attention from family members when suffering from pain) as well as the positive factors that can be relied on for support during treatment. The Minnesota Multiphasic Personality Inventory may be useful to help determine the presence of depression and other personal characteristics that may be helped by treatment (see Psychological Assessment, Section 196). In many cases, consultation with a psychologist will be helpful.

After establishing the patient's trust and desire to improve, it is often useful to draw up a therapeutic contract that lists the specific goals and steps in treatment.

MANAGEMENT. The overall goal in the management of chronic pain syndrome is to restore physical and psychological function, not necessarily to eliminate pain. Specific treatment goals are to restore sleep and nutrition while increasing physical activity, psychological well-being, and coping skills.

Most authorities agree that chronic pain syndrome should not be treated with narcotics or sedative-hypnotics, either on a scheduled long-term basis (impairs the psychological and physical goals of treatment), or on an as-needed basis (reinforces suffering behaviors).

Many chronic pain syndrome patients have already been taking narcotics or sedative-hypnotics for long periods of time, often in high doses. In these cases it is advisable to begin a detoxification program with a long-acting narcotic such as methadone at a total daily dose equal to 120% of the short-acting narcotic taken by the patient (Table 13–1). Because the analgesic effect of methadone lasts 6 hours, the daily dose must be split into four doses over the course of the day. Detoxification from longer acting sedative-hypnotics (e.g., diazepam) may be accomplished with phenobarbital (Table 13–2), but successful detoxification from the shorter acting benzodiazepines (e.g., alprazolam or lorazepam) is difficult with phenobarbital.[2] Carbamazepine, 200 mg twice daily, has been used with some success in those using shorter acting benzodiazepines.[5] To assist in detoxification, the clinician should also use maximal doses of anti-

TABLE 13–1. NARCOTIC CONVERSIONS

Drug (Trade Name)	Dose (mg) Equal to 1 Narcotic Equivalent (= 10 mg Oral Methadone)	
	Oral	IM
Butorphanol (Stadol)	—	2.0
Buprenorphine (Buprenex)	—	0.3
Codeine	200.0	130.0
Diacetylmorphine (Heroin)	—	3.0
Hydromorphine (Dilaudid)	7.5	1.5
Meperidine (Demerol)	400.0	100.0
Methadone (Dolophine)	10.0	8.0
Morphine	60.0	10.0
Oxycodone (Percodan)	30.0	15.0
Oxymorphone (Numorphan)	—	1.5
Pentazocine (Talwin)	180.0	60.0
Propoxyphene hydrochloride (Darvon)[1]	260.0	—
Propoxyphene napsylate (Darvon-N)[1]	400.0	—

[1]For propoxyphenhydrochloride replacement, 40 mg methadone in 24 hours is the maximum dose.

TABLE 13–2. SEDATIVE/HYPNOTIC/TRANQUILIZER CONVERSIONS

Drug (Trade Name)	Dose (mg) Equal to 1 Barbiturate Equivalent (= 30 mg Oral Phenobarbital)
Benzodiazepines[1]	
Alprazolam (Xanax)	1.0
Chlordiazepoxide (Librium)	25.0
Clonazepam (Klonopin)	4.0
Clorazepate (Tranxene)	15.0
Diazepam (Valium)	10.0
Flurazepam (Dalmane)	15.0
Lorazepam (Ativan)	2.0
Oxazepam (Serax)	10.0
Barbiturates	
Amobarbitol (Tuinal)	100.0
Butabarbitol (Butisol)	100.0
Butalbital (Fiorinal)	100.0
Pentobarbital (Nembutal)	100.0
Secobarbital (Seconal)	100.0
Phenobarbital (Phenobarbital)	30.0
Other	
Meprobamate (Miltown)	400.0
Ethyl alcohol (100 proof)	90.0 ml

[1]Patients taking large doses of benzodiazepines may not tolerate conversion to phenobarbital (see text).

inflammatory medications, acetaminophen, and hydroxyzine. Medications may be given in tablet forms, though a patient-blinded liquid taper using a vehicle for dissolved medication (cherry syrup or an antacid) with a masking agent (e.g., liquid multivitamin) may be most effective. Medications are given only on a fixed time schedule, not on an as-needed basis, with methadone or phenobarbital tapered by 10% per day. An optimal schedule for tapering carbamazepine has not been described.

Detoxification may be easiest in an inpatient setting, where access to other medications and providers can be controlled and symptoms of withdrawal monitored. Nevertheless, a motivated patient can be detoxified on an outpatient basis with one physician managing the medications. Toxicology screens, done with the patient's permission, are useful. If at all possible, detoxification should occur when the patient is not experiencing other significant medical or social stresses. Family members and friends should be involved in both the treatment program and education about preventing relapse. If patients are abusing ethanol or illicit drugs, the clinician should manage this problem first, usually with the help of a specialist in alcohol and drug abuse.

Detoxification is only one part of the treatment plan.[3] A sedating tricyclic antidepressant (e.g., doxepin or amitriptyline) may restore sleep, improve nutrition, and enhance analgesia. Psychological counseling to increase the patient's coping skills may improve well-being. Family counseling may also be necessary to reduce the environmental reinforcers of suffering behaviors. Dietary avoidance of excessive caffeine and sugar may help avoid mood swings. Twelve-step recovery programs available in most communities (e.g., Alcoholics Anonymous, Narcotics Anonymous) may help prevent relapses in selected patients. A specifically prescribed and graded exercise program, reinforced by the patient keeping a diary of daily activities, may restore the flexibility, strength, and aerobic fitness lost after prolonged rest and disuse (see Prescription of Physical Activity, Section 72).

Physical modalities such as heat and cold, massage, and transcutaneous electrical stimulation are less useful in chronic pain syndrome than in the treatment of acute pain resulting from tissue damage or irritation.[3]

To prevent the development of the chronic pain syndrome, the clinician should accurately diagnose all acute injuries, thoroughly explain to patients the nature of the injury and the estimated recovery date, specifically prescribe doses and frequencies of activity and medications, and schedule prompt follow-up.

When patients with chronic pain syndrome respond poorly to treatment, they should be referred to a program specializing in chronic pain. There are 212 centers and clinics in 41 states that offer services on an inpatient or outpatient basis (listed in *Medical and Health Information Directory,* vol. 3, ed. 5. Backus K, Furtaw JC, Eds. Gale Research Inc., Detroit, 1991, pp. xiv, 419–425).

Cross-references: Assessment of Physical Activity (Section 72), Low Back Pain (Section 108), The Difficult Patient (Section 195).

REFERENCES

1. Bonica JJ. General considerations of chronic pain. In Bonica JJ, Ed. The Management of Pain. Lea & Febiger, Philadelphia, 1990, pp. 180–196.
    A two-volume text that covers all aspects of chronic pain.

2. Butter SH, Murphey TM. Use and abuse of drugs in chronic non-cancerous pain states. In Loeser JD, Eagen KJ, Eds. Managing the Chronic Pain Patient: Theory and Practice at the University of Washington Multidisciplinary Pain Center. Raven Press, New York, 1989, pp. 1162–1168.
    One center's approach to the management of chronic pain.

3. Cardenas DD, Eagan KJ. Management of chronic pain. In Kottke FJ, Stillwell GK, Lehmann JF, Eds. Krusen's Handbook of Physical Medicine and Rehabilitation, 4th ed. W.B. Saunders, Philadelphia, 1990, pp. 1162–1168.
    Another approach to management in a comprehensive physical medicine and rehabilitation text.

4. International Association for the Study of Pain. Classification of chronic pain: Description of chronic pain syndromes and definitions of pain states [Merskey H, Ed.]. Pain (suppl 3) 1986; S1.
    Discusses the multidisciplinary efforts to further understand chronic pain.

5. Ries RK, Roy-Byrne PP, Ward NG, Neppe V, Cullison S. Carbamazepine treatment for benzodiazepine withdrawal. Am J Psychiatry 1989;146:536–537.
    Case studies using carbamazepine.

14 AIDS

Problem

THOMAS G. COONEY

EPIDEMIOLOGY/NATURAL HISTORY. It is estimated that more than 1 million persons in the United States may be infected with human immunodeficiency virus (HIV). Over 200,000 cases of acquired immunodeficiency syndrome (AIDS) have been reported in the United States, and 130,000 people have died of AIDS. Most persons with HIV infection are asymptomatic or mildly symptomatic and will be managed in the ambulatory setting.

Although a variety of staging systems exist, the most useful system clinically divides HIV infection into three stages: (1) an acute phase, often asymptomatic or associated with a mononucleosis-like syndrome, that lasts for weeks; (2) a chronic phase lasting 5 to 10 years, during which a state of immunodeficiency evolves, often with few or no symptoms; and (3) an advanced, highly symptomatic stage, corresponding to ARC (AIDS-related complex) and AIDS. Occurrence of the latter two stages correlates closely with depressed CD4 cell counts (250–800 cells/mm^3 in the chronic phase, <250–300 cells/mm^3 in ARC or AIDS).

CHRONIC PHASE

SYMPTOMS AND SIGNS. Only during the later portion of the chronic phase do patients begin to experience symptoms and exhibit signs of HIV infection. Some of the earliest problems are due to problems with humoral (B-cell) immunity. Examples include recurrent sinusitis; recurrent bacterial pneumonia, often bacteremic and most commonly due to *Streptococcus pneumoniae;* immune thrombocytopenia purpura; and an inflammatory demyelinating polyneuropathy. Other early manifestations include dermatomal herpes zoster, *Mycobacterium tuberculosis* infection, and syphilis. Although not unique to HIV-infected patients, tuberculosis and syphilis have atypical presentations and follow accelerated courses in the setting of HIV infection. Kaposi's sarcoma occurs in both early and late stages of the disease. As CD4 counts drop below 250 to 300 cells/mm^3, patients may note symptoms such as fatigue and fever; oral candidiasis and hairy leukoplakia may appear, and, in women, recurrent vaginal candidiasis. A wide variety of cutaneous disorders, including seborrheic dermatitis, folliculitis, and dermatophyte infections, may appear at this time.

CLINICAL APPROACH. During the chronic phase of HIV infection, efforts should focus on collecting a complete data base and periodic monitoring for disease progression as evidenced by changes in laboratory tests (e.g., CD4 counts, anemia) or the occurrence of symptoms.

A complete medical history should emphasize a number of areas. Of particular importance are constitutional symptoms such as fever, weight loss, fatigue, and night sweats; pulmonary symptoms such as cough and shortness of breath; gastrointestinal symptoms such as diarrhea and odynophagia; neurologic symptoms such as headaches; and dermatologic lesions such as rashes. Other important areas to assess are risk behaviors (e.g., sexual history, intravenous [IV] drug use); prior infections, particularly tuberculosis, tuberculin skin test results, hepatitis, and syphilis; a travel or residence history suggesting exposure to fungal diseases such as histoplasmosis or coccidiodomycosis; and, in women, a detailed gynecologic history, including menstrual history, types of birth control measures used, pelvic infections, and Papanicolaou smear results.

The physical examination should include weight measurements and careful ocular, oral, skin, lymph node, neurologic, and pelvic/genitourinary examinations with attention to evidence of HIV-related complications.

Laboratory tests are ordered to determine the stage and severity of illness and to screen for secondary conditions or complications. A number of tests should be performed as part of the baseline evaluation. These include a complete blood cell (CBC) count with differential, liver function tests, hepatitis panel (A, B, and C), toxoplasmosis serology, syphilis serology, and a chemistry panel that includes blood urea nitrogen, creatinine, and glucose. Additionally, all patients should have a tuberculin skin test along with an anergy panel (e.g., mumps, SK/SD, *Candida*) and chest radiography. Women with HIV infection should have pelvic examinations and Papanicolaou smears at least yearly, and screening for gonorrhea and *Chlamydia* is advisable. Finally, the CD4 count should be determined in all patients. The optimal intervals for CD4 testing are unknown, but the following schedule is generally accepted. If the initial CD4 cell count is above 600 cells/mm^3, testing is repeated in 6 months. As the CD4 count approaches 500 cells/mm^3, it is repeated every 3 months. If the CD4 falls below 500 cells/mm^3, it is repeated and confirmed in 1 week. After zidovudine (azidothymidine, AZT) therapy has been initiated (see below), monitoring returns to every 6 months until the CD4 count falls below 300 cells/mm^3, when the interval decreases to 3 months. Whether to monitor the CD4 count below 200 cells/mm^3 is controversial. Though initially not recommended, the practice is increasing as certain complications (e.g., disseminated *Mycobacterium avium-intracellulare* infections) seem to occur only with very low (<50 cells/mm^3) CD4 counts.

MANAGEMENT. During the initial assessment and subsequent follow-up, preventive health care, education, and counseling are a major focus. Vaccinations should be administered, including influenza vaccine (yearly) and pneumococcal vaccine (see Adult Immunization, Section 10). Based on test results for hepatitis B virus, HBV vaccine should be considered for those at risk. Because of the striking prevalence of tuberculosis in HIV-infected individuals, chemoprophylaxis is indicated for all at-risk individuals (see Tuberculosis Screening, Section 60). A purified protein derivative (PPD) test that produces induration 5 mm or more in diameter should be considered positive and managed accordingly. Chemoprophylaxis should also be considered for selected anergic individuals, including those with a prior positive PPD, a chest radiograph suggesting prior tuberculosis, or those with extensive exposure to individuals with active disease. Education and counseling should focus on health promotion, including nutrition, exercise, and avoiding substance abuse, including alcohol and cigarettes. Safe sexual practices, IV drug use, and, in females, contraception and the risk of maternal-fetal HIV transmission must be addressed.

Attention should be paid to the patient's social and emotional support systems. Legal and ethical issues related to ultimate disability and death should be discussed, including advance directives, durable power of attorney, and wills.

Two additional interventions are routine in the chronic phase: initiation of antiretroviral therapy and prophylaxis against *Pneumocystis carinii* pneumonia. Zidovudine and didanosine (ddI) are the only antiretroviral drugs available for general use. AZT is indicated for any HIV-infected adult with a CD4 count below 500 cells/mm^3. Contraindications include a white blood cell (WBC) count below 1000/mm^3, an absolute neutrophil count below 500/mm^3, and a hemoglobin value below 8 g/dl. The dosage is 500 to 600 mg per day in five to six divided doses. Dose reductions are necessary if toxic hematologic effects develop; however, doses less than 300 mg/day have not been shown to be effective. If patients become anemic, alternatives include transfusions and, more recently, erythropoietin. No proven alternatives exist to manage neutropenia beyond dose reductions. The CBC count should be monitored every 2 weeks for 2 months, then every 1 to 3 months, depending on the most recent hemoglobin and WBC values and whether other drugs are used that might increase hematologic toxic effects. A rise in the mean corpuscular volume (unrelated to B$_{12}$ or folate deficiency) is usually seen by 6 months. Other common side effects of zidovudine include nausea, headache, and sleep disturbances; these usually can be managed without dose reductions. Myopathy and myositis are much less common but may require cessation of therapy.

The indications for ddI include intolerance of AZT or AZT failure. A definition of AZT failure is lacking but corresponds to the development of a major opportunistic infection or 50% reduction in baseline CD4 counts after beginning AZT. The major toxicities of didanosine are pancreatitis and peripheral neuropathy. Dosages are based on body weight. Preliminary data indicate that combination therapy (AZT/ddI or AZT/DdC) may be a useful alternative.

The risk of *P. carinii* pneumonia rises markedly when CD4 counts drop below 200 to 250 cells/mm^3. Primary prophylaxis is now recommended for pa-

TABLE 14–1. *PNEUMOCYSTIS CARINII* PNEUMONIA PROPHYLAXIS

Drug	Dose	Advantage	Disadvantage	Cost ($)/Month[1]
Trimethoprim-sulfamethoxazole	160 mg/800 mg tablets; 1 q.d., 3 days/week	Inexpensive, systemic	Toxicity: rash, fever, GI, hematologic	1.80
Dapsone	50–100 mg q.d.	Inexpensive, systemic	Toxicity: rash, fever, methemo-globinemia, hemolytic anemia	2.70–5.40
Pentamidine	300 mg via nebulizer monthly	Compliance	Expensive; special equipment and space needed; appreciable failure rate	124.31

[1]Average wholesale price, 1991 *Drug Topics Red Book.*

tients with counts below 200 cells/mm^3, as is secondary prophylaxis for any HIV-infected patient who has had an episode of *P. carinii* pneumonia. Three options are available (Table 14–1). Recent trials have shown that systematic therapy is superior to inhaled pentamidine.

ADVANCED, SYMPTOMATIC STAGE

SYMPTOMS AND SIGNS.   With advancing HIV disease (CD4 count ≤200–250 cells/mm^3), a number of symptoms and signs develop that may suggest serious underlying problems such as opportunistic infections or malignancies.

Oral lesions are common at this stage. Oral candidiasis presents as movable white plaques on any oral mucosal surface and, less commonly, as an atrophic form with smooth red patches. Hairy leukoplakia, thought to be caused by Epstein-Barr virus, manifests as a white thickening of the oral mucosa, usually the tongue, often with vertical folds or corrugations. Severe gingivitis and periodontitis are also seen. Red or purple macules, papules, or nodules occur with Kaposi's sarcoma.

Ocular findings include the hard exudates of HIV retinopathy and the exudates and hemorrhages associated with cytomegalovirus (CMV) retinitis. The most common symptoms suggesting CMV retinitis are "floaters" and decreasing visual acuity.

Respiratory symptoms such as cough, chest pain, and dyspnea are highly suggestive of opportunistic infection or HIV-associated malignancy in patients with advanced HIV infection. Pneumothorax can be a manifestation of *P. carinii* pneumonia.

Gastrointestinal symptoms are common. Odynophagia is usually caused by candidal esophagitis but may be caused by CMV or herpes simplex. Diarrhea is a troubling problem in many patients. Identifiable pathogens include protozoa (e.g., *Giardia*, crytosporidia, microsporidia), viruses (e.g., CMV), bacteria (e.g., *Shigella*), and mycobacteria. Jaundice may be caused by liver disease or biliary disease. Examples of the former include infections such as *M. aviumintracellulare* (MAI), infiltration with Kaposi's sarcoma or lymphoma, or hepatotoxicity due to drugs (e.g., sulfa-containing drugs). CMV and cryptosporidia both may cause biliary disease.

Neurologic and psychiatric symptoms and signs occur with increasing frequency as disease progresses. Broadly, such symptoms and signs may cause an encephalopathy syndrome (fever, headache, confusion); may produce focal deficits (e.g., hemiparesis, visual field cuts) with or without seizures; psychiatric syndromes such as depression, mania, or psychosis; spinal cord or peripheral nerve diseases (e.g., vacuolar myelopathy, peripheral neuropathy); and meningitis (fever, headache).

Finally, constitutional symptoms such as fever, malaise, anorexia, and weight loss may accompany many of the above symptom complexes or occur alone. The HIV wasting syndrome is characterized by the presence of two of the following three symptoms: recurrent fever, weight loss (>10% of body weight), and diarrhea (>1 month).

CLINICAL APPROACH.   Several important principles govern the clinical approach to advanced-stage HIV disease. First, it is common for patients to have several infections or complications simultaneously. Second, the natural history and clinical presentation of the disease are changing constantly owing to antiretroviral therapy and the use of prophylaxis. Third, diagnostic strategies must be tailored to individual patients, taking into account the stage of their disease, the likelihood of finding a treatable cause for the symptoms (based both on efficacy of therapy and on the ability of the patient to tolerate the treatment), and patient preferences.

In patients with visual symptoms, a careful ocular and funduscopic examination should be performed and ophthalmology consultation sought if any findings are present (e.g., decreased visual acuity, retinal lesions). The diagnosis of CMV retinitis is based on the appearance of the retina and does not require culture of CMV.

Oral lesions are usually diagnosed from their visual appearance, although examination of potassium hydroxide–stained specimens may help differentiate oral candidiasis from hairy leukoplakia. Usually, only the index Kaposi's sarcoma lesion will require biopsy confirmation (i.e., to provide an AIDS-defining diagnosis).

The initial test in evaluating respiratory symptoms is chest radiography. If there is a segmental or lobar infiltrate, the clinician should obtain sputum and blood samples for culture of bacterial pathogens. If the radiograph is normal, noninvasive evaluations of lactate dehydrogenase, the lung diffusing capacity of carbon monoxide, the alveolar-arterial oxygen gradient, and the erythrocyte sedimentation rate can, in combination, be used to stratify patients into groups at high or low risk for opportunistic infections.[4] Patients with diffuse infiltrates on chest radiographs or with abnormal findings on noninvasive tests should have sputum induced for detection of *P. carinii* and other opportunistic pathogens, including *M. tuberculosis*. If the sputum is normal or if the induced sputum test is unavailable, bronchoscopy with bronchoalveolar lavage should be performed.

In the presence of oral candidiasis, odynophagia can be assumed to be due to *Candida* esophagitis. In its absence, or if the odynophagia fails to improve with appropriate therapy, upper gastrointestinal endoscopy should be performed; barium studies generally have a lower diagnostic yield. Diarrhea lasting longer than 1 week should prompt collection of stool specimens for identification of ova and parasites, enteric pathogens, mycobacteria, cryptosporidia, and *Clostridium difficile*. If negative, further evaluation may include colonoscopy, particularly if CMV infection is suspected. Extensive small bowel disease due to cryptosporidia, *Giardia,* or microsporidia may be suggested by an abnormal D-xylose absorption test; a small bowel biopsy would be indicated. Liver tests (i.e., alkaline phosphatase, bilirubin, etc.) and imaging modalities such as ultrasound and computed tomography (CT) should be used to assess symptoms and signs of hepatobiliary disease. Blood cultures (two sets) are useful if MAI infection is suspected. Unexplained large increases in alkaline phosphatase levels are an indication for liver biopsy, if the clinician expects to use the results to guide management.

After a careful neurologic examination, examination of the cerebrospinal fluid (CSF) and CT or magnetic resonance imaging (MRI) are the most useful diagnostic tests to evaluate neurologic symptoms. Cryptococcal meningitis is most reliably diagnosed from the presence of cryptococcal antigen in the CSF (sensitivity $\geq 90\%$); the serum cryptococcal antigen assay is similarly positive. The CSF may be otherwise entirely normal. Seizures or local neurologic symptoms and signs warrant CT or MRI. In general, MRI is more sensitive but less specific than CT for the various infections or neoplastic causes. A diagnosis of toxoplasmosis encephalitis is based on the CT or MRI appearance; serologic tests neither confirm nor exclude this diagnosis. Biopsy is indicated only if the lesion is solitary on MRI, if there is no response to a trial of toxoplasmosis therapy, or if patient factors (e.g., IV drug abuse) suggest a cryptococcoma or tuberculoma.

Considerable caution must be exercised in diagnosing the HIV wasting syndrome as there are numerous other causes for fever, weight loss, and diarrhea. Sustained fevers strongly suggest an opportunistic infection or lymphoma and should be carefully evaluated; useful diagnostic tests include liver tests, blood cultures for MAI, and chest radiography. Other tests are dictated by the presence of specific symptoms. Weight loss requires an assessment of the patient's caloric intake. If inadequate, the clinician should determine if it is due to early satiety or anorexia. Early satiety suggests an intra-abdominal process. Anorexia may be due to drugs, depression, dementia, or dysphagia. Weight loss in a patient with adequate caloric intake suggests an underlying opportunistic infection or cancer; the workup is similar to that for fever. The evaluation of diarrhea was discussed earlier.

MANAGEMENT. Table 14–2 lists some of the drugs used in the outpatient management of advanced HIV disease. After placement of an indwelling central venous catheter and administration of an induction dose of ganciclovir,

TABLE 14–2. OUTPATIENT THERAPY FOR COMMON INFECTIOUS COMPLICATIONS OF AIDS[1]

Clinical Disease	Antimicrobial Agent	Administration	Daily Cost ($)[2]
Pneumocystis pneumonia	Trimethoprim-sulfamethoxazole	Trimethoprim, 15–20 mg/kg, and sulfamethoxazole, 75–100 mg/kg, daily in 3–4 divided doses PO for 21 days	1.20
	Trimethoprim-dapsone	300 mg trimethoprim q.6h. and 100 mg dapsone q.d. for 21 days	2.10
Candidiasis Oral	Nystatin	Two 500,000 U tab t.i.d.	0.90
	Clotrimazole	10-mg troche 5×/day for 14 days; dissolve slowly in mouth	3.21
Esophageal	Ketoconazole	200–600 mg q.d. for 14–21 days	2.18–6.54
	Fluconazole	100 mg q.d. for 14–21 days	6.87
Herpes simplex—mucocutaneous	Acyclovir	400 mg t.i.d.	4.26
Cytomegalovirus	Ganciclovir	6 mg/kg IV q.d., 5 days/week after induction	34.80
Cryptococcosis-meningitis	Fluconazole	200 mg/day	11.25
Toxoplasmosis-meningitis	Pyrimethamine and sulfadiazine	25 mg 2×/week 500 mg 2×/week	0.27 0.11

[1]These recommendations apply to mild infections or to maintenance therapy. Management of serious infections may require hospitalization and alternative medications.

[2]Average wholesale price, 1991 *Drug Topics Red Book.*

further therapy for CMV retinitis is conducted on an outpatient basis. Neutropenia is the major side effect, usually requiring that AZT be stopped. The role of foscarnet, a new agent, is being defined, but it may offer a survival advantage over ganciclovir.

Oral candidiasis can be managed with intraoral therapy, but as the disease progresses, systemic therapy may be needed. Because of absorption problems, increased doses of ketoconazole may be needed or, alternatively, fluconazole. Esophageal candidiasis requires systemic therapy; chronic suppressive therapy may be necessary.

Mild cases of *P. carinii* pneumonia ($Pao_2 > 70$ mm Hg) may be managed with outpatient oral therapy. More severe cases initially require admission for parenteral therapy, including adjunctive corticosteroids. Therapy may be completed on an outpatient basis.

After acute therapy, both CNS toxoplasmosis and cryptococcosis require chronic suppressive therapy.

MAI infection may be managed on a outpatient basis. Initial therapy should include four drugs: ciprofloxacin, 750 mg b.i.d.; clofazimine, 100 mg q.d.; ethambutol, 15 mg/kg/day; and rifampin, 600 mg q.d. If no response is seen in 6 weeks, amikacin may be added. Dose-limiting toxic effects and treatment failures are common.

The use of AZT in patients with advanced HIV infection is problematic. First, toxicity is enhanced by many other drugs used at this stage. Second, no good definition of AZT failure exists. The decision to continue AZT or to switch to alternative antiretroviral therapies (including combinations) will be based on emerging data.

FOLLOW-UP.   The complexity of management of late-stage HIV disease precludes simple guidelines for follow-up. In general, symptomatic patients are seen at least monthly. CD4 counts below 50 cells/mm³ indicate very advanced disease and the possibility of serious morbidity or mortality. Opportunistic infections such as CMV retinitis, CNS toxoplasmosis, and disseminated MAI infection are associated with median survivals of less than 1 year.

Cross-references: Death of Clinic Patients (Section 6), Diagnosis and Management of Drug Abuse (Section 8), Adult Immunizations (Section 10), Seborrheic Dermatitis (Section 29), Tuberculosis Screening (Section 60).

REFERENCES

1. Barnes PF, Block AB, Davidson PT, Snider DE. Tuberculosis in patients with human immunodeficiency virus infection. N Engl J Med 1991;324:1644–1650.
   Comprehensive review of the problems of diagnosis and treatment; indications for chemoprophylaxis.

2. Freedberg KA, Tosteson ANA, Cohen CJ, Cotton DJ. Primary prophylaxis for pneumocystis pneumonia in HIV-infected people with CD4 counts below 200/mm³: A cost effectiveness analysis. J AIDS 1991;4:521–531.
   Trimethoprim-sulfa drugs and dapsone are clearly superior.

3. Horsburgh CR. Mycobacterium avium complex infection in the acquired immunodeficiency syndrome. N Engl J Med 1991;324:1332–1338.
    A practical approach to diagnosis and treatment.

4. Katz MH, Baron RB, Grady D. Risk stratification of ambulatory patients suspected of pneumocystis pneumonia. Arch Intern Med 1991;151:105–110.
    Chest radiography, LDH, ESR, and oral lesions (e.g., candidiasis) can be used to stratify the risk of *P. carinii* pneumonia in outpatients with respiratory symptoms.

5. Musher DM, Hamill RJ, Baughn RE. Effect of human immunodeficiency virus infection on the course of syphilis and on the response to treatment. Ann Intern Med 1990;113:872–881.
    In-depth review of the unique problems that arise in diagnosing and managing syphilis in HIV-infected patients.

15 OBESITY

Problem

MARY ELLEN GILLES

EPIDEMIOLOGY.   Obesity affects one-fourth of adults in the United States. Slightly over 0.1% of the population is morbidly obese, defined as more than 100 lb overweight. The prevalence of obesity is inversely related to socioeconomic status, is higher among women and less educated people, and increases with age.

Body mass index (weight [kg] divided by height squared [m²]) correlates well with more precise measures of body fat. Health risks increase with moderate obesity, defined as a body mass index greater than 30. The Metropolitan Life height and weight tables, based on actuarial data, define desirable weight as that associated with the lowest mortality for a given height (Table 15–1). Obesity is defined as 120% of desirable weight.

Specific adverse health risks of obesity include cardiovascular disease, hypertension, hyperlipidemia, non-insulin-dependent diabetes mellitus, hypoventilation, sleep apnea, gallbladder disease, and degenerative joint disease. Low testosterone levels in men and abnormal menstrual cycles in women may accompany obesity. Obesity has been linked to prostate and colorectal cancer in men and cancers of the endometrium, uterus, gallbladder, cervix, ovary, and breast in women.

ETIOLOGY.   Although incompletely understood, obesity represents a nutrient imbalance with more energy stored than expended. The tendency toward obesity is partly inherited, but environmental factors play a role.

TABLE 15–1. METROPOLITAN HEIGHT AND WEIGHT TABLES

Height		Weight (lb)		
Feet	Inches	Small Frame	Medium Frame	Large Frame
Men				
5	2	128–134	131–141	138–150
5	3	130–136	133–143	140–153
5	4	132–138	135–145	142–156
5	5	134–140	137–148	144–160
5	6	136–142	139–151	146–164
5	7	138–145	142–154	149–168
5	8	140–148	145–157	152–172
5	9	142–151	148–160	155–176
5	10	144–154	151–163	158–180
5	11	146–157	154–166	161–184
6	0	149–160	157–170	164–188
6	1	152–164	160–174	168–192
6	2	155–168	164–178	172–197
6	3	158–172	167–182	176–202
6	4	162–176	171–187	181–207
Women				
4	10	102–111	109–121	118–131
4	11	103–113	111–123	120–134
5	0	104–115	113–126	122–137
5	1	106–118	115–129	125–140
5	2	108–121	118–132	128–143
5	3	111–124	121–135	131–147
5	4	114–127	124–138	134–151
5	5	117–130	127–141	137–155
5	6	120–133	130–144	140–159
5	7	123–136	133–147	143–163
5	8	126–139	136–150	146–167
5	9	129–142	139–153	149–170
5	10	132–145	142–156	152–173
5	11	135–148	145–159	155–176
6	0	138–151	148–162	158–179

Source: Lauter SA, Healey LA. Metropolitan height and weight tables. In Viaz SL, Ed. A Practical Guide to Clinical Management. W.B. Saunders, Philadelphia, 1992. Reproduced by permission.

Specific medical disorders cause obesity in less than 1% of cases. These conditions include Cushing's syndrome, hypothyroidism, Stein-Leventhal syndrome, insulinoma, gonadal failure, hypothalamic disturbances (neoplasm, trauma, infection), and the use of certain drugs (e.g., phenothiazines, cyproheptadine). Screening for these disorders in the absence of symptoms is unwarranted.

CLINICAL APPROACH.   During the physical examination the degree of obesity may be estimated by calculating the body mass index or by using height and weight tables. The presence of obesity and its health implications should be discussed with the patient. It may be helpful to determine the pattern of fat distribution, because abdominal obesity is associated with a higher frequency of comorbid conditions and premature death than is gluteal obesity. Abdominal obesity is present when the waist-to-hip-circumference ratio exceeds 0.95 for men and 0.85 for women.

MANAGEMENT.   Dietary manipulation is essential to weight loss programs. A registered dietitian can educate the patient and develop menus that are nutritionally adequate and compatible with the patient's life-style. Types of diets include balanced calorie-restricted, low-carbohydrate, high-carbohydrate, fad, and very low-calorie diets.

Balanced calorie-restricted diets (1000–1800 calories per day) eliminate high-calorie foods and emphasize healthy food selections. Low-carbohydrate diets induce a mild ketosis, which suppresses appetite, but may cause volume depletion, hyperuricemia, and increased serum cholesterol levels. High-carbohydrate, low-fat diets reduce serum lipid levels, require more time to chew and swallow, and promote satiety. Fad diets severely restrict food choices or make unfounded claims of unique weight-reducing properties of certain foods. Very low-calorie diets (300–800 calories per day) produce more rapid weight loss than conventional diets and preserve lean body mass compared with complete fasting. Very low-calorie diets may be indicated for morbidly obese adults but should be supervised by physicians experienced in their use.

Although weight loss by exercise alone is difficult, regular exercise does help patients maintain weight loss. Before prescribing exercise, the clinician should evaluate the patient for any conditions that require activity modification. Exercise should begin at low levels and be gradually increased. To lose weight and body fat, the American College of Sports Medicine recommends a minimum of 20 minutes of exercise three times weekly at an intensity to expend 300 calories per session (see Prescription of Physical Activity, Section 72).

Behavioral treatment for obesity identifies stimuli that lead to excessive eating and applies measures to produce and maintain appropriate eating behavior. Behavioral treatment, available through individual therapy or community group programs, together with caloric restriction and exercise is the most promising approach to long-term weight control and improved health.

Pharmacotherapy is not recommended for weight reduction. Appetite suppressants produce weight loss, but weight is commonly regained after discontinuation, and habituation and abuse are potential problems. Thyroid hormone supplementation is indicated only for patients with established hypothyroidism.

Antiobesity surgeries, jejunoileal bypass or gastric restrictive procedures, may have significant long-term complications and should be reserved for the morbidly obese in whom weight loss cannot be achieved with intensive nonsurgical measures.

FOLLOW-UP.   Regular follow-up visits provide support and monitor coexisting medical conditions as weight loss occurs. Blood pressure, serum cholesterol levels, and glucose regulation may improve with modest weight loss even if ideal body weight is not achieved.

Cross-references: Sleep Apnea Syndromes (Section 64), Assessment of Physical Activity (Section 72).

REFERENCES

1. Elliot DL, Goldberg L, Girard DE. Obesity: Pathophysiology and practical management. J Gen Intern Med 1987;2:188–198.

    Discusses proposed mechanisms of obesity, evaluates available treatments, and presents practical treatment recommendations.

2. Gilles ME, Pecoraro RE, Fihn SD. A clinical review of obesity. Med Rounds 1989;2:223–234.

    Review of prevalence, pathogenesis, and health risks of obesity, with an emphasis on treatment options.

3. Lew EA, Garfinkel L. Variations in mortality by weight among 750,000 men and women. J Chronic Dis 1979;32:563–576.

    Prospective study relating mortality to body weight. Mortality from cardiovascular disease, certain cancers, and diabetes mellitus was increased in overweight individuals. The lowest mortality was found in those of average weight and 10% to 20% below average weight.

4. Metropolitan Life Insurance Co. 1983 Metropolitan height and weight tables. Stat Bull Metropolitan Insur Co 1983;64:2–9.

    Tables indicate weight associated with the lowest mortality for a given height among a large sample of insured persons.

5. Wing RR, Jeffrey RW. Outpatient treatments of obesity: A comparison of methodology and clinical results. Int J Obes 1979;3:261–279.

    Meta-analysis of 145 articles comparing outpatient treatments for obesity. Diet, exercise, behavioral therapy, and drugs all produced modest weight losses without significant differences among them, but recidivism was the rule.

16 FEVER

Problem

BENJAMIN A. LIPSKY

EPIDEMIOLOGY.   Most studies of fever have focused on fever of unknown origin or fever occurring in hospitalized populations. Outpatient studies have mainly been conducted in emergency rooms, where about 5% of patients (range, 4% to 21% in published studies) are febrile (usually defined as an oral temperature $\geq$ 100°F or 38°C); about 30% of these patients are subsequently hospitalized.

ETIOLOGY.   Infections are the cause of fever in most ambulatory patients. Acute febrile illnesses of less than 2 weeks' duration are common, usually are uncomplicated, resolve spontaneously, and do not require a specific diagnosis. Bacterial infections and other more serious disorders require diagnostic evaluation and therapy. In immunocompetent hosts, fever is far more likely to be due to a common disease than to a rare one.

The most frequent infectious causes of fever are viral syndromes, pharyngitis, urinary tract infections, cellulitis, pneumonia, and gastrointestinal infections (e.g., bacterial diarrhea, diverticulitis, hepatobiliary infections). Noninfectious causes of fever include malignancies, inflammatory disorders (connective tissue or granulomatous diseases), drug reactions, and thromboembolic or neurologic events. The relative prevalence of these causes is highly dependent on the age of the population studied and the practice setting. Fevers caused by neoplasms generally last several weeks, do not abate following antimicrobial therapy, and respond promptly to anti-inflammatory agents such as naproxen. In one small study the sensitivity of the "naproxen test" was 0.93 and the specificity was 1.0. Viral syndromes and upper respiratory tract infections are uncommon causes of fever in adults over 60 years old (<5%) compared with those under 60 (about 40%).[2] Forty percent of febrile outpatients over 60 have an identifiable focal or systemic (i.e., bacteremic) bacterial infection.[5] Older outpatients presenting with fever are more likely to have a life-threatening illness (e.g., pneumonia, biliary tract infection, diverticulitis) and to require hospitalization.[2]

In 50% to 80% of patients, the initial evaluation identifies a localized source of the fever,[4] although the diagnosis is subsequently revised in 15% of patients. Occult bacterial infection is found in about one-third of adult outpatients whose fever was initially unexplained.[3,4] In parenteral drug abusers, fever is most often caused by pneumonia (about one-third of cases) and endocarditis (about one-sixth of cases); less frequent causes include pyrogen reactions, skin and soft tissue infections, and pyelonephritis. Endocarditis is more likely in those who inject cocaine, have a history of cardiac disorders or weight loss, or have a cardiac murmur or petechiae.

CLINICAL APPROACH. The clinician should inquire about localizing symptoms and, when appropriate, about recent travel, exposure to animals, unusual occupations or avocations, prescription and illicit drug use, risk factors for AIDS, unusual dietary exposures, and exposure to other sick individuals. The examination should focus on the skin and mucous membranes, lymph nodes, ocular fundi, heart and lung sounds, and palpation of the abdomen. Neither the fever's pattern nor its height are diagnostically reliable, though higher temperatures are more common in bacterial infections, especially in the elderly.[5] Dissociation of the body temperature and the pulse rate (Faget's sign) is of little diagnostic value. Fever lasting more than 2 weeks is unusual in common viral syndromes and most pyogenic infections and suggests subacute or chronic infections (e.g., tuberculosis, endocarditis) or noninfectious disorders.

Two studies have validated an index designed to predict occult bacterial infection in adult outpatients presenting with fever. The independent risk factors were age $\geq$50 years; diabetes mellitus; WBC count $\geq$15,000; neutrophil band count $\geq$1500; and erythrocyte sedimentation rate $\geq$ 30.[3,4] Patients who lack all of these features rarely need empirical antibiotic therapy or hospitalization.[3] Among febrile adult outpatients, bacteremia is present in 10% to 15% of patients in whom blood cultures are done.[1,4,5] In one study, less than 1% of those who were not hospitalized were bacteremic.[1] Blood cultures should usually be done only in patients who are to be hospitalized or in whom subacute bacterial endocarditis is suspected. Because urinary and lower respiratory tract infections account for about half of bacterial infections, urinalysis and chest roentgenography are often diagnostically helpful. Other diagnostic tests are indicated only when signs or symptoms suggest a localized infection, and in some elderly or cognitively impaired patients.

MANAGEMENT.   Hospitalization should be considered for febrile outpatients who are vulnerable hosts (e.g., the elderly, immunocompromised, or those with a serious underlying disease), who appear toxic (e.g., exhibit rigors, hypotension, prostration, extreme pyrexia, CNS dysfunction, cardiopulmonary compromise), or in drug-abusing, elderly, or chronically ill patients who have no obvious localizing findings. The predictive index discussed above may also help determine who should be hospitalized. Antibiotics are usually indicated only when a bacterial infection is suspected. Empirical antibiotic administration to a patient with fever of uncertain cause usually does more harm than good. If a therapeutic trial is elected for a patient with a prolonged febrile illness, the choice of antibiotic should be as narrow-spectrum as possible. Except in patients with temperatures above 40°C or those with severe cardiac or catabolic diseases, antipyretic therapy is unnecessary, potentially deleterious, and diagnostically confusing.

FOLLOW-UP.   Most patients with fever caused by conditions other than a viral respiratory syndrome should be seen (or telephoned) for follow-up in about 3 days. About 15% of febrile patients initially sent home from an emergency room will subsequently require hospitalization.

REFERENCES

1. Eisenberg JM, Rose JD, Weinstein AJ. Routine blood cultures from febrile outpatients: Use in detecting bacteremia. JAMA 1976;236:2863–2865.

    Blood cultures were done in 37% of febrile emergency room patients; bacteremia was present in 10% of those who were hospitalized, but only one of 124 patients not admitted.

2. Keating HJ, Klimek JJ, Levine DS, Kiernan FJ. Effect of aging on the clinical significance of fever in ambulatory adult patients. J Am Geriatr Soc 1984;32:282–287.

    In a retrospective analysis of adults seen in an emergency room, 93% of febrile patients older than 60 had an illness requiring hospitalization, and 32% of them had a focal or systemic bacterial infection.

3. Leibovici L, Cohen O, Wysenbeek AJ. Occult bacterial infection in adults with unexplained fever: Validation of a diagnostic index. Arch Intern Med 1990;150:1270–1272.

    The index developed by Mellors, when prospectively applied within 12 hours of hospitalization to 113 adults with fever without an obvious source, accurately identified patients for whom hospitalization was unnecessary.

4. Mellors JW, Horwitz RI, Harvey MR, Horwitz SM. A simple index to identify occult bacterial infection in adults with acute unexplained fever. Arch Intern Med 1987;147:666–671.

   Of 880 acutely febrile patients presenting to the medicine section of an emergency room, 85% had localizing symptoms or signs. In the remaining 15% of patients, five features were found to be significant independent predictors of occult bacterial infection (see text).

5. Wasserman M, Levinstein M, Keller E, Lee S, Yoshikawa TT. Utility of fever, white blood cells, and differential count in predicting bacterial infections in the elderly. J Am Geriatr Soc 1989;37:537–543.

   In 221 patients 70 years old or older who were seen in an emergency room, fever ≥ 37.5°C, leukocytosis (≥14,500/mm³), and bandemia (>6%) were each associated with the presence of a bacterial infection.

17 WEIGHT LOSS

Problem

STEVEN R. McGEE

EPIDEMIOLOGY.   In a survey of elderly male outpatients, 8% claimed a recent weight loss of more than 5 lb.[3] Careful evaluation failed to substantiate weight loss in one-half.

ETIOLOGY.   Weight loss reflects either diuresis, decreased food intake, or the increased caloric requirements of malabsorption, glucosuria or hypermetabolism. Physical disease is diagnosed in 65% of weight loss cases. Psychiatric diagnoses, such as depression, anorexia nervosa, and schizophrenia, account for 10% of cases. The diagnosis remains unknown in 25% despite at least 1 year of follow-up.

The most common physical causes are cancer (19%–37% of cases) and gastrointestinal disorders (15% of cases). Common gastrointestinal causes include peptic ulcer disease and malabsorption. Cancer cachexia results from anorexia, decreased food intake, and a small but significantly increased basal metabolic rate. The amount of weight lost depends on tumor location: sarcoma and breast cancers cause small amounts of weight loss; prostate, colon, and lung cancers cause intermediate weight loss; and stomach and pancreatic cancers cause significant weight loss.

Ultimately, most chronic illnesses can produce weight loss. Weight loss induced by tuberculosis, for example, sometimes mimics cancer cachexia. The historical label of "consumption" for both diseases reflects this diagnostic confusion, which still occurs when biopsies of masses or lymph nodes are not cultured for mycobacteria. The cachexia of chronic lung disease results from anorexia and hypermetabolism. Cardiac cachexia, which occurs in long-standing congestive heart failure, represents the combined effect of anorexia (unpalatable diet, digoxin, potassium therapy), early satiety (hepatomegaly, ascites), malabsorption of neutral fats, and hypermetabolism. Painful diabetic polyneuropathies produce profound but temporary anorexia, muscle wasting, and weight loss.

Most patients with cachectic diseases have symptomatic clues that help the physician isolate the cause of weight loss. For example, weight-losing patients with peptic ulcer disease experience abdominal pain. Endocrine disorders, in contrast, may produce isolated weight loss. Addison's disease and hypercalcemic disorders cause weight loss and decreased appetite; hyperthyroidism and hyperglycemia produce weight loss and increased appetite.

CLINICAL APPROACH.   Inspection of the patient's belt and clothing, chart review, discussions with the patient's family, and sequential clinic visits provide evidence of weight loss. Many patients, despite claims to the contrary, do not have weight loss. In addition, the chart review may disclose some patients with serious illnesses who do not report their weight loss. After a complete history and physical examination, diagnostic studies include serum electrolytes, glucose, creatinine, calcium, liver function tests, stool guaiac cards, CBC count and chest radiography. Further workup is guided by symptoms (for example, an upper gastrointestinal series in the patient with epigastric pain). Because occult disease is rare, the physician should avoid long diagnostic searches in the absence of directing symptoms. Physical diseases declare themselves within 6 months, although almost all diagnoses are made during the initial evaluation.

MANAGEMENT.   See discussion in following section.

Cross-reference: Anorexia (Section 18).

REFERENCES

1. DeWys WD, Begg C, Lavin PT, Band PR, Bennett JM, Bertino JR, Cohen MH, Douglass HO. Prognostic effect of weight loss prior to chemotherapy in cancer patients. Am J Med 1980;69:491–497.
    Discusses the epidemiology and adverse effects of weight loss in a variety of tumor types and stages.

2. Estes NA, Levine HJ. Cardiac cachexia. Med Grand Rounds 1982;1:188–200.
    Overview of the many factors involved in cardiac cachexia.

3. Marton KI, Sox HC, Krupp JR. Involuntary weight loss: Diagnostic and prognostic significance. Ann Intern Med 1981;95:568–574.
    Best prospective analysis of weight loss. Patients with nausea, vomiting, recent changes in appetite, or a change in cough were more likely to have a physical cause for weight loss; nonsmokers and those without a change in activity despite weight loss were less likely to have a physical cause.

4. Pitlik SD, Fainstein V, Bodey GP. Tuberculosis mimicking cancer—a reminder. Am J Med 1984;76:822–825.
    The most common diagnosis was tuberculosis of the lung or lymph nodes.

5. Rabinovitz M, Pitlik SD, Leifer M, Garty M, Rosenfeld JB. Unintentional weight loss: A retrospective analysis of 154 cases. Arch Intern Med 1986;146:186–187.
    Confirms Marton's findings that the diagnosis is usually made with simple procedures during an initial evaluation; 23% remained undiagnosed despite a mean follow-up interval of 30 months.

18 ANOREXIA

Problem

STEVEN R. McGEE

EPIDEMIOLOGY.   Anorexia, or loss of appetite, may be associated with many different acute and chronic diseases or may occur in the absence of physical disease. Point prevalence rates in the elderly approach 20%.

ETIOLOGY.   In the hypothalamus, the nerves that control desire for food are linked to those that control the autonomic and endocrine responses to food. Stimulation of the hypothalamic ventromedial nucleus causes anorexia and catabolic responses (decreased gastric acid production, increased glycogenolysis and increased free fatty acids), while stimulation of the lateral hypothalamus produces the opposite response. Within the CNS, opioid peptides promote feeding; serotonin, corticotropin-releasing factor, and dopamine inhibit feeding. Peripheral hormones (e.g., insulin, cholecystokinin, estradiol, bombesin) provide feedback to the hypothalamus and inhibit feeding.

This information, largely derived from animal experiments, may provide insight into human appetite disorders. For example, anorexia accompanies most catabolic diseases, such as cancer and chronic infections. Appetite increases after oophorectomy, when estrogen levels are low. Naloxone (an opioid antagonist) and fenfluramine (serotonin agonist) produce anorexia, while cyproheptadine (serotonin antagonist) causes increased appetite and weight. Finally, many antihypertensive, antidepressant, and neuroleptic medications alter appetite, perhaps through changes in these central neurotransmitters.

Other factors that may cause anorexia include (1) abnormal taste and smell—both the aging process and multiple medications (e.g., captopril, antibiotics, and carbamazepine) alter these senses (see Section 52, Abnormal Taste and Smell); (2) learned food aversions—cancer patients subconsciously associate unpleasant experiences, such as chemotherapy, with food ingested during that experience; (3) medications—digoxin, for example, may cause profound anorexia even when drug levels are within therapeutic range; and (4) depression.

Some chronic wasting illnesses, however, may mimic depression and produce *vegetative* symptoms (anorexia, fatigue, weight loss, insomnia) without *nonphysical* symptoms of depression (low self-esteem, guilt, suicidal feelings). These patients are not depressed and usually do not benefit from antidepressants.

CLINICAL APPROACH.   The clinician should distinguish "anorexia" from "early satiety" (in which the appetite is initially normal but promptly disappears after ingestion of unusually small amounts of food) and from "sitophobia" (in which eating provokes unpleasant symptoms such as abdominal angina, dumping, or odynophagia). During the evaluation of anorexia, the physician should constantly search for a responsible medication, inquire into the possibility of depression, and investigate the patient's ability to prepare, taste, smell, and chew food. After a complete history, physical examination, and routine laboratory tests, the diagnostic search should not go beyond that recommended for involuntary weight loss (see Section 17).

MANAGEMENT.   General principles include (1) treating the underlying specific physical or psychiatric illnesses, (2) limiting unpalatable dietary restrictions, and (3) increasing the patient's socialization during meals. Flavor enhancers may benefit those with decreased taste and smell. Specific drugs that increase appetite include marijuana (which produces too many side effects for chronic use), the serotonin antagonist cyproheptadine, and, in patients with cachexia from cancer or AIDS, the progesterone derivative megestrol acetate.

Cross-references: Weight Loss (Section 17), Abnormal Taste and Smell (Section 52).

REFERENCES

1. Banks T. Digitalis cachexia. N Engl J Med 1974;290:746.
    Profound anorexia occurred in six patients, two of whom were being evaluated for occult malignancy. After withdrawal of digoxin, normal appetite returned.

2. Morley JE, Silver AJ. Review: Anorexia in the elderly. Neurobiol Aging 1988;9:9–16.
    Overview of pathophysiology of anorexia in elderly. Several related articles in this issue deal with anorexia.

3. Noble RE. Effect of cyproheptadine on appetite and weight gain in adults. JAMA 1969;209:2054–2055.
    In a double-blind, randomized, placebo-controlled trial, cyproheptadine increased appetite and produced weight gain in underweight adults.

4. Tchekmedyian NS, Hickman M, Heber D. Treatment of anorexia and weight loss with megestrol acetate in patients with cancer or acquired immunodeficiency syndrome. Semin Oncol 1991;18:35–42.
    Reviews the available data. Megestrol acetate may promote appetite and weight gain with few side effects.

5. Theologides A. Anorexins, asthenins, and cachectins in cancer. Am J Med 1986;81:696–698.
    A humoral substance causes cancer anorexia: The leading candidate is cachectin/tumor necrosis factor.

19 DYSPNEA

Problem

STEVEN R. McGEE

EPIDEMIOLOGY. Dyspnea refers to the discomfort associated with labored breathing. In one recent series, dyspnea accounted for 15% of admissions to a general medical service.[2]

ETIOLOGY. Although the precise mechanism of dyspnea is unknown, it commonly occurs when (1) ventilatory capacity is reduced (by obstructive or restrictive pulmonary disease), or (2) inadequate oxygen delivery to muscle produces lactic acidosis and increased ventilatory demands (as in cardiac disease, pulmonary vascular disease, pulmonary parenchymal disease, or anemia). Four diagnoses account for 70% of cases of chronic dyspnea: asthma, chronic obstructive pulmonary disease (COPD), interstitial lung disease, and cardiomyopathy.[1] Common causes of acute dyspnea include, in addition to the above diagnoses, pneumonia, pleural effusion, lung cancer, and pulmonary embolus.

Dyspnea occurs during the tachypnea phase of **Cheyne-Stokes respirations,** which result from low cardiac output or extensive disease of the cerebral cortex. **Orthopnea** describes the abrupt dyspnea that develops in the supine position and promptly disappears after the subject sits up or flexes the head. It occurs in both cardiac and pulmonary disease. **Paroxysmal nocturnal dyspnea,** in contrast, wakes the patient after 1 to 2 hours of sound sleep and lasts minutes despite sitting up or walking around (the patient experiences pulmonary edema). Paroxysmal nocturnal dyspnea is specific for cardiomyopathy and elevated left atrial pressure, although it may be confused with other causes of nocturnal dyspnea such as Cheyne-Stokes respiration (which often first appears during sleep), sleep apnea, asthma, or reflux esophagitis and aspiration. Dyspnea that occurs with sitting but is relieved by lying down (the opposite of orthopnea) is called **platypnea.** Most affected patients have intrapulmonary or intracardiac right-to-left shunts. **Trepopnea** describes the dyspnea that occurs in one lateral decubitus position and spares the other. Causes include cardiomegaly (less dyspnea with the right side down), unilateral parenchymal lung disease (less dyspnea with the good lung down), and mediastinal or endobronchial tumors.

CLINICAL APPROACH. Acute dyspnea usually requires urgent hospitalization, evaluation, and management. One exception is the patient with asthma, who is sometimes effectively treated in the emergency department.

Chronic dyspnea is usually managed in the outpatient clinic. A careful history and physical examination, combined with a chest roentgenography, will yield the correct diagnosis in 70% of cases.[1] Sections 68 and 79 review the common findings in patients with asthma, COPD, or congestive heart failure. In addition to the classic symptoms and signs of congestive heart failure, an abnormal blood pressure response to the bedside Valsalva maneuver will uncover the cardiac contributions to dyspnea even in patients with known pulmonary disease.[3]

The most useful diagnostic tests after chest roentgenography are pulmonary function tests. In patients whose baseline pulmonary function tests are unrevealing, a methacholine challenge may disclose asthma. Cardiopulmonary exercise testing is indicated when patients experience dyspnea that remains unexplained or is out of proportion to objective findings. This test defines the relative contributions of cardiac and pulmonary disease to the patient's dyspnea (e.g., in patients who have disorders in both systems) and also identifies patients with deconditioning or who have psychogenic dyspnea.

MANAGEMENT.   Therapy for the underlying condition alleviates dyspnea in 80% of cases.[1] Unfortunately, some diseases respond poorly to specific therapy. Examples include severe COPD and interstitial fibrosis. The following types of symptomatic treatment may benefit such patients: (1) home oxygen therapy—reduces dyspnea, hypoxic symptoms (confusion, headache, sleeplessness), and improves survival in patients with severe chronic hypoxemia ($Po_2 < 55$ mm Hg), (2) pursed lip breathing and leaning forward—improves lung mechanics and reduces dyspnea in patients with COPD, (3) muscle training with a simple home inspiratory resistance device—improves muscle strength and reduces dyspnea in severe COPD, and (4) a cold air stream directed against the face (e.g., a fan)—decreases breathlessness both in normal subjects made dyspneic (by inspiratory resistance or hypercapnia) and in many patients. Finally, controlled trials demonstrate that codeine, alcohol, and promethazine all reduce dyspnea and improve exercise tolerance; however, because the benefits are meager and the potential for drowsiness and addiction are great, these drugs are not recommended.

Cross-reference: Pulmonary Function Testing (Section 69).

REFERENCES

1. Pratter MR, Curley FJ, Dubois J, Irwin RS. Cause and evaluation of chronic dyspnea in a pulmonary disease clinic. Arch Intern Med 1989;149:2277–2282.

    Prospective evaluation of 89 consecutive patients referred to a pulmonary subspecialty clinic with chronic dyspnea (mean duration of dyspnea, 2.9 years). The diagnosis was made in 100%.

2. Schmitt BP, Kushner MS, Wiener SL. The diagnostic usefulness of the history of the patient with dyspnea. J Gen Intern Med 1986;1:386–393.

    146 consecutive hospital admissions for dyspnea. The initial diagnosis (obtained by a 5–15 minute history) correlated with the final diagnosis in 74% of cases.

3. Zema MJ, Masters AP, Margouleff D. Dyspnea: The heart or lungs? Differentiation at bed-
    side by use of the simple Valsalva maneuver. Chest 1984;85:59–64.
    In 37 patients with COPD and dyspnea, an abnormal response to the Valsalva maneuver predicted left
    ventricular dysfunction (detected by radionuclide ventriculography) with a sensitivity of 0.88 and spec-
    ificity of 0.90.

20 DIZZINESS

Problem

STEVEN R. McGEE

EPIDEMIOLOGY.   General practitioners evaluate two-thirds of all patients
with dizziness, the fifth most common complaint among patients older than 65
years. Dizziness is more common in women and the elderly. One-year prevalence rates approach 20% in those older than 60 years.

ETIOLOGY.   Peripheral vestibular disorders, the hyperventilation syndrome,
and multiple sensory deficits account for 74% of dizziness (Table 20–1). **Benign
positional vertigo** produces short (less than 1 minute) episodes of vertigo
brought on by head movements; over 50% of affected patients have sustained
a previous ear trauma or infection. Neurologic examination, other than the
Nylen-Barany test, is normal. **Vestibular neuronitis,** also called acute vestibu-

TABLE 20–1.   ETIOLOGY OF DIZZINESS

Etiology of Dizziness		% of Cases
Peripheral vestibular disorders		38
Benign positional vertigo	12	
Vestibular neuronitis	10	
Meniere's disease	4	
Other	12	
Hyperventilation syndrome		23
Multiple sensory deficits		13
Other		17
Unknown		9

Source: Drachman DA, Hart CW. An approach to the dizzy patient. Neurology 1972;22:323–334.
Adapted with permission.

lopathy or acute labyrinthitis, causes acute temporary vertigo, nausea, and vomiting. Most patients are young and have experienced a recent viral illness. **Basilar vertebral insufficiency,** an uncommon cause seen in elderly patients with known cerebrovascular disease, produces acute dizziness associated with diplopia, dysarthria, Horner's syndrome, and motor or sensory abnormalities. **Multiple sensory deficits** are combinations of poor vision, neuropathy, orthopedic deformity, or mild vestibular deficits that progressively diminish the patient's orientation to the environment. Affected patients are typically elderly, often diabetic, and experience no dizziness at rest but vague unsteadiness during walking and turning.

Other causes of dizziness include cardiovascular disorders (e.g., carotid sinus hypersensitivity; see Section 75, Syncope), various toxins (welder's fumes, carbon monoxide, hydrocarbon solvents), and medications (quinine, alcohol, and antihypertensive, anticonvulsant, antidepressant, or cardiovascular medications). In 10% to 15% of cases no cause can be identified despite extensive evaluation. Recent studies demonstrate no association between untreated hypertension and dizziness.

CLINICAL APPROACH.   The most useful diagnostic test, in both primary care and sophisticated referral centers, is a careful history, which yields the diagnosis in over 70% of cases. The physician should review the patient's own description of dizziness, its duration and precipitants, the patient's medications, and any symptoms of neurologic or cardiac disease. Categories of dizziness include (1) vertigo, a definite rotatory sensation in the head, which implies vestibular or, rarely, brain stem disease; (2) the sensation of impending faint or loss of consciousness, which implies hypotension; and (3) unsteadiness, not in the head, which implies cerebellar or proprioceptive disorders. Unfortunately, the symptoms in 40% of patients, some with multiple sensory deficits or hyperventilation syndrome, are too vague or diverse to classify neatly.

The physical examination carefully reviews the ears, heart, and nervous system (proprioception, cranial nerves, and cerebellum). Nystagmus is normal if it is present only on extreme lateral gaze but indicates vestibular disease if it is rotatory, and suggests brain stem disease if it is purely vertical, horizontal, or worse in the abducting eye. In all patients, the clinician should perform tests intended to provoke the patient's dizziness, including (1) postural blood pressure determinations, (2) hyperventilation (30 breaths/min for 3 minutes), (3) Nylen-Barany (Hallpike-Dix) maneuvers, and (4) a sudden turn when walking (if dizziness appears during this test and is relieved by a touch of the examiner's finger, multiple sensory deficits may be present). The Nylen-Barany maneuvers evaluate dizziness brought on by head movements. With the physician's assistance, the seated patient turns his head to one side and quickly lies down so that his head hangs over the table edge. If vertigo appears after a pause of 2 to 20 seconds (latency), then dies away after seconds (adaptation) and is less prominent during immediate repeat testing (fatigability), the patient has common benign (peripheral) positional vertigo. The rare patient with central positional vertigo due to brain stem or cerebellar causes experiences milder vertigo without latency, adaptation, or fatigability during this test.

An audiogram is necessary in any patient with associated hearing loss or tinnitus to screen for Meniere's disease and acoustic neuroma. The results of bithermal caloric studies and electronystagmography, although frequently abnormal, merely support diagnoses obvious from the history and physical examination.[1]

MANAGEMENT.   Some cardiovascular disorders, such as carotid sinus hypersensitivity, require specific therapy. Postural hypotension improves with support hose and reduction of responsible medications. Multiple sensory deficits are partially offset by correct eyeglass prescriptions, use of nightlights at home, and a referral to a physical therapist for a cane or other appropriate ambulatory aids.

Patients with acute or chronic vertigo benefit from specific rehabilitative exercises. Seated at home, the patient lies down quickly to one side to provoke vertigo repeatedly until it disappears.[2] Anticholinergic or antihistamine medications may also help (Table 20–2), although no confirmatory trial in humans has been reported and most recommendations are derived from animal studies, human caloric responses, and tradition. Benzodiazepines are recommended for severe sustained vertigo (e.g., vestibular neuronitis) but are ineffective in controlled trials of episodic positional vertigo. Scopolamine or dimenhydrinate are traditionally prescribed for motion sickness and meclizine for chronic positional vertigo, though all may be interchangeable. Because medications may retard CNS adaptation to vertigo and prolong recovery, they should not be used for long periods.

FOLLOW-UP.   Vestibular neuronitis resolves after 10 to 14 days. Benign positional vertigo resolves after weeks or months, or infrequently years. Dizzy patients rarely need hospitalization or referral and are not at increased risk of

TABLE 20–2. ANTIVERTIGO MEDICATIONS

Drug	Dose	Cost ($ per 3 Days)[1]
Anticholinergic Scopolamine (Transderm Scop)	0.5 mg transdermal patch q.3d.	3.05
Antihistamine Dimenhydrinate[2] (Dramamine)	50 mg PO q.6h., PRN	0.24 (generic) 3.00
Meclizine[2] (Antivert)	25 mg PO q.6h., PRN	0.30 (generic) 5.16

[1]Average wholesale price, 1991 *Drug Topics Red Book.*
[2]Available over the counter.

death or institutionalization. If vertigo is disabling and unresponsive to treatment, a neurology or otolaryngology referral is indicated.

Cross-reference: Hyperventilation Syndrome (Section 190).

REFERENCES

1. Baloh RW, Sloane PD, Honrubia V. Quantitative vestibular function testing in elderly patients with dizziness. Ear Nose Throat J 1989;68:935–939.

    Electronystagmograms, abnormal in 65% of patients, contributed little to assessment from history and physical examination. The test added new information in only four of seventy-five patients, all with unsuspected bilateral vestibular disease.

2. Brandt T, Daroff RB. Physical therapy for benign paroxysmal positional vertigo. Arch Otolaryngol 1980;106:484–485.

    Describes exercises that produced relief in 66 of 67 patients with benign positional vertigo, usually within 7 to 10 days.

3. Drachman DA, Hart CW. An approach to the dizzy patient. Neurology 1972;22:323–334.

    Classic prospective evaluation of 104 dizzy patients; history, physical examination, and provocative testing uncover most of the final diagnoses. Illustrates Nylen-Barany test.

4. Fisher CM. Vertigo in cerebrovascular disease. Arch Otolaryngol 1967;85:529–534.

    Seventy-seven percent of basilar vertebral ischemia patients experienced dizziness: in 75%, dizziness and other neurologic symptoms (e.g., diplopia) occur together; in 25%, dizziness is the sole initial symptom, although other revealing neurologic symptoms appear within 6 weeks.

5. Heckerling PS, Leikin JB, Maturen A, Perkins JT. Predictors of occult carbon monoxide poisoning in patients with headache and dizziness. Ann Intern Med 1987;107:174–176.

    Three percent of cases of headache and dizziness resulted from carbon monoxide poisoning. Risk factors included the use of gas stoves or heaters, an affected cohabitant, faulty heating equipment, and cigarette smoking.

21 FATIGUE

Problem

STEVEN R. McGEE

EPIDEMIOLOGY.   In the internist's office, fatigue is one of the most common chief complaints, with a point prevalence of 24% and an annual incidence of 3% to 7%. Fatigue is more common in women than in men.

ETIOLOGY.   Evaluation of fatigue identifies a physical cause in 20% to 40% of affected patients, a psychiatric cause in 50% to 65%, and no cause in 10% to 30%. The leading physical causes are infections (especially viral diseases), metabolic disorders (thyroid disease, hypokalemia), and medications (sedatives, diuretics, beta blockers, antihistamines, psychotropic medications). Although fatigue may persist long after infections with Epstein-Barr (EBV) and influenza viruses have resolved, the exact role of the virus is unclear, because some studies suggest that those with prolonged recovery were depression prone even before their infection. The most common psychiatric disorders are depression, anxiety, and somatization disorder. The evaluation of fatigue present for less than 4 weeks yields a physical diagnosis in 70% of cases, while fatigue exceeding 4 months leads to a psychiatric diagnosis in 76%.

Only 5% of patients with chronic fatigue satisfy the criteria of the chronic fatigue syndrome, a disorder characterized by fatigue persisting longer than 6 months, the absence of known physical causes of fatigue, and the presence of sore throat, lymphadenopathy, myalgia, headache, and sleep disturbance, among other associated symptoms.[1] Early studies attempted to link this syndrome to chronic EBV infection, but subsequent work has demonstrated that abnormal EBV serology is very nonspecific and no such association exists for most, if not all, patients.

In one study, 70% of patients with chronic fatigue also experienced diffuse musculoskeletal pain, had multiple tender muscle points on examination, and otherwise met the diagnostic criteria for fibromyalgia (see Section 122, Fibromyalgia).

CLINICAL APPROACH.   The physician should carefully distinguish the patient's complaint of fatigue from the exertional dyspnea of cardiopulmonary disease, the muscle weakness of neuromuscular disease (myasthenia gravis, multiple sclerosis, polymyositis), and the daytime hypersomnolence of sleep apnea (usually associated with morning headache and nighttime snoring and apnea). The finding of weakness or fever on physical examination requires a different diagnostic approach (see Section 16, Fever, and Section 139, Muscular Weakness).

If the cause of fatigue is not obvious after the initial history and physical examination, recommended laboratory testing includes a CBC count, electrolytes, glucose, calcium, creatinine, thyroxine, liver function tests, and erythrocyte sedimentation rate. Such routine testing, however, provides clues to the diagnosis of chronic fatigue in only 5% of patients. Other tests, including EBV serology, are appropriate only when directed by suggestive signs and symptoms. No specific EMG, muscle biopsy, or muscle enzyme defects have ever been identified in patients with fatigue.

The physician should address with all patients the possibility of excessive life stresses, substance abuse, risk factors for HIV infection, and symptoms of depression and anxiety. Even in patients with physical disease, depression or anxiety may contribute significantly to fatigue.

MANAGEMENT.   Double-blind, placebo-controlled, randomized trials have shown that acyclovir or combined liver extract–folate–vitamin B_{12} injections are no better than placebo in the chronic fatigue syndrome, and that the placebo effect is powerful in these patients. Amantadine has a meager benefit for the disabling fatigue of multiple sclerosis, but its use for fatigue remains restricted to this group of patients.

Specific therapy may benefit patients with known physical or psychiatric disease. For patients with fatigue of unknown cause, one logical approach includes the following: (1) consider withdrawal of medications suspected as a cause, (2) prescribe moderate, not excessive, exercise (see Section 72), (3) reduce stresses in the patient's life, and (4) consider empirical antidepressant medications. This approach is untested, but a similar disorder, fibromyalgia, does improve with very low doses of tricyclic medications. Nonsedating antidepressants are probably best, unless insomnia is a significant problem.

FOLLOW-UP.   Patients with fatigue are not at increased risk of hospitalization or death but do have a significantly greater number of clinic visits than nonfatigued patients. Most patients remain employed. Chronic fatigue tends to wax and wane over years and may remit; some 30% to 50% of affected patients show improvement at 1-year follow-up.

Cross-references: Fibromyalgia (Section 122), Screening for Depression (Section 187), Generalized Anxiety (Section 188), Somatization (Section 191).

REFERENCES

1. Holmes GP, Kaplan JE, Gantz NM, Komaroff AL, Schonberger LB, et al. Chronic fatigue syndrome: A working case definition. Ann Intern Med 1988;108:387–389.
    Reviews the two major and fourteen minor criteria for the diagnosis of chronic fatigue syndrome, and discusses its tenuous relationship to EBV infection.

2. Kroenke K. Chronic fatigue: Frequency, causes, evaluation, and management. Compr Ther 1989;15(7):3–7.
    Best overall review.

3. Kroenke K, Wood DR, Mangelsdorff AD, Meier NJ, Powell JB. Chronic fatigue in primary care: Prevalence, patient characteristics, and outcome. JAMA 1988;260:929–934.
    Prospective analysis of 102 patients with chronic fatigue (>1 month). Laboratory testing was unhelpful in diagnosis, and most fatigued patients had high depression or anxiety ratings.

4. Morrison JD. Fatigue as a presenting complaint in family practice. J Fam Pract 1980; 10:795–801.
    The longer the fatigue, the more likely is a psychiatric diagnosis.

5. Swartz MN. The chronic fatigue syndrome—One entity or many? N Engl J Med 1988; 319:1726–1728.
    Outstanding historical review.

IV CHAPTER

DISORDERS OF THE SKIN

22 PRINCIPLES OF DERMATOLOGIC DIAGNOSIS AND THERAPY

JAN V. HIRSCHMANN

DIAGNOSIS

The ability to diagnose dermatologic disorders depends heavily on visual recognition of patterns of skin abnormalities, a skill that requires considerable knowledge and experience. Still, even for the expert, a systematic approach to the history and the physical examination is necessary for an accurate appraisal of cutaneous problems. The clinician should inquire about the duration and evolution of the disorder, including any relationship to season, ambient temperature, occupation, travel, animal exposure, hobbies, other illnesses, and drug use (including illicit drugs and over-the-counter medications) and about similar skin diseases in family or other contacts. Especially important is information about previous or current treatment, not only because it may indicate the efficacy of such therapy, but also because certain treatments may alter the appearance of the skin lesions. For example, topical corticosteroids often significantly diminish the erythema and scaling of a superficial fungal infection, making it more difficult to identify. Sometimes, treatment will replace one disease with another. For example, topical neomycin erroneously given for a mild, self-limited eruption may result in a contact dermatitis to that antibiotic, which is the problem that the clinician sees, rather than the initial rash that has spontaneously resolved. The symptoms of dermatologic disease to elicit are mainly pruritus, pain, or paresthesias in the skin, but because some skin lesions may be manifestations of a systemic disease, in certain circumstances it is important to inquire about other problems, such as weight loss, fever, arthralgias, and the like.

The clinician should scrupulously examine the entire skin surface (including the scalp, nails, axillae, and anogenital area), the conjunctivae, and the oral cavity. The examiner should use the dermatologic terminology of macule, papule, nodule, and so forth to characterize the abnormalities seen. Other important elements to note are the color, palpable features (such as consistency, temperature, and tenderness), and the shape (e.g., round, oval, annular) of the individual lesions. If several lesions are present, the clinician should identify their arrangement (grouped or widespread) and distribution (e.g., symmetric, on sun-exposed areas, on extensor surfaces). Many dermatologic diseases have such typical patterns of skin involvement that the location of the lesions is among the most important identifying characteristics. The use of a hand lens may reveal important information unappreciated by the naked eye.

Scratching pruritic areas frequently alters or destroys the original lesions, leaving nonspecific excoriations as the only finding. Similarly, certain topical therapies may so change the appearance of a skin disorder that it is unrecognizable. In these circumstances, other features, such as the distribution of the eruption, may suggest the proper diagnosis. Most helpful diagnostically are undisturbed ("primary") lesions.

TOPICAL THERAPY

WET DRESSINGS.   Wet dressings are often useful for acute conditions where erythema, vesicles, crusting, pruritus, and oozing are present. They cool through evaporation, reducing itching and causing vasoconstriction of the dilated vessels found in acute inflammation. Because of capillary action, moistened crust and superficial dead skin adhere to the dressing, the removal of which provides gentle debridement. Tap water alone may suffice, but aluminum acetate (Burow's) solution, one packet or tablet dissolved in 2 cups of cool or lukewarm water, is more drying and has mild antimicrobial activity. Items found in most households, such as washcloths, towels, or sheets, are excellent dressings when applied loosely in two to three layers (wet, but not dripping) to the affected area and changed every 5 minutes for a period of about 20 minutes three to five times a day. Longer use may cause skin maceration. Wet dressings are rarely necessary for more than 24 to 48 hours.

MOISTURIZERS.   Certain preparations help the epidermis retain the moisture necessary to keep the skin's surface smooth and soft. They are especially useful in patients with xerosis (dry skin), a common problem in the elderly, and in those with atopic eczema.

Moisturizers may be occlusive or humectants. The occlusive types create a partially permeable barrier that helps the skin retain its moisture. They are creams or ointments that contain emulsions of oil in water or water in oil. When the amount of oil exceeds the amount of water by a certain amount, the formulation changes from a pourable cream to a semisolid ointment. Oil-in-water emulsions that are useful moisturizers include hydrophilic ointment (e.g., generic or Cetaphil Lotion, Keri Lotion, Lubriderm Cream, Nivea Cream). Water-in-oil emulsions that rehydrate the skin include cold creams and lanolin preparations (e.g., generic or Eucerin). Oil-in-water emulsions are less greasy and more easily removed, but water-in-oil emulsions provide better lubrication and occlusion. Water-absorbent ointment bases contain no water but will absorb it and become water-in-oil emulsions. Examples are hydrophilic petrolatum (generic) and anhydrous lanolin (e.g., generic or Aquaphor). All these occlusive moisturizers are nonprescription drugs.

Humectants, when absorbed, help the skin retain moisture. Examples include urea, available as a 10% lotion (e.g., Nutraplus, Carmol-10) or a 20% cream (Carmol-20), and lactic acid (Lac-Hydrin). These preparations are especially useful for dry, scaly conditions such as atopic dermatitis.

Patients with dry skin should use one of these moisturizing agents several times a day, particularly after washing the hands or bathing, when the agent should be applied to damp but not dripping skin. They will help the water present on the skin surface to penetrate into the epidermis rather than evaporating. When moisturizers are put over dry skin, little water is added, but they will help protect the epidermis from further loss.

TOPICAL CORTICOSTEROIDS. In general, creams and lotions, which are more drying than ointments, are appropriate for acute or subacute inflammatory disorders characterized by oozing, erythema, crusting, and vesiculation. Ointments are superior for chronic, dry, scaling, and lichenified conditions and are better absorbed than creams. Because creams and lotions blend into the skin readily and do not have the greasy feel of ointments, however, they are often more acceptable to patients. Lotions are especially useful in hairy areas, where creams and ointments are difficult to apply.

The absorption of topical corticosteroids varies markedly according to the site on the skin, being much greater where the skin is thin, such as on the face and scrotum. Absorption is also increased severalfold with well-hydrated skin. Therefore, when possible, patients should moisten the area to be treated by bathing or briefly soaking the area before applying the medication. Some disorders that respond poorly to conventional topical corticosteroid therapy may improve when a cream preparation is covered with occlusive dressings. An ointment is not ordinarily used under occlusion because it is more likely to produce folliculitis and maceration. The patient should apply the cream to moist skin and cover the area for a minimum of 6 hours (overnight use is usually most convenient) with a plastic wrap such as Saran Wrap for large areas, plastic gloves for hands, plastic bags for the hands or feet, and a bathing cap for the scalp. The edges should be sealed with tape, elastic bandages, or items of clothing such as underwear or panty hose, depending on the area being treated.

Topical corticosteroids, of which there are many types, vary considerably in potency. It is useful to learn one or two in each group. In general, therapy should begin with a medium-strength formulation for mild to moderately severe conditions, with the most potent types reserved for very severe or refractory disorders. In chronic dermatoses, a lower strength corticosteroid is often appropriate for maintenance therapy after the condition has responded to a more potent preparation. With the chronic use of the strong corticosteroids, especially when applied under occlusion, atrophy, telangiectasias, and striae may develop. The face, axillae, and genital areas are particularly susceptible, and ordinarily only low-potency preparations are indicated for long-term treatment of these areas. The following list includes a few of the available topical corticosteroids according to their potency. Trade names are included to help identify the products, but those preparations available as generic prescriptions are marked by an asterisk. In each category, the medications are in approximate descending order of strength, although frequently the difference, if any, is slight.

Very High Potency
Clobetasol propionate cream, ointment, solution 0.05% (Temovate)
*Betamethasone dipropionate cream, ointment 0.05% (Diprolene)

High Potency
Betamethasone dipropionate cream, ointment 0.05% (Diprosone) (different vehicle than
  Diprolene)
Fluocinonide cream*, ointment, lotion 0.05% (Lidex)
Halcinonide cream 0.1% (Halog)
*Betamethasone valerate ointment 0.1% (Valisone)

Intermediate Potency
*Fluocinolone acetonide cream 0.2%, ointment 0.025% (Synalar)
*Triamcinolone acetonide ointment 0.1% (Aristocort, Kenalog)
*Betamethasone valerate cream, lotion 0.1% (Valisone)
*Triamcinolone acetonide cream 0.025% (Aristocort)

Low Potency
Desonide cream 0.05% (Tridesilon)
*Hydrocortisone cream, ointment, lotion 1.0%, 2.5%

FREQUENCY AND AMOUNT OF APPLICATION.   With topical corticosteroids, twice daily application nearly always suffices; more frequent use is rarely more effective. With some disorders, particularly for maintenance therapy of chronic conditions, a single treatment a day is adequate. Patients should apply the medication in a thin layer to the skin; thick applications are wasteful, because only the material directly touching the skin has any therapeutic benefit. It takes about 30 g of topical medication to cover the entire body for one application, with the following approximate amounts:

	Monthly Amount (b.i.d.)
Head, both hands, buttocks (each area): 2 g	120 g
Neck, genitals, feet (each area): 1 g	60 g
Both arms: 4 g	240 g
Trunk: 8 g	480 g
Both legs: 10 g	600 g

REFERENCES

1. Arndt KA. Manual of Dermatologic Therapeutics: With Essentials of Diagnosis, 4th ed. Little, Brown, Boston, 1989.
   A superb, concise, and practical summary of the management of common dermatologic disorders.

2. Sams WM, Lynch PJ. Principles and Practice of Dermatology. Churchill Livingstone, New York, 1990.
   An excellent medium-sized textbook, appropriate for primary care clinicians. Numerous first-rate clinical photographs, in color.

23 PRURITUS

Symptom

JAN V. HIRSCHMANN

EPIDEMIOLOGY.   Although pruritus is the most common symptom in dermatologic diseases, its prevalence in the general population is unknown.

ETIOLOGY.   Often, skin lesions are present that clarify the cause of itching. Common skin diseases typically associated with pruritus are xerosis (dry skin), scabies, pediculosis, urticaria, atopic or contact dermatitis, insect bites, fiberglass dermatitis, and fungal infections. When no skin lesions are present except excoriations, the cause may be a systemic disorder (primarily uremia), cholestasis from drugs, primary biliary cirrhosis or extrahepatic biliary obstruction, lymphomas (especially Hodgkin's disease), polycythemia vera, and, perhaps, thyroid disease. About 15% of patients with itching but no diagnostic skin lesions will have an associated systemic disease at initial evaluation; lymphoma will emerge as a cause on follow-up in a very small number. About 65% of patients in whom no cause is found will continue to have pruritus for years.

CLINICAL APPROACH.   The history should elicit information about the nature and duration of the itching, the precipitating factors, the patient's occupation and hobbies, previous therapy, medications taken, similar symptoms in close contacts, systemic symptoms like weight loss, and the travel history. The pruritus of Hodgkin's disease is frequently burning in quality and typically occurs on the legs. The itching of polycythemia vera is often "prickling" and tends to develop when the patient abruptly cools off after emerging from a warm bath or shower. The itching of scabies is particularly intense at night. Xerosis is especially likely in the older patient, particularly following frequent bathing or during the winter months, when indoor heating reduces the ambient humidity.

The physical examination should include a thorough examination of the entire cutaneous surface, including the genitalia. Burrows of scabies tend to occur in the interdigital webs, volar wrists, axillae, umbilicus, and genital areas. Xerosis is indicated by dryness of the skin, fine platelike scaling, and delicate fissuring with erythema. Stroking the back firmly with the blunt end of a pen and examining the area for a wheal 2 to 3 minutes later will reveal dermographism, an accentuated wheal-and-flare response, that can cause itching (see Section 34, Urticaria). The examination should also include palpation for abdominal masses, hepatosplenomegaly, and lymph node enlargement in those with no obvious cause of the itching.

If no primary skin lesions are present, the cause of pruritus is inapparent, and the condition has not responded to a 2-week trial of treatment for xerosis (see below), a reasonable laboratory evaluation includes a complete blood cell (CBC) count (to detect polycythemia, iron deficiency anemia, or leukemia), determination of alkaline phosphatase levels (to seek evidence of cholestasis) and thyrotropin, thyroxine, and triiodothyronine levels (to detect hypo- or hyperthyroidism), and chest radiography (to detect mediastinal lymph node enlargement in lymphomas, metastatic disease, or evidence of primary pulmonary neoplasm). If this workup is unrevealing, further testing in the absence of other evidence of systemic disease is probably unrewarding.

MANAGEMENT.   For xerosis, infrequent bathing, the use of mild soaps such as Dove or Tone, the generous application of emollients such as Aquaphor or Carmol 20 (urea cream 20%), and humidification of dry air in heated environments are useful measures.

Antihistamines are helpful for some but not all forms of pruritus. They are the drugs of choice for symptomatic dermographism. Hydroxyzine (25–50 mg t.i.d.) is a reasonable agent that is also sedating—a helpful feature for those with nocturnal itching. Doxepin, an antidepressant and a potent antihistamine, is a good alternative, especially for those with chronic symptoms that have led to depression.

Patients with uremic pruritus may benefit from ultraviolet B therapy, parathyroidectomy (in those with secondary hyperparathyroidism), oral activated charcoal (6 g/day), or oral cholestyramine (5 g b.i.d.). The itching of cholestasis may improve with cholestyramine, 4 g one to three times a day; occasionally, ultraviolet B light treatment is helpful.

REFERENCES

1. Denman ST. A review of pruritus. J Am Acad Dermatol 1986;14:375–392.
   A thorough review.

2. Rosenbaum M. Pruritus of unknown origin. Hosp Pract 1988;23:19–26.
   A practical approach to patients with itching of no obvious cause.

24 CORNS AND CALLUSES

Problem

JAN V. HIRSCHMANN

EPIDEMIOLOGY. Corns and calluses are common hyperkeratotic lesions of the feet that arise from chronic trauma to areas of pressure over bony prominences. The most frequent cause is poorly fitting shoes, but sometimes an abnormal gait or an unusual bony architecture of the feet is responsible.

SYMPTOMS AND SIGNS. When symptomatic, corns and calluses cause pain on pressure. Corns are small, well-defined areas of skin thickening with a central hyperlucency; they are most common around the fifth toe. Sometimes they occur as a whitish hyperkeratosis in the toe webs ("soft corns"). Calluses are larger and less well-delineated areas of skin thickening and hardness that usually develop under the first and fifth metatarsal heads.

CLINICAL APPROACH. Paring the surface of corns will reveal a central clear area ("nucleus") that disappears with deeper cuts, while shaving plantar warts (often confused with corns) will demonstrate black and red specks representing thrombosed capillaries. Furthermore, warts tend to be painful with lateral pressure, corns with vertical pressure. Some patients, particularly the elderly, have hyperkeratotic, fissured areas on the heel that seem to occur from a combination of severely dry skin and pressure. These are not calluses in the usual sense, and they respond best to aggressive hydration of the skin with emollients.

MANAGEMENT. The pain produced by the thickened skin will abate after the surface of corns and calluses has been pared with a scalpel blade. Patients can often achieve good results by applying a 40% salicylic acid plaster every night, soaking the area in water the following morning, and then abrading the surface with a pumice stone, emery board, or callus file. These lesions return unless the underlying problem, such as ill-fitting footwear, is corrected. For difficult or recurrent lesions, consultation with a podiatrist may be helpful.

25 WARTS

Problem

JAN V. HIRSCHMANN

EPIDEMIOLOGY. Warts result from intraepidermal infection with human papillomaviruses. DNA hybridization techniques have identified over 50 types of these viruses, many associated with different clinical appearances of the warts. They are most common in childhood, with a peak incidence at ages 12 to 16, but may occur at any age. Infection develops by contact with another affected person or by autoinoculation from a site elsewhere on the body; the wart appears 1 to 12 months later, most commonly after about 2 to 3 months.

SYMPTOMS AND SIGNS. Warts are usually asymptomatic unless present in areas of frequent pressure, especially on the plantar surfaces. They are usually categorized by their location or appearance. A common wart (verruca vulgaris) is a papule with an irregular surface that tends to occur on the hands and fingers, often in the periungual area. A flat wart (verruca plana) is a slightly elevated, flat-topped papule primarily found on the face, neck, forearms, and hands. Plantar warts are flat or elevated, thickened lesions that interrupt the skin lines (unlike calluses); often have black or red dots on the surface, representing thrombosed capillaries; and usually are surrounded by a collar of thickened skin. Filiform warts are small, slender papules, usually present on the neck or face. Anogenital warts (condylomata accuminata) are typically soft, moist, hyperplastic lesions found primarily on the foreskin and head of the penis in men, on the labia in women, and in the anal and urethral openings in both sexes.

Warts may demonstrate the Koebner phenomenon, the tendency to appear in areas of trauma. This characteristic explains some configurations of warts, such as their linear arrangement where a previous scratch has occurred.

CLINICAL APPROACH. The clinical appearance is usually diagnostic; occasionally, a biopsy is necessary. Since about 65% of warts spontaneously disappear in 2 years, not all require treatment.

MANAGEMENT. The simplest treatment of most warts is cryotherapy with liquid nitrogen applied for 5 to 30 seconds with a cotton applicator or by spray from a special instrument. The wart and a 1-mm rim of normal surrounding skin should turn white with freezing. Repeating the liquid nitrogen freezing after the area defrosts probably yields greater success than a single treatment. A blister, sometimes hemorrhagic, may form but is unnecessary for effective therapy. An alternative approach, especially for warts on the hands or feet, is a salicylic acid–lactic acid paint (e.g., Duofilm) applied daily. This treatment is more effective if the area of the wart is soaked in hot water and gently abraded with an emery board before the solution is applied. Improvement usually begins in 1 to 2 weeks, and 70% to 85% of patients are cured by 3 months.

REFERENCE

1. Cobb MW. Human papillomavirus infection. J Am Acad Dermatol 1990;22:547–566.
    A complete review of the cutaneous manifestations of human papillomaviruses, with excellent color photographs.

26 SUPERFICIAL FUNGAL INFECTIONS

Problem

JAN V. HIRSCHMANN

DERMATOPHYTE INFECTIONS

EPIDEMIOLOGY.   Dermatophytes, fungi that can invade the hair, skin, and nails of living hosts, belong to the genera *Epidermophyton, Microsporum,* and *Trichophyton.* Some species are confined to humans; others live in the soil or on other animals and infect humans who come in contact with these sources. About 10% of adults with apparently normal skin on their feet harbor dermatophytes; an additional 5% to 10% have clinical disease of the feet (tinea pedis) due to these organisms, primarily in the interdigital toe spaces.

SYMPTOMS AND SIGNS.   The most common manifestations of tinea pedis are boggy whiteness and fissuring in the toe webs, especially the fourth interspace. A second form is characterized by redness and dry scaling of the sole and lower portion of the dorsal foot ("moccasin distribution"). Sometimes erythema and vesicles or bullae develop, the roofs of which are found to contain fungi on microscopic examination. Onychomycosis, also called tinea unguium, is a dermatophyte infection of the nails and is very common on the toenails. It causes yellow, opaque, thickened nails that may crumble easily and often have extensive hyperkeratosis and debris beneath, with separation of the nail plate from the nail bed (onycholysis). Often both feet are infected with fungi, and when concomitant hand involvement occurs, inexplicably only one hand is typically affected ("two feet, one hand disease").

Dermatophyte infections elsewhere on the skin usually occur as patches of erythema and scaling with raised red borders and central clearing. Tinea cruris involves the upper thighs and pubic area but spares the scrotum in men. On the trunk (tinea corporis) usually only one lesion develops. Infection may also occur on the face (tinea facei) and the scalp (tinea capitis), the latter usually in children.

CLINICAL APPROACH.   Examination of skin or nail scrapings immersed in potassium hydroxide (KOH) 10% to 30% and gently heated is a very sensitive and specific test but requires experience for reliable interpretation. Positive preparations demonstrate translucent, septate hyphae, often with individual barrel-shaped segments that represent arthrospores. The different genera of dermatophytes are indistinguishable by this test, but scrapings inoculated onto fungal media will yield the organism and allow specific identification. Cultures are usually unnecessary, however, if the KOH preparation is positive, unless the history or epidemiologic setting suggests an unusual organism.

MANAGEMENT.   Most cases of tinea pedis, tinea corporis, tinea facei, and tinea cruris respond to topical antifungals applied twice a day for about 4 weeks. Available agents, all equally effective against both dermatophytes and *Candida* spp., include ciclopirox (Loprox), clotrimazole (Lotrimin, Mycelex), econazole (Spectazole), ketoconazole (Nizoral), miconazole (Micatin, Monistat-Derm), oxiconazole (Oxistat), and sulconazole (Exelderm). Clotrimazole and miconazole are available without prescription.

With extensive disease, involvement of the hands, or scalp infection, oral griseofulvin is the drug of choice. It is a very safe medication; the traditional teaching that it is significantly hepatotoxic or that its use requires monitoring of liver function is untrue. The usual daily dose is 500 mg of the ultra-micro-sized form given for 1 to 2 months, depending on clinical response. Oral ketoconazole, equally effective but not superior for most cases, is occasionally necessary for those who cannot tolerate or do not respond to griseofulvin. The usual dose is 200 mg/day. Hepatic injury rarely occurs (incidence: about 1 in 10,000), usually early in the course of therapy.

Fingernail infection commonly responds to griseofulvin, 750 mg to 1 g/day for 4 to 12 months. Toenail involvement is much more resistant, especially in the elderly, and many clinicians attempt treatment only in younger patients, giving griseofulvin, 1 g/day for 12 to 18 months. Topical treatment of toenails is not very effective, but surgical removal of the nail with destruction of the nail matrix by phenol to prevent regrowth eliminates the infection and is sometimes indicated for symptomatic disease. For many patients, careful nail trimming and filing with an emery board or nail file, while not curative, relieves any discomfort caused by the dystrophic nail.

FOLLOW-UP.   Dermatophyte infection, especially tinea pedis, often recurs, and many patients learn to resume therapy when symptoms or signs reappear. Patients receiving ketoconazole should know the symptoms of hepatotoxicity, stop treatment if they appear, and seek prompt medical attention.

TINEA (PITYRIASIS) VERSICOLOR

EPIDEMIOLOGY.   Tinea, or pityriasis, versicolor is due to a yeast that is a normal skin organism and resides primarily on the face, neck, and upper trunk. This fungus has several names, *Pityrosporon ovale, P. orbiculare,* or *Malassezia furfur.* In some people the oval yeast forms become filamentous and cause the cutaneous lesions of tinea versicolor. This disorder occurs in up to 50% of people in tropical climates, compared to 5% of residents in dry, temperate areas. Systemic corticosteroid therapy, Cushing's disease, compromised cell-mediated immunity, and pregnancy may increase the incidence.

SYMPTOMS AND SIGNS.   Most patients are asymptomatic, but mild pruritus occasionally occurs. Many patients complain of the altered pigmentation that the characteristic macular lesions cause: in dark-skinned patients (including whites with suntans) they are often hypopigmented; in those with light complexions they are usually darker than the surrounding skin. The colors of the macules range from white to brown (*versicolor*). The borders are well delineated, but individual macules often coalesce to form larger patches. Gentle scratching will produce a fine scale. The areas most involved are the trunk and neck, although lesions may occur on the abdomen, upper arms, and genital area.

CLINICAL APPROACH.   KOH preparations of skin scrapings establish the diagnosis by demonstrating abundant yeasts and hyphae ("spaghetti and meatballs"). Parker's Blue-Black Ink will stain them blue, making their identification easier. Culturing this organism, which requires special media, is of no diagnostic value because it is normally present on the skin.

MANAGEMENT.   Treatment is usually successful but relapse is common unless the agents are continued. Selenium sulfide suspension (Selsun) applied overnight from the chin to the waist and from the shoulders to the wrists and then rinsed off is effective. Re-treatment 1 week later and repeated every few weeks as necessary will usually control this disorder. If this program causes skin irritation, the shampoo may be rinsed off 5 to 15 minutes after application and the treatment repeated for 3 consecutive days. The use of topical antifungals like clotrimazole is also effective but more expensive. The scaling resolves quickly, but the pigmentary changes may not disappear for weeks to months.

FOLLOW-UP.   Patients can learn to re-treat any relapses, which should respond to the same agent used before, without further visits to the clinician.

CANDIDA INFECTIONS

EPIDEMIOLOGY.   *Candida* spp. are normal inhabitants of the alimentary tract, but not the skin. *Candida* infections most commonly seen in ambulatory care are thrush, perleche, intertriginous candidiasis, and vulvovaginitis (see Section 166, Vaginitis). Conditions predisposing to thrush are diabetes, decreased saliva (as in Sjögren's syndrome), recent broad-spectrum antibacterial therapy, or diminished cell-mediated immunity, especially AIDS. Perleche (angular cheilitis) usually occurs in older patients with increased moisture and maceration at the angles of the mouth, especially from poorly fitting dentures or drooling because of neurologic disorders. *Candida* is commonly, but not universally, present in the characteristically red and fissured lesions. Intertriginous candidiasis usually occurs in the skin folds of obese people.

SYMPTOMS AND SIGNS.   Thrush is characterized clinically by whitish plaques, usually resting on an erythematous base and found on the tongue, buccal mucosa, gums, or palate. The plaques may be asymptomatic or may cause soreness of the mouth. Perleche causes soreness of the angles of the mouth, where moisture, erythema, and fissuring are present. Intertriginous candidiasis can occur in any body fold, especially beneath pendulous breasts, between folds of fat on the abdomen, or in the groin. Erythema, moisture, and whitish debris are present, often with an irregular peeling edge and with pustules or reddish papules outside this border ("satellite lesions").

CLINICAL APPROACH.   Scraping the oral lesions of thrush with a tongue blade, smearing the material onto a slide, and examining it under a microscope will establish the diagnosis. Gram stains, easier than a KOH preparation for most people to interpret, disclose large gram-positive yeasts and pseudohyphae characteristic of the organism. Cultures are not indicated because *Candida* spp. are part of the normal mouth flora. For skin lesions, KOH preparations or Gram stains will reveal the fungi. If these are positive, cultures are usually unnecessary.

MANAGEMENT.   Nystatin, 4 to 6 ml (400,000 to 600,000 units) q.i.d., swished around in the mouth for several minutes and then swallowed, is very effective when given for 1 to 2 weeks. Clotrimazole troches (10 mg) dissolved slowly in the mouth and swallowed 5 times a day also work. For very severe or refractory disease, oral ketoconazole (200 mg/day for 2 weeks) may be required. Perleche usually responds to topical antifungal creams effective against *Candida* spp., such as clotrimazole b.i.d. Correction of predisposing factors, such as poorly fitting dentures, is important to prevent recurrences. Intertriginous candidiasis can be treated with topical creams as well. Weight loss for obese patients, keeping the area dry, and wearing loose-fitting clothing are helpful measures. Some patients with intertriginous inflammation do not have a fungal infection. Such cases usually respond to topical corticosteroids, such as hydrocortisone 1% for the groin or axilla and more potent agents such as triamcinolone 0.1% for other areas.

REFERENCES

1. Crislip MA, Edwards JE. Candidiasis. Infect Dis Clin North Am 1989;3:103–133.
    A thorough review of both superficial and deep infections due to *Candida* spp.

2. Lesher JL, Smith JG. Antifungal agents in dermatology. J Am Acad Dermatol 1987;17:383–394.
A detailed discussion of topical and systemic agents.

27 SCABIES AND LICE

Problem

JAN V. HIRSCHMANN

SCABIES

EPIDEMIOLOGY.   *Sarcoptes scabiei* var. *hominis* is an obligate human parasite that usually cannot survive for more than a few days off the human skin. Close physical contact, especially sexual relations, allows person-to-person transmission of the mites. Family outbreaks are common.

SYMPTOMS AND SIGNS.   In previously uninfected patients, symptoms begin about 4 to 6 weeks after infestation. Generalized pruritus, characteristically worse at night, is the most prominent symptom. Burrows—short, wavy lines, especially likely to occur between fingers, on the penis, or on the flexor areas of the wrist—are usually the earliest lesions, but may not develop or may disappear after vigorous scratching. Other common sites are the nipples, umbilicus, buttocks, or axillae. The head is usually spared but may be involved, particularly in children and in elderly or bedridden patients. Frequently the major or only lesions are excoriations and erythematous papules. Occasionally vesicles, bullae, or nodules occur. Pustules develop in areas of secondary infection, which is especially likely to occur in hot, humid climates.

CLINICAL APPROACH.   The definitive diagnosis depends on finding mites, their eggs, or feces on skin samples, best obtained by applying a drop of mineral oil over burrows or papules and scraping with a scalpel blade. This material, placed on a slide, is examined under low power on a microscope. Because the number of mites on the skin of an infested person is small, frequently no definitive findings are present and the clinical diagnosis depends on the patient's response to empirical antiscabetic therapy.

MANAGEMENT.   Lindane 1% (Kwell) remains effective therapy in the United States when applied as a lotion to cover the body from the head to the soles of the feet, left on for 8 to 12 hours, and then washed off. If new lesions develop, a second treatment 10 days later is necessary. Permethrin 5% cream (Elimite) applied in the same manner as lindane is an effective but not superior alternative in the United States. Close contacts should receive simultaneous therapy, but special treatment of clothing is probably unnecessary.

FOLLOW-UP. Pruritus often persists for 2 to 4 weeks and is not an indication for re-treatment. For this symptom, antihistamines such as hydroxyzine, 25 mg t.i.d., or topical corticosteroids may be useful. For intolerable itching a short course of systemic corticosteroids—for example, 40 mg prednisone for 5 to 7 days, then tapered off over the following week—will provide relief.

LICE

EPIDEMIOLOGY. Body lice reside mostly in clothing, where they lay eggs and from which they emerge, mostly at night, to feed on the host's blood. Therefore, they usually infest those with poor personal hygiene who do not wash or change clothes frequently. Head lice live in the scalp, attached to hair, on which they lay their eggs. They infest mostly children. They are probably transmitted from person to person by close head contact or the sharing of hats, combs, and brushes. Pubic lice live mostly in the hairs of the pubic area but can also reside in the beard, eyelashes, scalp, or axilla. Close body contact, commonly sexual activity, transmits the lice; fomites such as bed clothing or towels may occasionally be responsible, but pubic lice survive only about 12 hours off the host.

SYMPTOMS AND SIGNS. The most common symptom in all forms of infestation is pruritus. Patients may notice the lice on their bodies or have the sense of movement on their skin as the lice migrate. Excoriations are frequent; some patients develop secondary skin infections with purulent lesions, tender lymph nodes, fever, and malaise ("feeling lousy"). With head lice the scalp usually reveals excoriations and crusts, and the posterior cervical lymph nodes may be enlarged. With pubic lice, some patients have asymptomatic maculae caerulae ("sky-blue spots") 1/2 to 1 cm in diameter in the area of infestation, probably representing the host's blood pigments altered by the lice's saliva.

CLINICAL APPROACH. The diagnosis of louse infestation depends on detecting the lice or their eggs (nits), which are brown or white and, in the case of pubic or head lice, are cemented to the hairs. In the scalp they may resemble dandruff but are not easily movable along the hair shaft. Microscopic examination of a plucked hair with an attached nit that is covered by a drop of oil will reveal the egg and developing embryo. Because neither lice nor nits are usually present on the skin with body lice infestation, the diagnosis typically rests on finding them in the patient's clothing, usually along the seams.

MANAGEMENT. Lindane is effective for all lice. For head lice, lindane shampoo left on for 10 minutes or the lotion left on overnight and then rinsed off is effective. An alternative therapy is permethrin cream rinse (NIX) left on for 10 minutes, then washed off. After these treatments, all nits should be removed with a comb or tweezers ("nitpicking"). All household contacts should be treated at the same time. For pubic lice, lindane lotion left on for 12 hours and then washed off is effective. All sex partners should also be treated. Permethrin cream rinse is equally efficacious.

Because body lice live on clothing, the patient's skin does not usually require treatment, but if lice or nits are present, lindane lotion left on for 12 hours and then rinsed off is appropriate. The patient's clothes should be laundered with hot water or dry-cleaned.

FOLLOW-UP.   Reexamination of patients about 1 week after treatment for head and pubic lice will determine the efficacy of therapy. If viable nits or live lice are present, re-treatment is necessary.

REFERENCE

1.   Elgart ML. Scabies. Pediculosis. Dermatol Clin North Am 1990;8:219–228; 253–263.
     Good reviews of both entities.

28 ECZEMA

Problem

JAN V. HIRSCHMANN

Eczema (or "dermatitis") is a pattern of skin inflammation with the clinical features of erythema, itching, scaling, lichenification, papules, and vesicles in various combinations. Several distinctive forms exist, but some cases defy simple classification. The types commonly seen are atopic eczema, asteatotic eczema, nummular eczema, pompholyx (hand and foot eczema), prurigo nodularis, lichen simplex chronicus, venous eczema (stasis dermatitis), and contact dermatitis. The overall prevalence of all forms of eczema is about 18 per 1000 in the United States.

ATOPIC ECZEMA

EPIDEMIOLOGY.   The prevalence of atopic eczema in the United States is about 7 per 1000. It typically begins in childhood, usually before 5 years of age, and commonly subsides by adulthood, although in some patients it recurs after years of quiescence. Only occasionally does the disease begin after age 30.

SYMPTOMS AND SIGNS. In adults the usual lesions are dry, lichenified, and hyperpigmented patches in flexor areas of the elbows and knees, wrists, neck, ankles, and around the eyes. With exacerbations erythematous papules and vesicles may develop, sometimes diffusely over the body. Itching is the major symptom.

CLINICAL APPROACH. The clinician should seek and eliminate factors that exacerbate the disease, such as extremes of temperature, sweating, irritating clothing (especially silk and wool), and harsh soaps. Although atopic patients have a lower prevalence of contact dermatitis than the general population, unexplained worsening, particularly in well-delimited areas of topical therapy, should suggest the possibility of sensitivity to the agent being applied.

MANAGEMENT. Because dry skin is a major component of atopic eczema, an important element of treatment is adequate cutaneous hydration. Immediately after bathing or washing their hands, patients should pat the skin (not rub it) with a towel and apply emollients such as Aquaphor or Eucerin to the damp, not dripping, skin. In addition, they should use these agents several times a day to keep the skin moist. Potent topical corticosteroids such as betamethasone valerate 0.1% applied two to three times a day are the mainstay of treatment and should be prescribed as ointments since creams are more drying. For stubborn lesions, topical corticosteroid creams applied under occlusion, usually done most conveniently at night, may be helpful. Systemic corticosteroids given in short courses are sometimes necessary for severe, widespread exacerbations, but chronic use is rarely appropriate. *Staphylococcus aureus* is very commonly present on eczematous skin in all phases of the disease, but when its presence indicates infection rather than colonization is often unclear. Treatment is appropriate for pustules or cellulitis; many dermatologists, however, prescribe systemic antistaphylococcal agents such as dicloxacillin or erythromycin, 250 to 500 mg q.i.d., for widespread exudative lesions as well. The evidence of benefit for this practice is weak.

FOLLOW-UP. During exacerbations clinicians should see patients frequently until the problem subsides. Hospitalization is occasionally necessary for adequate therapy, and often a brief stay results in rapid improvement.

ASTEATOTIC ECZEMA (ECZEMA CRAQUELE)

EPIDEMIOLOGY. Asteatotic eczema occurs primarily in the elderly and seems to reflect decreased skin lipids. The drying effect of indoor heating during winter, frequent bathing, and diuretic therapy for edema are common initiating or exacerbating factors.

SYMPTOMS AND SIGNS. The lesions may be asymptomatic or pruritic. They occur primarily on the anterior legs as areas of dryness, scaling, and a fine fissuring of the skin resembling the cracks seen in china porcelain. Erythema may be diffuse in the involved area or most prominent along the edges of the fissures, from which clear fluid may exude. Asteatotic eczema may also involve the backs of the hands and fingertips, where dryness, cracking, and a shrunken appearance are common.

MANAGEMENT.   Emollients such as Aquaphor, Eucerin, or 20% urea cream provide the necessary hydration. Topical corticosteroids such as triamcinolone ointment 0.1% applied twice daily are also helpful. Patients should use bland soaps containing cold cream, such as Dove or Tone, and avoid excessive bathing.

NUMMULAR ECZEMA

EPIDEMIOLOGY.   Nummular eczema has a prevalence in the United States of about 2 per 1000, primarily in adults over 50. Men are more often affected than women.

SYMPTOMS AND SIGNS.   The lesions may be asymptomatic or pruritic. They are rounded (nummular means "coinlike"), erythematous plaques, sometimes with a central clear area. The plaques contain vesicles, exudation, and crusting, or dry scaling. Although they may be single, sparse, or widespread, the lesions are discrete, with normal intervening skin. They most commonly appear on the back and legs, but can also involve the hands and arms.

MANAGEMENT.   Emollients may be helpful for dry skin, but the major treatment is a potent corticosteroid ointment such as betamethasone valerate 0.1%. Lesions often respond slowly, and higher potency preparations such as clobetasol propionate (Temovate) may be necessary. New lesions form unpredictably. Often, patients have periods of disease activity for weeks to months, and then the disorder subsides, sometimes to relapse later. In others, mild disease may become extensive without any clear explanation, although dry humidity, especially during the winter months, and exposure to irritating substances on the skin may sometimes be provocative factors.

POMPHOLYX (DYSHIDROTIC ECZEMA)

EPIDEMIOLOGY.   The prevalence of this eczema is about 2 per 1000 in the United States, with most cases beginning before age 40.

SYMPTOMS AND SIGNS.   Pompholyx usually involves the hands alone, although sometimes both hands and feet are affected and occasionally the eczema is confined to the feet. The main symptom is itching; the major sign is the presence of tiny deep-seated vesicles that look like tapioca pudding and occur symmetrically on the palms, soles, and the borders of the fingers. The vesicles may coalesce to form bullae. Sometimes the main finding is dryness, cracking, and scaling of the palms, soles, and digits.

CLINICAL APPROACH.   When pompholyx is unilateral, particularly on the foot, a KOH examination of the roofs of vesicles or scrapings from a scaly area is necessary to exclude a dermatophyte infection. A careful history should help ensure that contact dermatitis (for example, from an unprescribed topical preparation) is not the cause or an exacerbating factor of the eczema.

MANAGEMENT.   For acute weeping lesions, wet dressings of aluminum acetate (Burow's) solution applied over the affected area three to four times a day may be soothing. Potent topical corticosteroids are usually necessary to control the inflammation, and oral antihistamines such as hydroxyzine may be useful for the pruritus. A short course of oral corticosteroids is occasionally appropriate for severe disease. Patients should avoid irritating substances such as detergents, polishes, and cleansing agents. With prolonged exposure to water, which removes skin lipids, they should wear rubber or, preferably, vinyl gloves with cotton liners beneath. For dry work and gardening, leather or heavy fabric gloves are advisable, and patients should wear warm gloves during cold, dry weather, which worsens the eczema. They should use little soap when hand washing. Because rings often exacerbate dermatitis by trapping irritating substances beneath them, patients should remove rings during housework and before hand washing and should clean them frequently on the inside.

PRURIGO NODULARIS

EPIDEMIOLOGY.   Prurigo nodularis (nodular prurigo, "picker's nodules") is most common in middle-age subjects, especially women.

SYMPTOMS AND SIGNS.   Intense pruritus is the major complaint, and the urge to scratch is overwhelming. Early lesions are papules but they become firm, reddish or purple 1- to 3-cm nodules, with an excoriated surface. They occur primarily on the arms and back, but not in the interscapular area, where the patient cannot readily reach. On regression, hyper- or hypopigmented scars may remain.

MANAGEMENT.   Treatment can be very difficult. Oral antihistamines such as hydroxyzine (25 mg t.i.d.) may diminish the pruritus. Potent corticosteroids in ointments such as betamethasone valerate 0.1% or in tape form (Cordran) may help, but intralesional corticosteroid injection may be the most effective therapy. Some patients benefit from ultraviolet light treatments or liquid nitrogen cryotherapy.

LICHEN SIMPLEX CHRONICUS ("NEURODERMATITIS")

EPIDEMIOLOGY.   This disorder may occur at any age but is most common between 30 and 50 years of age. It is more frequent in women than in men.

SYMPTOMS AND SIGNS.   Lichen simplex chronicus occurs from repeated scratching or rubbing of the skin. The most common sites are the back or sides of the neck, the ankles, the lateral aspect of the lower legs, the upper thighs, and the anogenital region. The affected areas are markedly pruritic and exhibit lichenification and erythema, or sometimes hyperpigmentation.

CLINICAL APPROACH.   Other entities to consider include contact dermatitis and psoriasis.

MANAGEMENT.   A potent corticosteroid ointment such as betamethasone valerate 0.1% applied twice daily or the daily application of Cordran tape usually suffices, but intralesional injection of corticosteroids may be indicated in refractory cases.

VENOUS ECZEMA ("STASIS DERMATITIS")

EPIDEMIOLOGY.   Venous eczema is a complication of venous insufficiency of the legs, a disorder most common in the elderly, especially women.

SYMPTOMS AND SIGNS.   Venous eczema may be asymptomatic or may cause pruritus or burning discomfort. It may also be the site of entry for streptococci that cause cellulitis. It almost always occurs around the malleoli, especially the medial ones, but it may extend up the leg. It consists of erythematous scaling, often with exudation, crusts, and superficial ulcerations. Signs of venous hypertension are present, including varicosities, hemosiderin pigmentation, edema, venous ulcers, and dilated venules.

MANAGEMENT.   Burow's (aluminum acetate) wet dressings applied for 20 minutes three to four times a day are useful for acute weeping dermatitis. Topical corticosteroid creams, such as triamcinolone 0.1% applied twice daily, will usually relieve the eczema. Treatment of the venous hypertension with leg elevation and the use of elastic support stockings is crucial to control the edema and prevent future exacerbations.

CONTACT DERMATITIS

EPIDEMIOLOGY.   Contact dermatitis, which may occur from irritating substances or because of allergy to a material, is frequent, especially on the hands and in certain occupations. Contact allergy may develop as a reaction to topical medications, the most common agents being neomycin, lanolin, and topical anesthetics like benzocaine.

SYMPTOMS AND SIGNS.   With first exposure to the agent, the eruption may occur several days later; in those sensitized by previous contact, it usually appears 12 to 48 hours after exposure. Pruritus is the main complaint. Acute lesions show vesicles, oozing, erythema, and crusting. Chronic lesions are scaly, lichenified, and fissured. The diagnosis may be obvious from the history, but physical findings suggesting a contact cause are straight borders or lines, or a configuration conforming to some object touching the skin, such as a band around the wrist from an allergy to a component of a watchband. Failure of another skin disorder to improve despite apparently adequate topical therapy should suggest the possibility of contact allergy to an element of the treatment.

Clinical Approach. After the dermatitis resolves, skin testing to confirm the diagnosis and the identity of the contact allergen may be indicated.

Management. Removal of the responsible agent is crucial. The dermatitis should respond to topical corticosteroids.

REFERENCES

1. Epstein E. Hand dermatitis: Practical management and current concepts. J Am Acad Dermatol 1984;10:395–424.
   A practical guide to the management of hand dermatitis, with good instructions for patients to use.
2. Rook A, Wilkinson DS, Ebling FJG, Champion RH, Burton JL, Eds. Textbook of Dermatology. Blackwell, Oxford, 1986; pp. 367–533.
   Superb clinical discussions of the various eczemas. The best dermatology textbook in English.

29 SEBORRHEIC DERMATITIS

Problem

JAN V. HIRSCHMANN

Epidemiology. Seborrheic dermatitis, a chronic disorder probably caused by overgrowth of a normal skin yeast, *Pityrosporon orbiculare,* is rare before puberty and usually begins in adults between 18 and 40 years of age. It is more common in males and is especially frequent in patients with Parkinson's disease and in those with AIDS, in whom it is often very severe.

Symptoms and Signs. Seborrheic dermatitis occurs predominantly on the scalp, face, and upper trunk. These areas have abundant sebaceous glands, and the sebum produced contains the lipids necessary for *P. orbiculare* to grow. Erythema and scaling, often of a "greasy" nature, are the most common findings. In the scalp the scaling is usually diffuse, often with patches of redness and thick, sometimes weeping crusts. Common areas of facial involvement are the forehead, eyebrows, the skin around the nasal alae, the external auditory canal, and postauricular region. In those with mustaches or beards, yellowish white scales may adhere to the hairs, and the skin surrounding the follicles is often red. Blepharitis—inflammation of the eyelid margins—commonly occurs.

On the trunk, yellowish brown or red patches of scaling may occur on the presternal or interscapular regions. Seborrheic dermatitis may also involve the axillary, submammary, or groin areas, typically as patches of bright, moist erythema with mild scaling.

MANAGEMENT.   For scalp involvement, selenium sulfide shampoo applied for 5 to 10 minutes before rinsing is usually effective when used daily or less often as necessary. Alternative shampoos include those containing zinc pyrithione (e.g., Head and Shoulders), salicylic acid–sulfur (e.g., Ionil) or tar (e.g., Ionil T, Zetar). Topical corticosteroid lotions (e.g., fluocinolone) used twice daily are helpful for those with substantial inflammation or a poor response to a shampoo alone. Removal of thick crusts often requires nighttime application of keratolytic medications such as Baker's P&S (phenol and saline) or Keralyt (6% salicylic acid), covering the scalp with a shower cap overnight, and shampooing in the morning.

Seborrheic dermatitis elsewhere usually responds to topical corticosteroids—hydrocortisone 1% on the face and groin, more potent agents (e.g., triamcinolone 0.025%), if necessary, on the trunk. Patients with recalcitrant disease, especially those with AIDS, may require topical ketoconazole twice a day (instead of, or in addition to, corticosteroids) or even oral ketoconazole (200 mg/day) to achieve control. For most immunocompetent hosts, topical corticosteroids seem slightly better and much less expensive than topical ketoconazole, although refractory disease sometimes requires combined topical treatment with both agents.

Involvement of the eyelid margins usually subsides with the use of hot compresses, debridement with a cotton-tipped applicator stick, and washing with baby shampoo, or use of 10% sodium sulfacetamide ophthalmic ointment (Sulamyd) two to four times a day.

FOLLOW-UP.   Seborrheic dermatitis is a chronic disease that usually relapses quickly when treatment ends. Most patients learn to manage their disease, resuming therapy when the symptoms and signs recur, and need infrequent return visits for this problem. The chronic use of hydrocortisone on the face and elsewhere is safe, as is the use of potent corticosteroids on the scalp.

Cross-references: AIDS (Section 14), Redness of the Eye (Section 37), Otitis Media and Externa (Section 56).

REFERENCES

1.   Bergbrant IM, Faergemann J. The role of *Pityrosporum ovale* in seborrheic dermatitis. Semin Dermatol 1990;9:262–268.
     A thorough review of the microbiology of this organism and evidence of its role in seborrheic dermatitis.

2.   Stratigos JD, Antoniou C, Katsambas A, et al. Ketoconazole 2% cream versus hydrocortisone 1% cream in the treatment of seborrheic dermatitis. J Am Acad Dermatol 1988;19:850–853.
     In a double-blind trial, hydrocortisone had a better result than ketoconazole (clinical response, 94% vs. 81%).

30 HERPES ZOSTER

Problem

JAN V. HIRSCHMANN

EPIDEMIOLOGY. About 10% to 20% of all people have herpes zoster during their lifetimes. The incidence increases with age from less than 50 per 100,000 person-years for those less than 15 years old to more than 400 per 100,000 person-years for people over 74. The average age of patients with herpes zoster is about 45. The presence of cancer modestly increases the risk, while immunocompromising conditions such as Hodgkin's disease, AIDS, or organ transplantation are associated with incidences as high as 10% to 30% per year. A second attack occurs in about 5% of patients.

SYMPTOMS AND SIGNS. A prodrome of burning, tingling pain, and hyperesthesia in a dermatome is frequent and may last for a few days (occasionally as long as a week or more) before skin lesions appear. The lesions begin as erythematous papules that transform into vesicles, with contents that are originally clear but later turn yellow and turbid, or occasionally bloody. Darkening of the roofs is frequent, and the skin may become black, representing focal gangrene. The vesicles usually evolve over 4 to 7 days before crusts appear. The crusts fall off several days later, leaving scars in many patients.

Herpes zoster occurs in the thoracic dermatomes in 60% of patients and involves the cranial nerves in about 15%, usually the trigeminal nerve in one of its three subsegments—ophthalmic, maxillary, or mandibular. About 20% of those with herpes zoster of the trigeminal nerve have eye involvement; most of these (85%) have Hutchinson's sign (lesions on the tip of the nose). The cervical dermatomes are affected in 10%, the lumbar in 10%, and the sacral in 5%. Rather than involvement of a single dermatome, in many patients adjacent dermatomes are involved. Immunocompetent patients often have scattered lesions distant from the original dermatome. Only the presence of numerous extradermatomal lesions (at least twenty-five) qualifies as clinically significant dissemination, which is virtually always confined to severely immunocompromised patients. In these patients, evidence of cutaneous dissemination begins about 6 to 10 days after the original lesions appear; involvement of organs such as lung, liver, or brain occurs in only about 10% of untreated immunocompromised patients with disseminated disease.

Postherpetic neuralgia, generally defined as pain lasting more than 1 month, occurs in 10% to 60% of patients overall, is more frequent in older patients, especially those over 60 years of age, and may be more common in immunocompromised patients. The distribution of the dermatomes involved reflects that of herpes zoster in general, except that postherpetic neuralgia is uncommon in the lumbar area.

CLINICAL APPROACH.   The appearance of papules, vesicles, and pustules in a dermatomal distribution is virtually pathognomonic of herpes zoster. Viral cultures and immunofluorescent or electron microscopic techniques can confirm the diagnosis but rarely are necessary. In confusing cases a simple diagnostic test is the Tzanck smear, in which material is scraped from the base of vesicles, pustules, or erosions, placed on a slide, and treated with Wright's stain. Characteristic nuclear changes, including enlargement and multinucleation, are found in 91% of patients with varicella or zoster but do not distinguish this entity from herpes simplex. Because herpes zoster may be an early complication of AIDS, patients with risk factors for this disease should undergo testing for anti-HIV antibody. Herpes zoster is rarely a sign of occult malignancy; without other clinical evidence, further tests are unnecessary.

Patients with herpes zoster are contagious to people who have not had varicella in the past. By age 20, about 90% of the population is immune. During the first trimester of pregnancy, varicella causes congenital abnormalities in about 10% of fetuses. This infection is especially risky close to the time of delivery (with onset of disease from 5 days before to 2 days after), when infant mortality is 20% to 30%. Patients with herpes zoster should carefully avoid contact with pregnant women and immunocompromised patients who have not had varicella; in them, the disease can be severe.

MANAGEMENT.   Herpes zoster ordinarily requires no topical therapy, although wet dressings may be useful for exudative lesions. Painful disease may require narcotics. In most immunocompetent patients acyclovir has little clinical benefit and does not decrease the frequency of postherpetic neuralgia. In patients with ophthalmic involvement, however, oral acyclovir reduces the incidence and severity of the most common eye complications if treatment is begun within 7 days of the appearance of skin lesions. For those with normal renal function the recommended oral dose is 800 mg five times a day for 10 days; the same regimen is appropriate for immunocompromised patients with herpes zoster at any cutaneous site. Patients with severe disease may require hospitalization and IV acyclovir.

In immunocompetent patients, oral corticosteroids may reduce the frequency of postherpetic neuralgia, although their use is controversial. Candidates are patients older than 50 with painful lesions. A recommended regimen is prednisone, 60 mg/day for 1 week, 30 mg/day for the second week, and 15 mg/day for the third week. Dissemination of herpes zoster rarely, if ever, occurs with this treatment.

For patients with postherpetic neuralgia—either a steady or lancinating pain in the dermatome that lasts for more than 1 month—the most effective treatment is amitriptyline begun at 25 mg q.h.s., with the dose increased by 25 mg every 2 to 5 days until pain subsides or side effects preclude further use. In one study, 75 mg (range, 25–137.5 mg) was the median daily dose necessary to provide good to excellent pain relief, a goal achieved in about two-thirds of patients. Topical capsaicin (Zostrix) applied three times daily furnishes some benefit in about 80% of patients, but often the effect is only modest.

Cross-references: AIDS (Section 14), Redness of the Eye (Section 37).

REFERENCES

1. Liesegang TJ. The varicella-zoster virus: Systemic and ocular features. J Am Acad Dermatol 1984;11:165–191.
    A superb review, with excellent color photographs of the cutaneous and ocular findings.
2. Watson PN, Evans RJ. Postherpetic neuralgia: A review. Arch Neurol 1986;43:836–840.
    A sensible, detailed assessment of the published information.

31 ACNE

Problem

JAN V. HIRSCHMANN

EPIDEMIOLOGY.   Acne is virtually universal during adolescence, with peak incidences at age 14 to 17 years in girls, 16 to 19 years in boys. Occasionally, especially in girls, acne begins before other features of puberty appear. In about 85% of patients acne is mild; in 15% it is more troublesome. Acne usually disappears in the late teens or early 20s, but in a few people, especially women, it continues until age 40 or beyond. Occasionally acne begins in the early 20s or later. The distribution and the severity of acne tend to be similar in family members, suggesting a heredity component to this disease. Acne frequently worsens just before or during menstruation, but diet seems unimportant. Moderate exposure to sunlight is usually beneficial; excessive sweating in tropical climates, however, may worsen the disease.

SYMPTOMS AND SIGNS.   The face is nearly always involved, and patients usually have lesions on the chest and back as well. Most have several types of cutaneous abnormalities in varying combinations, including both noninflammatory (open comedones [blackheads], closed comedones [whiteheads] and inflammatory (papules, pustules, nodules, cysts) lesions. Scarring is frequent in severe disease, causing hypertrophic lesions, depressed areas (icepick scars), or small regions of increased or decreased pigmentation, especially in those with dark skin.

CLINICAL APPROACH. The diagnosis of acne is evident on physical examination. Clinicians should inquire about medications that can precipitate or exacerbate acne, including androgenic hormones, anabolic steroids, topical or systemic corticosteroids, phenobarbital, isoniazid, lithium, and cyclosporin. Cosmetics, oily hair products, and occupational exposure to cutting oils (e.g., in machinists) can also cause or worsen the disease.

MANAGEMENT. Medications used to treat acne alter one or more of the four major etiologic factors in acne: (1) increased sebum production, resulting from the effects of endogenous androgenic hormones; (2) hypercornification of the follicular orifice, causing duct obstruction; (3) colonization of the pilosebaceous duct with *Proprionibacterium acnes;* and (4) inflammation, perhaps in response to microbial products of *P. acnes.* Most cases of mild acne respond to topical agents. Benzoyl peroxide, which decreases the population of *P. acnes* and diminishes the inflammatory response to it, is used twice daily or less frequently to produce mild erythema and dryness. Topical antibiotics, either clindamycin or erythromycin, which also reduce the numbers of *P. acnes* are effective in about 70% of patients. Tretinoin (Retin A) decreases ductal hypercornification and possibly colonization with *P. acnes;* when applied overnight it is very useful, especially in those with predominantly comedonal acne. These topical agents may be given alone or in combination—tretinoin at night, benzoyl peroxide or topical antibiotics in the morning—but should not be applied at the same time. These medications require at least 3 months of use to attain their optimal effect, although improvement is usually evident by 2 to 3 weeks.

For moderate or severe involvement, oral tetracycline, 500 mg b.i.d., is effective and well tolerated. Patients should use it for at least 6 months to achieve maximum benefit. Long-term administration (several years) appears safe and effective. For those unable to tolerate tetracycline, erythromycin, 500 mg b.i.d., or sulfamethoxazole-trimethoprim, one double-strength tablet once or twice daily, are acceptable alternatives. Patients who do not respond to these measures or who have very severe acne should consult a dermatologist, who might consider estrogens or prednisone in females or isotretinoin, a very potent medication with dramatic effects on acne, in both sexes. Local measures sometimes helpful are gentle removal of blackheads and whiteheads by a comedone extractor and drainage, and intralesional corticosteroids or cryotherapy for cysts.

FOLLOW-UP. During early therapy, monthly review may be wise to monitor improvement, reassure patients, and offer encouragement. Later, follow-up every 3 to 4 months usually suffices.

REFERENCES

1. Cunliffe WJ. Acne. Year Book Medical Publishers, Chicago, 1989, 391 pp.
   A thorough and practical book on acne, with superb color photographs.
2. Pochi PE. The pathogenesis and treatment of acne. Annu Rev Med 1990;41:187–198.
   A brief overview.

32 PSORIASIS

Problem

JAN V. HIRSCHMANN

EPIDEMIOLOGY.   Psoriasis occurs in about 1.5% of American adults of both sexes. Onset typically occurs in the 20s and is somewhat earlier in women than in men. A family history is common.

SYMPTOMS AND SIGNS.   The most common form of psoriasis consists of well-defined plaques of white to silver scale of varying thickness, adherent to an erythematous base. The scales tend to occur in one or more of the following areas: lower back, including the gluteal cleft; the scalp; the extensor surfaces of the elbows and knees; and in the genital area. Where scale is removed, bleeding points may occur (Auspitz's sign). The appearance of lesions about 1 to 2 weeks after trauma to a previously uninvolved area (Koebner's phenomenon) is common; paradoxically, many note that injury to an area of psoriasis may result in improvement. Nail changes occur in 25% to 50% of patients, especially those over 40, and include pitting, separation of the nail from the nail bed (onycholysis), subungual hyperkeratosis, splinter hemorrhages, areas of salmon-pink discoloration under the nail, and opaque yellowing. The palms and soles may have thick hyperkeratosis and pustules.

Some patients develop widespread small, scaling papules called guttate ("droplike") psoriasis; another uncommon form is erythrodermic psoriasis, which is characterized by confluent erythema and fine scaling involving nearly the entire skin surface.

About 10% of patients with psoriasis develop arthritis. The arthritis may be (1) predominantly a sacroiliitis or spondylitis; (2) a symmetric polyarthritis resembling rheumatoid arthritis and mostly affecting the hands; (3) arthritis mutilans, a form associated with osteolysis of the phalanges; (4) distal interphalangeal joint involvement; or (5) asymmetric oligoarthritis affecting the distal or proximal interphalangeal joints, often with swelling of a single digit.

MANAGEMENT.   Emollients may be helpful for areas of excessive dryness. For mild plaque psoriasis, topical corticosteroids may control the disease. Hydrocortisone 1% or 2.5% is recommended for the face, genitals, and axillae; more potent agents such as triamcinolone ointment 0.025% to 0.1% or even stronger preparations are appropriate for other areas. Patients often become resistant to corticosteroids despite an initial response. Coal tar formulations such as Estar gel may be used daily or twice daily, combined or alternated with corticosteroids. For very thick plaques, the overnight use of Keralyt gel (6%

salicylic acid) will help remove thick, adherent scales and allow daily corticosteroid therapy to be more effective.

An excellent, simple alternative treatment for chronic plaque psoriasis is anthralin (dithranol) in a cream base (Drithrocreme). Available in strengths of 0.1%, 0.25%, 0.5%, and 1.0%, it can be applied to affected skin for 20 to 30 minutes a day and then washed off. Beginning with 0.1% or 0.25%, the strength can be increased every few days to weeks if the response is slow or absent. This preparation often induces remissions for several weeks to months. Its main side effects are a burning sensation (which suggests too potent a concentration or too lengthy an application) and purplish brown skin staining. This discoloration, which is not a reason for discontinuing the medication, fades quickly when the treatment ends, which should occur when the plaques have disappeared. Anthralin can then be resumed at the earliest signs of recurrence.

Scalp psoriasis is often difficult to manage. A tar shampoo such as Zetar or T-gel is frequently effective for mild involvement. For more severe or inflammatory disease the addition of a corticosteroid lotion or solution (e.g., fluocinolone [Synalar] or betamethasone valerate [Valisone] twice daily is recommended. The most potent topical corticosteroid currently available, clobetasol propionate 0.05% scalp application (Temovate), used twice daily for several weeks is effective for severe disease. Whether long-term use of clobetasol causes adverse effects such as cutaneous atrophy is unknown, and some experts recommend intermittent use alternating with rest periods of at least 1 week between each 2-week treatment course. Chronic use of the lower potency corticosteroids on the scalp, however, seems safe. Overnight treatment with salicylic acid gel 6% (Keralyt) or Baker's P&S (phenol and saline) applied to a wet scalp and covered by a shower cap will help loosen very thick scale, and the patient can then shampoo with a tar preparation, followed by application of a corticosteroid solution when the scalp is still wet to increase absorption. An alternative is to use anthralin (Drithroscalp) overnight, followed by a tar shampoo. This preparation can cause a brownish discoloration of blonde, gray, or white hair.

Nail psoriasis is generally unresponsive to topical therapy. Application of a corticosteroid ointment (e.g., betamethasone valerate) to affected skin around the nail may help a little. Keeping the nails trimmed and removing the subungual debris may be the most that can be achieved.

When patients have widespread disease or fail to respond to the simple measures outlined above, they should see a dermatologist, who can offer more complicated therapy such as ultraviolet light treatment or systemic agents such as methotrexate.

Cross-reference: General Approach to Arthritic Symptoms (Section 107).

REFERENCES

1. Buxton PK. Psoriasis. Br Med J 1987;295:904–906.

2. Going SM. Treatment of psoriasis. Br Med J 1987;295:984–986.
    Brief overviews, with a distinctive British flavor, from a series of simple but rewarding articles on skin diseases titled "ABC of Dermatology," later published in book form.

3. Roenigk HH, Maibach HI, Eds. Psoriasis. Marcel Dekker, New York, 1991.
    The quality varies markedly in this book, but there are good chapters on the clinical manifestations and treatment of this complex disease.

33 MALIGNANT MELANOMA

Problem

JAN V. HIRSCHMANN

Among the primary skin cancers that primary care clinicians are likely to see—basal cell carcinomas, squamous cell carcinomas, and malignant melanomas—only melanomas cause significant mortality. Whether widespread screening of asymptomatic people for this disorder is worthwhile remains uncertain. When clinicians encounter pigmented lesions because of patients' concerns or during routine examinations, however, they should know about the epidemiologic and clinical features that help distinguish lesions deserving further dermatologic evaluation from those that are not worrisome.

EPIDEMIOLOGY.   In the United States the incidence of malignant melanoma is currently increasing faster than the incidence of any other cancer. The annual incidence is about 12 per 100,000 people, but it is higher in the Southwest. Available evidence strongly implicates sunlight as an important etiologic factor, especially infrequent, brief, intense exposures leading to sunburns rather than regular, protracted exposure. Darkly pigmented people have a much lower risk than fair-skinned ones; for example, among blacks in the United States the incidence is about 0.8 per 100,000. In the caucasian population, significant risk factors, reflecting the importance of skin melanin as a protective factor, are red or blonde hair, blue eyes, a tendency to freckle, and an inability to tan. A history of melanoma increases the risk of developing another one ninefold, and a family history increases the risk eightfold.

SYMPTOMS AND SIGNS.   Some melanomas cause itching, bleeding, crusting, or inflammation, but most patients have no symptoms except, perhaps, a concern about a lesion's identity, enlargement, or changed appearance. Nearly all melanomas are pigmented. Features that help distinguish these cancers from other pigmented lesions are summarized by the mnemonic ABCDE: asymmetry in shape (one half unlike the other), border is irregular (edges scalloped), color is a haphazard variety of hues (blue, red, white, gray in a brown to black lesion), diameter is large (>6 mm), and elevation is usually present, with surface distortion obvious or detectable by side lighting. Another scheme to suggest which pigmented lesions are worrisome is a seven-point checklist:

Major features:

1. Change in size
2. Irregular edge
3. Irregular pigmentation

Minor features:

4. 7 mm or more in diameter
5. Inflammation
6. Oozing, crusting, or bleeding
7. Altered sensation, usually itching

The authors of this list suggest referral to dermatologist when patients have any major feature; the concurrent presence of any minor feature increases the likelihood that melanoma is present. The sensitivity and specificity of these criteria are unknown.

Four basic types of melanomas occur: superficial spreading (about 60%–80% of melanomas in the United States), nodular (10%–20%), acral lentiginous (5%), and lentigo maligna (5%). Superficial spreading melanoma tends to occur on the legs of females and the backs of males. About 50% of patients report a preexisting, apparently benign lesion at the site. These tumors have a lengthy radial growth phase (lateral extension of the cancer) that may last from months to years before vertical growth (invasion into deeper structures) occurs and clinically detectable nodules form. In nodular melanoma the vertical growth phase is present when the lesion is first clinically apparent. It is a raised pigmented nodule with normal surrounding skin. Acral lentiginous melanomas involve the palms, soles, or subungual areas, often manifesting initially as a pigmented macule that later becomes nodular. This is the most frequent form of melanoma in blacks. Lentigo maligna melanoma occurs mostly on the face in elderly people. It begins as a slow-growing area of macular pigmentation, typically on the temple or cheek, sometimes with central regression. At this stage it is called lentigo maligna and is a melanoma in situ with malignant-appearing cells that have not invaded from the epidermis into the dermis. When such penetration occurs, with papule formation, the lesion is called lentigo maligna melanoma.

CLINICAL APPROACH. Clinicians should inspect and palpate the areas around suspicious lesions, to detect satellite metastases, and the regional lymph nodes, to detect lymphatic involvement. A careful search of the remaining skin surface for other intracutaneous metastases and palpation of the liver and spleen complete the preliminary assessment before the patient is referred to a dermatologist for further evaluation. Routine laboratory or radiographic studies are not warranted at this stage in the absence of suggestive symptoms or signs.

MANAGEMENT.   Although primary care clinicians generally do not manage patients with malignant melanoma, they should know about some important issues. The melanoma staging system identifies three stages: I—localized disease, II—regional lymph node involvement, III—distant metastases. Overall 5-year survival rates for these are about 90%, 60%, and 0%, respectively. For stage I lesions the most important prognostic feature is the depth of tumor, measured in millimeters from the granular layer of the epidermis to the deepest penetration into the dermis or subcutaneous tissue. Five-year survival rates, figured according to the thickness of the tumor, are 96% to 99% for tumors less than 0.76 mm, 87% to 94% for tumors 0.76 to 1.5 mm, 66% to 77% for tumors 1.51 to 4.0 mm, and less than 50% for tumors larger than 4.0 mm. Factors other than tumor depth that suggest a poor prognosis include lesions on the head, neck, trunk, hands, and feet; age older than 50; male sex; and ulceration of the lesion.

Excisional biopsy is the treatment of choice. For thin melanomas (<1 mm), a 1-cm margin is adequate; for thicker lesions, margins of 1 to 3 cm are appropriate. Elective regional dissection of clinically normal lymph nodes is controversial, but regional lymph node dissection is clearly indicated for patients with histologically involved nodes (stage II).

FOLLOW-UP.   A common practice is evaluation monthly for 3 months, every 3 months for up to 2 years, every 6 months to 5 years, and annually thereafter. Lengthy follow-up is necessary because about 2.5% of affected patients first experience recurrence more than 10 years after removal of a malignant melanoma, most commonly at the original site or in its draining lymph node area. Furthermore, about 5% of patients will develop a second primary melanoma. Accordingly, at each visit the clinician should examine the excision site, the regional lymph nodes, and the remainder of the skin surface.

REFERENCES

1. Ho VC, Sober AJ. Therapy for cutaneous melanoma: An update. J Am Acad Dermatol 1990;22:159–176.

    A thorough discussion of the management of melanoma.

2. MacKie RM. Skin Cancer. Year Book Medical Publishers, Chicago, 1989, 346 pp.

    An excellent book that discusses both benign and malignant skin tumors. Superb color illustrations of clinical and histologic material.

34 URTICARIA

Problem

JAN V. HIRSCHMANN

EPIDEMIOLOGY.   Urticaria occurs once or more in the lifetime of about 20% of the population. Most attacks are acute, short-lived, and frequently provoked by identifiable causes, such as medications or food (e.g., nuts, seafood, eggs). In chronic urticaria, defined as lasting more than 6 weeks, a cause usually remains undiscovered. Some forms of urticaria, called physical urticaria, are due to physical stimuli, usually easily discernible from the history, including cold (cold urticaria), exercise or heat (cholinergic urticaria), or sunlight (solar urticaria). Dermographism, an exaggerated wheal-and-flare response to stroking the skin, is present in 4% to 5% of the general population, but only a minority of affected people have symptoms.

SYMPTOMS AND SIGNS.   Urticaria usually occurs as raised, erythematous, pruritic plaques with sharply defined borders and often whitish centers. Individual lesions typically last up to 12 hours, although new ones may continue to appear. Those remaining unchanged for more than 24 hours (especially if associated with arthralgias and accompanied by scaling, purpura, or pigmentation on resolution) should suggest the diagnosis of urticarial vasculitis, a disorder with different diagnostic and therapeutic implications. Lesions of the physical urticarias usually disappear within one half-hour of the provoking stimuli, and one form, cholinergic urticaria, has a distinctive morphology: tiny (1–3-mm) papular wheals with surrounding erythema. Patients with symptomatic dermographism (most commonly young adults) typically have attacks of itching and subsequent wheals from scratching that may be provoked by heat or pressure from various sources such as tight clothing, sitting, or working with tools.

CLINICAL APPROACH.   A detailed history searching for such provocative factors as food or drug intake and physical stimuli is the most important investigation. If a cause is discovered, it is usually evident in the history. In chronic urticaria, no cause is apparent in 90% of cases, and laboratory tests are rarely rewarding. Stroking the back firmly with the blunt end of a pen and examining the area 1 to 3 minutes later for an accentuated wheal-and-flare reaction will confirm the diagnosis of dermographism in patients with a suggestive history. The wheal is 2 mm or more in diameter, and erythema of 5 to 10 mm in width spreads out from it. The wheal reaches its maximum size in 6 to 7 minutes and fades within 10 to 15 minutes.

MANAGEMENT.   Antihistamines are the mainstay of treatment. Hydroxyzine, 25 mg three to six times a day, is an excellent agent. When drowsiness is

105

a significant complication, a nonsedating antihistamine such as terfenadine, 60 mg b.i.d., is a useful substitute. Doxepin begun in doses of 10 mg t.i.d. is another effective alternative. At these low doses dryness of the mouth and sedation may not occur; at higher amounts these side effects, though common, often diminish with time. With refractory cases, particularly for patients with symptomatic dermographism, the addition of an H_2 receptor blocker like cimetidine, 300 mg q.i.d., or ranitidine, 150 mg b.i.d., may be helpful. Patients with chronic urticaria should avoid aspirin, which may provoke or worsen attacks.

FOLLOW-UP.   Acute urticaria usually resolves in 1 to 2 weeks and, by definition, abates within 6 weeks. Chronic urticaria usually subsides over several months, but occasionally the condition is much more protracted.

REFERENCES

1.   Casale TB, Sampson HA, Hanifin J, et al. Guide to physical urticarias. J Allergy Clin Immunol 1988;82:758–763.
   An excellent, brief summary.

2.   Champion RH. Acute and chronic urticaria. Semin Dermatol 1987;6:286–291.
   A succinct overview that emphasizes the importance of history in detecting a cause.

DISORDERS OF THE EYE

35 SCREENING FOR GLAUCOMA

Screening

HOWARD BARNEBEY

EPIDEMIOLOGY. Glaucoma can be defined as a progressive anterior optic neuropathy that frequently develops in patients with elevated eye pressure. This new definition emphasizes the optic nerve and its appearance and does not emphasize intraocular pressure (IOP) as much as older definitions. Most studies screening for glaucoma have used elevated IOP to identify people at risk for the development of glaucoma. In fact, 2% to 4% of the population have elevated IOP (IOP > 21 mm Hg).

Screening for glaucoma traditionally depended on IOP measurement. Unfortunately, IOP as a sole predictor of glaucoma lacks both sensitivity (50%–70%) and specificity (30%), thus limiting its usefulness as a sole screening strategy.

In addition, the IOP normally fluctuates throughout the day. Even in patients with suspected glaucoma who have known elevations in IOP, there is a one in five chance that IOP will be normal on a single reading. Screening sensitivity is dramatically improved by ophthalmoscopic evaluation of the optic disc, which focuses on the finding of a large cup-disc ratio (i.e., ≥0.6), vertical elongation of the cup, or loss of rim inferiorly or superiorly.

RATIONALE FOR SCREENING. Early diagnosis and treatment can prevent or minimize progressive optic nerve atrophy and visual loss. Because the disease is relatively common, with a presymptomatic stage, and there are benefits from treatment, it is a suitable condition for screening programs.

Unfortunately, no single test has adequate predictive power to identify all glaucoma suspects. One approach, however, which combines tonometry (IOP measurement) with optic disc evaluation (ophthalmoscopy), will detect the most affected people. Most studies have suggested that screening for glaucoma

107

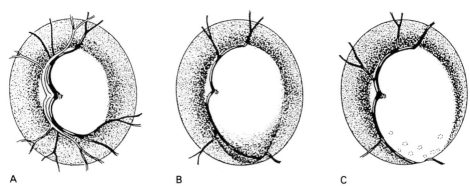

A   B   C

FIGURE 35–1. Appearance of normal and glaucomatous optic cup. *A*. Prominent cup:disc ratio (0.5) in normal patient. *B*. Glaucomatous optic atrophy with focal loss at inferior rim of disc. Note kinking of retinal vessel. *C*. Glaucomatous optic atrophy with further loss of inferior rim. Note "bayonetting" of retinal vessels indicating absence of rim tissue. Also visible is the lamina cribrosa demonstrating deepening of cup. (From Shields MB. Textbook of Glaucoma. Williams & Wilkins, Baltimore, 1987, with permission.)

be directed toward high-risk populations, including the elderly (>50 years old), blacks, diabetics, high myopes, and those with a family history of glaucoma.

ACTION.   Once high-risk individuals have been identified and screened, referral to an ophthalmologist is required.

Cross-reference: Glaucoma (Section 40).

REFERENCES

1.   Sommer A, Tielsch JM, Katz J, Quigley HA, Gottsch JD, Javitt JC, Martone JF, Royall RM, Witt KA, Ezrine S. Racial differences in the cause-specific prevalence of blindness in east Baltimore. N Engl J Med 1991;325:1412–1417.

Primary open-angle glaucoma accounted for 19% of all blindness among blacks; it was six times as frequent among blacks as whites and began 10 years earlier.

2.   Tielsch JM, Sommer A, Katz J, Royall RM, Quigley HA, Javitt J. Racial variations in the prevalence of primary open-angle glaucoma. The Baltimore Eye Survey. JAMA 1991; 266:369–374.

The prevalence of primary open-angle glaucoma among blacks ranged from about 1% in 40 - 49-year olds to 11% of those 80 or older; prevalence among blacks was 4 to 5 times higher than among whites.

Also see Section 40, Glaucoma.

36 VISUAL IMPAIRMENT

Screening

KENNETH E. HAMRICK

EPIDEMIOLOGY. Among individuals 40 years of age and older in the United States, the prevalence of visual impairment (i.e., Snellen acuity between 20/40 and 20/200) is about 3%, and the prevalence of legal blindness (i.e., best corrected visual acuity is worse than 20/200) is about 2%. The prevalence of blindness and visual impairment increases dramatically with age, from 1.7% among persons 40 to 49 years old to 12.5% among those aged 70 to 79 years. Blacks tend to have higher rates of visual impairment in all age categories except 80 years and older, at which point whites equal or pass blacks in the rate of blindness. Males and females develop visual impairment and blindness at equal rates.

Cataracts account for about 20% of cases of visual impairment and affect 15% of those older than 52 years. The prevalence of open-angle glaucoma, the leading cause of legal blindness, is 3.3%. Age-related macular degeneration, another important cause of legal blindness, affects 1.6% of people aged 52 to 64 years, 11% of those aged 65 to 74 years, and 27.9% of those aged 75 to 85 years.

RATIONALE. More than 50% of patients with visual impairment would benefit from proper correction of refractive error. Most cataracts are amenable to surgical extraction, with excellent visual results. Early detection and treatment of glaucoma may prevent blindness. Macular photocoagulation studies have demonstrated the benefits of laser treatment of neovascular membranes that otherwise lead to disciform macular scars and legal blindness. The benefits of laser treatment in preventing visual impairment and blindness from proliferative diabetic retinopathy are well substantiated.

STRATEGY. The clinician should screen the visual acuity of one eye at a time, using a Snellen chart 20 feet from the patient or a Snellen near equivalent chart 14 inches from the patient. The patient should wear his or her best available correction (e.g., bifocals, reading glasses) for the distance tested. Reduced acuity may be due to any of the conditions mentioned above. Pinhole acuity or squinting may improve vision in patients with refractive error, whereas pathologic acuity loss due to cataracts, macular degeneration, glaucoma, and diabetic retinopathy is not improved.

Factors associated with an increased risk of developing serious ocular disease include age over 65, diabetes, glaucoma, and a history of ocular trauma, infection, or chronic eye condition requiring follow-up.

ACTION.   To allow timely referral of treatable conditions and proper rehabilitation of the visually impaired, appropriate referral patterns should be established. Depending on the circumstances, referrals to optometrists, general
ophthalmologists, glaucoma and retinal specialists, or rehabilitation or low vision practitioners may be suitable.

REFERENCES

1.   DeSylvia DA. Low vision and aging. Optom Vis Sci 1990;67:319–322.
     Describes functional losses, visual needs, low vision solutions, and rehabilitation suggestions for the
     visually impaired.
2.   Kini MM, Leibowitz HM, Colton T, Nickerson RJ, Ganley J, Dawber TR. Prevalence of
     senile cataract, diabetic retinopathy, senile macular degeneration, and open-angle glaucoma
     in the Framingham Eye Study. Am J Ophthalmol 1978;85:28–34.
     Epidemiology of the major causes of blindness in the elderly.
3.   Macular Photocoagulation Study Group. Argon laser photocoagulation for senile macular
     degeneration: Results of a randomized clinical trial. Arch Ophthalmol 1982;100:912–918.
     Describes the treatment benefits of laser photocoagulation and the follow-up of patients with macular
     degeneration.
4.   Strahlman E, Ford D, Whelton P, Sommer A. Vision screening in a primary care setting: A
     missed opportunity? Arch Intern Med 1990;150:2159–2164.
     Describes effective screening for serious eye disease in an internal medicine setting.
5.   Tielsch JM, Sommer A, Witt K, Katz J, Royall RM. Blindness and visual impairment in an
     American urban population: The Baltimore Eye Survey. Arch Ophthalmol 1990;108:286–
     290.
     Delineates the prevalence of blindness and visual impairment and their epidemiologic significance.

37 REDNESS OF THE EYE

Symptom

STEPHAN D. FIHN

EPIDEMIOLOGY/ETIOLOGY.   After changes in visual acuity, redness of the
eye is the most common ocular problem encountered by primary care providers. Redness of the eye is nonspecific. Causes can be separated into those related to disorders of the globe, those related to disorders of the surrounding
soft tissue and supporting structures, and trauma (Table 37–1).
    Disorders affecting the eye itself include conjunctivitis, keratitis, scleritis/
episcleritis, uveitis, keratoconjunctivitis sicca, and acute angle closure glau-

TABLE 37–1. DIFFERENTIAL DIAGNOSIS OF A RED EYE

Ocular Problem	Vision	Pain, Photophobia	Pupils	Intraocular Pressure	Discharge/ Smear	Conjunctival Injection	Cornea	Referral	Comments
Conjunctivitis Bacterial	Normal	Minimal to absent	Normal	Normal	Purulent/ neutrophilic	Diffuse	Normal	No, unless unresponsive to treatment	Eyes stick together
Viral	Normal	Minimal to absent	Normal	Normal	Watery/ lymphocytic	Diffuse/ follicular infiltrates	Normal	No	Associated URI; preauricular lymph node enlargement
Allergic	Normal	Minimal to absent	Normal	Normal	Stringy/ eosinophilic	Minimal	Normal	No	Associated atopy, itching, puffy eyes
Keratitis Infectious	Diminished, depends on extent and area of corneal involvement	Yes, less prominent in herpes and zoster	Usually normal	Normal	Possibly mild	Diffuse	Opacified ulcer, hypopyon, dendritic ulcer	Yes	
Abrasions	Usually mild blurring	Yes, sharp foreign body sensation	Normal	Normal	Tearing	Diffuse	Epithelial defects	Yes	
Iritis	Mild to moderate blurring	Yes	Miotic	Normal	No	Circumcorneal	Hazy, keratic precipitates	Yes	May have associated systemic disease
Glaucoma	Marked blurring	Yes, acute onset	Mid-dilated and fixed	Increased	No	Diffuse with circumcorneal prominence	Hazy with decreased light reflex	Yes	May complain of nausea and vomiting, headaches, colored halos

Source: Adapted from Bauman R, Fihn SD. The red eye. Med Rounds 1989;2:267–278. Reproduced by permission.

coma. Conjunctivitis is the most frequent cause of a red eye and is usually a result of viral or bacterial infection or allergy (see Section 43, Conjunctivitis). Keratitis may result from wearing contact lens for excessive periods of time or from corneal exposure due to seventh cranial nerve paralysis or ectropion. Keratitis can be also caused by primary or recurrent herpes simplex virus (HSV) infection, varicella-zoster, or less commonly, by other viruses such as measles, mumps, rubella, or Epstein-Barr virus.

Episcleritis is an inflammation of the episclera, the thin vascular layer covering the sclera. The etiology is uncertain but may be allergic. Scleritis is a more severe problem associated with systemic inflammatory disease such as rheumatoid arthritis, polyarteritis nodosa, systemic lupus, and Wegener's granulomatosis.

Inflammation of the uveal tract (iris, ciliary body, and choroid) may be anterior (iritis, iridocyclitis), posterior (choroiditis, chorioretinitis), or diffuse. Most cases are idiopathic, especially anterior uveitis. Uveitis occurs in 25% to 40% of patients with ankylosing spondylitis, 20% to 30% of those with Reiter's syndrome, and 20% to 25% of those with sarcoidosis. Acute iridocyclitis is common in young women with sarcoidosis, especially those with erythema nodosum, whereas chronic iridocyclitis occurs more commonly in elderly patients. Rarely, uveitis results from an infection—toxoplasmosis, histoplasmosis, candidiasis, tuberculosis, cytomegalovirus (CMV), HSV, or syphilis; the posterior uveal tract is most commonly involved. CMV retinitis is a significant cause of visual loss in patients with acquired immunodeficiency syndrome (AIDS).

Keratoconjunctivitis sicca (dry eyes) occurs in 16% of persons older than age 80 and among patients with connective tissue diseases (see Section 38, Dry Eyes and Excessive Tearing).

Acute angle closure glaucoma may be precipitated by pupillary dilation from entering a dark room or by the use of mydriatics or anticholinergics, and can rapidly lead to blindness (see Section 40, Glaucoma).

Redness of the eye may also be due to inflammation of the sebaceous glands in the tarsal plate (meibomian glands) or the glands along the margin of the eyelid (glands of Zeis or Moll). A **hordeolum** is a localized abscess most commonly caused by staphylococci. When the glands of Zeis or Moll are involved, it is called an external hordeolum or, more commonly, a stye. When the meibomian glands are involved, a larger abscess, termed an internal hordeolum, occurs. Blepharitis is a common inflammatory condition of the eyelid margins caused by infection (usually staphylococci) or by seborrhea.

Cellulitis may also redden the structures around the eye. Orbital cellulitis results from direct spread from the sinuses, trauma, or conjunctivitis.

Subconjunctival hemorrhage is a common and benign cause of a red eye that can be disconcerting to patients.

CLINICAL APPROACH.   The presence of ocular pain or impaired visual acuity suggests a serious disorder (e.g., keratitis, iritis, or acute angle closure glaucoma). Conjunctivitis typically causes burning and itching, while iritis and glaucoma cause a deep throbbing pain. Corneal injury is accompanied by a sharp foreign body sensation. The details of any ocular trauma should be obtained as well as information on the use of contact lenses or ophthalmic preparations. The presence of an underlying systemic disease such as rheumatoid arthritis or sarcoidosis may point to specific ocular disorders.

Visual acuity should always be documented with the use of a Snellen chart and corrective lenses, if available, or a pinhole card. Examination of the eye should begin with inspection of the globe and the periorbital structures, and pupillary reflexes. Although anisocoria can be a normal variant, the pupils should be round and equal unless there is a history of surgery or trauma. Most corneal opacities are obvious, but epithelial defects may require fluorescein staining for identification. Measurement of intraocular pressure helps to diagnose glaucoma but should be avoided if there is a purulent discharge or the possibility of globe perforation.

In **viral conjunctivitis** the discharge is watery, and conjunctival hyperemia is accompanied by follicular infiltrates (focal lymphoid hyperplasia) on the tarsal conjunctiva (creating a mild foreign body sensation and tearing). Conjunctival hyperemia tends to be most prominent at the fornices and decreases toward the limbus. Signs of an upper respiratory infections and preauricular adenopathy may be present. **Allergic conjunctivitis** commonly occurs in atopic patients or those exposed to allergens such as animal dander or eye preparations such as contact lens solutions. Patients complain of itching and tearing that is often bilateral. The discharge is typically watery to mucoid with a stringy consistency. Chemosis and swollen eyelids may be prominent. Conjunctival hyperemia tends to be mild as compared to viral or bacterial conjunctivitis. The discharge of **bacterial conjunctivitis** is copious and purulent, and patients complain of adherent eyelids upon awakening. Blepharitis may coexist, especially with a staphylococcal infection. The presence of pain, visual changes, pupillary abnormalities, or a ciliary flush (circumcorneal vessel dilation) suggests a diagnosis other than conjunctivitis.

Keratitis commonly produces visual impairment and pain made worse by lid movement, except when caused by HSV or zoster, which produce less pain and tearing. Pupils are normal unless there is an associated uveitis, in which case they may be miotic. Penlight examination reveals a hazy appearance of the cornea with loss of the normal corneal light reflex. Visualization of epithelial disruption is enhanced by touching a sterile fluorescein-impregnated strip to the wet conjunctiva in the lower fornices and having the patient blink. Bacterial infection may cause a hypopyon (collection of inflammatory cells in the anterior chamber) or centrally located ulcers. Herpes keratitis is usually unilateral with associated conjunctivitis and cutaneous vesicles. Corneal ulcerations are rare, although recurrent herpes may produce dendritic (branching) ulcers that are enhanced by staining with fluorescein.

Patients with **episcleritis** typically present with a unilateral red eye and excessive tearing, photophobia, and mild ocular discomfort. Visual acuity and pupillary examination are normal. Unlike conjunctivitis, episcleritis does not involve the palpebral conjunctiva. In **scleritis**, there is moderate to severe pain, excessive tearing, photophobia, and violaceous discoloration of the sclera. Visual acuity may be reduced if there is associated corneal or retinal involvement.

Patients with **keratoconjunctivitis sicca** often complain of a gritty sensation in the eye as well as burning, redness, mild pain and itching, and a mucoid discharge. Many patients note a paradoxic increase in tearing. The eye may appear grossly normal but is often red with a stringy mucoid discharge.

Unlike chronic open angle glaucoma, which is usually asymptomatic, **acute angle closure glaucoma** causes severe eye pain, headache, nausea and vomiting, and impaired vision. Patients may note colored halos around lights due to the corneal edema. The conjunctiva is injected, with prominent perilimbal vessels (ciliary flush) producing a violet hue. The pupils are characteristically mid-dilated and minimally reactive and appear hazy. Intraocular pressure is elevated, usually greater than 40 mmHg (normal, 12–20 mmHg). The depth of the anterior chamber can be estimated by shining a penlight from the temporal side of the head, parallel to the plane of the iris. If two-thirds or more of the nasal iris is in shadow, the anterior chamber is probably shallow and the angle narrowed.

An **internal hordeolum** is characterized by localized swelling, erythema, and pain. **Blepharitis** commonly manifests with crusting, scaling, erythema, and swelling of the eyelid.

Periorbital cellulitis, better termed preseptal cellulitis, involves the eyelid and surrounding skin. It is prevented from extending to the globe by the fibrous orbital septum. The globe itself is usually not red unless there is associated conjunctivitis. Patients with **orbital cellulitis** often are systemically ill and have erythema and chemosis of the lids and globe, as well as pain on eye movement that may be restricted from the swelling.

Trauma to the eye is usually apparent from the history and examination.

MANAGEMENT.   Mild conjunctivitis and blepharitis can usually be managed by the primary care provider (see Section 43, Conjunctivitis), as can keratoconjunctivitis sicca (see Section 38, Dry Eyes and Excessive Tearing). Any patient with ocular pain, visual disturbance, or pupillary abnormalities should be examined as soon as possible by an ophthalmologist.

FOLLOW-UP.   Patients with conjunctivitis who have not improved within 48 hours should be reexamined.

Cross-references: Eye Pain (Section 39), Glaucoma (Section 40), Foreign Bodies and Corneal Abrasions (Section 42), Conjunctivitis (Section 43).

REFERENCES

1. Bauman R, Fihn SD. The red eye. Med Rounds 1989;2:267–278.
    A thorough and practical review for the primary care provider.

2. Chalupa E, Swarbrick HA, Holden BA, Sjostrand J. Severe corneal infections associated with contact lens wear. Ophthalmology 1987;94:17–22.

Describes the hazards of wearing contact lens, particularly soft lens, for extended periods. Steroid use was a significant predisposing factor. Most infections were caused by *Pseudomonas* strains.

3. Gardner TW, Shock D. Handbook of Ophthalmology: A Practical Guide. Appleton & Lange, Norwalk, Conn., 1987.
    Indeed, a practical guide.

4. Spalton DJ, Hitchings RA, Hunter PA. Atlas of Clinical Ophthalmology. J.B. Lippincott, Philadelphia, 1984.
    An excellent atlas.

38 DRY EYES AND EXCESSIVE TEARING

Symptom

THOMAS D. LINDQUIST

EPIDEMIOLOGY/ETIOLOGY. Keratoconjunctivitis sicca, or aqueous-deficient dry eye, is an often overlooked condition that affects 20% to 25% of patients visiting eye clinics. The prevalence is greatest between 40 and 60 years of age, with a 6:1 female-male predominance.

Keratoconjunctivitis sicca most commonly is caused by lymphocytic infiltration and fibrosis of the lacrimal gland but may, on occasion, be associated with sarcoidosis, rheumatoid arthritis, or other connective tissue disease.

SYMPTOMS AND SIGNS. The symptoms are typically worse upon awakening and include burning, grittiness, or foreign body sensation, discharge in the inner canthus or lower cul-de-sac, redness of the eye, blurred vision, and difficulty opening the eyelids. Paradoxically, patients frequently describe *excessive* tearing due to a relative response to drying of the cornea.

Signs include sticky, ropy discharge, dilated bulbar conjunctival vessels (particularly within the interpalpebral fissure), filaments, punctate epithelial defects, and keratinization. Filaments are discrete strands of mucus intertwined with desquamated cells and cellular debris that dangle from an attachment to the corneal epithelium.

CLINICAL APPROACH. Drying causes a loss of the smooth refractive surface of the tear film and an irregular light reflex. Epithelial abnormalities are best elucidated by rose bengal or fluorescein staining of the epithelium. Drying, keratinization, filaments, and mucous plaques are readily seen with rose bengal. Frank epithelial defects stain brilliantly with fluorescein.

Tear production can be measured by Schirmer tests, in which a Whatman No. 41 filter paper, 5 mm in width, is placed for 5 minutes at the junction of the lateral and middle thirds of the lower lid. The inferior conjunctival cul-de-sac must be dried gently with a cotton applicator before testing. The length of the wet portion of the filter paper is measured after 5 minutes. Less than 5 mm of wetting is always suggestive of significant tear dysfunction. A normal test result in the unanesthetized eye is 15 mm or more of wetting; with topical anesthesia it is 10 mm or more of wetting.

Although a tearing eye may be a nuisance to the patient, it never causes permanent visual loss, whereas absence of tears may lead to keratinization of the corneal and conjunctival epithelium. Epiphora is a condition in which drainage of tears through the lacrimal system is faulty, with the result that tears overflow onto the cheek. This condition should be evaluated by an ophthalmologist.

MANAGEMENT.   A tear substitute should be prescribed, but many preparations contain preservatives (e.g., thimerosol and benzalkonium chloride) that cause hypersensitivity reactions when used frequently. Nonpreserved tear preparations are now commercially available in varying viscosities (Refresh, Hypotears PF, Celluvisc). Application of a nonpreserved tear substitute ointment at bedtime is highly recommended. Patients who continue to have symptoms and signs despite frequent supplemental lubrication should be referred to an ophthalmologist for punctal occlusion. Severe tear deficiency may even require lateral tarsorrhaphy to decrease the exposed surface area and retard evaporation.

FOLLOW-UP.   Patients with severe dry eyes should be followed by an ophthalmologist at 4- to 6-month intervals as they are at greater risk for persistent epithelial defects, infectious ulcers, and stromal melting.

REFERENCES

1. Baum JL. Systemic disease associated with tear deficiencies. Int Ophthalmol Clin 1973; 13:157–184.
    A thorough review of systemic diseases associated with tear deficiency.

2. Holly FJ, Lemp MA. Tear physiology and dry eyes. Surv Ophthalmol 1977;22:69–87.
    The dry eye syndromes can be divided as follows: aqueous tear deficiency, mucin deficiency, lipid abnormalities, lid surfacing abnormalities, and epitheliopathies.

3. van Bijsterveld OP. Diagnostic tests in the sicca syndrome. Arch Ophthalmol 1969;82:10–14.
    Emphasizes the role of rose bengal 1% in the diagnosis of dry-eye conditions.

39 EYE PAIN

Symptom

JAMES C. ORCUTT

ETIOLOGY. Pain in or around the eye occurs in one of four patterns: ocular pain, pain with eye movement, orbital pain, and referred pain.

Ocular pain generally is accompanied by additional ocular symptoms: foreign body sensation, decreased visual acuity, pupillary abnormalities, redness of the eye, or visual halos. Common causes are corneal abrasion (see Section 42, Foreign Bodies and Corneal Abrasion), acute angle closure glaucoma (see Section 40, Glaucoma), and iritis (see Section 37, Redness of the Eye). Ocular pain may stimulate the vagal reflex, producing nausea and vomiting. Chronic open angle glaucoma is rarely painful (see Section 40, Glaucoma).

Pain with eye movements can be due to optic neuritis, sinusitis, or idiopathic inflammation of the extraocular muscles (pseudotumor). Except in cases of pseudotumor, the pain is usually mild. Associated diplopia suggests pseudotumor, whereas associated impairment in vision with a noninflamed eye suggests optic neuritis.

Orbital pain is usually severe, constant, boring, localized behind the eye, and associated with proptosis. Primary orbital inflammation (pseudotumor), orbital hemorrhage, and orbital cellulitis are common causes. Because orbital malignancies are occasionally painful, the presence of pain does not help differentiate malignancies from other cause of orbital pain. Fleeting, shooting, sharp, stabbing pains lasting 1 to 5 seconds and unaccompanied by eye signs or symptoms are generally unassociated with pathology.

Referred pain is the most common cause of ocular pain. The pain is generally diffusely related to the eyes, brow, and forehead, or, in rare cases, is dermatomal. A common cause of diffuse referred pain is one of the common headaches (see Section 140, Headache); in such cases the eye examination is normal. Pain referred in a dermatomal pattern may be caused by nasopharyngeal carcinomas, intracranial aneurysms, cavernous sinus tumors, or herpes zoster infections. Dermatomal referred pain may be accompanied by other signs of cranial nerve involvement such as diplopia, numbness, or ptosis.

CLINICAL APPROACH. An eye examination including visual acuity, pupil evaluation, extraocular movements, external examination, cranial nerve examination, fluorescein staining, IOP, and funduscopy is required. The absence of specific findings would be most compatible with a diagnosis of referred pain. Additional diagnostic tests depend on the type of eye pain: for example, patients with pain on eye movement and a normal eye examination should be evaluated for sinusitis (see Section 57, Sinusitis); patients with referred pain and no ocular findings should be further evaluated for the causes of headache (see Section 140, Headache).

MANAGEMENT.   Various sections in this chapter review the management of red eye, conjunctivitis, blepharitis, foreign body, and corneal abrasion. Patients describing fleeting pain who have a normal eye examination should be reassured. In general, all patients with ocular pain, painful eye movements (unless due to sinusitis), orbital pain, or abnormal findings on an eye examination should be referred to an ophthalmologist.

FOLLOW-UP.   If the initial examination is unremarkable, a follow-up appointment should be scheduled for 2 to 4 weeks to monitor for any new ocular findings.

Cross-references: Redness of the Eye (Section 37), Foreign Bodies and Corneal Abrasions (Section 42), Conjunctivitis (Section 43), Sinusitis (Section 57), Headache (Section 140).

REFERENCES

1. Hitchings RA. The symptoms of ocular pain. Trans Ophthalmol Soc UK 1980;100:257–259. Discusses pathophysiology of eye pain; part of a four-article symposium on eye pain.

2. Kalina RE, Orcutt JC. Ocular and periocular pain. In Bonica JJ, Ed. The Management of Pain in Clinical Practice, 2nd ed., vol. 1. Lea & Febiger, Philadelphia, 1990, pp. 759-768. Up-to-date review of diagnosis and management.

40 GLAUCOMA

Problem

HOWARD BARNEBEY

EPIDEMIOLOGY.   Approximately 1% to 2% of the U.S. population will develop glaucoma. There is an increased prevalence among the elderly, myopic (near-sighted) people, blacks, diabetics, and hypertensives.

SYMPTOMS AND SIGNS.   **Open-angle glaucoma** is asymptomatic until quite late in the disease, when complaints of visual loss may occur. **Angle closure glaucoma** is less common than open-angle glaucoma but often is symptomatic, causing blurred vision, eye pain, headache, and even nausea and vomiting. Clinical examination reveals a red eye, corneal edema, and a mid-dilated pupil. The IOP is often quite high (>45 mm Hg).

MANAGEMENT.   Once open-angle glaucoma is detected, treatment to lower the IOP initially includes medications (Table 40–1), sometimes followed by laser treatments and surgery.

Angle closure glaucoma is a true emergency and requires the immediate lowering of IOP with medications, followed by laser iridectomy. Once an iridec-

TABLE 40–1.   MEDICAL MANAGEMENT OF GLAUCOMA

Medication	Mechanism	Side Effects	Cost ($)[1]
Beta blockers Timoptic Betagan Betoptic Optipranolol	Decrease aqueous secretion	Ocular: punctate keratitis, corneal anesthesia Other: bronchospasm, congestive heart failure, arrhythmias, mood changes, impotence	 11.96 10.84 14.06 10.79
Miotics Pilocarpine Ocusert Isoptocarbachol Pilopine Gel	Improve aqueous outflow	Ocular: constrict pupil, dim vision, decreased night vision, retinal tear/ detachment Other: headache, nausea, diarrhea, sweating, bronchospasm	4.00 (15 ml) 3.83 (7 days) 12.50 (15 ml) 18.13 (5 g)
Adrenergic agonists Propine Epinephrine	Improve aqueous outflow	Ocular: local erythma, allergy Other: hypertension, tachycardia, headache	11.48 9.23
Carbonic anhydrase inhibitors Diamox Neptazane Daranide	Decrease aqueous secretion	Paresthesias, lethargy, nausea, diarrhea, anorexia, mental depression, renal stones, aplastic anemia	0.31 (250 mg) 0.63 (50 mg) 0.41 (50 mg)

[1]Average wholesale cost per 5 ml, unless otherwise noted, 1991 *Drug Topics Red Book.*

tomy has been performed and the attack broken, the glaucoma can be considered "cured."

FOLLOW-UP.   Once stable, the patient needs to be monitored three or four times per year. Particular attention should be directed to any side effects from medication, which may not be apparent during the initial part of the treatment.

REFERENCES

1. Becker. Shaffer's Diagnosis and Therapy of the Glaucomas. C.V. Mosby, St. Louis, 1989.
2. Shields MB, Ritch R, Eds. The Glaucomas. C.V. Mosby, St. Louis, 1989.
    Two excellent textbooks.

41 CATARACTS

Problem

THOMAS D. LINDQUIST

EPIDEMIOLOGY.   A cataract is an opacity of the natural lens of the eye. The most common cause of cataract formation is related to the normal aging process, and some degree of clouding of the lens can be expected in persons over age 70. Other causes of cataract formation may be (1) congenital, from hereditary, infectious, or inflammatory causes, (2) traumatic, (3) metabolic, as in diabetes mellitus, (4) toxic, as in steroid use, or (5) secondary to ocular inflammation or intraocular disease.

SYMPTOMS AND SIGNS.   The principal symptom of an acquired cataract is a gradual decrease in vision unassociated with pain or inflammation. Monocular diplopia, photophobia, and the complaint of glare are other symptoms. Signs of a cataract are best seen with the slit-lamp biomicroscope following pupillary dilation; however, direct ophthalmoscopy does allow estimation of the degree of media opacity. The principal types of lens opacities are nuclear, cortical, or subcapsular. A nuclear cataract is a yellow or brunescent opacity of the lens nucleus; a cortical cataract frequently forms radial opacities in a spokelike pattern, whereas a posterior subcapsular cataract appears as a granular opacity just anterior to the posterior capsule itself. Posterior subcapsular cataract is the most visually disabling for its density and size, because it anatomically approximates the nodal point of the eye and also frequently involves the visual axis early. A mature cataract is white, does not allow visualization of the ocular fundus, and causes reversible blindness in the affected eye.

CLINICAL APPROACH. Patients should be asked about their continued ability to read, drive, and perform other daily activities. An acquired cataract warrants surgical extraction only when it significantly interferes with the patient's vision.

A hypermature cataract may leak lens protein through an intact capsule, resulting in a secondary glaucoma in which macrophages distended with lens material obstruct the trabecular meshwork. Prompt cataract extraction is indicated.

MANAGEMENT. Acquired cataracts are usually removed by extracapsular extraction or phacoemulsification, leaving the posterior capsule intact. A posterior chamber intraocular lens is preferred for optical correction of aphakia in adults without proliferative diabetic retinopathy or chronic uveitis. Severe complications of this surgery include endophthalmitis and expulsive choroidal hemorrhage but occur in less than 0.1% of patients.

FOLLOW-UP. Following cataract surgery, patients are treated with topical antibiotics until the surface reepithelializes, and with topical steroids until intraocular inflammation resolves. The wound is secure by 6 weeks postoperatively, when patients may resume normal activities.

REFERENCES

1. Jaffe NS. Cataract Surgery and Its Complications, 4th ed. C.V. Mosby, St. Louis, 1984.
   Describes preoperative workup, surgical technique and complications of cataract surgery.

2. Lane SS, Kopietz LA, Lindquist TD, Leavenworth N. Treatment of phacolytic glaucoma with extracapsular cataract extraction. Ophthalmology 1988;95:749–53.
   Phacolytic glaucoma may be treated by extracapsular cataract extraction with implantation of a posterior chamber intraocular lens.

3. Lindquist TD, Lindstrom RL, Eds. Ophthalmic Surgery. Year Book Medical Publishers, Chicago, 1990.
   Illustrates and describes extracapsular cataract and phacoemulcification techniques, intraocular lens insertion, and epikeratoplasty technique.

42 FOREIGN BODIES AND CORNEAL ABRASIONS

Problem

THOMAS D. LINDQUIST

EPIDEMIOLOGY.   Each year, over 1 million people sustain eye injuries; over 90% of these are preventable. Corneal abrasions are frequently caused by branches, fingernails, paper cuts, or contact lenses. Foreign bodies on the surface of the cornea account for about 25% of all eye injuries. Most intraocular foreign bodies are caused by small particles penetrating the cornea or sclera; the majority are released from the striking of metal on metal.

SYMPTOMS AND SIGNS.   Symptoms of a corneal foreign body may vary from minimal discomfort to severe pain. The patient may sense a foreign body and usually inaccurately localizes it to the outer portion of the upper eyelid. Corneal abrasions are associated with intense pain, photophobia, ciliary injection, and tearing. A corneal abrasion may be visualized readily by instillation of a sterile 2% fluorescein solution that stains the denuded epithelium. A corneal foreign body may be seen by careful inspection, preferably aided by magnification with a loupe or direct ophthalmoscope when a slit-lamp is unavailable.

CLINICAL APPROACH.   Corneal foreign bodies should be removed entirely to allow reepithelialization and to minimize pain. An attempt should be made to remove a corneal foreign body by irrigation before removing it with a spud or the tip of a needle (see Section 45, Foreign Body Removal).

The conjunctiva and cornea should be examined carefully for a possible penetrating injury with an intraocular foreign body. A small conjunctival hemorrhage or a suspicious corneal lesion requires slit-lamp examination and indirect ophthalmoscopy of the fundus by an ophthalmologist. Roentgenography or computed tomography of the orbit is indicated in suspected cases of penetrating injuries to rule out intraocular foreign bodies. Retained iron foreign bodies slowly oxidize within the eye to form an irreversible ferrous compound that results in gradual vision loss (siderosis). Retention of copper particles (chalcosis) is much more rapidly injurious to the eye, but the tissue reaction is reversible if the copper particle is removed. Retention of an intraocular foreign body must be ruled out in any patient who develops uveitis following an eye injury.

MANAGEMENT.   Treatment of a corneal abrasion with or without prior foreign body removal should include topical antibiotic solution. Sulfacetamide, tobramycin, or trimethoprim/polymyxin-B solutions provide broad antibacterial coverage. A cycloplegic such as cyclogyl 1% or homatropine 5% may be instilled for patient comfort if there is ciliary injection or photophobia. Topical atropine 1% may have a duration as long as 2 weeks and therefore should not be used acutely. A pressure dressing may be applied to immobilize the eyelids but should not be used if it causes discomfort. Patching does not increase the rate of reepithelialization.

FOLLOW-UP.   As any foreign body may introduce microorganisms, the eyes should be examined daily until the epithelium resurfaces.

Cross-references: Eye Pain (Section 39), Foreign Body Removal (Section 45).

REFERENCES

1. De Juan E Jr, Sternberg P Jr, Michels RG. Penetrating ocular injuries. Ophthalmology 1983;90:1318–1322.
    Initial acuity after injury correlated closely with the final visual outcome.

2. Lobes LA Jr, Grand MG, Reece J, Penkrot RJ. Computerized axial tomography in the detection of intraocular foreign bodies. Ophthalmology 1981;88:26–29.
    CT is particularly useful in evaluating multiple foreign bodies, foreign bodies adjacent to the ocular wall, and, in some cases, to distinguish metallic from nonmetallic foreign bodies.

3. Schein OD, Hibberd PL, Shingleton BJ, Kunzweiler T, Franbach DA, Seddon JM, Fontan NL, Vinger PF. The spectrum and burden of ocular injury. Ophthalmology 1988;95:300–305.
    Only 10% of injured individuals were wearing protective eyewear; many injuries could be prevented.

43 CONJUNCTIVITIS

Problem

THOMAS D. LINDQUIST

EPIDEMIOLOGY/ETIOLOGY.   Conjunctivitis is the most common eye disease worldwide. It is characterized by inflammation with cellular infiltration and exudation. The cause may be bacterial, viral, allergic, toxic, mechanical, or parasitic.

SYMPTOMS AND SIGNS.   The onset is usually insidious. Patients complain of foreign body sensation, itching, and burning. Discomfort from infectious causes is most severe upon awakening: the eyelids are swollen and the eyelashes matted. The conjunctiva is diffusely injected, in contrast to the perilimbal flush more characteristic of iritis or uveitis or the sectorial injection seen with episcleritis or scleritis.

CLINICAL APPROACH. **Bacterial conjunctivitis** is accompanied by an acute purulent or mucopurulent discharge. *Streptococcus pneumoniae* and *Haemophilus aegyptius* can each occur in epidemics and may be associated with small petechial subconjunctival hemorrhages. Most cases of bacterial conjunctivitis are self-limited, with the exception of those caused by *Neisseria* spp.

Viral conjunctivitis is accompanied by a follicular response except in infants less than 6 to 8 weeks old, who have an immature immune system. The conjunctival follicle is a smooth elevation of the conjunctiva representing a lymphocytic response with an active germinal center. Whereas follicles represent a specific response, the conjunctival papillary response is a nonspecific conjunctival sign that can result from any type of inflammation. Papillae are characterized by a central fibrovascular core with the vessel breaking into a fine spokelike pattern on reaching the surface. In viral conjunctivitis a preauricular node is usually palpable and may be quite prominent and tender. The infection usually begins in one eye and often spreads to involve the other eye, although the first eye is always more severely affected. Adenovirus is the most common cause of acute conjunctivitis and is associated with copious tearing, minimal mucopurulent discharge, swollen lids, and significant injection. Epidemic keratoconjunctivitis, caused by adenovirus types 8 and 19, is associated with keratitis in 80% of cases, leading to severe photophobia and foreign body sensation. Small granular subepithelial corneal opacities may develop that may be visually significant and persist for months to years following resolution of the conjunctivitis. Because epidemic keratoconjunctivitis is spread with ease through fomites, patients should restrict possible exposure to others for 2 weeks.

Primary herpesvirus conjunctivitis may be associated with vesicles on the eyelids and may progress to involve the cornea. Because most people have antibodies to HSV type 1 by 15 years of age, herpetic blepharoconjunctivitis in adults usually represents recurrent disease.

Adult inclusion conjunctivitis (caused by *Chlamydia trachomatis*) is generally transmitted to the eyes from the genital area. It is frequently unilateral and associated with large follicles, foreign body sensation, and conjunctival injection. A conjunctival scraping should be sent for immunofluorescence and culture to establish the diagnosis.

Lyme disease may be associated with follicular conjunctivitis and keratitis.

Allergic conjunctivitis is characterized by bilaterality, recurrences, and marked itching. A papillary conjunctival response is seen, with only a mild mucoid discharge. Conjunctival scrapings frequently reveal eosinophils. Soft contact lens wearers may develop giant papillary conjunctivitis that is most prominent on the upper tarsal plate.

MANAGEMENT. Mild bacterial conjunctivitis generally resolves within 1 to 3 days when treated with broad-spectrum topical antibiotics such as sulfacetamide 10% or trimethoprim/polymyxin-B, which may be given q.i.d. for 5 to 7 days or until the conjunctivitis resolves. Bacterial conjunctivitis with copious purulent discharge or corneal ulceration should be cultured and Gram and Giemsa stains performed; referral to an ophthalmologist is recommended. Topical steroids should be avoided in infectious conjunctivitis.

Adenovirus conjunctivitis is usually self-limited. Cool compresses bring relief; prophylactic topical antibiotic solution may be given but is unnecessary. Patients with herpetic conjunctivitis should be referred to an ophthalmologist and treated with topical trifluridine (Viroptic) or vidarabine (Vira-A). Inclusion conjunctivitis requires systemic treatment with tetracycline or doxycycline for 3 weeks in adults.

Allergic conjunctivitis may be treated with cool compresses, systemic antihistamines, and topical decongestant-antihistamines or with disodium cromoglycate 4% q.i.d. for chronic conditions.

Cross-reference: Redness of the Eye (Section 37).

REFERENCES

1. O'Day DM, Guyer B, Hierholzer JC. Clinical and laboratory evaluation of epidemic keratoconjunctivitis due to adenovirus types 8 and 19. Am J Ophthalmol 1976;81:207–215.
    Considerable variability in disease severity may be seen in patients with epidemic keratoconjunctivitis due to adenovirus types 8 and 19.

2. Rapoza PA, Quinn TC, Terry AC, Gottsch JD, Kiessling LA, Taylor HR. A systematic approach to the diagnosis and treatment of chronic conjunctivitis. Am J Ophthalmol 1990;109:138–142.
    The proper approach to diagnosing chronic conjunctivitis is outlined.

3. Sheppard JD, Kowalski RP, Meyer MP, Amortegui AJ, Slifkin M. Immunodiagnosis of adult chlamydial conjunctivitis. Ophthalmology 1988;95:434–443.
    Direct monoclonal fluorescent antibody and enzyme and immunosorbent assays for chlamydial antigens are available to supplement culture and Giemsa staining.

4. Steere AC, Bartenhagen NH, Craft JE, Hutchinson GJ, Newman JH, Rahn DW, Sigal LH, Spieler PN, Stenn KS, Malawista SE. The early clinical manifestations of Lyme disease. Ann Intern Med 1983;99:76–82.
    Conjunctivitis is the most commonly reported ocular complication of Lyme disease; its incidence was 10% in this series.

44 DIABETIC RETINOPATHY

Problem

THOMAS H. MATSKO

EPIDEMIOLOGY. Diabetic retinopathy is one of the leading causes of new blindness worldwide and the leading cause of blindness in those 20 to 64 years old in the United States. Diabetic retinopathy is traditionally considered as nonproliferative or background retinopathy (characterized by microaneurysms, dilated veins, hard exudates, cotton wool spots, and retinal hemorrhages) and proliferative retinopathy (characterized by neovascular vessel formation on the optic nerve or retina). The incidence and severity of diabetic retinopathy are strongly related to the patient's age at diagnosis, the duration of diabetes, the type of diabetes, and whether insulin is required for glycemic control (Table 44–1). The severity of diabetic retinopathy also correlates with increased glycosylated hemoglobin levels, increased systolic blood pressure, and the presence of proteinuria. Approximately 25% of the diabetic population have some form of diabetic retinopathy, while 5% have the more severe proliferative retinopathy.

SYMPTOMS AND SIGNS. Diabetic retinopathy is a disease of the retinal capillaries that is most pronounced around the optic nerve and macula of the eye. Some patients remain asymptomatic despite widespread retinal damage and the high risk of severe visual loss, because the disease may spare the macula until late in the course. Vision loss may result from macular edema, ischemic maculopathy, vitreous hemorrhage from neovascularization, or traction retinal detachment from fibrosis and contraction of neovascular membranes.

TABLE 44–1. FREQUENCY OF DIABETIC RETINOPATHY (DR), BY DIABETIC SUBGROUP

Age at Diabetes Diagnosis (yr)	Duration (yr)	Frequency (%)	
		Any DR	*Proliferative DR*
<30	5	20	0
	15	90	25
	>20	100	>50
>30, no insulin	2	23	3
	15	57	4
	>20	60	15
>30, insulin	2	30	15
	15	84	20
	>20	90	25

The first clinically observable changes are microaneurysms (MA), seen as red dots in the back of the eye. Further damage leads to leakage from capillaries and whitish deposits of lipoproteins (hard exudates) and hemorrhages in the retina. Disease progression results in dilated capillaries known as intraretinal microvascular abnormalities (IRMA), dilation and beading of the major retinal veins, and nerve fiber layer infarcts (cotton wool spots, CWS). Severe retinal ischemia may induce retinal neovascularization, seen as fine vessels growing in patches on or around the disc (NVD) or elsewhere in the fundus (NVE). All of these changes are readily visible with the direct ophthalmoscope unless the patient has cataracts or other media opacities.

CLINICAL APPROACH. The physician should inquire about changes in central, peripheral, color, and night vision and should examine the fundus at each visit. Fears about inducing angle closure glaucoma by dilating a patient's pupils are unfounded, as this condition is rare and requires anatomic variations predisposing the patient to this condition. One drop of neosynephrine 2.5% or tropicamide 1% solution in the eye produces adequate dilation after 15 minutes in most patients, although tropicamide results in more significant blurring, especially of near vision. Any patient with visual complaints or retinal lesions on examination should be referred to an ophthalmologist.

Patients without signs or symptoms of eye disease should be seen by an ophthalmologist 5 years after the diagnosis of diabetes if onset is before age 31, and at the time of diagnosis in older patients. Women who develop diabetes during pregnancy should be examined by an ophthalmologist at the time of diagnosis and every 3 months thereafter until delivery.

MANAGEMENT. There is no evidence that tight control of blood sugar levels will halt or reverse the progression of existing diabetic retinopathy. Rapidly bringing a diabetic whose blood sugars are out of control into euglycemia may cause a florid onset or the fulminant progression of diabetic retinopathy.

Laser photocoagulation effectively prolongs retention of central vision. In patients with macular edema, fluorescein angiography identifies leaking sites in the macula, which are then photocoagulated. High-risk proliferative disease may regress following panretinal or "scatter" photocoagulation, a technique of applying 1200 to 1600 burns over the entire retina outside the macular area. In some patients the disease continues to progress and further laser treatment is needed.

Vitrectomy may be required in patients with persistent dense vitreous hemorrhage, progression of neovascularization in spite of maximal laser treatment, or traction retinal detachment threatening vision.

FOLLOW-UP. Ophthalmic follow-up intervals vary from yearly examinations for patients who show no diabetic retinopathy or only minimal changes, to monthly or weekly examinations for patients with severe changes threatening vision. At each visit a dilated fundus examination by means of binocular indirect ophthalmoscopy is essential, and adjuncts such as photography and fluorescein angiography may be needed. With adequate follow-up and appropriate treatment, most diabetics will retain useful vision for their lifetime.

Cross-references: Ophthalmoscopy (Section 46), Diabetes Mellitus (Section 157).

REFERENCES

1. Bresnick GH. Background diabetic retinopathy. In Ryan SJ, Ed. Retina, vol. 2. C.V. Mosby, St. Louis, 1989, pp. 327–366.
2. Davis MD. Proliferative diabetic retinopathy. In Ryan SJ, Ed. Retina, vol. 2. C.V. Mosby, St. Louis, 1989, pp. 367–402.
3. Frank RE. Etiologic mechanisms in diabetic retinopathy. In Ryan SJ, Ed. Retina, vol. 2. C.V. Mosby, St. Louis, 1989, pp. 301–326.
    Good, detailed discussions of diabetic eye disease with extensive references, though aimed at the ophthalmologist. Includes many photographs of clinical and pathologic specimens.
4. Klein R, Klein BEK, Moss SE, Davis MD, DeMets DL. The Wisconsin Epidemological Study of Diabetic Retinopathy: II. Prevalence and risk of diabetic retinopathy when age at diagnosis is less than 30 years. III. Prevalence and risk of diabetic retinopathy when age at diagnosis is 30 or more years. Arch Ophthalmol 1984;102:520–532.
    Large epidemiologic study of diabetic retinopathy.
5. Kohner EM. The evolution and natural history of diabetic retinopathy. Int Ophthalmol Clin 1978;18(4):1–16.
    Good overview.

45 FOREIGN BODY REMOVAL

Procedure

THOMAS D. LINDQUIST

RATIONALE.   All corneal foreign bodies should be removed entirely to allow reepithelialization, minimize pain, and remove contaminated material.

METHODS.   Slit-lamp examination is the optimal means of assessing the depth of a foreign body. Foreign bodies or corneal abrasions involving only the epithelium do not leave a scar. Scarring results from injuries deep to Bowman's layer. A full-thickness corneal foreign body should be removed by an ophthalmologist because it is likely to result in a shallow or flat anterior chamber unless the perforation site is sutured. Intraocular foreign bodies need to be removed in the operating room under an operating microscope.

An attempt to remove a conjunctival or corneal foreign body by irrigation using a syringe and sterile saline solution should be tried initially. If a corneal foreign body cannot be removed by irrigation, it should be removed with a sharp instrument rather than a cotton applicator, which can significantly damage the corneal epithelium. A sterile spud or a 25- or 27-gauge needle on a tuberculin syringe should be used. The instrument should be held tangential to the cornea such that the cornea would not be perforated if the patient lunged forward. The spud is used to gently elevate the foreign body off the cornea. Corneal anesthesia is accomplished by use of topical proparacaine or tetracaine. A slit-lamp is best suited as it provides adequate illumination and magnification, but a binocular loupe may be used. Many emergency rooms are equipped with slit-lamps.

A rust ring may be present if an iron foreign body has been retained for several hours or days. This is best removed by an ophthalmologist with a battery-operated, slow-speed drill with a fairly rounded bur. Rust rings that cannot be removed readily at the first attempt can often be removed easily 24 hours later, after leukocytes have softened the surrounding corneal tissue.

Topical antibiotics should be used until the corneal surface reepithelializes. Topical cycloplegics may be given, depending on patient discomfort. The eye should be examined daily until it has healed to ensure a corneal ulcer has not developed.

REFERENCES

See Section 42, Foreign Bodies and Corneal Abrasions.

46 OPHTHALMOSCOPY

Procedure

CRAIG G. WELLS

INDICATIONS. Ophthalmoscopy may be useful during directed examinations in patients with visual symptoms, vascular disorders, and neurologic disease. Ophthalmoscopy by nonophthalmologists is not reliable,[3] and examination should be performed by an ophthalmologist if findings are critical or if a potentially blinding disorder such as diabetic retinopathy is under consideration. Guidelines for screening have been published.[1,2]

RATIONALE.   Ophthalmoscopy allows direct examination of the inside of the eye.

METHODS.   Pupillary dilation facilitates examination, improving clarity and field of view.

The pupil is dilated with either tropicamide 0.5% or phenylephrine 2.5%, or both in combination. Tropicamide is an anticholinergic agent that may blur near vision but produces dilation unaffected by the examining light. Phenylephrine does not blur vision but the pupil constricts with bright light, limiting the examination. A single drop is applied in the inferior conjunctival fornix with the patient's gaze directed upward.

After dilation, the patient's spectacles are removed. The examiner's right hand and right eye are used to examine the patient's right eye, and the left hand and left eye are used for the patient's left eye. A +6 (black numbers) lens at a distance of about 1 foot is used to examine the ocular media for opacities, which appear black in the red reflex. The patient's eye is then approached closely, and the ophthalmoscope lens power reduced until the optic disc is visualized. The examiner's middle finger rests on the malar eminence to stabilize the ophthalmoscope. Systematic inspection of the optic disc, retinal vessels, retinal background, and macula is then performed. Peripheral examination is facilitated by having the patient look in the direction the examiner wishes to see and by the examiner moving his head in order that the examiner's eye, the patient's pupil, and the part of the fundus in which inspection is desired are all on a straight line.

Opacities in the media may be due to corneal, lens, cataract, or vitreous pathology. Optic disc pallor indicates neuronal death from neurologic or vascular disease. Optic nerve edema obscures vessel borders at the disc margins and may be due to increased cerebrospinal fluid pressure, inflammation, or ischemia. Cupping greater than 50% of the optic nerve head width usually indicates glaucomatous damage. Abnormal neovascular blood vessels are in front of normal retinal vessels and frequently arranged in a spoked wheel pattern. Leakage of serum causes macular edema and waxy, yellow, "hard" exudates.

COMPLICATIONS.   Rarely, angle closure glaucoma is precipitated. Individuals at risk may be detected by shining a penlight parallel to the iris plane.

Cross-references: Screening for Glaucoma (Section 35), Visual Impairment (Section 36), Diabetic Retinopathy (Section 44), Diabetes Mellitus (Section 157).

REFERENCES

1.   American Academy of Ophthalmology. Comprehensive Adult Eye Examination: Preferred Practice Pattern. American Academy of Ophthalmology, San Francisco, 1989.

2. American Academy of Ophthalmology. Diabetic Retinopathy: Preferred Practice Pattern. American Academy of Ophthalmology, San Francisco, 1989.

   Two documents from an ophthamological society that review recommended intervals for screening and follow-up.

3. Sussman EJ, Tsiaras WG, Soper KA: Diagnosis of diabetic eye disease. JAMA 1982; 247:3231–3234.

   Nonophthalmologists frequently miss the diagnosis of diabetic retinopathy.

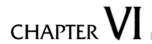

CHAPTER VI

DISORDERS OF THE EARS, NOSE, MOUTH, AND THROAT

47 DETECTION AND INITIAL MANAGEMENT OF ORAL CANCER

Screening

ALLEN D. HILLEL

EPIDEMIOLOGY. Malignant tumors of the oral cavity account for 3% of all new cancers per year and for 1.6% of cancer deaths per year. The disease occurs twice as often in men as in women. The most common histologic type is squamous cell carcinoma, which is almost always associated with a history of tobacco use (cigarette, cigar, pipe, or chewing tobacco). Other histologic types include melanoma and minor salivary gland cancers such as adenoid cystic, mucoepidermoid, and malignant mixed carcinomas.

RATIONALE. A thorough examination of the oral cavity should be conducted as part of a physical examination of all smokers and tobacco chewers. Teenagers should be included in this risk category because the widespread use of chewing tobacco has increased their incidence of oral cancer. While lesions on the lips are usually easily seen, lesions inside the mouth often remain asymptomatic and undetected until, as advanced lesions, bleeding or pain eventually occurs. Dentists discover oral cancers more often than physicians because they usually perform screening examinations before dental treatments and because a frequent presenting symptom of oral cancer is ill-fitting dentures.

STRATEGY. A thorough examination of the oral cavity requires a strong light, preferably a headlight that will allow the examiner to use a tongue blade in each hand. One systematic approach includes the following steps. (1) After the tongue blade has been inserted in the open mouth, the patient is instructed to close the mouth halfway, allowing the cheeks to relax for easy examination of the buccal mucosa and the buccal side of the alveolar ridges. (2) The mouth is widely opened to examine the lingual side of the alveolar ridges, the tongue, and the palate. (3) With appropriate positioning of the tongue, the anterior floor of the mouth, the undersurface and sides of the tongue, and the retromolar trigones (corner on each side where the tongue, jaw, and palate meet) are examined. (4) The tongue is depressed to view the anterior tonsillar pillars and the tonsillar fossae (or tonsils if present).

Squamous cell cancers usually present as ulcerations, although early lesions may appear as leukoplakia or erythroplakia. Tumors of salivary gland origin usually present as submucosal masses without ulceration.

ACTION. Patients with lesions that do not resolve within 7 to 10 days should be referred to a qualified specialist for further evaluation and biopsy.

Tumors are classified by site (lip, anterior tongue, buccal mucosa, alveolar ridge, hard palate, soft palate, or retromolar trigone) and graded T1 through T4 on the basis of size and invasion of adjacent structures. Treatment options for malignant lesions include surgery with or without adjuvant radiation therapy. Small tumors are often successfully treated by local resections. For advanced cases, recent advances in reconstructive surgery, including myocutaneous flaps, free flaps (with arterial and venous anastomoses), and bone grafts, offer excellent functional and cosmetic results.

Cross-reference: Periodic Health Assessment (Section 7).

REFERENCES

1. Baker SR. Malignant neoplasms of the oral cavity. In Cummings CW, et al, Eds. Otolaryngology—Head and Neck Surgery. C.V. Mosby, St. Louis, 1986.
    Reviews anatomy, description of lesions, and treatment.

2. Hillel AD, Fee WE. Malignant tumors of the palate. In English GM, Ed. Otolaryngology. Harper & Row, Philadelphia, 1982.
    Detailed account of palatal lesions, including non-squamous cell malignancies.

3. Sullivan MJ, Urken ML, Glenn MG, Baker SR. Free tissue transfer: Head and neck reconstruction. In Cummings CW, Ed. Otolaryngology—Head and Neck Surgery. Update II. C.V. Mosby, St. Louis, 1990.
    Overview of reconstruction for advanced oral cancers.

48 SCREENING FOR HEARING IMPAIRMENT

Screening

CYNTHIA MULROW

EPIDEMIOLOGY.   Hearing impairment is one of the three most common chronic health problems of elderly Americans. One-fourth of individuals over age 65 report problems with their hearing, and audiologically detectable hearing loss is present in more than one-third of individuals over age 65. Most are affected by presbyacusis, the bilateral high-frequency hearing loss that occurs with advancing age. The etiology of presbyacustic changes is not known, though exposure to occupational and environmental noise is thought to be a factor.

RATIONALE.   Adverse effects on physical, cognitive, emotional, and social function are associated with hearing loss. These effects are reversible with hearing aids. Simple accurate methods for screening exist, including portable audioscopy (the device costs approximately $400). Reported sensitivities for audioscopy range from 93% to 96%, specificities from 70% to 90%, and positive likelihood ratios from 3.1 to 9.4. Audioscopy allows concomitant examination of the ear for cerumen impactions, a relatively uncommon yet potentially significant cause of hearing impairment. In the absence of audioscopy, a whispered voice test may be used. Reported sensitivities and specificities are approximately 80% to 85% and positive likelihood ratios range from 3.8 to 6.7. Tuning fork tests are not recommended.

STRATEGY.   Primary care providers should screen for hearing impairment in elderly persons as part of their annual preventive health care examinations. Portable audioscopy should be considered the screening test of choice.

ACTION.   Persons who fail screening examinations should be referred to audiologists for audiometric evaluations and possible amplification interventions. Costs for formal audiometry and hearing aids vary depending on the type of aid (i.e., behind-the-ear, in-the-ear, programmable) but range from approximately $500 to $1000. Many vendors will refund the majority of these costs if the individual is not satisfied.

REFERENCES

1. Feller BA. Prevalence of selected impairments, United States, 1977. DHHS publication No. PHS 81-1562, pp. 1–11. National Center for Health Statistics, Washington, D.C., 1981.
    Describes prevalences of common disorders in elderly people.

2. Frank T, Peterson DR. Accuracy of a 40 dB HL audioscope® and audiometer screening for adults. Ear Hear 1987;8:180–183.
    Describes use and accuracy of portable audioscope.

3. Lichtenstein MJ, Bess FH, Logan SA. Validation of screening tools for identifying hearing-impaired elderly, in primary care. JAMA 1988;259:2875–2878.
    Describes screening protocol, including audioscopy, useful in the general practice setting.

4. Mulrow CD, Aguilar C, Endicott JE, et al. Quality of life changes and hearing impairment: Results of a randomized trial. Ann Intern Med 1990;113:188–194.
    Randomized trial documenting reversibility of hearing loss–associated social and emotional handicaps with hearing aids.

5. Mulrow CD, Aguilar C, Hill JA, et al. Association between hearing impairment and the quality of life of elderly individuals. J Am Geriatr Soc 1990;38:45–50.
    A cross-sectional study evaluating multiple handicaps associated with hearing loss in the elderly; also reviews past literature on the subject.

49 HICCOUGH (SINGULTUS)

Symptom

KATHLEEN H. MAKIELSKI

EPIDEMIOLOGY.   Hiccoughs are inspiratory sounds made by abrupt glottic closure associated with rhythmic spasms of the accessory respiratory muscles and diaphragm. Hiccoughs occur at any age (including during fetal life) and may last up to 60 years. There is a strong male predominance.

ETIOLOGY.   Hiccoughs result from a wide variety of conditions affecting a reflex arc that includes the vagus nerve as the afferent limb, brain stem centers, and the phrenic nerve as efferent limb. Causes may be peripheral (more often left-sided than right) or central. Lesions or postsurgical states of the abdomen, chest, or neck are common peripheral causes, especially when the disease is adjacent to the diaphragm or along the course of the phrenic or vagus nerves. Examples include gastric distention (common), esophagitis, pancreatic carcinoma, peritonitis, subphrenic abscess, myocardial infarction, pneumonia, and aortic aneurysm.

Examples of central causes include central nervous system (CNS) lesions (meningitis, stroke, tumor, trauma, multiple sclerosis), metabolic disorders (diabetes mellitus, gout, uremia, hypokalemia, hypocalcemia, hyponatremia), drugs (alcohol, general anesthetics, barbiturates, diazepam, midazolam, α-methyldopa, dexamethasone, methylprednisolone), and psychogenic disorders (more common in women).

A foreign body in the ear canal may also produce hiccoughs by stimulating the auricular branch of the vagus nerve.

CLINICAL APPROACH. Persistent hiccoughs (lasting more than 48 hours) suggest a serious underlying disease and require evaluation. The patient interview and physical examination should focus on the CNS, ears, throat, esophagus, chest, and abdomen, with a careful review of alcohol intake and medications. Diagnostic tests include chest radiography, electrocardiography, complete blood cell (CBC) count, electrolyte and blood glucose determinations, and liver and renal function tests.

MANAGEMENT. There is no single most effective treatment, and few controlled trials exist. One reasonable approach is to start with mechanical stimulation of the pharynx or esophagus, which attempts to interrupt the reflex arc. Any of the following may be tried.

1. Have the patient swallow a tablespoon of granulated sugar.
2. Pass a catheter into the patient's nasopharynx.
3. Massage the soft palate or apply traction to tongue.
4. Pass a nasogastric tube.

If these steps are ineffective and the diagnostic evaluation fails to reveal a treatable disorder, specific pharmacologic treatment may benefit the patient, probably by acting on the CNS hiccough center. Treatment is largely empirical. Successes have been reported with anesthetics, anticonvulsants, calcium channel blockers, dopamine antagonists, γ-aminobutyric acid agonists, hypnotics, muscle relaxants, narcotics, sedatives, tranquilizers, and tricyclic antidepressants. Response to treatment may require hours or days. Reasonable initial choices are chlorpromazine (50 mg given intravenously [IV], then 25–50 mg given orally [PO] q.6h.) or metoclopramide (10 mg PO q.4h. for 10 days).

Hypnosis, acupuncture, and digital rectal massage are also reported to be effective, but no controlled data exist.

Severe cases refractory to all pharmacologic options should be referred to an anesthesiologist for anesthetic infiltration of the left phrenic nerve. If hiccoughs recur after anesthetic blocks, a phrenic nerve crush (usually on the left side, rarely bilateral) may be effective but should only be considered if the anesthetic block produced at least transient relief without adversely affecting pulmonary function.

Complications of severe, protracted hiccoughs include vomiting, dehydration, weight loss, fatigue, surgical wound dehiscence, and death.

REFERENCES

1. Jones JS, et al. Persistent hiccups as an unusual manifestation of hyponatremia. J Emerg Med 1987;5:283–287.
   A concise review, with an emphasis on the etiology and a description of the hiccough reflex.

2. Lewis JH. Hiccups: Causes and cures. J Clin Gastroenterol 1985;7:539–552.
    Detailed review, including specific treatment regimens.

3. Nathan MD, et al. Intractable hiccups. Laryngoscope 1980;90:1612–1618.
    Reviews etiology and treatment of hiccoughs.

50 HOARSENESS

Symptom

KATHLEEN H. MAKIELSKI

EPIDEMIOLOGY/ETIOLOGY.   Hoarseness occurs when the vocal cords vibrate abnormally. It is one of the most common symptoms of laryngeal disease. Hoarseness may result from local disorders (i.e., in the larynx) or from vocal cord paralysis, which occurs when lesions affect nerves innervating the larynx (i.e., lesions in the brain stem, or along the vagus, superior or recurrent laryngeal nerves).

Among the local causes of vocal cord dysfunction, viral laryngitis and voice abuse are the most common causes of acute hoarseness seen by general practitioners. Other important local lesions include laryngeal cancer (most commonly squamous cell carcinoma), benign mass lesions (papillomas, polyps, nodules), inflammatory diseases (gastroesophageal reflux), trauma or irritants (endotracheal intubation, tobacco), and other functional disorders (spastic dysphonia, presbyphonia). Examples of disorders causing vocal cord paralysis include brain stem strokes; parapharyngeal neoplasms (deep lobe parotid tumors, glomus tumors); neck or chest trauma (blunt, penetrating, or surgical); neoplasms of the esophagus, lung, thyroid, or larynx; neuropathy (diabetic, heavy metal); cardiomegaly; and aortic aneurysm. Bilateral vocal cord paralysis is most often secondary to thyroid surgery in adults and CNS lesions in children. Unilateral vocal cord paralysis is more common on the left side, where the thoracic course of the recurrent laryngeal nerve is longer. In one study of 181 patients hospitalized because of vocal cord paralysis, evaluation revealed cancer in 20% (lung, esophageal, jugular foramen tumors), blunt injury to the nerves from cardiomegaly, aortic aneurysm, or other causes in 23%, surgical damage to the nerves (thyroid, neck surgery) in 23%, inflammatory and CNS lesions in 14%, and no identifiable cause in 20%.[1]

Clinical Approach.   The patient interview should focus on the duration of the hoarseness (persistent and progressive hoarseness is more ominous than intermittent symptoms), recent respiratory tract infections (viral, tubercular, fungal), tobacco and alcohol abuse (laryngeal cancer is extremely rare in non-smokers), and other symptoms suggestive of malignancy (neck mass, referred otalgia, aspiration, dysphagia, odynophagia, stridor, previous lung cancer, weight loss) or gastroesophageal reflux (sensation of lump in the throat, nocturnal cough, sore throat, frequent throat clearing). Other important clues in the history are previous endotracheal intubation (especially if prolonged), surgery or trauma in the neck or chest, symptoms of hypothyroidism (weight gain, cold intolerance), diabetes mellitus, rheumatoid arthritis (which may cause cricoarytenoid arthritis), and patterns of voice use and abuse (public speaking, singing, shouting).

Although most cases of hoarseness are self-limited (e.g., viral infections, voice abuse) or respond to initial therapy (e.g., treatment of reflux esophagitis), hoarseness lasting longer than 6 to 8 weeks requires an examination of the larynx, especially in smokers, who are at risk for developing squamous cell carcinoma. To examine the larynx, an indirect mirror or Hopkins (rigid) fiberoptic telescope suffices in most patients. Others may require evaluation with a flexible fiberoptic scope. The clinician should note the quality of voice, mobility of the vocal cords and arytenoids, and the presence of lesions or inflammation. Mass lesions of the larynx often require direct (operative) laryngoscopy for diagnosis.

If the laryngeal examination reveals vocal cord paralysis, appropriate diagnostic tests include direct (operative) endoscopy, chest radiography, barium swallow, and, if the cause is still unexplained, computed tomography (CT) or magnetic resonance imaging (MRI) of the chest, neck, and skull base.

Management.   The patient with acute hoarseness should stop smoking and rest the voice. Humidification of air and drinking hot tea with sugar are often recommended, although evidence directly supporting their efficacy is lacking. If the patient has symptoms suggestive of acid-induced laryngitis (e.g., heartburn, nocturnal cough), treatment with antacids or H_2 receptor antagonists is appropriate.

An otolaryngologist often assists in the management of patients with chronic hoarseness. The cure rate for laryngeal cancers detected early is high, and there is an excellent chance of saving the voice. A speech pathologist may help manage functional voice disorders.

Patients with unilateral vocal cord paralysis may compensate over several months and recover a more normal voice, although Teflon injection of the paralyzed cord is sometimes indicated (i.e., uncompensated breathy voice or risk for severe aspiration). When bilateral vocal cord paralysis is present, tracheotomy is usually necessary to prevent airway obstruction.

Cross-references: Smoking Cessation (Section 11), Dysphagia and Heartburn (Section 97).

REFERENCES

1. Maisel RH, Ogura JH. Evaluation and treatment of vocal cord paralysis. Laryngoscope 1974;84:302–316.
    Discusses the evaluation and final diagnoses in 181 patients with vocal cord paralysis (see text).

2. Vaughan CW. Diagnosis and treatment of organic voice disorders. N Engl J Med 1982; 307:863–866.
    Reviews the management of laryngitis, vocal fold nodes, polyps, neoplasia, and vocal cord paralysis.

3. Vaughan CW. The hoarse patient: When to refer. Hosp Pract 1989 (April 30); 24:21–29.
    Discusses the pathophysiology of disorders causing a "rough" voice, a "weak and breathy" voice, and a voice with altered pitch or resonance.

4. Ward PH, Berci G. Observations on the pathogenesis of chronic non-specific pharyngitis and laryngitis. Laryngoscope 1982;92:1377–1382.
    Discusses the role of gastroesophageal reflux in chronic laryngitis.

51 TINNITUS

Symptom

KATHLEEN C.Y. SIE

EPIDEMIOLOGY.   Tinnitus refers to the perception of sound in the absence of an appropriate acoustic stimulus. Although estimates of the prevalence of tinnitus are misleading, a 1968 survey by the National Center for Health Statistics found that 32% of adults in the United States complained of tinnitus at least once; 6.4% described tinnitus that was severe or debilitating. The prevalence of tinnitus increases with age until 70 years, after which it decreases.

ETIOLOGY.   The most common type of tinnitus is continuous, high-pitched, and nonpulsatile. This type of tinnitus is usually bilateral and associated with sensorineural hearing loss due to noise exposure, presbycusis, or other causes. This "head noise" tends to be most bothersome in a quiet setting, when the patient is trying to rest or relax. Other common causes of tinnitus are middle and external ear disease, such as middle ear effusions, negative middle ear pressure, tympanic membrane perforation, and cerumen impaction. Inner ear disorders such as Meniere's syndrome (fluctuating hearing loss, aural fullness, and vertigo), ototoxicity (Table 51–1), and neurosyphilis can also cause tinnitus. Drug-induced tinnitus is generally dose-related, reversible after cessation of the offending agent, and not always associated with hearing loss. Tinnitus associated with aspirin ingestion usually occurs with doses of greater than 4 g/

TABLE 51–1. DRUGS THAT CAUSE OR EXACERBATE TINNITUS

Alcohol
Aspirin
Caffeine
Cocaine
Heavy metals
Marijuana
Oral contraceptives
Quinine
Tobacco

day and usually resolves within 2 to 3 days after aspirin is discontinued. Tinnitus may also be a manifestation of cerebellopontine angle lesions. In these cases the tinnitus is usually unilateral and may be continuous or pulsatile, with associated asymmetric hearing loss, vertigo, or facial numbness. The most common cerebellopontine angle tumor is the acoustic neuroma, a benign neoplasm originating from Schwann cells, that causes tinnitus in up to 90% of affected patients. Other cerebellopontine tumors include meningiomas, cholesterol granulomas, primary cholesteatomas, and metastases. Temporomandibular joint syndrome can also be associated with tinnitus. Depression is known to exacerbate the perceived severity of tinnitus.

Pulsatile tinnitus refers to tinnitus synchronous with the patient's pulse. It is usually unilateral and implies a vascular etiology. The differential diagnosis includes glomus tumors, arteriovenous shunts, carotid artery disease, and vascular malformations of the internal auditory canal or middle ear. Palatal myoclonus may cause a unilateral tinnitus that is synchronous with palatal contractions. Myoclonus of the stapedial or tensor tympani muscles can also cause tinnitus. Venous hums from intracranial hypertension or an abnormal jugular bulb may produce a low-pitched machinery sound.

On physical examination, tinnitus can be classified as subjective or objective, although this distinction is not often clinically useful. Objective tinnitus is audible to both the patient and the examiner, implying a vibratory source of the sound such as vascular abnormalities.

CLINICAL APPROACH. The patient interview should identify the quality (ringing, humming, roaring, pulsatile), pitch (high, low), fluctuation, location (unilateral, bilateral), and relationship to activity (chewing, Valsalva maneuver, breathing, pulse) of the tinnitus, as well as its effect on equilibrium. The patient should also be asked about past noise exposure, infections (particularly meningitis), head injury, and medications (especially over-the-counter preparations containing aspirin).

Tinnitus can be evaluated in the outpatient department unless the patient has signs of increased intracranial pressure (e.g., papilledema). Clinical examination of the head and neck should include pneumatic otoscopy, auscultation of the carotid arteries, and assessment of cranial nerve and cerebellar function.

All patients who complain of bothersome tinnitus should undergo audiography with speech discrimination testing. Audiometric findings of asymmetric sensorineural hearing loss or disproportionately poor speech discrimination suggests the possibility of a retrocochlear lesion such as an acoustic neuroma. Depending on the clinician's level of suspicion for such a lesion, further tests may include stapedial reflex testing and auditory brain stem–evoked responses. Patients with asymmetric hearing loss and no other evidence of retrocochlear pathology may be followed with serial audiograms every 6 to 12 months. Progressive hearing loss or the development of retrocochlear findings (i.e., disproportionately poor speech discrimination or roll-over, prolonged wave I–V interpeak latency on auditory brain stem response, stapedial reflex decay) should prompt further evaluation for a retrocochlear process. Fine-cut CT of the internal auditory canal with contrast agent enhancement or MRI with gadolinium is necessary to demonstrate lesions of the internal auditory canal. MRI is the most sensitive imaging modality for demonstrating acoustic neuromas.

If the clinician sees a vascular mass in the middle ear medial to the tympanic membrane or palpates a neck mass suggestive of a glomus tumor, computed tomography (CT) and angiography may be necessary.

MANAGEMENT.   Management of the patient with tinnitus should include identification and treatment of underlying pathology, identification of associated problems (e.g., hearing loss), assessment of symptom severity, and symptom suppression. Mass lesions such as acoustic neuromas and glomus tumors generally must be excised, although poor surgical candidates may sometimes be treated with radiation therapy. Otitis media or cerumen impaction should be treated (see Section 56, Otitis Media and Externa, and Section 58, Cerumen Removal), and ototoxic medications should be discontinued if possible.

If no treatable cause of tinnitus is identified, patients should be reassured that the tinnitus is benign. Management of these patients generally includes habituation (tinnitus becomes less bothersome with time without specific treatment) or masking (static from tuning a radio between stations helps some patients sleep). Antidepressants and anticonvulsants are generally ineffective in the treatment of tinnitus, although patients with signs and symptoms of depression should be appropriately evaluated and treated.

FOLLOW-UP.   Patients complaining of tinnitus with symmetric sensorineural hearing loss and no treatable cause should undergo periodic audiography every 1 to 2 years initially to detect progression of hearing loss or the development of retrocochlear signs. If the hearing loss remains stable over 2 to 4 years, they may be followed less frequently. Patients with unilateral tinnitus, asymmetric hearing loss, pulsatile tinnitus, or vestibular symptoms should be referred to an otolaryngologist for further evaluation. Patients with asymmetric sensorineural hearing loss in whom acoustic neuroma has been ruled out should be reevaluated every 6 to 12 months. Progression of asymmetric sensorineural hearing loss should prompt reassessment to rule out a retrocochlear process.

Cross-references: Otitis/Media and Externa (Section 56), Cerumen Removal (Section 58), Screening for Depression (Section 187), Management of Depression (Section 192).

REFERENCES

1. Hazell JW. Tinnitus: II. Surgical management of conditions associated with tinnitus and somatosounds. J Otolaryngol 1990;19:6–10.
    Discusses surgical options for some of the more unusual causes of tinnitus, i.e., palatal myoclonus, stapedial myoclonus, etc.

2. Hazell JW. Tinnitus: III. The practical management of sensorineural tinnitus. J Otolaryngol 1990;19:11–18.
    A comprehensive discussion of management strategies, including a decision algorithm used in a large tinnitus clinic.

3. McFadden D. Tinnitus: Facts, Theories, and Treatment. National Academy Press, Washington, D.C., 1982.
    Excellent review.

52 ABNORMAL TASTE AND SMELL

Symptom

JOHN B. STIMSON

EPIDEMIOLOGY.   More than 2 million Americans suffered from disorders of taste and smell in 1979.[4]

ETIOLOGY.   Taste is mediated by specialized taste buds served by cranial nerves VII, IX, and X and spread over the tongue, soft palate, pharynx, larynx, epiglottis, uvula, and upper one-third of the esophagus. There are four types of receptors, responding to salty, sweet, bitter, and sour substances. Nuances of taste are provided by olfaction, which appears to have unlimited capacity for recognition of distinct odors. As a result, the symptom of diminished or absent taste most commonly results from loss of smell (anosmia) rather than loss of taste (ageusia). Olfactory receptors are confined to a 2- to 3-cm area at the top of the nasal cavities, and their afferents are transmitted by cranial nerve I through the cribriform plate of the ethmoid bone. Because the olfactory system is spatially confined, mechanical or structural problems, such as tumors, air flow obstruction, trauma, or mucosal disruption, are much more likely to cause anosmia than ageusia. Conditions affecting taste more often are systemic (e.g., drug effect, uremia, hepatitis) and more commonly produce distorted taste (dysgeusia) than absence of the sensation.

Table 52-1 lists the causes of abnormal taste or smell organized by the anatomic level of the defect. In two recent series of patients evaluated for anosmia, 30% to 34% had nasal and sinus inflammatory conditions (allergic rhinitis, sinusitis, or polyps), 16% to 30% of cases followed a viral infection, and 10% of cases followed head injury.[1,5] No similar data exist for disorders of taste.

TABLE 52–1. CAUSES OF ABNORMAL TASTE AND SMELL

Level of Defect	Smell Disorders	Taste Disorders

Substance delivery	Nasal obstruction
	  Nasal polyps
	  Mucosal edema (rhinitis)
	  Sinusitis
	  Adenoid hypertrophy
	Air flow diversion
	  Laryngectomy
	  Tracheostomy	

Mucosa	Dryness
	  Sjögren's syndrome
	  Smoking
	Destruction
	  Viral infections
	  Leprosy
	  Ozena
	  Caustic exposure (e.g., ammonia)
		Sjögren's syndrome
		Smoking
		Radiation therapy
		Dysautonomia
		Viral infections
		Thermal burn

Receptor abnormality	Absence
	  Kallmann's syndrome
	    (hypogonadotropic hypogonadism
	    with anosmia)	

Peripheral nerve	Head injury
	Craniotomy
	Post-subarachnoid hemorrhage
	Meningitis
	(Tumor)
		Bell's palsy (unilateral
		  and usually
		  asymptomatic)

Central nervous system	Meningioma or other tumor Parkinson's disease Multiple sclerosis	
Systemic	Vitamin B_{12} deficiency Myxedema Depression	Drugs[1] Hepatitis Uremia Malignancy Pregnancy Myxedema Addison's disease Deficiencies of zinc or niacin

[1]Some common examples are griseofulvin, amitryptiline, antithyroid drugs, chlorambucil, cholestyramine, penicillamine, procarbazine, vincristine, vinblastine, angiotensin-converting enzyme inhibitors, and propafenone.

CLINICAL APPROACH.   Inquiry should focus on recent upper respiratory tract infections, rhinitis or sinusitis, medications, and symptoms of systemic conditions such as uremia, hepatitis, pregnancy, hypothyroidism, and depression. A history of head injury or other CNS disease (Parkinson's disease, multiple sclerosis, subarachnoid hemorrhage) is important in the evaluation of anosmia. Fluctuating anosmia strongly suggests nasal or sinus inflammatory disease. A taste disorder with inordinate anorexia should bring malignancy to mind.

The nasal examination should evaluate airway patency and look for evidence for infection and the presence of allergic discoloration (pallor), polyps, and moisture. Oral examination should include assessment for adequate salivation, poor dentition, glossitis, or purulent postnasal drainage. If uncertainty exists about the presence of polyps or sinusitis, endoscopic nasal examination or computed tomography (CT) of the sinuses may be indicated. Although less expensive than CT, traditional radiography of the sinuses is insensitive. Physical examination may provide clues to systemic conditions such as liver disease, endocrine disorders, or malignancies.

Selected laboratory tests to exclude pregnancy, vitamin B_{12} deficiency, hypothyroidism, and liver or kidney dysfunction are appropriate in the proper clinical setting. The presence of more than 10% eosinophils on a Hansel's-stained smear of nasal secretions supports the diagnosis of nasal or sinus inflammatory disease.

Testing of taste or smell in a symptomatic patient is probably of little value in a primary care setting unless confusion exists between ageusia and anosmia, or there is suspicion of malingering. Smell is tested by presenting aromatic substances and odorless controls (water) in a patient-blinded fashion and testing one nostril at a time. Pungent or irritating substances such as ammonia or oil of wintergreen are best avoided because they stimulate trigeminal nerve endings and can be misleading. Taste testing is probably unnecessary.

MANAGEMENT.   Cases of recent onset and no evident cause may resolve spontaneously, and it is often sensible to defer a detailed evaluation for 1 to 2 months. Allergic rhinitis and sinusitis frequently coexist and often respond to a combination of antibiotics, intranasal steroids, and a short course of oral corticosteroids, although results are sometimes temporary. Nasal polyps or obstructing adenoids can be removed surgically. Vitamin B_{12} deficiency and hypothyroidism are easily treatable. The diagnosis of an untreatable cause of taste or smell dysfunction, such as anosmia following head injury, has value in limiting further costly workup and patient concern. Potentially offending medications, such as angiotensin-converting enzyme inhibitors, should be stopped on a trial basis. Smokers are advised to stop smoking prior to extensive evaluation. Conditions due to mucosal dryness (Sjögren's syndrome, radiation effects, dysautonomia) do not respond to moisturizing agents, but patients with Sjögren's syndrome may respond to specific therapy.[3] Lastly, zinc-deficient patients frequently are ageusic, but this condition is rare, and the widespread use of zinc supplements in the treatment of idiopathic ageusia has not been beneficial.[2]

Patients with permanent anosmia have lost the warning function of olfaction. They should be advised to install smoke detectors in their homes, to avoid natural gas appliances, and to date all groceries to prevent consumption of spoiled foods.

Cross-references: Smoking Cessation (Section 11), Anorexia (Section 18), Sinusitis (Section 57).

REFERENCES

1. Davidson TM, Jalowayski A, Murphy L, Jacobs RD. Evaluation and treatment of smell dysfunction. West J Med 1987;146:434–438.
    Series from a smell disorder clinic.

2. Henkin RI, Schecter PJ, Friedewald WT, Demets DL, Raff M. A double blind study of the effects of zinc sulfate on taste and smell dysfunction. Am J Med Sci 1976;272:285–299.
    No significant benefit occurred with zinc supplements.

3. Henkin RI, Talal N, Larson AL, Mattern CFT. Abnormalities of taste and smell in Sjögren's syndrome. Ann Intern Med 1972;76:375–383.
    No benefit was derived from moisturizing agents, but steroids or irradiation helped if they increased salivary flow.

4. Schiffman SS. Taste and smell in disease. N Engl J Med 1983;308:1275–1279, 1337–1343.
    Excellent overview.

5. Scott AE. Clinical characteristics of taste and smell disorders. Ear Nose Throat J 1989;68:297–315.
    General review summarizing practical experience in a taste and smell dysfunction clinic.

53 DENTAL DISEASE

Problem

MARK M. SCHUBERT

EPIDEMIOLOGY/ETIOLOGY.   The two most common dental diseases are decay and periodontal disease. Untreated disease may lead to loss of the involved teeth or, especially in immunocompromised patients, extension of infection into surrounding bone and soft tissue. Additionally, patients with valvular heart disease and dental infections are at risk for bacterial endocarditis. The most important dental infections are (1) dental caries, which may spread to the dental pulp (causing severe pain) or further into periapical tissues, and (2) acute periodontal abscesses.

The oral microflora is extremely complex and consists of at least thirty-five to forty species of aerobic and anaerobic bacteria and fungal organisms. The predominant organisms depend on whether the problem is an orofacial odontogenic infection (polymicrobial, with obligate anaerobes comprising 65% of isolates), dental caries (gram-positive facultative anaerobes or microaerophilic cocci), pulpal infection (anaerobes), or periodontal infections (anaerobic gram-negative rods and motile forms, including spirochetes).

SIGNS AND SYMPTOMS.   *Dental Caries.*   Decay is initially asymptomatic and appears as a darkly stained cavitation of the tooth surface. Decay can also proceed adjacent to existing restorations and under crowns. The involved tooth structure is soft or leathery when examined with a dental explorer. As decay deepens and approaches the pulp, the tooth becomes sensitive to hot and cold as well as sweet foods (which rapidly increase bacterial acid production). When bacteria invade the pulp, constant severe pain occurs. Stimulated pain that lasts for a few seconds is generally referred to as "reversible pulpitis," indicating that decay removal and placement of dental restoration will allow healing of pulpal tissues. However, stimulated pain that lasts longer than 30 to 60 seconds indicates more severe pulpal disease that generally will require root canal therapy or extraction to cure. Although patients can initially localize pain to the involved tooth, this becomes more difficult as disease progresses. Periapical infection makes the tooth sensitive to percussion. Radiographically, carious tooth structure and periapical infections appear as radiolucent changes, though radiolucent dental filling materials and normal anatomic structures can have a similar radiographic appearance.

Gingivitis and Periodontitis.   These are low-grade localized infections that usually are asymptomatic but can cause symptoms of gingival pain and tooth sensitivity to hot and cold and sweets. Gingivitis refers to infection of the gingiva, while periodontitis denotes infection that results in the loss of supporting bone and ligaments for the teeth. The first sign of gingivitis is gingival bleeding, usually associated with localized erythema and edema. Although erythema and edema may be absent with periodontitis, probing of the involved periodontal pocket causes bleeding or, in severe cases, reveals pus. Progressive periodontitis deepens the periodontal pockets (normal, 2–3 mm), increases bone loss, loosens the involved teeth, and increases the risk of an acute periodontal abscess. Gingivitis and periodontitis can be the source of bacteremia and cause endocarditis or fevers of unknown origin.

Orofacial Odontogenic Infections.   Acute odontogenic infections produce localized and painful soft tissue swelling (sometimes with cellulitis or fluctuance) with associated fever, local lymphadenitis, leukocytosis, and an increased erythrocyte sedimentation rate. Accumulated pus from periapical infections usually perforates bone and drains into the mouth, but may track along tissue planes and spread to deeper facial spaces, most commonly the sublingual, submandibular, pterygomandibular, and buccal spaces, less commonly the temporal, masseteric, parotid, lateral pharyngeal, and retropharyngeal spaces. Deep space infections that spread into pharyngeal spaces can cause significant trismus and compromise the airway and thus constitute a medical emergency requiring immediate treatment. Periodontal abscesses may also cause deep space infections.

CLINICAL APPROACH. The diagnosis of dental caries and periodontal disease depends on the patient's symptoms, clinical examination (caries detection, periodontal probing, percussion, and palpation), tests to determine pulp vitality (e.g., cold and hot testing and electrical stimulation of teeth), and radiographic examination. Pulp vitality tests determine the pain responsiveness of pulpal tissue, a measure of tooth vitality.

A number of nondental conditions may produce facial pain and mimic odontologic pathology. Maxillary sinusitis can cause toothache symptoms in upper posterior teeth. Myofascial pain arising in the muscles of mastication, especially the masseter muscles, can cause pain referred to dental structures. Angina pectoris may be referred to the jaw, most commonly the mandible, but maxillary pain has also been reported. Other conditions to be considered are trigeminal neuralgia and atypical orofacial pain. Local and metastatic tumors may produce radiolucencies that are confused with pathology of dental origin.

MANAGEMENT. The prevention of dental infectious diseases depends on consistent removal of dental plaque from teeth and gingival tissue. The treatment of established odontogenic infections requires instrumentation or surgical techniques, including decay removal, root canal therapy, tooth extraction, periodontal curettage, or, in the case of acute abscesses, incision and drainage. In addition to tooth brushing and flossing to remove plaque, topical antimicrobial rinses (tetracycline, chlorhexidine, povidone iodine, etc.) can be beneficial.

Most of the microorganisms implicated in orofacial infections, including anaerobes, are susceptible to penicillin. Because of its excellent absorption and high serum levels, amoxicillin is especially effective. Erythromycin has similar antimicrobial activity and is used in patients allergic to penicillin. When beta-lactamase–producing anaerobes are suspected (e.g., serious orofacial odontogenic infections), metronidazole is an excellent alternative.

Antibiotic prophylaxis (see Section 218, Preoperative Infectious Disease Problems) is necessary before invasive dental procedures are undertaken in patients at risk for bacterial endocarditis or with intravascular dialysis catheters in place. Similar recommendations for patients with prosthetic implants, especially joint implants, have not been clearly established.

Patients who are at particular risk for medical complications from dental disease and who would benefit from referral to an oral surgeon or a specialist include patients at risk for bacterial endocarditis, patients with indwelling venous access lines for dialysis, immunocompromised patients (e.g., HIV-infected patients, patients scheduled to receive cancer chemotherapy or high-dose systemic steroids, organ transplant recipients, and so forth), and patients who are to receive radiation therapy to the jaws and oral cavity.

Cross-references: Sinusitis (Section 57), Myofascial Pain Syndromes (Section 123), Preoperative Infectious Disease Problems (Section 218).

REFERENCES

1. Dajani AS, Bisno AL, Chung KJ, et al. Prevention of bacterial endocarditis: Recommendations by the American Heart Association by the Committee on Rheumatic Fever, Endocarditis, and Kawasaki Disease. JAMA 1990;264:2919–2922.
   Most recent recommendations.

2. Kureishi A, Chow AW. The tender tooth: Dentoalveolar, pericoronal, and periodontal infections. Infect Dis Clin North Am 1988;2:163–182.
   Discusses clinical and pathologic features of dental caries, pulpitis, periapical abcess, pericoronitis, and periodontal infections.

3. Moenning JE, Nelson CL, Kohler RB. The microbiology and chemotherapy of odontogenic infections. J Oral Maxillofac Surg 1989;47:976–985.
   Reviews rationale for the use of recommended antibiotics.

4. Odell PF. Infections of the fascial spaces of the neck. J Otolaryngol 1990;19:201–205.
   Reviews anatomy, microbiology, and treatment of these life-threatening infections.

54 PHARYNGITIS

Problem

ROBERT M. CENTOR

EPIDEMIOLOGY/ETIOLOGY.   Pharyngitis leads to more than 16 million office visits each year, accounting for 2.5% of all visits to primary care physicians. In adult patients with sore throat, pharyngeal cultures are positive for group A beta-hemolytic streptococci in about 10% of cases seen in an office practice setting and in about 25% of cases seen in an emergency (or urgent) care setting.

Other probable causes include *Arcanobacterium haemolyticum* (formerly *Corynebacterium haemolyticum*), non-group A streptococci (especially group C), a variety of viral infections, *Chlamydia trachomatis* (or perhaps *C. pneumoniae*, the TWAR agent), *Mycoplasma pneumoniae*, and *Neisseria gonorrhoeae*.

SYMPTOMS AND SIGNS.   The most common symptoms are difficulty swallowing, fever, cough, and coryza. Patients who have severe pain on swallowing or fever are more likely to have a group A beta-hemolytic streptococcal infection, while both cough and coryza occur more often with viral infections. On examination, findings of pharyngeal exudates and/or redness, fever, and swollen anterior cervical nodes all support the diagnosis of strep throat.

CLINICAL APPROACH.   Four clinical variables (absence of cough, history of fever, exudates, and swollen, tender anterior cervical nodes) help one estimate the probability of strep throat (Table 54–1). This initial screen allows the clinician to select a group of patients who need no further evaluation, i.e., patients with a very low probability of having streptococcal pharyngitis. Many physicians prescribe antibiotics for high probability patients ($\geq$38% probability of strep) without performing any diagnostic tests.

Rapid antigen tests have a sensitivity of 80% and a specificity of 98% for strep throat. The clinician should confidently treat patients with positive test results. In those with negative test results, however, a throat culture may be beneficial (to detect the 20% of strep throat patients who have negative tests). This strategy, while having a higher cost, greatly decreases the probability of missing strep throat and decreases the possibility of rheumatic fever.

MANAGEMENT.   Penicillin is the drug of choice for suspected streptococcal pharyngitis (either a single IM injection of penicillin G benzathine, 1.2 million units, or a full 10-day course of penicillin V potassium, 125–250 mg PO q.i.d. or 250–500 mg PO b.i.d.). For patients allergic to penicillin, erythromycin is the drug of choice.

At the current time no other common cause of sore throats requires treatment. Some clinicians use erythromycin to treat patients with pharyngitis, reasoning that it has activity against other causes of pharyngitis such as *Chlamydia* spp. and *Mycoplasma*. Currently no data support or refute this practice.

Patients often receive symptomatic benefit from a variety of minor pain and cold preparations.

**TABLE 54–1.   ESTIMATING THE PROBABILITY OF GROUP A
STREPTOCOCCAL PHARYNGITIS**

Prevalence	10%[1]	20%[2]
Strep score[3]		
0	1%	3%
1	4%	8%
2	9%	18%
3	21%	38%
4	43%	62%

[1]Most office practices.

[2]Most emergency rooms.

[3]Points for strep score come from four clinical variables (one point each): lack of a cough; presence of tonsillar exudates; presence of swollen, tender anterior cervical nodes; recent history of fever.

FOLLOW-UP.   Follow-up of patients with sore throats is generally unnecessary. Most patients' symptoms are self-limited. If symptoms persist, the clinician may consider retesting for group A beta-hemolytic streptococci and, if noncompliance is suspected, treating the patient with parenteral penicillin. Alternatively, a penicillinase-resistant antibiotic may be used to cover beta-lactamase-producing organisms.[3]

Because asymptomatic carriers require no treatment, routinely culturing patients after resolution of symptoms is unnecessary.

Cross-reference: Upper Respiratory Infection (Section 66).

REFERENCES

1. Belsey RE, Hale DC, Marcy SM. Rapid office tests: How useful? Patient Care 1990;24:103–125.
    Recent compilation of available rapid antigen tests, with data on the majority of strep test kits currently on the market.

2. Centor RM, Meier FA, Dalton HP. Throat cultures and rapid tests for diagnosis of group A streptococcal pharyngitis in adults. In Sox HC Jr, Ed. Common Diagnostic Tests: Use and Interpretation, 2nd ed. American College of Physicians, Philadelphia, 1990, p. 253.
    A comprehensive review, revised from the 1986 *Annals of Internal Medicine* article by the same authors.

3. Kaplan EL, Johnson DR. Eradication of group A streptococci from the upper respiratory tract by amoxicillin with clavulanate after oral penicillin V treatment failure. J Pediatr 1988;113:400–403.
    A study of the management of "treatment failure."

4. Meier FA, Centor RM, Graham L, Dalton HP. Clinical and microbiological evidence for endemic pharyngitis among adults due to group C streptococci. Arch Intern Med 1990;150:825–829.
    Evidence for group C streptococci causing pharyngitis.

55 EPISTAXIS

Problem

MICHAEL G. GLENN

EPIDEMIOLOGY.   Nosebleeds are common and affect more than 60% of adults, though only one-tenth of these individuals seek medical attention. Severe or refractory bleeding is rare. Nosebleeds are considerably more common in cold, dry climates.

ETIOLOGY.   The most common cause of epistaxis is venous bleeding due to dryness and crusting of the anterior nasal septum (Kissselbach's plexus). Irritation and bleeding at this site is commonly exacerbated by nose-picking. Uncontrolled hypertension, blood clotting disorders, sinonasal infections, and tumors of the nose and paranasal sinuses may all cause epistaxis. Aspirin, nonsteroidal anti-inflammatory drugs, and chronic alcohol abuse may cause a minor coagulopathy that contributes to persistent or recurrent epistaxis.

CLINICAL APPROACH.   Although patients often exaggerate the amount of blood lost during nosebleeds, clinicians should estimate the amount of blood lost and the frequency and duration of each episode. In addition, the patient interview should identify provoking factors (bending, lifting, or straining), any previous history of easy bruising or bleeding at other sites, the patient's medications (including over-the-counter preparations containing aspirin), and whether there is a family history of bleeding, especially bleeding associated with routine surgical procedures.

The physical examination focuses on measurement of any orthostatic changes in vital signs and on evaluation for dried blood or active bleeding sites. The anterior nasal septum, the lateral floor of the nose posteriorly, and the area just below the middle turbinate on the posterolateral wall of the nose should all be inspected. The use of a decongestant spray will facilitate a complete examination. If there is ongoing bleeding, headlight illumination and suction with a small-tipped suction catheter is helpful, if available. Laboratory testing includes a hematocrit, prothrombin time, a partial thromboplastin time, and a platelet count.

MANAGEMENT.   *No Active Bleeding.*   If an old bleeding site is apparent, cautery with silver nitrate following topical anesthetization with lidocaine is useful. The patient should moisturize the nasal mucosa by frequent use of a nasal saline spray and humidification of the household environment. Patients should discontinue nasal decongestant or steroid sprays. To prevent recurrent bleeding, management of hypertension and any reversible clotting disorders is essential.

Active Bleeding.   Direct pressure on the nasal alae against the nasal septum, maintained for 5 minutes with the head elevated to decrease venous pressure, should stop most bleeding. Patients should learn to do this for themselves in future episodes. Intranasal packing with ointment-impregnated gauze or with specially designed balloon devices is indicated only when direct pressure fails. Packing should remain in place for 3 days and should be accompanied by antibiotic prophylaxis directed toward *S. aureus*. Otolaryngology consultation is necessary if anterior packing fails to control bleeding or if pressure alone fails to stop the bleeding in an immunocompromised or thrombocytopenic patient (in whom intranasal packing is best avoided).

FOLLOW-UP.   Hypertensive patients should have their blood pressure measured and treated appropriately. Patients with persistent bleeding, especially if unilateral, should be referred to an otolaryngologist to exclude tumors or other anatomic abnormalities.

Cross-references: Essential Hypertension (Section 86), Sinusitis (Section 57), Bleeding (Section 197).

REFERENCES

1. Jackson KR, Jackson RT. Factors associated with active, refractory epistaxis. Arch Otolaryngol Head Neck Surg 1988;114:862–865.

    Evaluation of patients referred because of refractory bleeding. Good diagrams of most likely bleeding sites.

2. Schaitkin B, Strauss M, Houck JR. Epistaxis: Medical versus surgical therapy. A comparison of efficacy, complications, and economic considerations. Laryngoscope 1987;97:1392–1396.

    Convincing rebuttal to earlier studies that advocated immediate surgery. Surgical intervention was reserved for (1) failure of nonsurgical techniques to control hemorrhage, (2) patients with impending complications of packing, or (3) those who rebleed within 6 months of packing removal.

3. Welsh LW, Welsh JJ, Scogna JE, Gregor FA. Role of angiography in the management of refractory epistaxis. Ann Otol Rhinol Laryngol 1990;99:69–73.

    Good presentation of vascular anatomy. Angiography should be considered when packing or surgical ligation fails.

56 OTITIS MEDIA AND EXTERNA

Problem

ANDREW F. INGLIS, JR.

OTITIS MEDIA

Epidemiology/Etiology.   **Acute otitis media** is an acute bacterial middle ear infection with a mucopurulent effusion. Usual organisms are *Streptococcus pneumoniae, Haemophilus influenzae, Streptococcus pyogenes,* and *Moraxella catarrhalis.* Acute otitis media is extremely common in children but relatively rare in adults. **Otitis media with effusion** refers to a middle ear effusion, sometimes sterile, that persists for several weeks to months. **Chronic otitis media** is an active or smoldering infection, present for weeks to years, associated with a foul-smelling otorrhea that drains through a tympanic membrane perforation. A mixed infection of enteric gram-negative rods, *Staphylococcus aureus,* and anaerobes is usually present. Chronic otitis media may be caused or accompanied by an epithelial cyst (cholesteatoma), which if left untreated will expand to fill the middle ear and mastoid, injuring associated structures such as the ossicular chain, facial nerve, dural sinuses, or brain. All forms of otitis media are more common in patients with a predilection for eustachian tube dysfunction; risk factors include Native American or Southeast Asian race, cleft palate (repaired or not), nasopharyngeal carcinoma, ciliary dysmotility syndromes, and immunocompromise.

SYMPTOMS AND SIGNS. Patients with acute otitis media initially experience symptoms of an upper respiratory infection (rhinorrhea, sore throat, cough) associated with a growing ear pressure sensation. This is followed by fever, severe otalgia, and hearing loss, sometimes with vertigo or unsteady gait. The tympanic membrane is usually bulging and displays dilated blood vessels on a cream or yellow background. In contrast, the finding of prominent blood vessels on an otherwise normal tympanic membrane is normal, not to be confused with acute otitis media. Pneumatic otoscopy reveals reduced tympanic membrane mobility. The tympanic membrane may spontaneously rupture, with profuse otorrhea and rapid reduction of otalgia. Otitis media with effusion, which may follow acute otitis media, causes a sensation of aural pressure and hearing loss. The tympanic membrane is usually thickened, slightly retracted, opaque, and hypomobile. If the diagnosis is in doubt, a tympanogram should be obtained. Chronic otitis media may follow ear surgery. Examination reveals a perforated tympanic membrane with thick, foul otorrhea that becomes copious during exacerbations. Granulation tissue from the middle ear may obscure the perforation or cholesteatoma.

CLINICAL APPROACH. The initial approach to suspected acute otitis media and otitis media with effusion is empirical antibiotic administration; no further tests are necessary. In immunocompromised patients, however, the potential pathogens are too diverse to allow accurate prediction of infecting organisms, and middle ear culture by tympanocentesis should precede antibiotic treatment. In chronic otitis media, a hearing screen or formal audiogram should precede therapy. The therapeutic goals in these patients are to sterilize the middle ear and mastoid cavity, either medically or surgically, to exclude cholesteatoma, and ideally to restore the integrity of the tympanic membrane.

MANAGEMENT. Acute otitis media and otitis media with effusion usually respond to a 2-week course of amoxicillin or trimethoprim-sulfamethoxazole (Table 56–1). If the effusion persists, a 1-week trial of prednisone with a 3-week trial of amoxicillin plus clavulanate is appropriate.

In chronic otitis media, the ear should be gently cleaned with miniature cotton swabs or a No. 6 French nasotracheal suction catheter set on low suction. Appropriate antibiotics include both ototopical preparations (e.g., a suspension of polymyxin, neomycin, and hydrocortisone) and an antistaphylococcal oral agent such as cephalexin. Patients in whom this regimen fails should have the drainage cultured and may require an antipseudomonal agent such as ciprofloxacin. Patients should use ototopical antibiotics only as long as the otorrhea persists, because sustained treatment of noninflamed ears may result in ototoxicity.

TABLE 56–1.   OTITIS MEDIA AND OTITIS EXTERNA: SUGGESTED TREATMENT

Drug	Dose and Duration	Cost ($)[1]
Acute Otitis Media		
Amoxicillin	500 mg t.i.d. × 10 days	7.50
Trimethoprim-sulfamethoxazole	1 DS b.i.d. × 10 days	6.00
Amoxicillin-clavulanate	500 mg t.i.d. × 10 days	62.10
Cefuroxime axetil	250 mg b.i.d. × 10 days	49.00
Cefixime	400 mg q.d. × 10 days	46.80
Otitis Media with Effusion[2]		
Trimethoprim-sulfamethoxazole	1 DS b.i.d. × 21 days	12.60
or		
Amoxicillin-clavulanate	250 mg t.i.d. × 21 days	95.76
plus		
prednisone	1 mg/kg × 7 days	2.10[4]
Chronic Otitis Media		
Systemic		
Cephalexin	250 mg q.i.d. × 14 days	57.68
Amoxicillin-clavulanate	250 mg t.i.d. × 14 days	63.84
Ciprofloxicin	500 mg b.i.d. × 14 days	71.40
Ototopical[3]		
Polymyxin B sulfate–neomycin sulfate–hydrocortisone suspension	4 gtts t.i.d. × 5–10 days	2.85 for 10 ml
Gentamicin ophthalmic solution	Same as above	10.32 for 5 ml
Tobramycin ophthalmic solution	Same as above	12.81 for 5 ml

[1]Average wholesale price, 1991 *Drug Topics Red Book,* for duration listed unless otherwise noted.
[2]Efficacy of antibiotic/steroid combination established in children; trials in adults lacking.
[3]The potential for ototoxicity exists with prolonged use; patients should be instructed to stop administering drops when otorrhea resolves.
[4]Cost for 60 mg/day × 7 days.

FOLLOW-UP.   Patients with acute otitis media should be instructed to call back if otalgia and fever do not improve within 2 to 3 days; many subsequently respond to broader spectrum antibiotics such as amoxicillin-clavulanate, cefixime, or cefuroxime. The physician should examine all patients again in 2 to 4 weeks to ensure that the middle ear effusion has resolved. Patients with otitis media with effusion should be seen monthly. If the effusion does not clear in 2 to 3 months despite antibiotic therapy, the patient should be referred to an otolaryngologist for consideration of tympanostomy tube placement and to exclude nasopharyngeal carcinoma. Patients with chronic otitis media should return in 1 month, sooner if there is otalgia. Patients who do not respond, who have tympanic perforations, or who have membrane abnormalities suggestive of a cholesteatoma should be referred to an otolaryngologist.

OTITIS EXTERNA

EPIDEMIOLOGY/ETIOLOGY.   Otitis externa usually refers to a bacterial infection of the external auditory canal. Predisposing factors include a humid climate, ear trauma, collapse or stenosis of the canal, or overly vigorous cleaning of the naturally bactericidal cerumen. Conditions that mimic bacterial otitis externa include eczema of the external auditory canal and fungal, herpetic, and necrotizing (malignant) otitis externa. Malignant otitis externa is a life-threatening pseudomonal infection that occurs in diabetic or immunocompromised hosts and is marked by granulation tissue in the external auditory canal and periostitis of the skull base, often with cranial nerve palsies.

SYMPTOMS AND SIGNS.   Pruritus typically precedes mild to excruciating otalgia in bacterial otitis externa. Manipulation of the pinna is painful. There is a scant amount of discharge and debris. Edema is usually present and may occlude the canal and produce hearing loss.

CLINICAL APPROACH.   The diagnosis is based on the combined findings of severe otalgia, auricular tenderness, swelling and erythema of the skin in the canal, and a scant, cheesy discharge. Denudation of the skin of the canal or adjacent meatus with little edema suggests an atopic or eczematoid process. If the pinna itself is inflamed or swollen, the diagnosis is most likely perichondritis, cellulitis, or erysipelas; otologic consultation is indicated. Microscopic examination of ear canal scrapings may reveal hyphal elements in fungal otitis externa. Vesicular lesions suggest herpetic otitis externa. The history should carefully identify diabetic or immunocompromised patients to exclude the possibility of necrotizing (malignant) otitis externa. If granulation tissue (which appears as fleshy, friable, polypoid tissue) is present in the canal, the blood glucose level should be measured.

Copious otorrhea with a slightly macerated or erythematous canal suggests chronic otitis media with a tympanic membrane perforation.

MANAGEMENT.   Simple pruritus of the external auditory canal responds to topical hydrocortisone cream, applied with a swab three times daily as needed. In bacterial otitis externa, a narcotic-containing pain medicine, including oxycodone or meperidine, may be necessary. Mild cases are treated with a homemade preparation of 50% isopropyl alcohol (as a drying agent) and 50% vinegar (to create a hostile pH for *Pseudomonas*) applied three times daily for 1 to 2 weeks. In more severe cases, a polymyxin-neomycin-hydrocortisone otic solution should be substituted. If the integrity of the tympanic membrane is in doubt, the suspension form should be used.

If edema of the external auditory canal skin does not completely occlude the lumen, the canal should be gently cleaned with a miniature cotton swab or a soft No. 6 French nasotracheal suction catheter set on low suction. An ear wick (e.g., a Pope Oto-wick) should be inserted when swelling obstructs the canal lumen.

Vesicles should be cultured for viruses; herpes oticus may benefit from oral acyclovir. Fungal infections can be treated with topical amphotericin B lotion.

Necrotizing (malignant) otitis externa requires prolonged (6 weeks or more) courses of parenteral antipseudomonal antibiotics or ciprofloxacin. An otologic consult should be obtained whenever it is suspected.

FOLLOW-UP.   Mild cases of bacterial otitis externa that respond to topical therapy do not require follow-up. In more severe cases, ear wicks should be replaced daily and the external auditory canal cleaned until the swelling sub-sides enough to allow ototopical drops to penetrate. If there is no response after a few days, one should consider culturing the ear and changing the antibiotic to a topical ophthalmic solution of either gentamicin or tobramycin. Cutaneous allergic reactions to neomycin are common and must be considered in cases that fail to respond.

Cross-references: Eczema (Section 28), Herpes Zoster (Section 30), Upper Respiratory Infection (Section 66).

REFERENCES

1. Pelton SI, Klein JO. The draining ear, otitis media and externa. Infect Dis Clin North Am 1988;2:117–129.
    A detailed review of these diseases, which are sometimes difficult to differentiate.
2. Rubin J, Yu VL. Malignant external otitis: Insights into pathogenesis, clinical manifesta-tions, diagnosis, and therapy. Am J Med 1988;85:391–398.
    A good clinical guide for this very difficult disease.

57 SINUSITIS

Problem

PAUL G. RAMSEY

EPIDEMIOLOGY.   The bacterial causes of acute and chronic maxillary sinusi-tis have been established by sinus puncture technique. *Haemophilus influen-zae, Streptococcus pneumoniae,* and *Moraxella catarrhalis* are the primary agents causing acute sinusitis (symptom duration < 4–6 weeks), and oral an-aerobic organisms cause chronic sinusitis (symptom duration > 2–3 months). Sinusitis can be categorized according to the anatomy of the paranasal sinuses. **Maxillary sinusitis** is the most common (approximately 1% of "colds" are com-plicated by acute maxillary sinusitis), but complications are rare. Bacterial in-fections of the **frontal, ethmoid,** and **sphenoid sinuses** are less common but may be associated with serious complications. Multiple conditions predispose to the development of sinusitis, including viral upper respiratory tract infection (URI symptoms persisting more than 7 days suggest sinusitis), mechanical problems such as deviated nasal septum and nasal polyps, cigarette smoking, allergies, cystic fibrosis, AIDS, and adjacent odontogenic infections. Immunosuppressed patients are prone to develop complications of sinusitis related to unusual organisms (e.g., fungal infections in diabetes).

SYMPTOMS AND SIGNS. The clinical features of sinusitis depend on the anatomic location. Maxillary sinusitis is often associated with cough and a purulent nasal discharge. Facial pain aggravated by stooping occurs less frequently, and headache and fever occur in only a minority of patients. The only sensitive physical signs are the presence of purulent nasal discharge and abnormal findings on sinus transillumination (see below). Acute frontal sinusitis is associated with fever, tenderness over the frontal sinus, and purulent nasal discharge. Puffy edema over the forehead suggests a diagnosis of subperiosteal abscess ("Potts' puffy tumor"). Ethmoiditis may be associated with orbital complications, including edema of the eyelid, ophthalmoplegia, chemosis, and proptosis. The most common initial symptom in patients with sphenoid sinusitis is headache. Pain is often unilateral and may involve the frontal, temporal, or occipital regions. Patients with sphenoid sinusitis may have unexplained tenderness over the vertex of the skull or over the mastoids. Fever is present in the majority of patients with acute sphenoiditis but may be absent in patients with chronic infection. Acute sphenoiditis may be associated with serious complications such as cavernous sinus thrombosis, acute pituitary insufficiency, and meningitis.

CLINICAL APPROACH. Most suspected cases of acute maxillary sinusitis can be diagnosed by sinus transillumination. The finding of an opaque maxillary sinus correlates with active purulent infection as determined by sinus puncture. Radiologic examination, however, remains the most sensitive and specific test. A single Waters's view provides the most specific and least expensive examination of the maxillary sinuses. Findings of opacity, air-fluid level, or mucosal thickening greater than 8 mm correlate with purulent material and microbial pathogens found by sinus puncture. Radiologic examination is essential for diagnosing frontal, ethmoid, and sphenoid sinusitis. When complications related to sinusitis are suspected, CT is a sensitive and specific examination. Direct sinus aspiration is the only procedure that provides accurate information concerning microbial etiology but is not necessary for uncomplicated cases of maxillary sinusitis. Nasal swab cultures are *not* useful because the results do not correlate with cultures obtained by direct sinus aspiration.

MANAGEMENT. Outpatient acquired acute maxillary sinusitis should be treated with a 10-day course of an oral antibiotic. Trimethoprim-sulfamethoxazole (1 double-strength tab PO b.i.d.), amoxicillin-clavulanate (250 mg PO t.i.d.), or cefuroxime (250 mg PO b.i.d.) are effective. There is no documented role for oral decongestants. Oxymetazoline hydrochloride (Afrin) nasal spray (one spray in each nostril t.i.d.) may be useful for symptoms, but its use should be limited to 2 or 3 days maximum. For patients with chronic maxillary sinusitis, management efforts should be directed toward removing predisposing factors and consultation with an otolaryngologist for possible drainage procedures. There is no proven role for antibiotics in chronic maxillary sinusitis, although some clinicians recommend an extended course (e.g., 4–6 weeks) of an antibiotic by mouth directed against oral anaerobic flora. Patients with suspected complications of ethmoid, frontal, or sphenoid sinusitis should be admitted to the hospital for IV antibiotic therapy and additional management in consultation with an otolaryngologist.

FOLLOW-UP. No follow-up is generally needed for patients with acute maxillary sinusitis. Symptoms should resolve within several days of beginning antibiotic therapy, although cough may persist for 2 to 3 weeks following successful therapy. Following acute maxillary sinusitis, radiologic findings may not return to normal for 2 months, and follow-up x-rays are not needed unless symptoms become chronic.

Cross-references: Upper Respiratory Infection (Section 66), Headache (Section 140).

REFERENCES

1. Evans FO, Sydnor JB, Moore WEC, et al. Sinusitis of the maxillary antrum. N Engl J Med 1975;293:735–739.
   Clinical features and microbiology of acute maxillary sinusitis.

2. Frederick J, Braude AI. Anaerobic infection of the paranasal sinuses. N Engl J Med 1974;290:135–137.
   Microbiologic findings in patients with chronic sinusitis.

3. Hamory BH, Sande MA, Syndor A, et al. Etiology and antimicrobial therapy of acute maxillary sinusitis. J Infect Dis 1979;139:197–202.
   A follow-up article to the study by Evans et al.

4. Lew D, Southwick FS, Montgomery WW, et al. Sphenoid sinusitis: A review of 30 cases. N Engl J Med 1983;309:1149–1154.
   Clinical features of sphenoid sinusitis.

5. Ramsey PG, Weymuller. Complications of bacterial infection of the ears, paranasal sinuses and oropharynx in adults. Emerg Med Clin North Am 1985;3:143–160.
   Clinical features of complications related to sinusitis, and a management approach.

58 CERUMEN REMOVAL

Procedure

STEVEN R. McGEE

INDICATIONS/CONTRAINDICATIONS. Common indications for removal of cerumen, or ear wax, include conductive hearing loss and the sensation of ear fullness. Hearing loss may appear suddenly, especially after swimming or showering (the epithelial component of cerumen absorbs water, swells, and occludes the canal). Tinnitus, vertigo, or intractable cough also may resolve after cerumen removal. Indications in asymptomatic patients include preparation for audiologic evaluation or tympanic membrane examination. Otitis externa or prior tympanic membrane perforation are contraindications to ear syringing.

RATIONALE. Cerumen is a normal product of the apocrine and sebaceous glands located in the outer one-third of the external ear canal. Simple mendelian genetics determines the cerumen type; the dry type of cerumen, common in Asians and native Americans, is recessive to the wet sticky type, common in whites and blacks. Cerumen inhibits the growth of bacteria and fungi in vitro; patients with inadequate cerumen, such as those with seborrheic dermatitis, may experience repeated external ear infections. Normal migration of the underlying epithelium from the tympanic membrane toward the outer canal continuously clears cerumen from the canal. Movements of the mandibular condyle during chewing also promote the exit of cerumen. Despite these self-cleansing mechanisms, cerumen sometimes becomes impacted. Predisposing factors include older age, narrow external ear canals, use of cotton-tipped swabs, and certain professions such as anesthesiology in which occluding ear pieces are worn for prolonged periods. Impacted cerumen may contain hair and, because of associated desquamated epithelium, may appear to have a membranous lining.

METHODS. Three different techniques clear cerumen impaction: use of instruments, ear syringing, or suction. The physician may use dull ring curettes to tease the edges of the cerumen away from the canal wall. The cerumen block may then be removed with the curette or tiny forceps. Because the canal is extremely sensitive and susceptible to bleeding, the use of instruments requires direct visualization and great care. During ear syringing, the physician pulls the auricle up and back and directs a stream of body-temperature tap water against the posterosuperior canal wall. Small gaps in the cerumen blockage at this location frequently allow the flow of water to pass behind the cerumen and push it out from the inside. A basin held under the ear collects the returning stream.

159

TABLE 58–1.   CERUMEN-SOFTENING AGENTS

Chemical	Generic	OTC/Rx?[1]	Cost
Mixed glycerides of oleic acid	Olive oil	OTC	$4.00 per 480 ml
Triethanolamine	Cerumenex	Rx	$10.28 per 6 ml bottle[2]
Carbamide peroxide	Debrox drops	OTC	$3.93 per 15 ml bottle[2]
	Murine ear drops	OTC	$4.22 per 15 ml bottle[2]

[1]Over-the-counter or prescription drug.
[2]Average wholesale price, 1991 *Drug Topics Red Book*.

If the cerumen is hard and does not clear easily, the patient should use a cerumenolytic (Table 58–1) for 3 days before attempts at syringing are repeated. If the second attempt fails, the patient should be referred to a specialist, who may use suctioning tools to clean the canal.

Controlled clinical trials demonstrate that olive oil, used to soften ear wax for over 100 years, is as effective as proprietary cerumenolytics. Other specialists recommend a light mineral oil, such as baby oil. Most ear drops are applied twice a day (the exception is Cerumenex, which the manufacturer recommends be given as a single dose). The patient retains each dose in the ear for 15 minutes, either by keeping the head tilted or by plugging the ear with cotton. A cerumenolytic's ability to dissolve wax in vitro correlates poorly with its clinical efficacy.

Cross-references: Dizziness (Section 20), Screening for Hearing Impairment (Section 48), Tinnitus (Section 51), Cough and Sputum (Section 63).

REFERENCES

1. Carne S. Ear syringing. Br Med J 1980;280:374–376.
    An illustrated guide to ear syringing.

2. Fraser JG. The efficacy of wax solvents: In vitro studies and a clinical trial. J Larygnol Otol 1970;84:1055–1064.
    Randomized double-blind controlled trial of cerumenolytics in elderly patients with bilateral cerumen impaction: olive oil was as effective as any other available medication.

3. Matsunaga E. The dimorphism in human normal cerumen. Ann Hum Genet 1962;25:273–286.
    The wet type of cerumen correlates with the presence of axillary odor, suggesting that the apocrine glands at both sites are genetically linked.

4. Raman R. Impacted ear wax: A cause for unexplained cough? Arch Otolaryngol Head Neck Surg 1986;112:679.
    After removal of cerumen impaction, three patients experienced relief of chronic nonproductive cough. The author postulates a reflex involving the auricular branch of the vagus nerve.

5. Editorial. Wax in the ear. Br Med J 1972;4:623–624.
    Brief but complete overview of the subject.

RESPIRATORY DISORDERS

59 SCREENING FOR OCCUPATIONAL LUNG DISEASE

Screening

WILLIAM S. BECKETT

EPIDEMIOLOGY.   Occupational exposures may cause any respiratory tract disorder except pulmonary arterial disease. The most common occupational lung diseases in the United States are industrial bronchitis, occupational asthma, bronchogenic carcinoma (related to asbestos or other carcinogens), asbestosis, silicosis, and coal workers' pneumoconiosis. Although not well documented, an estimated 5% to 15% of cases of new-onset adult asthma are probably occupationally related. Asbestosis is probably the most common cause of diffuse pulmonary fibrosis among elderly shipbuilders or construction workers who worked with large amounts of the substance.

The incubation period between exposure and disease varies from a few days, in the case of industrial bronchitis, to several decades, in the case of asbestos-related pleural mesothelioma. Occupational asthma develops after weeks to years of exposure (usually less than 5 years). The pneumoconioses, except for acute silicosis, occur 10 or more years after initial exposure to the dust.

RATIONALE.   Early detection is critical to limit exposure to toxins and halt progression to irreversible damage. Occupational asthma, for example, may resolve if exposure is removed early in the course, whereas disease frequently persists despite withdrawal of the offending agent in those exposed for long periods. Most chronic interstitial occupational diseases (e.g., silicosis, coal workers' pneumoconiosis, beryllium lung disease) progress long after exposure to the dust ceases.

The chest radiograph reveals most symptomatic chronic interstitial lung disease due to inhaled mineral dusts, although a few patients may have exercise-induced symptoms, diffuse fibrosis, and normal chest films. The combination of radiography and pulmonary function tests (spirometry, lung volumes, and diffusing capacity) has a higher sensitivity for detecting disease but is not specific for an occupational cause. In most cases, an occupational history of sufficient exposure to pathogenic dusts, consistent chest radiographs, and the exclusion of systemic diseases and drugs associated with interstitial lung disease such as rheumatoid arthritis, sarcoidosis, Sjögren's syndrome, chemotherapeutic agents, amiodarone, and nitrofurantoin provide a high degree of specificity without lung biopsy.

Certain chest radiographic findings are pathognomonic. Symmetric pleural plaques, with or without calcification, along the lateral chest wall and domes of the diaphragm are characteristic of asbestos exposure. Eggshell calcifications of hilar lymph nodes associated with small rounded opacities at the apices are characteristic of silicosis.

STRATEGY. The general internist should maintain a high index of suspicion for occupational lung disease in patients with any respiratory symptom. One logical approach includes the following steps: (1) define the type of disease present (e.g., asthma, pleural disease, interstitial fibrosis), (2) establish a differential diagnostic list, and (3) specifically question the patient about occupational exposures known to cause that disease. When patients can't recall specific exposures, the physician should obtain information from Material Safety Data Sheets, which employers legally must provide to employees or their physicians. A complete occupational history reviews all materials and length of exposure from all places of employment (summer jobs to the present time). Self-questionnaires are available, which the patient may complete at home or in the waiting room.[5]

Symptoms that suggest occupational disease include associated rhinitis and eye irritation (in the case of occupational asthma and bronchitis); the resolution or abatement of symptoms over weekends, holidays, and vacations, with recurrence after return to work; and the occurrence of similar illness in coworkers.

Spirometry performed before and after a work shift may miss delayed asthmatic responses. Self-administered peak expiratory flow measurements are more useful: the patient uses a portable hand-held peak flow meter every 4 hours for 2 weeks at work and 2 weeks away from work. Decrements in peak flow during work and increments during holidays establish a work-related etiology.

Based on information from cigarette smokers, screening chest radiography probably does not improve the survival of those exposed to other inhaled carcinogens (e.g., asbestos workers, uranium miners).

ACTION. Patients should understand the prognosis of their disease, that it is work related, and that they may apply for workers' compensation. Unless otherwise directed by the patient, communication with the employer should preserve patient confidentiality and include only whether the patient can work and if so, under what restrictions. If there is a possibility of immediate hazard to others in the workplace, the physician should promptly telephone the employer to alert others to the hazard. Some state and local health departments require the reporting of all or certain categories of occupational disease.[4] Most internists are unfamiliar with the procedures involved and may want to refer the patient to an occupational medicine specialist, who will in turn contact the employer to cooperate in preventive measures, visit the workplace, or notify OSHA or other appropriate public health officials of the presence of hazardous working conditions.

Respirators—protective devices worn over the face to prevent inhalation of toxins—become uncomfortable with prolonged use and are an inferior alternative to the use of safer materials or engineered ventilation systems. Respirators can be effective when used properly, but their selection and use should be monitored by knowledgeable industrial hygienists.

No specific therapy exists for most occupational lung diseases. Bronchodilators and corticosteroids benefit patients with occupational asthma (after complete withdrawal from exposure) and corticosteroids may help those with acute hypersensitivity pneumonitis. Patients with occupational lung disease should receive influenza and pneumococcal vaccines and should stop smoking.

Cross-references: Determining Disability: The Primary Physician's Role (Section 5), Periodic Health Assessment (Section 7), Adult Immunizations (Section 10), Dyspnea (Section 19), Asthma and Chronic Obstructive Pulmonary Disease (Section 68), Pulmonary Function Testing (Section 69).

REFERENCES

1. Becklake MD. Asbestos related disease of the lung and other organs: Their epidemiology and implications for clinical practice. Am Rev Respir Dis 1976;114:187–227.
   A superb clinician's review of the many issues involved in the clinical care of these patients.

2. Chan-Yeung M, Lam S. Occupational asthma. State of the art. Am Rev Respir Dis 1986; 133:686–703.
   Includes a listing of substances known to cause occupational asthma.

3. Cullen MR, Cherniack MG, Rosenstock L. Occupational medicine. N Engl J Med 1990;322:594–601, 675–883.
   Excellent review.

4. Freund D, Seligman PJ, Chorba TL, Safford SK, Drachman JG, Hull HF. Mandatory reporting of occupational diseases by clinicians. JAMA 1989;262:3041–3044.
   A state-by-state listing of which occupational diseases must be reported to health departments.

5. Occupational and Environmental Health Committee. Taking the occupational history. Ann Intern Med 1983;99:641–651.
   Contains a reproducible occupational history form designed to be self-administered.

60 TUBERCULOSIS SCREENING

Screening

JOYCE E. WIPF

EPIDEMIOLOGY. Following a steady decline in the previous 30 years, the incidence of tuberculosis in the United States began to rise in 1986, with 23,495 tuberculosis cases reported (9.1 per 100,000) in 1989. High-risk groups include individuals with human immunodeficiency virus (HIV) infection, drug and alcohol abusers, the homeless, immigrant minority groups, and confined populations such as those in nursing homes and prisons. The only acceptable screening method is the tuberculin skin test (PPD, purified protein derivative), a test that detects delayed or cell-mediated immunity to tuberculosis infection. An estimated 10 million Americans are infected (defined as asymptomatic tuberculin skin test positive). Eighty percent of active tuberculosis cases result from reactivation of latent infection in tuberculin reactors.

RATIONALE. The goals of screening are to identify infected individuals at high risk of developing active disease and to eventually eradicate tuberculosis by preventive treatment with isoniazid (INH). Active tuberculosis ultimately develops in about 10% of infected persons; actual probabilities vary between 5% over 5 years for recent (within 2 years) converters, and 0.1% per year for other reactors without additional risk factors. One year of INH therapy is over 90% effective in preventing activation of tuberculosis, although no studies of chemoprophylaxis efficacy in HIV-infected or immunocompromised patients are available. Studies to evaluate 6-month prophylaxis with INH are ongoing.

STRATEGY. The standard test is 5 tuberculin units of intermediate strength, administered intradermally with controls, and read at 48 to 72 hours. A positive test is defined as ≥ 10 mm diameter of induration at the site, or ≥ 5 mm in an HIV-infected person or close contact of a patient with tuberculosis. Positive controls are ≥ 10 mm induration for *Candida* and *Trichophyton,* and ≥ 5 mm erythema for mumps. Elderly persons who are negative on initial testing require a second test within 2 weeks because many will show a "booster" reaction. False-positive tuberculin reactions are usually 5 to 10 mm and due to mycobacteria other than *M. tuberculosis.* False-negative reactions (typically due to anergy and confirmed by negative control tests) occur in 15% of patients with proven active pulmonary tuberculosis and in up to 50% of those with miliary tuberculosis.

The Centers for Disease Control (CDC) and American Thoracic Society recommend tuberculin testing in the following groups:

1. Persons suspected of active tuberculosis
2. Close contacts of persons with known or suspected tuberculosis

3. HIV-infected individuals
4. Alcoholics or IV drug abusers
5. Residents of long-term care facilities and prisons
6. High-risk racial minorities (blacks, Asians, Latin Americans, native Americans)
7. Newly arrived immigrants, foreign workers
8. Nursing home and hospital employees
9. Persons with chronic medical conditions that may put them at increased risk (data limited for most): silicosis, previous gastrectomy, chronic renal failure, diabetes mellitus, immunosuppressive therapy or diseases, glucocorticoid therapy, myeloproliferative malignancies, and malnutrition

ACTION.   PPD test and control results should be recorded in the patient's chart. Periodic retesting is recommended only for nonreactors at high risk such as a household contact. Tuberculin reactors require evaluation for active tuberculosis. Six to 12 months of isoniazid, 300 mg/day, is recommended for the following asymptomatic tuberculin-reactive patients:

1. Household members and other close contacts of persons with tuberculosis ($\geq$5 mm reaction)
2. Persons with HIV infection ($\geq$5 mm reaction)
3. Newly infected persons (recent converters, within 2 years)
4. Persons with an abnormal chest radiograph in whom active tuberculosis has been excluded
5. Persons with associated medical conditions such as silicosis, diabetes mellitus, hematologic malignancies, end-stage renal disease, malnutrition, or those receiving chronic steroid or other immunosuppressive therapy
6. All other tuberculin reactors under the age of 35

These recommendations for chemoprophylaxis are debated, particularly in healthy young adults and patients with chronic diseases, in whom data on the risk of tuberculosis are limited. Compliance and abstinence from alcohol are important during INH therapy. Adverse reactions to INH include rash, nausea, malaise, fever, chills, and arthralgias. Because the risk of INH-associated hepatitis increases with age over 35, a monthly review of symptoms and periodic liver function tests are required.

Cross-references: Periodic Health Assessment (Section 7), AIDS (Section 14), Fever (Section 16).

REFERENCES

1. American Thoracic Society. The tuberculin skin test. Am Rev Respir Dis 1981;124:356–363.
    Reviews administration and interpretation of the tuberculin test; covers booster phenomenon and false-negative and false-positive reactions.
2. Centers for Disease Control. Screening for tuberculosis and tuberculosis infection in high risk populations, and the use of preventive therapy for tuberculosis infection in the United

States: Recommendations of the Advisory Committee for Elimination of Tuberculosis. MMWR 1990;39:153–156.

Summary of tuberculosis data and risks among ethnic groups; goals for eradication of tuberculosis.

3. Chaisson RE, Slutkin G. Tuberculosis and human immunodeficiency virus infection. J Infect Dis 1989;159:96–100.

Concise summary of association between tuberculosis and HIV infection, and of atypical and extrapulmonary forms of tuberculosis seen in HIV-infected patients.

4. Rose DN, Schechter CB, Silver AL. The age threshold for isoniazid chemoprophylaxis: A decision analysis for low risk tuberculin reactors. JAMA 1986;256:2709–2713.

Decision analysis concludes that prophylaxis is beneficial for tuberculin reactors of all ages, even low-risk individuals. Reviews issues in the debate on chemoprophylaxis.

5. Wipf JE, Lipsky BA. Tuberculosis screening and chemoprophylaxis: An update for clinicians. Med Rounds 1988;1:188–196.

Detailed review of the tuberculin test, mechanics of testing, and data on high-risk populations. Includes recommendations for testing and chemoprophylaxis with isoniazid and outlines the controversial aspects of chemoprophylaxis.

61 PLEURITIC CHEST PAIN

Symptom

DAVID H. INGBAR

EPIDEMIOLOGY.   Pleuritic chest pain often accompanies disorders of the chest wall, pleural space, or underlying lung. Its frequency is not well defined.

ETIOLOGY.   The causes of pleuritic pain can be classified by their anatomic origin. The chest wall may be the source of pain from muscular tears, muscle inflammation, costochondritis, fractured ribs, or neural inflammation (e.g., herpes zoster). Pleurodynia, a coxsackievirus infection, usually causes local chest wall myositis rather than a true pleuritis. Pleural disorders produce pain by involvement of the parietal pleura since the visceral pleura has very few pain fibers. These conditions include empyema, inflammatory effusions (such as in systemic lupus erythematosis or postpericardial injury syndromes), tuberculous pleurisy, metastatic or primary lung cancer with local involvement, mesothelioma, pneumothorax, and pulmonary embolism with infarction. Tumors that commonly involve the pleura are bronchogenic carcinoma and metastases from breast, pancreas, colon, and stomach primary sites. Pneumothoraces may be either spontaneous or induced secondarily by trauma or iatrogenic events. Spontaneous pneumothoraces occur either in patients with underlying lung diseases, including chronic obstructive pulmonary disease, eosinophilic granuloma, interstitial lung disease, lymphangioleiomyomatosis, or, if idiopathic, in those with multiple apical subpleural blebs. Abnormalities of the underlying lung, such as pneumonia, also may cause pleuritic pain.

CLINICAL APPROACH.   The evaluation focuses on the patient's age, the duration of the pain, and the accompanying symptoms and signs. In young, otherwise healthy individuals, pneumothorax, trauma, and pleurodynia are most common, but pulmonary emboli should always be a concern because of their life-threatening potential. Pleuritic chest pain often is one of the earliest presenting complaints of patients with lupus. Chronic pleuritic pain in an older individual with malaise or weight loss raises the concern of cancer, empyema, or tuberculosis.

Particular attention should be paid to suggestions of recent trauma, chronic infection, cancer, or polyserositis. Chest wall tenderness suggests a chest wall etiology but is not absolutely reliable. A pleural friction rub strongly supports the presence of pleural inflammation. Laboratory studies usually include a complete blood cell (CBC) count, platelet count, prothrombin time, activated partial thromboplastin time, and liver function tests. If the pain is unexplained, other tests, such as antinuclear antibody and rheumatoid factor assays, should be done. The electrocardiogram (ECG) may reveal pericarditis, a recent myocardial injury, or a pattern suggestive of pulmonary embolism (new right bundle-branch block, $S_1Q_3T_3$). Posteroanterior and lateral chest radiographs are essential for determining if a pneumothorax, parenchymal infiltrate, pleural thickening, adenopathy, or pleural fluid are present. In addition, the volume and mobility of pleural fluid on lateral decubitus chest radiographs determine its accessibility for diagnostic thoracentesis. If significant pleural fluid is present, thoracentesis should be performed (see Section 70, Thoracentesis).

If the clinical evaluation suggests pulmonary emboli, ventilation-perfusion (V/Q) lung scans and/or proximal leg vein studies (Doppler/ultrasound studies, impedance plethysmography, contrast or radionuclide venography) should be pursued. Pulmonary angiography should be performed when leg studies are negative and lung scans indeterminate, when there is a high risk of bleeding from anticoagulation, or when there is a discrepancy between the clinical suspicion and the lung scan result.

Because patients often restrict chest wall expansion on the side with pleuritic pain, atelectasis, decreased cough, and infection may result.

MANAGEMENT.   Pleuritic pain usually responds to aspirin or nonsteroidal anti-inflammatory agents. Specific therapy depends on the diagnosis. Empyemas must be treated with antibiotics and early drainage to prevent loculation and the subsequent need for open drainage with rib resection or decortication. Although small pneumothoraces may resolve spontaneously, most necessitate catheter or chest tube drainage. If pain is chronic and nonresponsive, then other measures such as local nerve blocks or nerve stimulators may be useful.

Cross-references: Pleural Effusion (Section 65), Thoracentesis (Section 70), Chest Pain (Section 74), Painful and Swollen Calf (Section 131).

REFERENCES

1. Branch WT, McNeil BJ. Analysis of the differential diagnosis and assessment of pleuritic chest pain in young adults. Am J Med 1983;75:671–679.

    Discusses the difficult distinction between pulmonary emboli and viral pleuritis, emphasizing the utility of pleural effusions, risks for deep vein thrombosis or physical signs of phlebitis as indicators for pursuing the diagnosis of pulmonary embolism.

2. Chernow B, Sahn SA. Carcinomatous involvement of the pleura: An analysis of 96 patients. Am J Med 1977;63:695–702.

    The best series dealing with this problem.

3. Chretien J, Bignon J, Hirsch A, Eds. The Pleura in Health and Disease. Vol. 2, in Lung Biology in Health and Disease. Marcel Dekker, New York, 1985.

    A two-volume comprehensive treatise on all aspects of pleural disease.

4. Conces DJ, Tarver RD, Gray WC, Pearcy EA. Treatment of pneumothoraces utilizing small caliber chest tubes. Chest 1988;94:55–57.

    Reviews the outpatient use of a small drainage catheter in spontaneous idiopathic pneumothorax, avoiding the necessity of chest tube therapy.

5. Hull RD, et al. Pulmonary embolism in outpatients with pleuritic chest pain. Arch Intern Med 1988;148:838–844.

    Pulmonary emboli are common (21%) in this setting, V/Q scans often are indeterminate, and a combination of V/Q scans and leg studies reduces the need for pulmonary angiography from 43% to 26% of the group.

6. Stelzner TH, King TE, Antony VB, Sahn SA. The pleuropulmonary manifestations of the postcardiac injury syndrome. Chest 1983;84:383–387.

    Reviews the features of the difficult-to-diagnose Dressler's and postpericardiotomy syndromes.

62 HEMOPTYSIS

Symptom

DAVID H. INGBAR

EPIDEMIOLOGY.   Hemoptysis was the presenting complaint of 10% to 15% of patients seen at chest clinics in the mid-1950s, but with the declining incidence of tuberculosis and bronchiectasis, now it probably represents only 1% to 5% of modern chest clinic referrals.

ETIOLOGY.   Hemoptysis occurs in many respiratory and systemic illnesses (Table 62–1). In addition, gastrointestinal and nasopharyngeal sources of bleeding are common and may be difficult to separate from true hemoptysis, which is defined as the coughing up of blood derived from the lungs or tracheobronchial tree. The most common causes of hemoptysis are bronchiectasis (often

TABLE 62–1.   ETIOLOGIES OF HEMOPTYSIS

Etiology	Incidence (%)	% of Cases with Bleeding	% Massive
Bronchogenic carcinoma	10–15	30–55	10
Bronchiectasis	20	25–45	30*
Pulmonary tuberculosis	25–40*	5–20	20*
Lung abscess	1–6	10–15	25*
Bronchial adenoma	1	40–55	10
COPD + exacerbation	10–20*	10*	<5*
Cardiovascular	1–7*	?	?
Arteriovenous malformation	10*	40	25*

*Estimate; little information is available in recent literature.

occurring in the setting of an exacerbation of chronic obstructive pulmonary disease [COPD] or an upper respiratory infection), tuberculosis, and lung cancer. Other important causes include lung infections (aspergilloma, necrotizing pneumonia, lung abscess), broncholithiasis, bullous emphysema, pulmonary embolism with infarction, pulmonary-renal syndromes (Wegener's granulomatosis, systemic lupus erythematosis, Goodpasture's syndrome), cystic fibrosis, mitral stenosis, drugs, trauma, and bleeding disorders and other entities listed in Table 62–1. The patient's age markedly affects the likelihood that hemoptysis results from cystic fibrosis, congenital anomalies (valvular lesions, sequestered lobe), or bronchogenic carcinoma.

Massive hemoptysis usually is defined as greater than 200 ml of expectorated blood per 24 hours. Tuberculosis, lung abscess, and bronchiectasis account for approximately 90% of cases of massive hemoptysis.

CLINICAL APPROACH.   Hemoptysis often signals the presence of a serious underlying disease that needs diagnosis and treatment; it is as well a potential warning sign of a life-threatening bleeding episode. The course of hemoptysis is very unpredictable; a small bleed may be the harbinger of a sudden massive bleed. Hemoptysis may be fatal due to asphyxiation rather than exsanguination, especially in patients with significant preexisting lung compromise.

The clinical evaluation should determine if the bleeding is from the lung or a gastrointestinal or nasopharyngea source. Clues to hematemesis include black oxidized blood, low pH, the presence of food particles, and a history of vomiting. Guaiac-positive stool does not differentiate whether a patient may have secondarily swallowed blood that has been coughed up. A careful ear, nose, and throat examination is important in all patients but especially in older smokers, who are at risk for head and neck carcinomas.

The clinician should inquire about associated cough, chest pain, fevers, weight loss, and the onset of hemoptysis relative to other symptoms, since each suggests a set of possible causes. Purulent sputum suggests pneumonia or abscess, whereas blood-streaked sputum occurs most commonly with cancer or bronchitis. Any drugs used (aspirin, anticoagulants, recreational drugs), travel, occupational history, and cigarette use are all important. Paragonimiasis, for example, the most common worldwide cause of hemoptysis, is suggested by a history of travel to Southeast Asia. Familial occurrence of hemoptysis, frequent prior episodes, or intracranial bleeding suggests the arteriovenous malformations of Osler-Weber-Rendu syndrome.

Clues to the etiology that should be sought on physical examination include telangiectasias (Osler-Weber-Rendu syndrome), heart murmur (mitral stenosis), clubbing (bronchiectasis, tumor, cystic fibrosis), nasal septal ulceration (Wegener's granulomatosis), and chest flow murmur (arteriovenous malformations). Laboratory studies should include a CBC with platelet count and differential; coagulation studies (prothrombin time, activated partial thromboplastin time, bleeding time); blood urea nitrogen and creatinine levels; urinalysis; chest radiography; arterial blood gases; and sputum for Gram stain and culture, along with tuberculosis and cytologic studies. The volume of bleeding should be quantified. If possible, pulmonary function testing should be performed after tuberculosis has been excluded to assess whether a patient might be a surgical candidate if the hemoptysis should become massive.

MANAGEMENT.   Several major management issues must be addressed. First, is the bleeding massive in quantity? In the outpatient setting, this is best assessed historically. Patients with massive hemoptysis have a high mortality and should be rapidly admitted to the hospital for aggressive diagnostic and therapeutic measures, including control of the airway, if necessary.

Second, where in the lungs is the bleeding coming from? Is the bleeding localized or diffuse? Diffuse bleeding, as in pulmonary-renal syndromes, excludes surgical or embolic therapy. If localized, where is the bleeding site? Physical examination and chest radiography often are misleading about the bleeding site, because blood may move to dependent areas such as the lower lobes. Virtually all patients with hemoptysis should be rapidly referred to a pulmonologist for evaluation and probable flexible fiberoptic bronchoscopy. This should be performed on all patients with hemoptysis not due to a known necrotizing pneumonia, even if there is only streaking of the sputum with blood. Early performance of bronchoscopy, while a patient is still actively bleeding, more frequently identifies a bleeding site but may not change the ultimate diagnosis or outcome. If the site of bleeding is known and bleeding becomes massive, a patient can more readily undergo emergency angiographic embolotherapy or surgery. In more elective situations, computed tomography (CT) of the chest may also be useful to uncover bronchiectasis, tumors, or other lesions.

One of the most difficult outpatient management issues is the chronic smoker or older individual who presents with small amounts of blood-streaked sputum in the setting of an upper respiratory infection or an exacerbation of COPD. Although it is easy to disregard the hemoptysis, there is a major risk of missing the diagnosis of lung cancer with endobronchial involvement. These patients should have sputum cytologies and fiberoptic bronchoscopy performed shortly after they recover from their intercurrent illness. Lung cancer most commonly manifests as small amounts of blood-streaked sputum occurring intermittently for more than 1 to 2 weeks in older individuals or smokers. These patients should be referred to an otolaryngologist for a careful fiberoptic examination for head and neck carcinomas. During the interim it is reasonable to use antibiotics to treat any component of infectious bronchitis and bronchiectasis in order to hasten their recovery.

Cross-references: Lower Respiratory Infection (Section 67), Bleeding (Section 197).

REFERENCES

1. Rogers RM. The management of massive hemoptysis in a patient with pulmonary TB. Chest 1976;70:519–526.
    Discusses the multiple ways that active and inactive tuberculosis can cause hemoptysis.

2. Weaver LJ, et al. Selection of patients with hemoptysis for fiberoptic bronchoscopy. Chest 1979;76:7–10.
    Cancer often manifests with several weeks of blood-streaked sputum.

3. Winter S, Ingbar DH. Massive hemoptysis: Pathogenesis and management. J Intensive Care 1988;3:11–29.
    A comprehensive review of this medical emergency.

63 COUGH AND SPUTUM

Symptom

SHAWN J. SKERRETT

EPIDEMIOLOGY.   Cough is a normal reflex that becomes symptomatic when it is unusually frequent or productive. In the 1978–1979 National Health Survey, cough was the fifth most common reason for consulting a physician and the second most common symptom, accounting for 2.5% of office visits. A chronic cough afflicts most smokers of more than a pack of cigarettes per day, and 8% to 22% of nonsmokers.

ETIOLOGY.   Involuntary coughing most often results from the stimulation of cough receptors in the larynx, trachea, or major bronchi but may follow irritation of the nose and paranasal sinuses, the external auditory canal, the pharynx, the diaphragm, the pleura, the pericardium, the esophagus, or the stomach.

Acute cough is accompanied by symptoms of respiratory tract infection in over 85% of cases. Chronic cough, variably defined as lasting at least 3 to 8 weeks, is often related to cigarette smoking. Among patients with chronic cough referred to pulmonologists, the most common causes are asthma (35%), postnasal drip (20%–50%), gastroesophageal reflux (5%–20%), recent respiratory infection (10%–15%), and chronic bronchitis (5%–12%). Other causes include exposure to dust or noxious gases, interstitial lung disease, bronchiectasis, neoplasm (primary or metastatic), recurrent aspiration, hair or cerumen in the external ear, congestive heart failure, drugs (particularly angiotensin-converting enzyme inhibitors and beta blockers), and psychiatric disorders. Up to 25% of cases of chronic cough have more than one cause. In 1% to 12% of cases no cause can be identified.

CLINICAL APPROACH. The history and physical examination will usually suggest the diagnosis. The history should focus on smoking habits, environmental exposures, the duration and character of the cough, and associated symptoms of respiratory, gastrointestinal, neurologic, and heart disease. The examination should be directed toward the ears, nose, throat, neck, chest, and heart.

An **asthmatic cough** may be productive or nonproductive and is typically paroxysmal and precipitated by exertion or specific environmental exposures (cold air, perfume, smoke, pollen, dander, etc.). Although usually accompanied by dyspnea and wheezing, cough may be the sole manifestation of asthma. **Postnasal drip** from allergic rhinitis, perennial nonallergic rhinitis, or sinusitis is suggested by a cough productive of scant mucoid or mucopurulent sputum, worse in the morning, often associated with a sensation of secretions draining down the posterior pharynx, and a need to frequently clear the throat. Nasal discharge and symptoms of sinus congestion (facial pain, headache) also occur, and examination of the nose and pharynx may reveal mucoid or mucopurulent secretions and a "cobblestone" appearance of the mucosa due to prominent submucosal lymphoid follicles. A persistent cough following a viral **respiratory tract infection** may have features of postnasal drip or asthma; bronchial hyperreactivity may persist for up to 7 weeks following infection. Most patients with **gastroesophageal reflux** admit to heartburn, a sour taste in the mouth, or morning hoarseness, but cough may be the only symptom. Although the cough in this setting is often nocturnal or postprandial, the absence of this pattern does not exclude reflux. **Chronic bronchitis** is defined by a productive cough on most days for at least 3 months of 2 or more consecutive years. Daily or recurrent production of purulent sputum is suggestive of **bronchiectasis. Lung cancer** may present with new or changing cough, but additional symptoms, such as hemoptysis, chest pain, dyspnea, and weight loss, are elicited in over 80% of cases. A dry cough precipitated by deep inhalation and associated with dyspnea on exertion is suggestive of **interstitial lung disease. Left ventricular failure** and

mitral stenosis may present with cough that is worse with exertion or supine posture. A history of neurologic, oropharyngeal, or esophageal disease or of coughing while eating should prompt consideration of **recurrent aspiration.**

When the history and examination findings do not suggest a diagnosis or grounds for a therapeutic trial, further evalution should include chest radiography and spirometry. Methacholine challenge testing is necessary to diagnose most cases of cough-variant asthma, but bronchial provocation studies should be delayed for 8 weeks after a respiratory tract infection. Esophageal reflux may be demonstrated by barium swallow or endoscopic evidence of esophagitis, but 24-hour esophageal pH monitoring is the most sensitive method. Laryngoscopy may reveal evidence of chronic laryngeal irritation, consistent with postnasal drip or recurrent aspiration. Sinus radiographs should be ordered in patients with chronic postnasal drip to exclude sinusitis. Fiberoptic bronchoscopy and cardiac studies may be indicated in selected cases.

MANAGEMENT.   The treatment of cough should be directed toward a specific diagnosis, such as asthma, chronic bronchitis, heartburn, or sinusitis. Oral bronchodilators are indicated as initial therapy for asthma if inhaled agents provoke coughing. Postnasal drip in the absence of infection is best treated with nasal inhalation of corticosteroids (e.g., beclomethasone, one puff in each nostril two to four times a day), with a long-acting oral decongestant-antihistamine combination added if necessary. Specific treatment is effective in 87% to 98% of patients with chronic cough.

Antitussive agents should be used with caution, as cough serves to protect the airway and expel secretions. Syrups, lozenges, and topical anesthetics may be helpful in the setting of dry or irritated pharyngeal mucosa. Among the centrally active antitussives (Table 63–1), opiates are the most effective, and dextromethorphan is a useful nonprescription agent.

Mucolytics and expectorants are of uncertain value in the management of chronic productive cough. The agents listed in Table 63–1 have been shown to produce subjective improvement in at least one controlled trial, but the benefits are slight and inconsistently demonstrated.

TABLE 63–1.   NONSPECIFIC TREATMENT OF COUGH

Class/Agent	Dose	Daily Cost ($)[1]
Central antitussives		
Codeine	20–60 mg q.i.d.	0.76
Propoxyphene	100 mg q.i.d.	0.40
Dextromethorphan[2]	15–30 mg q.i.d.	0.35
Diphenhydramine[2]	25–50 mg q.i.d.	0.08
Mucolytics, expectorants		
N-acetylcysteine	3–5 ml of 20% solution by aerosol t.i.d.–q.i.d.	7.71
Iodinated glycerol	60 mg q.i.d.	1.89
Guaifenesin[2]	400 mg q.i.d.	0.92

[1]Average wholesale price, lower daily dose listed, 1991 *Drug Topics Red Book.*
[2]Over-the-counter medications.

Cross-references: Sinusitis (Section 57), Screening for Occupational Lung Disease (Section 59), Lower Respiratory Infection (Section 67), Asthma and Chronic Obstructive Pulmonary Disease (Section 68), Dysphagia and Heartburn (Section 97).

REFERENCES

1. Braman SJ, Corrao WM. Cough: Differential diagnosis and treatment. Clin Chest Med 1987;8:177–188.
    A helpful review.
2. Goldszer RC, Lilly LS, Solomon HS. Prevalence of cough during angiotensin-converting enzyme inhibitor therapy. Am J Med 1988;85:887.
    Cough was reported in up to 25% of patients taking these commonly used drugs.
3. Irwin RS, Curley FJ, French CL. Chronic cough. The spectrum and frequency of causes, key components of the diagnostic evaluation, and outcome of specific therapy. Am Rev Respir Dis 1990;141:640–647.
    A specific diagnosis was made in 101 of 102 patients; directed treatment was successful in 98%.
4. Poe RH, Harder RV, Israel RH, Kallay MC. Chronic persistent cough: Experience in diagnosis and outcome using an anatomic diagnostic protocol. Chest 1989;95:723–728.
    A specific diagnosis was made in 88% of 139 patients; therapy was successful in 87%.
5. Editorial. Physiology and treatment of cough. Thorax 1990;45:425–430.
    A different perspective.

64 SLEEP APNEA SYNDROMES

Problem

RICHARD M. HOFFMAN

EPIDEMIOLOGY.   Sleep apnea syndromes affect an estimated 1% to 4% of adults, most commonly older men, and are characterized by frequent and prolonged cessation of breathing during sleep, fragmented sleep, and daytime hypersomnolence. In obstructive apnea (>80% of cases), anatomic or functional upper airway abnormalities cause cessation of air flow despite continuous inspiratory efforts. Obstructive apnea is associated with obesity, snoring, hypertension, hypothyroidism, and acromegaly. The pickwickian syndrome is a variant of obstructive apnea characterized by obesity and daytime hypoventilation. In central apnea (<5% of patients), abnormalities of the medullary respiratory center cause periodic cessation of both inspiratory efforts and air flow. Central apnea is associated with neurologic disorders, congestive heart failure, and nasal obstruction. The remaining patients have a mixed sleep apnea involving airway obstruction and respiratory center impairment.

SIGNS AND SYMPTOMS. Obstructive and mixed apneic episodes lead to repeated brief arousals from sleep (by EEG criteria) to resume breathing. This sleep deprivation leads to daytime hypersomnolence, the usual presenting symptom. In extreme cases, hypersomnolence may interfere with normal activities such as eating, talking, or driving. Snoring is always present in obstructive apnea, and sleeping partners often observe restlessness, gasping, choking, and apnea during sleep. Pure central apnea is often asymptomatic but may cause insomnia or awakenings due to dyspnea.

Common neuropsychiatric disturbances include anxiety, depression, sexual dysfunction, intellectual deterioration, and morning headaches. Cardiopulmonary complications, resulting from prolonged hypoxemia and hypercapnia, include systemic and pulmonary hypertension, biventricular failure, nocturnal angina, arrhythmias, conduction disturbances, and sudden death.

CLINICAL APPROACH. Sleep apnea should be suspected in patients with daytime hypersomnolence, observed sleep abnormalities, unexplained right heart failure, or polycythemia. Functional impairment should be described and aggravating factors identified, including weight gain, sleeping in a supine position, and the use of alcohol, narcotics, or sedatives at bedtime. The upper airway should be examined for hypertrophied tonsils or adenoids, macroglossia, a large pendulous uvula and droopy soft palate, mandibular abnormalities, and nasal obstruction.

Aside from thyroid functions, there are no specific routine tests for sleep apnea. A cardiopulmonary evaluation is recommended, including arterial blood gases, hematocrit, chest radiography, ECG, and, in selected patients, Holter monitoring and spirometry.

Diagnosing sleep apnea requires an objective evaluation of breathing during sleep. An overnight polysomnogram in a sleep laboratory documents apnea and assesses its severity. Polysomnography monitors sleep stages, respiratory air flow and effort, arterial oxygen saturation, cardiac rhythm, body position, periodic movements, and snoring. Screening test (tracheal sound recordings, ear oximetry, and Holter monitoring), ambulatory monitoring systems and daytime nap studies are less expensive and more convenient than polysomnography but have either limited accuracy in detecting apnea or difficulty distinguishing obstructive from central apnea. Data on the cost-effectiveness of these techniques are currently unavailable.

After obstructive sleep apnea has been confirmed, upper airway endoscopy, lateral head and neck films, and head CT may assist in determining the site of obstruction and in guiding treatment.

MANAGEMENT. Treatment should be dictated by the severity of clinical symptoms, polysomnographic abnormalities, and anatomic findings. In severe cases—those with cardiopulmonary complications or debilitating hypersomnolence—urgent tracheostomy or nasal continuous positive airway pressure (CPAP) is indicated. A tracheostomy effectively bypasses upper airway obstruction but entails significant medical and psychological morbidity. CPAP maintains upper airway patency and is a relatively well-tolerated, long-term treatment for obstructive and mixed sleep apnea. Surgical procedures such as tonsillectomy and adenoidectomy, removal of nasal polyps, repair of septal deviation, and mandibular advancement are effective in appropriate cases.

Treatment options for patients with mild to moderate hypersomnolence but no cardiopulmonary complications include CPAP, uvulopalatopharyngoplasty (surgical removal of redundant upper airway tissue; snoring is eliminated in over 80% patients, although apnea is significantly reduced in only 50%), prosthetic oral devices, and medications. Protryptiline, a nonsedating tricyclic agent, reduces hypersomnolence and improves nocturnal oxygenation in mild obstructive apnea, although anticholinergic side effects limit its use. Medroxyprogesterone acetate, a centrally acting respiratory stimulant, is used for the obesity-hypoventilation (pickwickian) syndrome. Acetazolamide, a carbonic anhydrase inhibitor that stimulates respiration by producing a metabolic acidosis, is used for central sleep apnea. The efficacy of drug therapy, however, remains uncertain because few studies have been controlled, sample size and follow-up have been limited, and outcomes assessed inconsistently.

General measures include eliminating respiratory depressants (alcohol, narcotics, and sedatives), encouraging weight loss, and advising patients to avoid sleeping in a supine position. (A tennis ball sewn into the back of a pyjama top can sometimes accomplish this.) Supplemental oxygen diminishes hypoxemia but occasionally prolongs apneic episodes; therefore, its initial use should be monitored by oximetry or polysomnography.

FOLLOW-UP.   All patients treated for sleep apnea require close follow-up to document lessened daytime hypersomnolence, improved neuropsychiatric functioning, improvement in cardiopulmonary complications, and decreased frequency and severity of apneic episodes. A repeat sleep study is sometimes necessary, particularly when CPAP is used.

Cross-reference: Asthma and Chronic Obstructive Pulmonary Disease (Section 68).

REFERENCES

1. American Thoracic Society. Indications and standards for cardiopulmonary sleep studies. Am Rev Respir Dis 1989;139:559–568.
    Current consensus opinions from the American Thoracic Society.

2. Sullivan CE, Issa FG. Obstructive sleep apnea. Clin Chest Med 1985;6:633–650.
    Summary of clinical features and treatment.

3. Thawley SE, Ed. Symposium on Sleep Apnea Disorders. Med Clin North Am 1985;69: 1121–1412.
    Extensive review of pathophysiology and therapy.

4. Wiggins RV, Schmidt-Nowara. Treatment of obstructive sleep apnea syndrome. West J Med 1987;147:561–568.
Concise review.

65 PLEURAL EFFUSION

Problem

DAVID H. INGBAR

EPIDEMIOLOGY.   There are few data on the prevalence of effusions in the many common outpatient clinical situations in which they occur (e.g., congestive heart failure [CHF], pneumonia). Of patients presenting to an emergency room with pneumococcal pneumonia, 10% initially have or develop an effusion. In viral or mycoplasmal pneumonia, 10% to 20% of patients will develop an effusion during the course of their illness.

SYMPTOMS AND SIGNS.   Although pleural fluid usually causes no symptoms unless the effusion is at least several liters, it can be an important indicator of an underlying lung or systemic abnormality. There may be associated pleuritic chest pain from involvement with inflammation or malignancy or, if the effusion is large, there may be shortness of breath from chest wall displacement and compression of the underlying lung. An effusion that is very large can displace the chest wall and respiratory muscles, causing easy fatigability.

Physical examination reveals dullness to percussion, decreased tactile fremitus, diminished breath sounds, and decreased transmitted breath sounds (whispered pectoriloquy, egophony). Large effusions may compress the underlying lung, creating focal crackles on deep inspiration immediately above the fluid. Other lung findings reflect the underlying cause of the effusion. Pulmonary function tests reveal a restrictive defect (decreased vital capacity and total lung capacity with a normal ratio of the forced expiratory volume in 1 second to the forced vital capacity [FEV_1/FVC ratio]), if the effusion is moderately large.

CLINICAL APPROACH.   Because the main significance of effusions is that they may indicate an underlying illness that requires specific diagnosis and treatment, the clinical examination should focus on symptoms of infection; rashes or joint findings (suggesting connective tissue disease); adenopathy, clubbing, or organomegaly (suggesting cancer); and elevated central venous pressure, an S_3 gallop, or edema (suggesting CHF). A review of old and recent chest radiographs, which may show as little as 100 to 200 ml of fluid, is essential in determining the chronicity and size of the effusion. Bilateral decubitus films reveal not only the amount of fluid and whether it is free-flowing, but also may reveal subdiaphragmatic effusions or underlying parenchymal disease. Lack of movement suggests the diagnoses of pleural mass, fibrosis, or loculated fluid from infection. Laboratory tests that should be performed in most patients without an obvious cause of their effusion include BUN, creatinine, thyroid function tests, antinuclear antibody, rheumatoid factor, sputum analysis for tuberculosis, and sputum cytologies.

If there is any doubt about the cause of the effusion and if thoracentesis is safe, a sample of pleural fluid should be obtained and analyzed for cell counts, lactate dehydrogenase (LDH), glucose, protein, amylase, cytology, Gram stain and culture (aerobic and anaerobic organisms), and pH. Most patients should undergo thoracentesis the initial evaluation, with the possible exception of patients with obvious CHF and a right-sided effusion. Even in patients with CHF, however, it is probably better to perform a small-volume diagnostic tap prior to aggressive diuresis, because diuresis may convert a transudate into an exudate. If the patient is febrile, thoracentesis should be aggressively pursued to exclude the presence of an empyema. Serum for glucose, LDH, and protein determinations should also be obtained simultaneously to calculate the pleural fluid:serum ratios of LDH and protein. These ratios determine whether the fluid is an exudate (LDH ratio > 0.6 or protein ratio > 0.5) or a transudate. Exudates are caused by many different diseases, whereas the causes of transudates are limited to CHF, hypothyroidism, nephrotic syndrome, severe hypoalbuminemia, and Meigs' syndrome. The finding of a transudate is reassuring since it makes cancer, infection, collagen vascular disease, and many other dangerous causes of effusions much less likely.

Some pleural fluid abnormalities may suggest an etiology or narrow the differential diagnosis. Bloody effusions ($>10^5$ RBCs/ml) suggest tumor, trauma, tuberculosis, or a leaking thoracic aortic aneurysm. A very low glucose ($<$ 10 g/dl) suggests that either empyema, tuberculosis, or rheumatoid arthritis is causing the effusion. Very low pH values occur from many causes but raise the question of a partially treated empyema or a parapneumonic effusion that is likely to loculate. Chylous effusions (triglyceride > 110 mg/dl) occur most commonly with traumatic thoracic duct damage or lymphoma.

Unexplained exudative effusions require pleural biopsy, especially if cancer or tuberculosis is being considered in the differential diagnosis. Thoracoscopy with visually guided biopsies has an even higher yield and may be required to diagnose mesothelioma. Bronchoscopy should be performed if there is volume loss in the lung on the side of the effusion, suggesting endobronchial obstruction from malignancy. Approximately 5% of effusions remain unexplained after careful assessment.

MANAGEMENT.   Appropriate treatment is determined by the symptoms (if any), cause, and rapidity of recurrence. Large, symptomatic effusions should be drained, initially by thoracentesis, with repeat radiography to assess the rate of recurrence. An empyema requires hospitalization, complete drainage, and appropriate parenteral antibiotic therapy. Whether a low pH, parapneumonic effusion without loculation and negative Gram stain and culture should be drained with a chest tube is controversial. Chest wall resection of metastatic or primary lung tumors involving the pleura usually is not attempted because of poor outcome. Symptomatic malignant effusions that recur despite intermittent large-volume thoracentesis (1–1.5 liters each) respond to pleurodesis with tetracycline in 50% to 70% of patients. Patients with bloody effusions due to trauma or pneumothorax should be completely drained because resulting adhesions may trap the lung and prevent expansion. Intrapleural instillation of thrombolytic agents may break up loculations and adhesions.

Cross-references: Pleuritic Chest Pain (Section 61), Pulmonary Function Testing (Section 69), Thoracentesis (Section 70).

REFERENCES

1. Chretien J, Hirsch A, Eds. Diseases of the Pleura. Masson Publishing, New York, 1983.
    A richly illustrated summary of European views with somewhat greater emphasis on cellular mechanisms and pathogenesis.

2. Lemmer JH, Botham MJ, Orringer MB. Modern management of adult thoracic empyema. J Thorac Cardiovasc Surg 1985;90:849–855.
    A review of 70 patients, emphasizing the role of early operative intervention.

3. Light RW. Pleural Diseases, 2nd ed. Lea & Febiger, Philadelphia, 1990.
    A comprehensive, well-written review of pleural diseases.

4. Sahn SA, Light RW. The sun should never set on a parapneumonic effusion. Chest 1989;95:945–946.
    Emphasizes the importance of looking aggressively for empyema when patients present with a parapneumonic effusion.

5. Wiener-Kronish JP, Matthay MA. Pleural effusions associated with hydrostatic and increased permeability pulmonary edema. Chest 1988;93:852–858.
    How effusions occur in heart failure or lung injury.

66 UPPER RESPIRATORY INFECTION

Problem

SHAWN J. SKERRETT

EPIDEMIOLOGY. Infections of the upper respiratory tract, including the overlapping clinical syndromes of the common cold, influenza, sinusitis, otitis media, pharyngitis, and laryngitis, are the most common acute illnesses of man. Adults average two to four colds per year, with exposure to children in the home an important risk factor. Colds occur year-round, with different viruses prominent in each season. Sinusitis and otitis media are infrequent complications of common colds, developing in fewer than 1% of cases in adults. Influenza occurs every winter, with overall attack rates of 10% to 20%; these rates are higher in epidemic and pandemic years. Lower respiratory tract complications of influenza, including tracheobronchitis and viral or bacterial pneumonia, develop in 10% of all patients, mainly in a high-risk group composed of persons over age 65, residents of chronic care facilities, and people with diabetes, immunodeficiencies, hemoglobinopathies, and chronic heart, lung, or kidney disease.

Although most upper respiratory tract infections do not come to medical attention, acute respiratory symptoms are the most common reasons for consulting a physician, accounting for 14% of outpatient physician contacts in 1980. Over 40% of time lost from work and school is due to acute respiratory illnesses.

The common cold is caused by rhinoviruses in 30% to 40% of cases in adults, coronavirus in 10% to 20%, other respiratory viruses in 10% to 20%, and unidentified agents in 30% to 40%. Laryngitis is viral in origin in over 90% of cases; the most common causes are influenza virus, rhinovirus, adenovirus, and parainfluenza virus. The etiologic agents of otitis, pharyngitis, and sinusitis are discussed in other chapters.

SYMPTOMS AND SIGNS. The clinical manifestations of the common cold are familiar to everyone. After a 2- to 5-day incubation period, the prototypic rhinovirus infection begins with a scratchy discomfort in the throat, followed by rhinorrhea (initially watery, then mucopurulent), nasal congestion, sneezing, and cough. Fever is rare, and low grade when present. The acute symptoms usually resolve within 7 days, but cough due to postnasal drip, viral tracheobronchitis, or bronchial hyperreactivity may persist for several weeks. Symptoms of sinusitis may include facial or dental pain, fever, anosmia, and purulent nasal discharge. Ear pain, drainage, and hearing loss are common manifestations of otitis media. Influenza may present with symptoms similar to the common cold, but nasal features are typically less prominent, while cough and systemic manifestations such as fever, malaise, headache, and myalgias are more severe. Most symptoms of uncomplicated influenza resolve within 7 days, but lassitude and cough may persist for weeks.

Examination of the patient with the common cold reveals erythema and crusting of the nares, erythema and edema of the nasal mucosa, and nasal discharge; mild pharyngeal injection may be seen. The presence of a pharyngeal exudate and tender cervical adenopathy is suggestive of bacterial pharyngitis, mononucleosis, or adenovirus infection; the latter often causes an associated conjunctivitis (pharyngoconjunctival fever). Vesicles on the palate suggest infection with coxsackievirus or herpes simplex virus. A purulent nasal discharge, facial tenderness, and opacification on transillumination are indicative of sinusitis. Otitis media is diagnosed from the presence of fluid in the middle ear, most reliably identified by an immobile tympanic membrane on pneumatic otoscopy.

CLINICAL APPROACH.   Most patients with upper respiratory infections are self-diagnosed; evaluation is directed at confirming the diagnosis and excluding complications. Allergic and vasomotor rhinitis may mimic the common cold but can be distinguished by the exposure history and chronicity, respectively. Influenza should be differentiated from the common cold on the basis of clinical features. A specific virologic diagnosis of colds and influenza is unnecessary. The clinical approaches to pharyngitis, otitis media, sinusitis, and pneumonia are discussed in separate sections.

MANAGEMENT.   The treatment of the common cold is aimed at relief of symptoms (Table 66–1). Sympathomimetics effectively relieve nasal congestion but do not reduce rhinorrhea. Topical decongestants are at least as effective as oral agents and have fewer side effects, but rebound symptoms may occur if topical decongestants are used for more than 3 or 4 days. Topical parasympatholytics, such as ipratropium bromide, appear to be effective in reducing nasal discharge but are not yet available for this indication. The use of antihistamines is controversial, but their anticholinergic effects may help dry unwanted secretions. Acetaminophen and aspirin are helpful for pain and fever. Multiple combination preparations should be avoided. There is no role for antibacterial antibiotics, and antiviral therapy for the common cold remains elusive. Although topical interferon-α_2 has shown prophylactic efficacy, its therapeutic activity has been disappointing, and irritation of the nasal mucosa has been a limiting side effect. Vitamin C, zinc, and countless folk remedies are popular but of unproven value.

Vaccination is effective in preventing influenza A and B and should be offered to all high-risk patients. Amantadine is effective in preventing influenza A and should be considered as a supplement to vaccination for prophylaxis in high-risk patients during an outbreak of influenza A. Amantadine also is effective as therapy for influenza A if given within 48 hours of the onset of symptoms, and therapeutic use should be considered in high-risk patients. The pro-

TABLE 66–1.   OVER-THE-COUNTER NASAL DECONGESTANTS (WITH REPRESENTATIVE DRUGS)

Medication	Dose	Cost ($)[1]
Topical Sympathomimetics		
Phenylephrine 0.5%	2–3 sprays or drops q.i.d.	
Dristan		3.39 (15 ml)
Neo-synephrine		3.25 (15 ml)
Vicks Sinex		3.10 (15 ml)
Naphazoline 0.05%	2–3 sprays or drops q.i.d.	
Privine		2.59 (15 ml)
Oxymetazoline 0.05%	2–3 sprays or drops b.i.d.	
Afrin		3.84 (15 ml)
Dristan Long Lasting		3.68 (15 ml)
Neo-synephrine 12 Hour		3.29 (15 ml)
Xylometazoline 0.1%	2–3 sprays or drops b.i.d.	
Otrivin		4.02 (15 ml)
Oral Sympathomimetics		
Pseudoephedrine	60 mg q.i.d. or 120 mg b.i.d.	
Sudafed		3.23 (24 tabs, 30 mg)
Sympathomimetic/Antihistamine Combinations		
Pseudoephedrine plus	60 mg q.i.d. or 120 mg b.i.d.	
Brompheniramine	6 mg q.i.d. or 12 mg b.i.d.	
Bromfed		4.93 (120 ml, 5 ml = 30/2[2])
Pseudoephedrine plus	60 mg q.i.d. or 120 mg b.i.d..	
Chlorpheniramine	4 mg q.i.d. or 8 mg b.i.d.	
Allerest Max Strength		3.50 (24 tabs, 30/2)
Sinarest Tabs		3.14 (20 tabs, 30/2)
Sudafed Plus		4.08 (24 tabs, 60/4)
Phenylpropanolamine plus	25 mg q.i.d. or 75 mg b.i.d.	
Brompheniramine	4–6 mg q.i.d. or 12 mg b.i.d.	
Dimetapp Tabs		3.74 (24 tabs, 25/4)
Phenylpropanolamine plus	25 mg q.i.d. or 75 mg b.i.d.	
Chlorpheniramine	4 mg q.i.d. or 8 mg b.i.d.	
Contac		6.25 (20 tabs, 25/4)
Coricidin		3.84 (24 tabs, 12.5/2[3])
Triaminic Cold Tabs		3.30 (24 tabs, 12.5/2[4])

[1]Average wholesale price, 1991 *Drug Topics Red Book.*
[2]30/2 means the tablet or dose listed contains 30 mg of the first medication listed and 2 mg of the second medication.
[3]Also contains 325 mg acetaminophen, 30 mg dextromethorphan.
[4]Also contains 325 mg acetaminophen.

phylactic dose is 200 mg/day through the period of exposure, and the therapeutic dose is 200 mg, followed by 100 mg/day for 5 days. The dose must be reduced for renal dysfunction and age over 65 years. Rimantadine has equal efficacy with fewer gastrointestinal and central nervous system (CNS) side effects, but is not yet available. The treatment of sinusitis, pharyngitis, and otitis are discussed elsewhere.

FOLLOW-UP.   Follow-up of the common cold is unneccessary unless patients develop symptoms of otitis or sinusitis. Patients with influenza, particularly the elderly, should be warned about lower respiratory tract symptoms (dyspnea, worsening cough, recurrence of fever) that suggest the development of pneumonia.

Cross-references: Adult Immunization (Section 10), Pharyngitis (Section 54), Otitis Media and Externa (Section 56), Sinusitis (Section 57), Cough and Sputum (Section 63), Lower Respiratory Infection (Section 67).

REFERENCES

1. Douglas RG. Prophylaxis and treatment of influenza. N Engl J Med 1990;322:443–450.
    Current recommendations for the use of vaccines and amantadine.

2. Lowenstein SR, Parrino TA. Management of the common cold. Adv Intern Med 1987;32:207–233.
    An engaging review of fact and fancy.

3. Macknin ML, Mathew S, Medendorp SV. Effect of inhaling heated vapor on symptoms of the common cold. JAMA 1990;264:989–991.
    Chicken soup revisited? A negative study.

4. Sperber SJ, Hayden FG. Chemotherapy of rhinovirus colds. Antimicrob Agents Chemother 1988;32:409–419.
    A review of past experience and future prospects.

67 LOWER RESPIRATORY INFECTION

Problem

SHAWN J. SKERRETT

EPIDEMIOLOGY/ETIOLOGY.   Lower respiratory infections include tracheobronchitis and pneumonia. In the United States, there are over 3 million cases of community-acquired pneumonia in adults each year, leading to more than 500,000 hospital admissions. Risk factors for lower respiratory infection include chronic airway disease (such as chronic bronchitis, bronchiectasis, or bronchogenic carcinoma), an aspiration diathesis (such as alcoholism or seizure disorder), recent upper respiratory infection (especially influenza), advanced age, and immunodeficiency.

Table 67–1 lists the common agents causing community-acquired pneumonia in hospitalized patients. *Mycoplasma, Chlamydia,* and viruses often cause relatively mild illnesses that are typically treated in the ambulatory setting, and may be underrepresented in the table. Acute tracheobronchitis is most often caused by viruses, followed by *Mycoplasma pneumoniae* and *Chlamydia pneumoniae.* Acute exacerbations of chronic bronchitis associated with purulent sputum are commonly due to *Haemophilus influenzae, Streptococcus pneumoniae,* and *Moraxella (Branhamella) catarrhalis.*

SYMPTOMS AND SIGNS. Acute tracheobronchitis presents with cough, often productive, and usually with concurrent or recent symptoms of upper respiratory infection. Examination may reveal rhonchi or wheezes, but there are no signs of pneumonia.

The cardinal symptoms of pneumonia are cough (75%–90% of cases, productive in 60%–70%) and fever (60%–70%). Dyspnea and chills each occur in about 50%, and chest pain in 30% to 40%. Most patients have fever, often with tachycardia and tachypnea. Chest examination findings are abnormal in over 90% of patients, revealing crackles, diminished breath sounds, rhonchi, and egophony, in decreasing order of frequency. Elderly patients may present with more subtle signs, such as an isolated alteration in mental status.

CLINICAL APPROACH. Routine laboratory tests should include chest radiography, CBC, and, when available, sputum for Gram stain and culture. Although most patients with fever, cough, and an infiltrate on chest radiographs are infected, a similar presentation can result from a variety of noninfectious processes such as pulmonary embolism, gastric aspiration, malignancy, drug toxicity, hypersensitivity, and vasculitis.

Clues to the cause of pneumonia may be found in the patient's medical history. Alcoholism, diabetes mellitus, and chronic renal failure are associated with colonization of the upper respiratory tract with gram-negative bacilli and *S. aureus,* and an increased risk of pneumonia due to these organisms (although pneumococcus is the most common agent in this group of patients). The lower

TABLE 67–1. ETIOLOGIC AGENTS OF COMMUNITY-ACQUIRED PNEUMONIA IN HOSPITALIZED PATIENTS

Organism	% of Cases
Streptococcus pneumoniae	10–50
Haemophilus influenzae	5–15
Viruses	5–15
Mycoplasma pneumoniae	2–15
Chlamydia pneumoniae	5–10
Legionella spp.	1–25
Mixed oral flora	3–15
Pneumocystis carinii	2–?
Gram-negative bacilli	1–8
Staphylococcus aureus	1–8
Unknown	30–50

respiratory tract of patients with COPD is often colonized with pneumococcus, *H. influenzae,* or *M. catarrhalis,* predisposing to infection with these agents. Neutropenia or defective neutrophil function predisposes to infection with gram-negative bacilli, *S. aureus,* and *Aspergillus.* Impaired humoral immunity, as may be found in multiple myeloma or chronic lymphocytic leukemia, leads to an increased risk of infection with encapsulated organisms such as pneumococcus and *H. influenzae.* Defective cell-mediated immunity, as in HIV infection, lymphoma, or corticosteroid therapy, increases the risk of infection with mycobacteria, *Legionella,* fungi, cytomegalovirus, and *Pneumocystis carinii.* Pneumonia in previously healthy young adults is usually caused by *Mycoplasma pneumoniae, Chlamydia pneumoniae,* a respiratory virus, pneumococcus, or *H. influenzae.*

The clinician should inquire about exposure to specific infectious agents. Illness in the community may suggest influenza or other virus, and exposure to sick children raises the possibility of *Mycoplasma* infection. Residence in a dormitory or barracks increases the risk of epidemic infection with *M. pneumoniae, C. pneumoniae, Neisseria meningitidis,* or adenovirus. Nursing home residents are at risk for outbreaks of influenza, respiratory syncytial virus, and tuberculosis, as well as staphylococcal and gram-negative infection. A travel history may suggest exposure to geographically restricted airborne fungi such as *Histoplasma* (Ohio, Mississippi, and Missouri river valleys), *Blastomyces* (central and southeastern United States), and *Coccidioides* (southwestern United States), or regionally distributed bacteria such as *Pseudomonas pseudomallei* (Southeast Asia) and *Legionella* (often resident in community water towers and hot water systems of old hotels). Also helpful is an occupational or recreational history of exposure to poultry or birds of the parrot family (psittacosis), domestic livestock such as cattle, sheep, and goats (Q fever, brucellosis, and anthrax), and wild rodents (tularemia and plague).

The typical acute pneumonia syndrome consisting of an abrupt onset of fever, chills, pleuritic chest pain, and cough productive of purulent sputum suggests infection with pyogenic bacteria such as pneumococcus, staphylococcus, or *H. influenzae.* The atypical pneumonia syndrome, defined by a more insidious onset, nonproductive cough, and prominent extrathoracic symptoms such as headache and myalgias, is commonly associated with *Mycoplasma, Chlamydia,* viruses, and Q fever (*Coxiella burnetti*). There is substantial overlap between these syndromes, however.

The chest radiograph may reveal evidence of endobronchial obstruction, such as mass lesions or volume loss. Lobar or segmental consolidation is usually due to a bacterial process, whereas bilateral mixed alveolar-interstitial infiltrates most likely represent viral or *Pneumocystis* infection. Nodular infiltrates suggest fungi, mycobacteria, *Legionella,* or *Nocardia.* Cavitation usually indicates infection with mixed anaerobes, gram-negative bacilli, *S. aureus,* hemolytic streptococci, fungi, or mycobacteria. Pleural effusions are evidence against viral or *Mycoplasma* infection. All parapneumonic effusions producing more than blunting of the costophrenic angle should be tapped to exclude empyema.

A sputum Gram stain with fewer than 10 squamous epithelial cells per low power field and a single predominant organism is very accurate in directing therapy. Unfortunately, a diagnostic Gram stain is available in less than 50% of patients with community-acquired pneumonia. Other rapid diagnostic methods, which detect microbial antigens or nucleic acids in respiratory specimens, are expensive and usually unnecessary in the outpatient setting. In patients with acute purulent bronchitis, microbiologic studies of sputum are necessary only if empirical therapy has failed.

MANAGEMENT. The indications for hospital admission include (1) features of severe illness, including hypotension (systolic blood pressure < 90 mm Hg), marked tachycardia (heart rate > 140), altered mental status, respiratory distress or hypoxemia (arterial Po_2 < 60 mm Hg or oxygen saturation <90% by pulse oximetry), evidence of a suppurative complication (such as empyema or metastatic infection), or severe hematologic or metabolic abnormalities (such as neutropenia, marked hyponatremia, or new azotemia); (2) a high risk for a complicated course because of immunodeficiency, postobstructive pneumonia, or suspected infection with particularly virulent organisms, such as *S. aureus* and gram-negative bacilli; and (3) suspicion of an opportunistic or unusual infections that warrants further diagnostic evaluation under observation. Further, hospital admission should be considered in patients over the age of 65 years, those with underlying chronic disease that may impair host defenses or pulmonary reserve (such as chronic renal insufficiency, diabetes mellitus, congestive heart failure, and COPD), and patients whose socioeconomic circumstances interfere with reliable treatment and follow-up.

The antibiotic treatment of pneumonia should be based on the sputum Gram stain, when possible. Empiric therapy can be directed toward the likely etiologic agents according to risk factors and clinical presentation, but erythromycin (500 mg q.i.d.) is usually the drug of choice in adults with nondiagnostic sputum. Antibiotics are unnecessary in most cases of acute bronchitis, but patients with underlying COPD and newly purulent sputum may benefit from treatment with ampicillin, trimethoprim-sulfamethoxazole, or tetracycline.

FOLLOW-UP. Treatment failures result from an incorrect presumptive etiologic diagnosis, obstruction to bronchial drainage, development of a suppurative complication such as empyema, or noncompliance. Patients should be seen routinely within 1 week and should be advised to return for increasing dyspnea or chest pain, alteration in mental status, or persistent fever after 3 days of treatment. All patients with pneumonia should undergo follow-up chest radiography 6 to 12 weeks after presentation to document complete resolution.

Cross-references: AIDS (Section 14), Pleural Effusion (Section 65), Upper Respiratory Infection (Section 66), Asthma and Chronic Obstructive Pulmonary Disease (Section 68).

REFERENCES

1. Boldy DAR, Skidmore SJ, Ayres JG. Acute bronchitis in the community: Clinical features, infective factors, changes in pulmonary function and bronchial reactivity to histamine. Respir Med 1990;84:377–385.

    A prospective study of 42 episodes in 40 patients without underlying lung disease. An etiology was identified in 12 episodes (viral or mycoplasmal in 11 of 12), and 37% of patients had reactive airways 6 weeks after presentation.

2. Fang G-D, Fine M, Orloff J, Arisumi D, Yu VL, Kapoor W, Grayston JT, Wang SP, Kohler R, Muder RR, Yee YC, Rihs JD, Vickers RM. New and emerging etiologies for community-acquired pneumonia with implications for therapy: A prospective multicenter study of 359 cases. Medicine (Baltimore) 1990;69:307–316.

    At three hospitals in Pittsburgh, the most common pathogens were pneumococcus, *H. influenzae, Legionella,* and *Chlamydia pneumoniae.* No specific pathogen was identified in 41% of patients.

3. Fine MJ, Smith DN, Singer DE. Hospitalization decision in patients with community-acquired pneumonia: A prospective cohort study. Am J Med 1990;89:713–721.

    Among 170 patients not severely ill at presentation, two or more of the following were predictive of a complicated course: age > 65 years, comorbid illness, temperature > 38.3°C, immunosuppression, and high-risk etiology (staphylococci, gram-negative bacilli, aspiration, or postobstructive).

4. Heckerling PS, Tape TG, Wigton RS, Hissong KK, Leiken JB, Ornato JP, Cameron JL, Racht EM. Clinical prediction rule for pulmonary infiltrates. Ann Intern Med 1990;113:664–670.

    Among patients with acute respiratory complaints, the following were independent predictors of radiographic infiltrates: temperature > 37.8°C, pulse > 100 beats/min, rales, decreased breath sounds, and the absence of asthma.

5. Macfarlane JT. Treatment of lower respiratory infections. Lancet 1987;2:1446–1449.

    A brief review.

68 ASTHMA AND CHRONIC OBSTRUCTIVE PULMONARY DISEASE

Problem

SHAWN J. SKERRETT

DEFINITIONS AND EPIDEMIOLOGY. Asthma is a clinical syndrome of episodic symptoms associated with reversible air flow obstruction and bronchial hyperreactivity. COPD is defined by progressive symptoms and irreversible air flow obstruction. The two major components of COPD are chronic bronchitis, defined by a productive cough on most days for at least 3 months in 2 consecutive years, and emphysema, defined anatomically by the destruction of alveolar walls and clinically by progressive air flow limitation, hyperexpansion, and reduced diffusing capacity for carbon monoxide (DL_{CO}). There is considerable overlap between asthma and COPD.

Asthma afflicts 3% to 5% of the adult population and accounts for 1% of outpatient visits. The mortality from asthma is rising, particularly among blacks and the elderly. COPD is found in 5% to 10% of the adult population, predominantly smokers, and is the fifth leading cause of death.

SYMPTOMS AND SIGNS.   Most patients with asthma have episodes of cough, wheeze, chest tightness, and dyspnea, separated by symptom-free intervals. Some patients have chronic symptoms punctuated by exacerbations, and cough may be the only manifestation. Common precipitating factors include airborne allergens and nonspecific stimuli such as cold air, irritants, and exercise. COPD typically presents as gradually progressive dyspnea on exertion, chronic productive cough, or both. Many patients with COPD have periodic exacerbations of symptoms, often associated with upper respiratory infections, changes in weather, or exposure to irritants.

The physical examination of the asthmatic patient with mild or absent symptoms may be normal. Diffuse wheezing is often apparent on chest auscultation, but may be detectable only on forced exhalation. An inspiratory to expiratory ratio of less than 1 may be the only indication of air flow obstruction. Evidence of atopy may be present, including skin rashes, coryza, nasal polyps, postnasal drip, serous otitis media, and tenderness and opacification of the sinuses. Examination during an acute asthma attack reveals agitation and respiratory distress; the patient may be unable to speak in complete sentences. Somnolence or confusion indicate exhaustion and impending ventilatory failure. Tachycardia and tachypnea are typically present, and a pulsus paradoxus (an inspiratory fall in systolic blood pressure of greater than 10 mm Hg) suggests severe obstruction. The use of accessory muscles (sternocleidomastoids and intercostals) to assist in breathing is another sign of a severe attack. Auscultation of the chest in this setting usually reveals diffuse wheezing, but a quiet chest is ominous, indicating very little air movement.

The physical signs of COPD include evidence of chronic air flow obstruction and the sequelae of ventilatory fatigue and hypoxemia. The patient with severe COPD typically sits upright, leaning forward onto supporting elbows to optimize lung mechanics and facilitate the use of accessory muscles. Pursed-lip breathing is common, and serves to maintain positive pressure in the large airways, thereby resisting collapse during active exhalation. Muscular wasting may result from the high caloric expenditure associated with the work of breathing in COPD, coupled with poor oral intake. Cyanosis may be due to hypoxemia, and plethora suggests compensatory erythrocytosis. The hyperexpanded chest has an increased anteroposterior diameter, and percussion demonstrates hyperresonance and low diaphragms. Auscultation typically reveals diminished breath sounds, rhonchi, wheezes or prolonged exhalation, and coarse crackles. Heart sounds are often distant and disguised by lung sounds in COPD, but a loud P_2 suggests pulmonary hypertension. Right ventricular failure is manifested by wide splitting of S_2, parasternal gallops, and tricuspid regurgitation. Other signs of cor pulmonale include elevated jugular venous pressure, tender hepatomegaly (pulsatile with prominent tricuspid regurgitation), ascites, and peripheral edema.

CLINICAL APPROACH.   In taking the history, the pattern of symptoms should be defined as progressive or intermittent, and any relation to time of day, day of week, or season should be noted. Precipitating factors and potentially contributory conditions such as sinusitis and gastroesophageal reflux should be identified. Patients should be questioned regarding smoking habits and exposure to other airborne pollutants at work, home, or play. A history of atopy and a family history of lung disease also may be relevant.

All patients with suspected air flow limitation should undergo pulmonary function testing. The diagnosis of asthma can be confirmed by the demonstration of air flow obstruction that is reversible over time or in response to bronchodilators. In contrast, COPD is associated with air flow obstruction that is progressive and predominantly irreversible. Substantial overlap exists: some patients with asthma develop chronic air flow obstruction ("asthmatic bronchitis"), and some patients with COPD have partially reversible air flow obstruction, or an "asthmatic" component. A low DLco in association with air flow obstruction is suggestive of emphysema. In patients with episodic symptoms compatible with asthma but in whom no evidence of air flow obstruction is found at the time of spirometry, a therapeutic trial of bronchodilators can be given or methacholine challenge testing can be used to identify bronchial hyperreactivity. A suspicion of exercise-induced asthma can be confirmed by spirometry immediately following exercise. The use of a hand-held peak flow meter at work and at home to record fluctuations in air flow throughout the day can be helpful in the diagnosis of occupational asthma and as a guide to management.

The chest radiograph may be of value in the evaluation of COPD. Flattened diaphragms, hyperlucency, and increased anteroposterior diameter are signs of air flow obstruction. Bullae and distal pruning of the vasculature suggest emphysema. Coarse reticular markings and peribronchial cuffing are consistent with chronic bronchitis. A descending right pulmonary artery greater than 16 mm in diameter suggests pulmonary hypertension, and an enlarged right ventricle and dilated azygos vein may be seen in cor pulmonale.

Blood studies in COPD may reveal erythrocytosis secondary to chronic hypoxemia or an elevated serum bicarbonate level in compensation for chronic respiratory acidosis. Eosinophilia is common in asthma. Arterial blood gases should be obtained in all patients with COPD and an FEV_1 of less than 1 to 1.5 liters or the clinical suspicion of hypoxemia or hypercarbia. Hereditary α_1-antitrypsin deficiency should be considered in nonsmoking patients with emphysema and smokers with accelerated or early-onset emphysema (fourth or fifth decade), particularly if the chest radiograph shows bullous changes that are predominantly located in the lower lobes.

The differential diagnosis of cough, wheeze, and dyspnea includes acute bronchitis, cystic fibrosis, bronchiectasis, upper airway obstruction, focal bronchial obstruction, interstitial lung disease, mitral stenosis, congestive heart failure, and pulmonary embolism. Viral respiratory tract infection can cause bronchial hyperreactivity that is indistinguishable from asthma but resolves within 8 weeks. Cystic fibrosis and other forms of bronchiectasis can usually be separated from asthma by the chronicity of symptoms, the copious production of purulent sputum, and abnormal chest radiographs. Upper respiratory obstruction typically causes stridor, in which wheezing is audible during both inspiration and exhalation, and can be differentiated from asthma in the pulmonary function laboratory by a flow-volume loop. Wheezing due to focal bronchial obstruction by tumor, foreign body, or stenosis is unilateral and often accompanied by radiographic abnormalities. Some interstitial lung diseases, such as sarcoidosis, eosinophilic granuloma, and lymphangioleiomyomatosis, may present with cough and wheeze, but these symptoms are usually accompanied by progressive dyspnea, auscultation of the chest often reveals crackles, the chest radiograph will show typical interstitial infiltrates, and pulmonary function tests will reveal a restrictive defect. Mitral stenosis and left ventricular failure can be distinguished by cardiac examination, and pulmonary embolism by the abrupt onset of dyspnea and other clinical features.

MANAGEMENT.   Asthma and COPD are not curable diseases. The goals of treatment are to relieve symptoms, improve functional status, prevent exacerbations, and prolong life. The components of management include (1) education regarding the nature of the disease and its treatment; (2) identification and avoidance of exacerbating factors such as allergens, irritants (including cigarette smoke and occupational exposures), drugs (such as aspirin and beta blockers), and infection; and (3) medication.

The bronchodilator and anti-inflammatory medications commonly given by inhalation to treat air flow obstruction are listed in Table 68–1. The effective administration of these medications requires that patients be instructed and repeatedly tested in the proper use of metered-dose inhalers. At the end of a normal tidal exhalation (functional residual capacity), the preshaken inhaler is held 4 cm from the open mouth and actuated once after initiation of a slow deep inhalation. At the end of inspiration the breath is held for 5 to 10 seconds, and tidal breathing is resumed. Each actuation (puff) should be separated by 1 minute. The use of a spacer should be considered in patients who have difficulty coordinating this procedure: the metered-dose inhaler is actuated into the spacer, then the patient takes a slow, deep breath and holds at total lung capacity for 5 to 10 seconds.

Most patients with asthma can be treated with an inhaled β_2-adrenergic agonist such as metaproterenol or albuterol used in response to symptoms and in anticipation of symptoms (before exercise, for example). An inhaled cortico-

TABLE 68–1. INHALED BRONCHODILATOR AND ANTI-INFLAMMATORY MEDICATIONS AVAILABLE IN METERED-DOSE INHALERS

Generic Name	Initial Dose	Brand Name	Cost/200 Puffs ($)[1]
β-Agonists			
Epinephrine	2 puffs q.4h.	Primatene	6.55
Isoproterenol	2 puffs q.4h.	Isuprel	15.17
Isoetharine	2 puffs q.4h.	Bronkometer	15.17
Metaproterenol	2 puffs q.4h.	Alupent	15.56
		Metaprel	8.76
Albuterol	2 puffs q.4–6h.	Ventolin	17.90
		Proventil	17.90
Terbutaline	2 puffs q.4–6h.	Brethaire	11.33
Bitolterol	2 puffs q.4–6h.	Tornalate	13.84
Pirbuterol	2 puffs q.4–6h.	Maxair	10.04
Anticholinergic			
Ipratropium	2 puffs q.6h.	Atrovent	21.44
Anti-inflammatory			
Cromolyn	2 puffs q.i.d.	Intal	47.69
Beclomethasone	2 puffs q.i.d.	Vanceril	23.61
Triamcinolone	2 puffs q.i.d.	Azmacort	25.20
Flunisolide	2 puffs b.i.d.	Aerobid	61.10

[1]Average wholesale price, 1991 *Drug Topics Red Book.*

steroid should be added if patients need to use β-adrenergic agonists on a daily basis, and can be given in doses up to 2 mg/day. Irritation of the throat and oral thrush can be avoided if the mouth is rinsed after the use of these agents. Cromolyn sodium is a helpful addition or alternative to inhaled corticosteroids, particularly in patients with allergic or exercise-induced asthma. Further benefit may be achieved in some patients by the addition of inhaled ipratropium bromide, high-dose β-adrenergic agonists delivered by nebulizer, or oral bronchodilators. Oral β-adrenergic agonists and oral theophylline are more toxic and less effective than inhaled bronchodilators, but have longer durations of action and may be particularly useful in patients with nocturnal symptoms. When symptoms are uncontrolled by the stepwise measures described above, oral prednisone (30–60 mg/day) should be added until full symptomatic recovery occurs, then tapered or stopped. If symptoms recur after discontinuation of corticosteroids, then prednisone should be maintained at the lowest effective daily or alternate-day dose and withdrawal attempted at a later date. Patients who cannot be weaned from oral corticosteroids should be referred to an allergist or pulmonologist for evaluation and consideration of alternative anti-inflammatory therapy.

Acute asthma attacks should be assessed by measurement of peak flow or FEV_1 and treated with oxygen and inhaled β-adrenergic agents delivered by nebulizer every 15 to 20 minutes. Subcutaneous epinephrine or terbutaline and inhaled anticholinergics may be effective in young adults who fail to respond to inhaled β-agonists, but theophylline probably adds toxicity without improving outcome. After one hour of treatment, further decisions should be based on clinical assessment and measurements of air flow: if peak flow or FEV_1 improves to greater than 70% of predicted, the patient can be discharged on bronchodilators; if air flow measurements are below 70% of predicted, the patient should be given oral or parenteral corticosteroids equivalent to 60 mg of prednisone. Patients with continued severe obstruction (air flow measurements < 40% of predicted) or evidence of ventilatory fatigue (e.g., somnolence or carbon dioxide retention) should be admitted. The decision to admit or continue outpatient treatment of patients with some clinical improvement and air flow measurements between 40% and 70% of predicted depends on the duration of the attack, the intensity of treatment before presentation, the severity of previous attacks, the time of day, and the reliability of supervision and follow-up.

Patients with COPD should be treated with inhaled bronchodilators on a regular schedule, even if no responsiveness to these agents is demonstrated by spirometry. Ipratropium bromide is a rational first choice in patients without a reversible component, but many patients prefer inhaled β-adrenergic agonists despite apparently fixed obstruction. The use of oral theophylline is controversial, but probably helpful in some patients. If a trial of theophylline is given, patients should be warned about potential toxic effects (such as gastrointestinal upset, palpitations, and agitation) and drug interactions (with cimetidine, phenytoin, and quinolones, for example). The theophylline dosage should be adjusted to maximum symptomatic benefit without side effects, usually found at a serum level of 10 to 15 mg/dl. Systemic corticosteroids (given as described above for asthma) are beneficial in acute exacerbations of COPD and in a minority of patients with stable COPD, particularly those with a reversible component. Inhaled corticosteroids are less effective for COPD than for asthma but should be tried in patients who are responsive to prednisone. Supplemental oxygen is the only treatment for COPD proven to prolong life. Continuous oxygen should be prescribed if the room air Pao_2 is 55 mm Hg or less or the arterial oxygen saturation (Sao_2) is 88% or less, or if the room air Pao_2 is 59 mm Hg or less or Sao_2 is 89% or less with cor pulmonale or polycythemia. Part-time oxygen should be given if there is evidence of significant desaturation during sleep or ambulation that can be corrected with supplemental oxygen. The need for supplemental oxygen should be reassessed after 1 to 3 months of therapy. Antibiotics such as trimethoprim-sulfamethoxazole (160/800 mg b.i.d.), amoxicillin (250–500 mg t.i.d.), and tetracycline (250–500 mg q.i.d.) may be effective in acute exacerbations of chronic bronchitis associated with purulent sputum. Low doses of codeine (10–30 mg t.i.d.) may be helpful in relieving severe chronic dyspnea, but side effects are often limiting, and there is a danger of depressed ventilatory drive.

Rehabilitation can assist patients with COPD in adapting to their progressive disability. Instruction in bronchial hygiene, pursed-lip breathing, and exercise conditioning; provision of devices such as shower chairs and electric carts to assist in daily activities; and attention to the psychosocial aspects of chronic disease can all be helpful. Smoking cessation is the single most important consideration in the management of COPD. Patients should receive a vaccination for influenza unless contraindicated.

FOLLOW-UP.   The interval between office visits for asthma and COPD will depend on the severity of symptoms, the frequency of exacerbations, and the complexity of treatment. Symptom control, the use of medications, and inhaler technique should be reviewed regularly. Patients with COPD should be monitored for evidence of hypoxemia and cor pulmonale, and spirometry should be repeated annually.

Asthma follows an unpredictable clinical course. The prognosis of COPD depends on the severity of air flow obstruction and the rate of decline in FEV_1. The 5-year survival of patients with an FEV_1 of less than 1 liter is approximately 50%, but substantial variation precludes accurate predictions of survival in individual patients.

Cross-references: Adult Immunization (Section 10), Smoking Cessation (Section 11), Screening for Occupational Lung Disease (Section 59), Cough and Sputum (Section 63), Upper Respiratory Infection (Section 66), Pulmonary Function Testing (Section 69), Dysphagia and Heartburn (Section 97).

REFERENCES

1.   Barnes PJ. A new approach to the treatment of asthma. N Engl J Med 1989;321:1517–1527.
     An excellent review emphasizing the inflammatory component of asthma.

2.   Dosman JA, Cockroft DW, Eds. Obstructive Lung Disease. Med Clin North Am 1990; 74:547–857.
     A collection of review articles on many aspects of asthma and COPD.

3.   George RB, Owens MW. Bronchial asthma. DM 1991;37:138–196.
     An excellent review of the pathophysiology, assessment, and treatment of asthma.

4.   Hodgkin JE, Ed. Chronic Obstructive Lung Disease. Clin Chest Med 1990;11:363–573.
     A dozen review articles on the subject.

5.   Mayo PH, Richman J, Harris HW. Results of a program to reduce admissions for adult asthma. Ann Intern Med 1990;112:864–871.
     In an inner city population of repeatedly hospitalized asthmatics, randomized referral to a special clinic emphasizing education, inhaled corticosteroids, and access to health care providers markedly reduced emergency visits and hospital admissions.

69 PULMONARY FUNCTION TESTING

Procedure

SHAWN J. SKERRETT

INDICATIONS/CONTRAINDICATIONS.   Common indications for pulmonary function testing include (1) the evaluation of patients with dyspnea, cough, or wheeze; (2) the screening of smokers for occult air flow obstruction or accelerated decline in FEV_1—markers for a high risk of developing COPD; (3) measuring bronchodilator responsiveness or the effect of corticosteroid treatment; (4) following the course of obstructive or restrictive defects; (5) monitoring of patients treated with potential pulmonary toxins, such as radiation or bleomycin; (6) preoperative evaluation; and (7) assessment of disability. The relative contraindications to pulmonary function testing include active airborne infection, and recent massive hemoptysis or pneumothorax.

RATIONALE.   Pulmonary function testing is used to identify air flow obstruction, restrictive defects in lung expansion, and abnormalities of the alveolar-capillary membrane. The measurements in common use include spirometry, peak expiratory flow rate, lung volumes, and the diffusing capacity of the lung for carbon monoxide (DLco). Normal values for pulmonary function tests are most accurately defined by the 95% confidence interval, or 1.64 SD from the predicted norm, but are commonly estimated as within 20% of the predicted value. Normal values for flow rates and volumes are influenced by sex, age, height, and race.

Spirometry, the measurement of air flow over time, is the simplest and most reproducible of these tests, and a variety of devices are available for use in the clinic. Figure 69–1 shows a normal spirogram, illustrating tidal breathing, a deep inhalation, and complete exhalation. The most useful spirometric measurements are the vital capacity (VC), the volume of air expelled by a slow (SVC) or forced (FVC) complete exhalation after full inhalation; and the forced expiratory volume in 1 second (FEV_1), the volume of air expelled in the first second of an FVC maneuver. Air flow obstruction is defined by a low FEV_1 and an FEV_1/FVC ratio below 0.75. Reduction in FEV_1 and FVC with a normal FEV_1/FVC ratio is consistent with a restrictive process, but this pattern may be seen in air flow obstruction if compression of large airways during forced exhalation reduces FVC and FEV_1 to a similar extent; in this case the SVC usually exceeds the FVC. A significant bronchodilator response is defined as a 15% improvement in FEV_1 or FVC measured 10 minutes after inhalation of a β-adrenergic agonist or 30 to 60 minutes after inhalation of ipratropium.

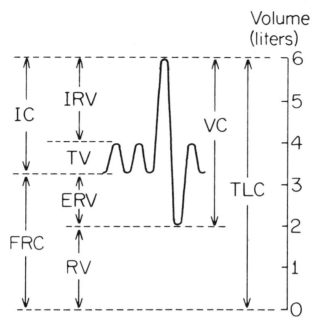

FIGURE 69–1. The normal spirogram and components of lung volume. (RV = residual volume, ERV = expiratory reserve volume, TV = tidal volume, IRV = inspiratory reserve volume, TLC = total lung capacity, VC = vital capacity, FRC = functional residual capacity, IC = inspiratory capacity. (Reproduced with permission from Culver B, Ed. The Respiratory System. University of Washington Health Sciences Academic Series, Seattle, 1990.)

Hand-held peak flow meters are a simple and inexpensive way to monitor air flow obstruction at home and in the clinic. The peak expiratory flow rate is linearly related to FEV_1, but more variable and effort dependent.

The measurement of lung volumes in the pulmonary function laboratory is required to define a restrictive defect. The four lung volumes and the four capacities they comprise are illustrated in Figure 69–1. These values are determined from spirometry and the measurement of functional residual capacity (FRC) by gas dilution or plethysmography. In the helium dilution method, the patient is connected to a closed circuit of helium at the end of a tidal breath (FRC), and allowed to breath to equilibrium; the helium concentration of exhaled gas will be diluted by FRC. In the nitrogen washout technique, the patient is connected to 100% oxygen at FRC and allowed to breath until nitrogen is no longer exhaled. FRC is calculated from the collected volume of expired nitrogen, assuming that nitrogen comprises 81% of alveolar gas. For plethysmography, the patient sits in an airtight chamber breathing through a mouthpiece, which is closed at FRC. The patient pants against the closed mouthpiece, and the resulting changes in thoracic volume and pressure are measured. The dilution methods measure communicating volume, which may underestimate total lung capacity in the presence of severe air flow obstruction with air trapping or bullous lung disease. Plethysmography measures the total volume of compressible air in the chest and is more accurate. A reduced total lung capacity defines a restrictive defect, found in interstitial lung disease, pulmonary resection, space-occupying intrathoracic abnormalities (such as pleural effusion, pneumonia, or tumor), chest wall defects, and neuromuscular disease. An elevated total lung capacity, residual volume, or total lung capacity–residual volume ratio suggests air trapping.

The diffusing capacity of carbon monoxide (DLco) is a useful indicator of alveolar-capillary gas exchange. The single-breath technique is most common: a known concentration of carbon monoxide is inhaled and held for 10 seconds, then the dilution of carbon monoxide is measured in the expired gas. DLco is low in conditions that reduce the surface area of the alveolar-capillary membrane (such as interstitial lung disease, pulmonary vascular disease, and emphysema) and when less hemoglobin is available for binding (as in anemia and in smokers with elevated carbon monoxide levels). An increased DLco may be seen with erythrocytosis, an elevated pulmonary blood volume (as in atrial septal defect or pregnancy), and alveolar hemorrhage.

Other tests commonly available in pulmonary function laboratories include measurements of inspiratory and expiratory pressures and maximum voluntary ventilation to evaluate respiratory muscle strength; methacholine challenge testing for the identification of bronchial hyperreactivity; and cardiopulmonary exercise testing to elicit oxygen desaturation, quantify impairment, and evaluate puzzling dyspnea.

METHODS.   Performance of the FVC maneuver with a spirometer should be explained and demonstrated. The patient is then instructed to inhale fully to inspiratory capacity, place his or her lips around the mouthpiece, and blow out forcefully until an acceptable end is reached: a plateau in the volume-time curve for at least 2 seconds with an exhalation of at least 6 seconds; an exhalation lasting more than 15 seconds without reaching a plateau; or, in the judgement of the clinician, the patient cannot or should not continue. Most patients require exhortation to complete the test. The use of nose clips is encouraged. After a brief rest, the test should be repeated until three satisfactory tracings are obtained. The largest FEV_1 and FVC are recorded, even if they come from different curves. The best two efforts should not differ by more than 5%. Common sources of error include hesitation, coughing, Valsalva maneuver, early termination, air leak, and an obstructed mouthpiece.

The measurement of peak expiratory flow with a peak flow meter requires a brief effort from full inhalation. The best of several measurements should be recorded.

COST/COMPLICATIONS.   Charges for spirometry range from $50 to $150, including interpretation. Charges for lung volume and DLco measurements are each in the range of $75 to $150. The FVC maneuver may precipitate coughing or bronchospasm.

Cross-references: Determining Disability (Section 5), Dyspnea (Section 19), Screening for Occupational Lung Disease (Section 59), Asthma and Chronic Obstructive Pulmonary Disease (Section 68), Preoperative Pulmonary Problems (Section 221).

REFERENCES

1. American Thoracic Society. Standardization of spirometry—1987 update. Am Rev Respir Dis 1987;136:1285–1298.
    Detailed recommendations regarding equipment, measurements, and interpretation.

2. Mahler DA, Ed. Pulmonary Function Testing. Clin Chest Med 1989;10:129–296.
    A collection of helpful and succinct reviews.

3. Nelson SB, Gardner RM, Crapo RO, Jensen RL. Performance evaluation of contemporary spirometers. Chest 1990;97:288–297.
    Only 35 of 62 devices were satisfactory; software problems were common.

4. Shapiro SM, Hendler JM, Ogirala RG, Aldrich TK, Shapiro MB. Evaluation of the accuracy of Assess and MiniWright peak flowmeters. Chest 1991;99:358–362.
    Two popular models performed well.

5. Zibrak JD, O'Donnel CR, Marton K. Indications for pulmonary function testing. Ann Intern Med 1990;112:763–771.
    A review of the role of pulmonary function testing in predicting postoperative outcomes, accompanied by a position paper from the American College of Physicians.

70 THORACENTESIS

Procedure

SHAWN J. SKERRETT

INDICATIONS/CONTRAINDICATIONS.   Diagnostic thoracentesis is indicated for the evaluation of pleural effusions of unknown etiology. Therapeutic thoracentesis is indicated for the reduction of large pleural effusions in dyspneic patients. The contraindications to thoracentesis include a bleeding diathesis, an uncooperative patient, infection of overlying skin, and a volume of pleural fluid too small to sample safely (<1 cm of fluid on a lateral decubitus radiograph). The risk of pneumothorax is particularly high in patients with one lung, bullous emphysema, or severe air flow obstruction.

RATIONALE.   The accumulation of detectable fluid in the pleural space is invariably abnormal. Prompt diagnostic thoracentesis is indicated, except when pleural effusions are found in the presence of obvious volume overload, such as uncompensated congestive heart failure or massive ascites. Aspiration of pleural fluid can yield a specific diagnosis of malignancy (cytology), infection (stains, culture), systemic lupus erythematosis (antinuclear antibody, lupus erythematosis [LE] cells), and esophageal rupture (low pH, high amylase). The finding of blood (cancer, infarction, trauma), chyle (lymphoma, disruption of thoracic duct, lymphangioleiomyomatosis), or urine (hydronephrosis) in the pleural space also has strong diagnostic implications. Less specific information may support a presumptive diagnosis and exclude other considerations, such as identifying a parapneumonic effusion as a sterile exudate, or proving an effusion to be transudative in a patient with heart failure. Diagnostic thoracentesis yields clinically helpful information in over 80% of cases. In one series of 86 patients, pleural aspiration yielded a specific diagnosis in 16%, a presumptive diagnosis in 51%, and useful but nondiagnostic information in an additional 16%.

Therapeutic thoracentesis may be helpful in relieving acute dyspnea in patients with large pleural effusions, particularly if a mediastinal shift is apparent on the chest radiograph. In patients with volume overload due to heart, liver, or renal failure, removal of pleural fluid may provide symptomatic relief while awaiting the effects of diuretic therapy or dialysis. Therapeutic thoracentesis also may be of temporary benefit in patients with malignant pleural effusions. When malignant effusions reaccumulate slowly, repeated aspiration offers an alternative to tube thoracostomy and pleurodesis.

METHODS.   The patient should be seated on the side of the examination table with his arms crossed over a pillow on a bedside table and his feet supported by a stool. After review of the chest radiograph and physical examination findings, the clinician should select a site in the posterior midclavicular line one intercostal space below the upper level of dullness, but not below the eighth interspace. Wearing sterile gloves and a mask, the clinician then prepares the skin with an iodine solution and affixes a sterile drape. A skin wheal is raised with 1% lidocaine using a 25-gauge needle on a small syringe. Then, with a second syringe containing 10 to 15 ml of lidocaine, the skin is penetrated with a 22-gauge, 1½- to 2-inch needle directed perpendicularly to the superior border of the rib. After the periosteum is anaesthetized, the needle is advanced over the rib (avoiding the neurovascular bundle under the adjacent rib), stopping every 1 to 2 mm to aspirate and inject. When pleural fluid is obtained, the needle is withdrawn. The track should be reentered with a 20- to 22-gauge, 1½- to 2-inch needle attached to a 50-ml syringe, and 30 to 50 ml of fluid aspirated for analysis. The placement of a plastic catheter over or through the insertion needle prior to aspirating fluid is unnecessary for diagnostic thoracentesis and may be associated with a higher complication rate. After the needle is withdrawn, a sterile dressing should be applied, and an expiration chest radiograph obtained to exclude a pneumothorax. The choice of pleural fluid studies will depend on the clinical situation but should always include protein, LDH, glucose, white cell count, and differential. Cultures and stains for microorganisms, cytology, amylase, lipid studies, and pH are indicated in selected circumstances (see Section 65, Pleural Effusion).

Large-volume (therapeutic) thoracentesis is most safely performed using a plastic catheter. The site is prepared in the manner described above, but once pleural fluid is obtained with the anesthetizing needle, a sterile curved clamp is placed on the needle at the skin surface before withdrawal, to mark the depth of insertion. A second clamp is placed at the same point on a 14-gauge Intracath needle attached to a 10-ml syringe, and this needle is inserted with the bevel downward until pleural fluid can be aspirated. The syringe is then disconnected and the hub of the needle occluded with a finger to prevent entry of air into the pleural space. The 16-gauge internal catheter is then threaded, angling the needle slightly downward. When the catheter is fully inserted, or when resistance is encountered, the needle is withdrawn and the needle guard mounted and taped to the chest. A 50-ml syringe with a three-way stopcock is attached to the catheter to aspirate fluid, which is then expelled through tubing connected to the side port of the stopcock (drainage may be accelerated by connecting the effluent tubing to a vacuum bottle). No more than 1 liter should be removed at a time to avoid reexpansion pulmonary edema. When drainage is complete, the needle and catheter are removed together (withdrawing the catheter through the needle may shear it off), a sterile dressing is applied, and a chest radiograph obtained.

COST/COMPLICATIONS. Thoracentesis is a potentially dangerous procedure that should not be attempted without experience or supervision. Among procedures performed by house staff, pneumothorax occurs in 10% to 15% of patients, cough, retching, or vasovagal hypotension in 5% to 10%, and subjective symptoms such as pain and anxiety in 30% to 50%. Technical problems, such as a dry or traumatic tap, occur in 20% to 25%. Other potential complications include hemothorax, hemoperitoneum, and puncture of the liver or spleen. The complication rate is significantly reduced if thoracentesis is performed under direct ultrasound guidance. The added expense of ultrasound is justified in patients with small or loculated effusions, and in patients in whom a pneumothorax may be catastrophic, such as those with one lung or poor pulmonary reserve. The cost of thoracentesis will depend on the diagnostic studies that are ordered ($50 to $250), the supplies that are used ($30 to $40), the professional fee for the procedure ($100 to $150), and the cost of radiographs or ultrasonography.

Cross-reference: Pleural Effusion (Section 65).

REFERENCES

1. Collins TR, Sahn SA. Thoracentesis: Clinical value, complications, technical problems, and patient experience. Chest 1987;91:817–822.

In a prospective study of 86 patients, thoracentesis yielded clinically useful information in 84%, but complications were common.

2. Grogan DR, Irwin RS, Channick R, Raptopoulos V, Curley FJ, Bartter T, Corwin W. Complications associated with thoracentesis: A prospective, randomized study comparing three different methods. Arch Intern Med 1990;150:873–877.
    Sonography-guided aspiration was associated with fewer complications than "blind" thoracentesis using needle-only or needle-catheter techniques.

3. Kohan JM, Poe RH, Israel RH, Kennedy JD, Benazzi RB, Kallay MC, Greenblatt DW. Value of chest ultrasonography versus decubitus roentgenography for thoracentesis. Am Rev Respir Dis 1986;133:1124–1126.
    Sonography was helpful in choosing sites for aspirating small effusions.

4. Light RW. Pleural Diseases, 2nd ed. Lea & Febiger, Philadelphia, 1990, pp. 295–304.
    An illustrated description of technique.

5. Sahn SA. The pleura. Am Rev Respir Dis 1988;138:184–234.
    An exhaustive review with a good discussion of the risks and benefits of thoracentesis.

71 ARTERIAL BLOOD GAS

Procedure

SHAWN J. SKERRETT

INDICATIONS/CONTRAINDICATIONS.   The most common indications for arterial blood sampling are suspected hypoxemia, hypercarbia, or acid-base disturbances. The evaluation of dyspnea, obtundation, cardiac arrhythmias, hypotension, vomiting, and renal failure are common clinical settings. There are no absolute contraindications, but relative contraindications include a bleeding diathesis and severe peripheral arterial disease.

RATIONALE.   Arterial blood is required for the accurate measurement of Po_2, Pco_2, and pH. Po_2 provides an indication of oxygen uptake by the blood but is an incomplete measure of oxygenation, which is determined by hemoglobin concentration, hemoglobin saturation, and tissue perfusion. Hypoxemia is usually defined as a Po_2 less than 80 mm Hg, but Po_2 normally falls with age. A simple approximation is to expect the Po_2 to be 1 mm Hg less than 80 for each year over 60. Pco_2 accurately reflects the balance of CO_2 production and elimination (ventilation) and is normally 35 to 45 mm Hg. The pH of arterial blood reflects the acid-base balance, but electrolytes must be measured simultaneously to characterize acid-base disturbances. The normal arterial pH is 7.35 to 7.45.

Automated blood gas analyzers measure Po_2, Pco_2, and pH directly, and calculate bicarbonate concentration. Most laboratories also measure hemoglobin concentration and estimate hemoglobin saturation. A co-oximeter is required to directly measure the various forms of hemoglobin, including oxyhemoglobin, deoxyhemoglobin, carboxyhemoglobin, and methemoglobin.

The most common sources of error in blood gas analysis occur in the collection and transportation of the sample. Active aspiration of blood during an attempted arterial puncture may result in venous admixture. If air bubbles are not removed, the partial pressures of gases in the blood will approach those of ambient air (Po_2, 150 mm Hg; Pco_2, 0 mm Hg), resulting in a fall in Pco_2 and an associated rise in pH. Dilution of the blood with heparin will reduce the measured Pco_2 and the hemoglobin concentration. A time delay or failure to transport the specimen on ice will permit continued cellular metabolism, particularly in the presence of leukocytosis or thrombocytosis, resulting in oxygen consumption, CO_2 production, and acidification. The laboratory must be notified of hypothermia or fever, as blood gases are measured at 37° C and must be corrected for in vivo conditions.

Pulse oximetry is a noninvasive, inexpensive alternative to arterial blood sampling for the measurement of hemoglobin saturation. Current instruments are accurate at saturations above 80%. The technique is limited by conditions that diminish vascular pulsations, such as cold, hypotension, peripheral vascular disease, or use of vasoconstrictors.

METHODS.   Arterial blood should be drawn from the radial, brachial, or femoral arteries, in descending order of preference. If the radial pulse is palpable, the adequacy of collateral circulation should be assessed with the modified Allen's test. The patient should be instructed to expel blood from the hand by making a tight fist. The clinician compresses the radial and ulnar arteries simultaneously, then asks the patient to relax (but not fully extend) the hand. If, after pressure is released from the ulnar artery, the color returns to normal within 10 seconds, the ulnar artery alone can supply the hand.

For radial artery puncture, the hand should be positioned with the wrist extended (a rolled towel or gauze is used for support) and the skin cleaned with alcohol or iodophore. A local anesthetic may be desirable if the operator is inexperienced or the patient is particularly anxious: a small wheal should be raised with 2% lidocaine, with care taken not to obscure the pulse. Heparin is drawn into a glass or low-friction plastic syringe through a 20-gauge needle, wetting the walls of the syringe. The needle should then be exchanged for a 22- to 23-gauge needle and the heparin expelled completely. With the examiner keeping a finger on the pulse, the skin should be punctured at a 30- to 60-degree angle and the needle slowly advanced until pulsatile blood fills the syringe (locating the artery is easier at a steeper angle, but through-and-through penetration and bleeding are less likely with a more oblique approach). The syringe should fill by arterial pressure, without aspiration. Once 2 to 3 ml of blood has been collected (sufficient to avoid significant dilution by residual heparin), the needle is withdrawn and firm pressure is applied to the artery for 5 minutes. Before transportation to the laboratory, the syringe should be free of air bubbles, sealed, and placed on ice.

COST/COMPLICATIONS.   The laboratory fee for blood gas analysis is in the range of $40 to $60, plus the charges for the procedure and supplies ($30 to $40). Local bleeding is common after inadequate compression. Distal ischemia is rare.

Cross-references: Dyspnea (Section 19), Sleep Apnea Syndromes (Section 64), Asthma and Chronic Obstructive Pulmonary Disease (Section 68), Hyperventilation Syndrome (Section 190).

REFERENCES

1.   Hansen JE, Simmons DH. A systematic error in determination of blood P_{CO_2}. Am Rev Respir Dis 1977;115:1061–1063.
     The effect of heparin.

2.   Hess CE, Nichols AB, Hunt WB, Suratt PM. Pseudohypoxemia secondary to leukemia and thrombocytosis. N Engl J Med 1979;301:361–363.
     Another source of error.

3.   Raffin TA. Indications for arterial blood gas analysis. Ann Intern Med 1986;105:390–398.
     A thoughtful review.

4.   Shapiro BA, Harrison RA, Cane RD, Templin R. Clinical Application of Blood Gases, 4th ed. Year Book Medical Publishers, Chicago, 1989, pp. 1–379.
     A good source for technical aspects and clinical interpretation.

5.   Vander Salm TJ. Arterial puncture. In Vander Salm TJ, Cutler BS, Wheeler HB, Eds. Atlas of Bedside Procedures, 2nd ed. Little, Brown & Co., Boston, 1988, pp. 113–117.
     An illustrated description.

CARDIOVASCULAR DISORDERS

72 ASSESSMENT OF PHYSICAL ACTIVITY

Screening

RICHARD M. HOFFMAN

EPIDEMIOLOGY. Approximately 40% of Americans are sedentary, and only 20% exercise at levels adequate for cardiopulmonary benefit. The young and persons in higher socioeconomic classes are the most active. Men and women participate equally in conditioning activities, though men more often engage in vigorous exercise. Surveys indicate that the most popular activities are walking, swimming, calisthenics, bicycling, and jogging. Activity levels often decline significantly in early adulthood and after marriage, job changes, moves, or recovery from serious illness or injury.

RATIONALE. Physical inactivity is a demonstrated risk factor for coronary heart disease, hypertension, and obesity. Regular activity can help lower blood pressure, control weight gain and non-insulin-dependent diabetes mellitus, prevent osteoporosis in postmenopausal women, and reduce anxiety and depression. Although the risk of sudden death increases transiently during exercise, the overall risk for sudden death is lower for the physically fit. Soft tissue injuries, tendinitis, and stress fractures occur more frequently with activity but are often preventable by avoiding excessive levels of activity, precipitous increases in activity, and the use of poor exercise technique or equipment. No studies have proven an association between physical activity and osteoarthritis.

STRATEGY. During all routine office visits, the physician should assess the patient's present activity level and its medical risks or benefits. Recommended baseline laboratory tests include serum electrolytes, hematocrit, ECG, and chest radiography. The use of graded exercise tests for screening purposes is

203

controversial, particularly for asymptomatic persons, because false-positive rates are high and true-positive tests do not accurately predict cardiac arrest during exercise.

ACTION. Physicians should counsel all patients to be physically active. An exercise prescription should specify the type, frequency, duration, and intensity of activity. Aerobic weight-bearing exercises (walking is ideal) two to four times a week for 30 minutes are recommended. Cardiovascular fitness requires exercising at 70% to 85% of the maximal heart rate (220 minus age). Exercise regimens should begin at 50% to 60% of maximal heart rate and increase every 2 weeks until the target heart rate is reached. Target heart rates for patients on beta blockers are based on maximal exercise heart rates. Sedentary and elderly persons should begin at lower levels and progress slowly. Exercise should not be too vigorous; signs of overexertion include prolonged postexercise tachycardia, nausea, vomiting, light-headedness, confusion, claudication, angina, or excessive dyspnea. Exercise should be avoided after consumption of alcohol or large meals, and during very hot or cold weather. Exercise prescriptions may need further modification depending on patient disability.

Patient compliance can be enhanced by presenting the health risks of inactivity and the benefits of exercise, selecting appropriate exercises, setting goals, encouraging social support, and providing positive reinforcement.

Cross-references: Periodic Health Assessment (Section 7), Chronic Pain Syndrome (Section 13), Obesity (Section 15), Essential Hypertension (Section 86), Exercise Tolerance Testing (Section 89), Osteoporosis (Section 117).

REFERENCES

1. Chisholm DM, Collis ML, Kulak LL, Davenport W, Gruber N. Physical activity readiness. Br Columbia Med J 1975;17:375–378.
    Questionnaire providing guidelines for exercise and medical evaluation, designed for patients.

2. Goldberg L, Elliot DL. Prescribing exercise. West J Med 1984;141:383–386.
    Discusses pre-exercise evaluation, exercise testing, contraindications to exercise, and specifics of exercise prescription and monitoring.

3. Harris SS, Caspersen CJ, DeFriese GH, Estes EH. Physical activity counseling for healthy adults as a primary preventive intervention in the clinical setting: Report for the U.S. Preventive Services Task Force. JAMA 1989;261:3590–3598.
    Concise review of risks and benefits of exercise and guidelines for counseling, with an excellent bibliography.

73 HYPERTENSION SCREENING

Screening

C. SCOTT SMITH

EPIDEMIOLOGY. The prevalence of hypertension in adults in the United States is conservatively estimated at 10% to 25% and increases with age. Blacks have a greater prevalence of hypertension than whites and also have more end-organ dysfunction for any given blood pressure. Up to one quarter of cardiovascular deaths may be at least in part attributable to "hypertensive" complications (stroke, congestive heart failure [CHF], accelerated hypertension).

RATIONALE. Blood pressure is a major, independent, treatable risk factor for cardiovascular disease. Risk increases in a direct linear relationship to the blood pressure, and there is no threshold level or critical point at which the risk accelerates. Although treatment guidelines are based on diastolic blood pressures, systolic pressure is a better independent predictor of stroke and cardiovascular events in most groups. Treatment of severe hypertension (diastolic BP > 115 mm Hg) has been shown to dramatically reduce the mortality and the incidence of cardiovascular complications. Treatment of moderate hypertension (diastolic BP 105–114 mm Hg) lessens end organ damage such as left ventricular hypertrophy. The benefits of treating mild hypertension (diastolic BP 90–104 mm Hg) accrue mainly from reducing fatal and nonfatal stroke (up to 40% reduction in most studies). Intervention trials have not shown a significant reduction in morbidity- or mortality-related ischemic heart disease from lowering mildly elevated blood pressure.

The exact level at which to initiate pharmacologic therapy remains controversial. The latest recommendations of the Joint National Committee on Evaluation, Detection, and Treatment of High Blood Pressure define hypertension as diastolic blood pressures exceeding 90 mm Hg. Even the most conservative recommendations begin therapy above diastolic blood pressures of 100 mm Hg (12%–15% of the American adult population).

Isolated systolic hypertension is defined as systolic blood pressure greater than 160 mm Hg. Recent evidence suggests that treatment of isolated systolic blood pressures greater than 160 mm Hg, at least in patients over 60 years old, may reduce the risk of stroke by about 40%.[4]

STRATEGY. Screening blood pressure should be recorded for all adults at each primary care visit, and at least every 2 years. This should be done with the patient sitting, after a brief rest, and with the arm supported at heart level. The pressure may be recorded without rolling the shirt sleeve up. Elevated values (see below) should be confirmed by more than one reading on three separate visits, at least 2 weeks apart. At least one of these readings should be done in a setting other than the office.

Blood pressure should be considered elevated if the average of the diastolic readings is 95 to 100 mm Hg diastolic or greater, *or* between 90 and 94 mm Hg if there is evidence of end-organ involvement (left ventricular hypertrophy, retinopathy, or nephropathy) or other significant coronary risk factors are present.

ACTION. If the patient is taking drugs that may cause elevations in blood pressure (e.g., oral contraceptives, estrogens, or nonsteroidal anti-inflammatories), the clinician should reevaluate their indications. Patients identified as hypertensive should be counseled to increase exercise, decrease weight and dietary salt, and limit alcohol consumption. Other cardiovascular risk factors should be evaluated and discussed if appropriate (smoking, hyperlipidemia). Pharmacologic treatment should be started immediately if the diastolic blood pressure is greater than or equal to 115 mm Hg. Otherwise, if after a 3- to 6-month trial of nonpharmacologic treatment as outlined above, the patient continues to maintain blood pressure at elevated levels, pharmacologic treatment should be instituted.

Cross-references: Periodic Health Assessment (Section 7), Diagnosis and Management of Alcoholism (Section 9), Obesity (Section 15), Assessment of Physical Activity (Section 72), Essential Hypertension (Section 86).

REFERENCES

1. Collins R, Peto R, MacMahon S, et al. Blood pressure, stroke and coronary artery disease: Part 2. Short term reduction in blood pressure. Overview of randomized drug trials in their epidemiologic context. Lancet 1990;335:827–838.
   An excellent review of the primary treatment trials in hypertension, showing little evidence for treating diastolic blood pressures below 100 mm Hg.

2. Frohlich ED, Grim C, Labarthe DR. Recommendation for human blood pressure determination by sphygmomanometers. Hypertension 1988;11:210A–222A.
   Definitive article on the technique of blood pressure measurement.

3. Joint National Committee on Detection, Evaluation, and Treatment of High Blood Pressure. The 1988 (fourth) Report of the Joint National Committee on Detection, Evaluation, and Treatment of High Blood Pressure. Arch Intern Med 1988;148:1023–1038.
   Established a national standard. Based on current thinking, their recommendations on when to initiate treatment may be too aggressive.

4. SHEP Cooperative Research Group. Prevention of stroke by antihypertensive drug treatment in older persons with isolated systolic hypertension. JAMA 1991;265:3255–3263. Editorial comment, pp. 3301–3302.
   See text.

74 CHEST PAIN

Symptom

DAVID H. HICKAM

EPIDEMIOLOGY.   Patients may describe chest discomfort with various words, including pain, pressure, tightness, fullness, or a burning sensation. Chest discomfort is more prevalent in older age groups. Angina pectoris refers to a syndrome of pain that usually is substernal in location and brought on by physical exertion. It is more frequent in patients who have coronary artery disease but can occur with other diseases, such as esophageal disorders. Unstable angina is the syndrome of anginal chest pain that is of recent onset or has become more frequent or severe in patients with chronic symptoms.

ETIOLOGY.   Causes of chest pain conventionally are classified into cardiovascular and noncardiovascular categories (Table 74–1). The etiologies that can be life-threatening if not treated immediately are in the cardiovascular category: acute myocardial infarction, unstable angina pectoris, and aortic dissection.

Among middle-aged and older adults who seek care for chest pain, approximately one-third have cardiac ischemia as the etiology, while another one-third have esophageal disease as the cause of discomfort.

CLINICAL APPROACH.   Most published studies of the yield of diagnostic evaluation of patients with chest pain have reported one of two types of patient

TABLE 74–1. CAUSES OF CHEST PAIN

Cardiovascular
Acute myocardial infarction
Atherosclerotic coronary artery disease, without acute infarction
Coronary artery spasm
Pericarditis
Aortic dissection
Aortic stenosis
Pulmonary embolism
Mitral valve prolapse

Noncardiovascular
Reflux esophagitis
Esophageal motor disorders
Pneumothorax
Pneumonia
Chest wall disorders
Chest trauma
Anxiety disorders, including hyperventilation

groups: patients who present to emergency rooms with pain of recent onset, or patients who have been referred for definitive evaluation because of recurrent chest pain. These studies have consistently shown that appropriate interpretation of the patient's history, physical examination findings, and initial electrocardiogram (ECG) usually reveals the correct cause of pain.

In patients with acute chest pain, the clinician first must estimate the probability that the pain is caused by cardiac ischemia. A study of emergency room patients with acute chest pain showed that initial decision-making can be based on the ECG.[2] Q waves or ST segment elevations (not known to be old) are specific enough for myocardial infarction that the physician should initiate management for this diagnosis when these findings are present, pending results of other tests. Although as many as 10% of patients with a normal ECG in the emergency room will subsequently be found to have a myocardial infarction, such patients have a low risk of serious complications.

If the ECG is neither completely normal nor shows the classic changes of an acute myocardial infarction, decisions should be based on the characteristics of the pain. Pain that is described as crushing, pressing, or tight is more likely to be ischemic than pain that is described as sharp or stabbing. Because the patient's description of symptoms is similar in unstable angina pectoris and acute myocardial infarction, the clinician should not try to distinguish these two syndromes from the history alone. There are no physical examination signs that are characteristic of cardiac ischemia. The probability of ischemia is lower in patients whose pain is fully reproduced by chest palpation, but in many cases this sign is not specific enough to be relied on.

Single serum cardiac enzyme levels have limited value for the initial assessment of patients with acute chest pain. Initial enzyme levels are insufficiently sensitive to exclude acute myocardial infarction, even in patients whose pain has lasted more than 12 hours. The false-positive rate of any of the enzyme tests (including isoenzyme determinations) is 10% or greater. Thus, in patients whose symptoms suggest a low probability of cardiac ischemia, an elevated serum enzyme level is likely to be a false-positive result. Serial ECGs and enzyme levels will establish whether the patient has acute myocardial infarction or unstable angina as the cause of ischemic-type chest pain.

Dissection of the thoracic aorta is rare but life-threatening. The history and physical examination are very useful for excluding this diagnosis. Nearly all patients with dissection of the proximal aorta will have a murmur of aortic regurgitation, pulse deficits, specific neurologic deficits, or a history of Marfan's syndrome. Most patients with dissection of the descending aorta are older than age 40 and have pain located in the posterior chest or a history of hypertension.

Chest pain occurs in most patients with acute pericarditis. The pain of pericarditis often can be differentiated from ischemic pain in being pleuritic, affected by body position, or described by the patient as sharp or stabbing. Some patients have ST segment elevation in multiple ECG leads, which can be confused with acute myocardial infarction. In pericarditis, the echocardiogram often shows a pericardial effusion. In the absence of an effusion, ventricular wall motion abnormalities suggest that ischemia is the more likely cause of pain.

Chest pain caused by pulmonary embolism is usually pleuritic, sharp, and located in the lateral chest. Pulmonary embolism may account for up to 20% of pleuritic chest pain. Pulmonary embolism is very unlikely in patients under age 40 who lack risk factors for thromboembolic disease. Because the perfusion lung scan is highly sensitive for pulmonary embolism, a completely normal test excludes the diagnosis. Because of a high false-positive rate, however, lung scans cannot be considered the reference standard for confirming pulmonary embolism (see Section 61, Pleuritic Chest Pain).

MANAGEMENT.   The most important initial decision in managing acute chest pain is whether to admit the patient to the hospital. Admission to a coronary care unit is appropriate when the probability of acute ischemia is greater than 10% or when aortic dissection is suspected. If the initial ECG changes are minimal, patients with suspected myocardial infarction can be safely managed in an intermediate care unit.

Patients with ECG changes characteristic of acute myocardial infarction are candidates for treatment with thrombolytic medication or coronary angioplasty. Because the effectiveness of these interventions decreases with increasing duration of the infarction, immediate consultation with a cardiologist should be obtained. The consultant may wish to perform coronary arteriography before proceeding with thrombolytic therapy.

Patients with acute myocardial infarction or unstable angina pectoris benefit from medical therapy that reduces cardiac workload and improves coronary perfusion. Sublingual nitroglycerin (0.4 mg every 5 minutes, as tolerated by the patient's blood pressure) is often beneficial while the patient is awaiting hospital admission.

Patients with aortic dissection require medical stabilization before definitive treatment. Patients with distal dissections associated with hypertension should have immediate treatment with intravenous (IV) antihypertensive agents in an intensive care unit (ICU). Pulmonary embolism also requires hospitalization for hemodynamic stabilization and initiation of anticoagulant therapy.

FOLLOW-UP.   If the patient is not admitted, outpatient follow-up should be scheduled for 2 to 3 days after the initial evaluation. Emergency room studies have found that approximately 5% of patients not hospitalized for acute chest pain will be found to have acute myocardial infarction on subsequent ECGs. If follow-up studies do not show myocardial infarction but the patient continues to have intermittent pain, the clinician should evaluate the patient for angina pectoris (see Section 78).

Cross-references: Pleuritic Chest Pain (Section 61), Angina (Section 78), Exercise Tolerance Testing (Section 89), Dysphagia and Heartburn (Section 97).

REFERENCES

1. DeSanctis RW, Doroghazi RM, Austen WG, et al. Aortic dissection. N Engl J Med 1987;317:1060–1067.
    General review of the diagnosis and management of aortic dissection.

2. Goldman L, Cook EF, Brand DA, et al. A computer protocol to predict myocardial infarction in emergency department patients with chest pain. N Engl J Med 1988;318:797–803.
    An algorithm for estimating the risk of acute myocardial infarction, developed from prospectively collected data on patients' symptoms and initial ECGs.

3. Hull RD, Raskob GE, Carter CJ, et al. Pulmonary embolism in outpatients with pleuritic chest pain. Arch Intern Med 1988;148:838–844.
    Describes an approach to evaluating clinical characteristics and test results in suspected cases of pulmonary embolism.

4. Lee TH, Cook F, Weisberg MC, et al. Impact of the availability of a prior electrocardiogram on the triage of the patient with acute chest pain. J Gen Intern Med 1990;5:381–388.
    Data on the clinical characteristics and relative usefulness of a prior ECG in patients who did and did not have acute myocardial infarction. A prior ECG improved the specificity of decisions to admit patients to the coronary care unit.

5. Lee TH, Rouan GW, Weisberg MC, et al. Sensitivity of routine clinical criteria for diagnosing myocardial infarction within 24 hours of hospitalization. Ann Intern Med 1987;106:181–186.
    Data on the basis for diagnosis in 1460 patients admitted for acute chest pain. In nearly all patients with acute myocardial infarction or unstable angina, the diagnosis can be made within 24 hours.

75 SYNCOPE

Symptom

WISHWA N. KAPOOR

EPIDEMIOLOGY.   Syncope is defined as a sudden transient loss of consciousness and postural tone that spontaneously resolves without electrical or chemical cardioversion. Syncope should be differentiated from other states of altered consciousness such as dizziness, vertigo, seizure, coma, and narcolepsy.

Syncope is a common problem in all age groups. It accounts for approximately 1% of hospital admissions and 3% of emergency room visits. Some 12% to 48% of healthy young adults have experienced loss of consciousness (about one-third of these instances follow trauma), though most do not seek medical attention. In people over age 75 years residing in long-term care institutions, the annual incidence of syncope is 6%, with 23% having had previous lifetime syncopal episodes.

ETIOLOGY. Syncope has a large differential diagnosis (Table 75–1). In approximately 60% of patients a cause is diagnosed; the cause is cardiac in about half of cases and noncardiac in half.

Vasodepressor (or vasovagal) syncope results from a sudden fall in blood pressure and is associated with autonomic symptoms such as pallor, nausea, sweating, bradycardia, and hyperventilation. This type of syncope often occurs in young individuals in response to fear or injury or prolonged standing, although it may occur without any identifiable predisposing factors.

Syncope may occur during urination (micturition syncope), defecation, cough, and swallowing, primarily because of exaggerated vasodilatory reflexes. Associated bradycardias or organic diseases are rarely found, with the exception of swallow syncope, which often results from bradyarrhythmias provoked by structural abnormalities of the lower esophagus.

Drugs (especially nitrates, beta blockers, and vasodilators) cause syncope by decreasing vascular volume or tone, provoking arrhythmias, or causing allergic or anaphylactic reactions.

A wide variety of conditions may result in orthostatic hypotension, including volume depletion, drugs, metabolic disorders (e.g., diabetes mellitus, adrenal insufficiency), and diseases of autonomic nervous systems (e.g., autonomic neuropathy, Shy-Drager syndrome).

Cerebrovascular disease is a rare cause of syncope. Examples are atherosclerotic disease, subclavian steal syndrome, and migraines (both common and basilar artery migraine).

TABLE 75–1.   ETIOLOGIES OF SYNCOPE

Noncardiac Diseases	Cardiac Diseases
Vasodepressor (vasovagal)*	Obstruction to flow
Situational*	Aortic stenosis
Micturition syncope	Hypertrophic cardiomyopathy
Defection syncope	Atrial myxoma
Cough syncope	Pulmonic stenosis
Swallow syncope	Pulmonary hypertension
Drug-induced syncope*	Pulmonary embolism
Orthostatic hypotension*	Myocardial infarct
Cerebrovascular disease	Cardiac tamponade
Carotid sinus syncope	Aortic dissection
Glossopharyngeal neuralgia	Arrhythmias*
Trigeminal neuralgia	Bradyarrhythmias
Seizure	Sinus node disease
Psychogenic	Second- and third-degree AV block
Anxiety disorder	Pacemaker malfunction
Panic disorder	Drug-induced bradyarrhythmias
Somatization	Tachyarrhythmias
Depression	Ventricular tachycardia
Hypoglycemia	Torsades de pointes (e.g., associated with congenital long QT syndromes or acquired QT prolongation)
	Supraventricular tachycardia

Source: Adapted from Amer J Med 1991;90:91–102, with permission.
*Most common causes.

Carotid sinus syncope is suspected in patients who lose consciousness following maneuvers that stretch or press the carotid sinus (e.g., a sudden turning of the head, shaving, or wearing a tight collar). Documentation of carotid sinus hypersensitivity (cardiac asystole $\geq$ 3 seconds or a drop in blood pressure $\geq$ 50 mm Hg in those without significant bradycardia) in those with a compatible clinical picture or recurrent unexplained syncope is diagnostic.

Psychiatric illnesses such as generalized anxiety, panic disorder, somatization disorder, and depression may all cause syncope, as may alcohol and abuse of drugs such as cocaine, hypnotics, and sedatives.

The various causes of cardiac syncope are noted in Table 75–1.

CLINICAL APPROACH.   The history and physical examination reveal the diagnosis in 50% to 85% of patients in whom it can be determined, and provide strong clues about several other etiologies (e.g., murmur of aortic stenosis) that guide further testing.

Routine blood tests are rarely abnormal or yield diagnostically helpful information in patients with syncope. A glucose tolerance test is not useful unless hypoglycemia is clinically suspected.

Arrhythmias are diagnosed by ECG, Holter monitoring, intermittent recorders, and electrophysiologic studies. A 12-lead ECG discloses the likely cause of syncope in 2% to 10% of patients (bradycardias, ventricular tachycardia, and supraventricular tachycardias) or may show an atrioventricular (AV) block or evidence of acute myocardial infarction. Exercise treadmill testing may detect exercise-induced tachyarrhythmias or bradyarrhythmias that occur after abrupt termination of exercise, but otherwise rarely leads to a cause of syncope.

Although widely used in the evaluation of syncope, prolonged ECG monitoring has several limitations. In only 4% of patients do symptoms and arrhythmias occur concurrently, establishing a probable cause of syncope; in approximately 17% symptoms occur in the absence of arrhythmias, excluding arrhythmias as a probable cause. The remaining 75% to 80% have no symptoms during monitoring; 15% of these, however, have arrhythmias. The causal relation between these arrhythmias and syncope is often uncertain. Extending the duration of monitoring up to 72 hours does not improve the diagnostic accuracy of ECG for symptomatic arrhythmias.

Patient-activated transtelephonic ECG recordings (e.g., loop monitors) document most arrhythmias during syncope, even if activated after the patient has regained consciousness, because at least 4 minutes of retrograde recording is possible and monitors can be worn for several weeks. Although 35% of patients wearing loop monitors report symptoms, the vast majority have a "normal" cardiac rhythm during symptoms, excluding arrhythmias as a cause.

Electrophysiologic testing should be reserved for patients with recurrent unexplained syncope who have organic heart disease (marked left ventricular [LV] dysfunction, hypertrophic cardiomyopathy, or severe coronary or valvular disease) and have undergone extensive noninvasive testing. Predictors of positive electrophysiologic studies include an ejection fraction of 0.40 or less, bundle-branch block, coronary disease, remote myocardial infarction, and injury with syncope. Electrophysiologic tests are abnormal in approximately 60% of patients with syncope who are studied and primarily reveal conduction system disease, ventricular and supraventricular tachycardia.

The upright tilt test is useful in documenting vasodepressor syncope, especially in patients with recurrent syncope of unknown etiology. A positive test is defined as reproduction of symptoms in association with hypotension or bradycardia. This test has been performed with or without concurrent use of isoproterenol. This test is positive in 75% to 88% of patients with recurrent, unexplained syncope. The specificity is reported to be above 85% although it is as low as 55% in young patients.

Routine echocardiography, stress testing, ventricular function studies, and cardiac catheterization are unnecessary except to clarify specific findings noted on the history and physical examination. Although signal-averaged ECGs that detect low-amplitude signals (late potentials) have a sensitivity of 73% to 89% and specificity of 80% to 90% for prediction of inducible sustained ventricular tachycardia, this test does not establish the diagnosis of syncope due to ventricular tachycardia.

Specialized autonomic function studies (e.g., blood pressure responses to Valsalva maneuver, catecholamine responses to stress, tests of sweating responses with a rise in temperature, and pupillary responses) are generally not needed in patients with orthostatic hypotension since clinical evaluation often provides clues to its etiology. EEG and head computed tomography (CT) are rarely useful, but they may be valuable when seizure is suspected clinically or there are associated focal neurologic symptoms.

MANAGEMENT. The decision to admit patients depends on the presence of comorbid illnesses and a consideration of possible causes. When a cause of syncope is apparent from the history, physical examination, and initial ECG, admission decisions can be made based on that cause (e.g., patients with gastrointestinal bleeding generally need to be admitted). In the remaining patients, admission is indicated if arrhythmic syncope is suspected, a fall has resulted in serious injury, or other serious causes are considered (such as aortic dissection cerebral hemorrhage or brain tumors).

Treatment depends on the specific cause of the syncope. Vasovagal syncope documented by a positive tilt test is treated with beta blockers, disopyramide, anticholinergic agents, or fludrocortisone plus salt.

FOLLOW-UP. Patients with cardiac causes of syncope have a markedly higher mortality and sudden death rates at 1 year and at 5 years than patients with syncope of noncardiac cause. Recurrence rates are as high as 12% to 15% per year and are similar whether the cause is cardiac or not.

Cross-references: Diagnosis and Management of Drug Abuse (Section 8), Diagnosis and Management of Alcoholism (Section 9), Dizziness (Section 20), Aortic Stenosis (Section 80), Chronic Ventricular Arrhythmias (Section 84), Ambulatory Cardiac Monitoring (Section 88), Cerebrovascular Disease (Section 141), Somatization (Section 191), Panic Disorder (Section 194).

REFERENCES

1. Kapoor WN. Evaluation and outcome of patients with syncope. Medicine 1990;69:160–175.
   A large prospective study of syncope. History and physical examination led to the diagnosis in most patients. Patients with a cardiac cause had a higher mortality.

2. Kapoor WN. Diagnostic evaluation of syncope. Am J Med 1991;90:91–106.
   An in-depth review of diagnostic tests for the evaluation of syncope.

3. Kapoor WN, Hammill SC, Gersh BJ. Diagnosis and natural history of syncope and the role of invasive electrophysiologic testing. Am J Cardiol 1989;63:730–734.
   Discussion of problems in diagnosis and the management of arrhythmias by electrophysiologic studies.

4. Kapoor WN, Bryant N. Evaluation of syncope by upright tilt table testing with isoproterenol: A nonspecific test. Ann Intern Med 1992;116:358–363.
   In a relatively young group of subjects tilt table testing was positive as often in patients with syncope as in controls.

76 PALPITATIONS

Symptom

BARBARA WEBER
WISHWA N. KAPOOR

EPIDEMIOLOGY.   Palpitations, the awareness of one's own heartbeat, are produced by a change in the rate, rhythm, or strength of cardiac contraction. Patients may describe palpitations as "fast heartbeats," "irregular heartbeats," "skipped heartbeats," "irregular heart rate," or "heart pounding." The incidence of this symptom in general medical practice is not accurately known, but may range between less than 1% to 8% per year.

ETIOLOGY.   The causes of palpitations range from isolated benign processes to serious cardiac diseases (Table 76–1). In a prospective study of 190 patients with palpitations, an etiology could be determined in 160 patients of which 51% were cardiac, 36% psychiatric, and 13% other causes.

CLINICAL APPROACH.   The clinical features of palpitations, such as the rapidity of onset and the frequency, duration, and regularity of the heartbeat, as well as any associated symptoms, help to characterize the cause and severity of the problem. For example, isolated forceful heartbeats following a pause frequently represent premature atrial or ventricular contractions. Abrupt runs of strong heartbeats suggest a paroxysmal reentrant tachycardia. A gradual on-

TABLE 76–1.   CAUSES OF PALPITATIONS

Habits (alcohol, caffeine, cocaine, tobacco)
Medications (sympathomimetic, anticholinergics, vasodilators)
Dehydration
Psychiatric (anxiety, panic disorder, somatization, emotional stress)
Metabolic (hypoglycemia, thyrotoxicosis, pheochromocytoma)
High-output states (anemia, fever, Paget's disease, pregnancy)
Increased stroke volume (valvular heart disease, exertion, cardiac and noncardiac
  arteriovenous shunts)
Pacemaker (diaphragmatic flutter, paced beats)
Prosthetic heart valve
Other cardiac diseases (cardiomegaly, mitral valve prolapse, myxoma)
Arrhythmias
  Isolated single palpitation
      Premature beats (atrial or ventricular)
      The beat after a compensatory pause
      The beat following a blocked beat
  Paroxysmal episodes
    Regular rhythm
      Supraventricular tachycardia
      Ventricular tachycardia
      Sick sinus syndrome
      Sinus bradycardia
    Irregular rhythm
      Paroxysmal atrial fibrillation
      Paroxysmal atrial tachycardia
      Multifocal atrial tachycardia
      Frequent premature ventricular contractions or premature atrial contractions

set and termination is more often associated with sinus (physiologic) tachycardia. Some patients learn to cough, drink ice water, or massage their neck (vagal maneuvers) to terminate palpitations, which suggests a supraventricular tachycardia as the cause.

The patient should be questioned about symptoms related to disorders that may cause palpitations, listed in Table 76–1, emphasizing psychiatric illnesses such as anxiety and panic disorders. The clinician should seek to identify high-risk patients who may require more intensive evaluation and management. Patients with underlying organic heart disease (coronary artery disease, CHF, valvular heart disease, hypertrophic cardiomyopathy) who experience recurrent palpitations are more likely to have arrhythmias. Although cohort studies of patients with palpitations are not available, patients with heart disease and complex ventricular ectopy appear to be at higher risk for sudden death.

Even though a patient's palpitations may have resolved, the vital signs may provide clues to their etiology. Orthostatic hypotension may indicate volume depletion. A fast, regular heart rate suggests supraventricular or sinus tachycardia, atrial flutter, or ventricular tachycardia. A rapid regular rate of 100 to 140 beats/min suggests sinus tachycardia and 150 beats/min suggests atrial flutter. A fast irregular rate may represent multifocal atrial tachycardia, atrial fibrillation, or atrial flutter with variable AV block. A slow heart rate results from sinus bradycardia, junctional rhythm, or complete heart block. Occasional irregularity of an otherwise regular pulse may represent premature contractions or atrial fibrillation.

When a diagnosis is not evident after clinical examination, helpful laboratory tests include a serum glucose, electrolytes, and a hemoglobin level. If these are normal, specialized tests such as thyroid function tests, serum and urine catecholamine levels, or echocardiography may be required to diagnose hyperthyroidism, pheochromocytoma, or underlying heart disease, respectively.

Although the yield of 12-lead ECG and rhythm strip is low, they may show specific arrhythmias (e.g., atrial fibrillation or premature ventricular contractions) or conduction system disease that prompts further evaluation such as electrophysiologic studies. The ECG may rarely show evidence of myocardial ischemia or infarction. If symptoms occur with exertion, an exercise ECG may be diagnostic.

Ambulatory ECG monitoring is often used to evaluate palpitations, despite a sensitivity of only 10% to 69% for symptomatic arrhythmias. Other limitations include a poor correlation between symptoms and arrhythmias, the frequent detection of brief asymptomatic arrhythmias unrelated to palpitations, and failure of intermittently symptomatic arrhythmias to occur during the monitoring period (see Section 88).

Although patient-activated transtelephonic monitoring (e.g., with loop monitors) is more likely to capture a rhythm during palpitations, data on its use for palpitations are scant.

Invasive electrophysiologic studies may be warranted in patients with unexplained recurrent palpitations who have organic heart disease, preexcitation syndrome, or conduction system disease (on 12-lead ECG), or to evaluate specific arrhythmias detected by noninvasive means.

MANAGEMENT.   Treatment of underlying disease should lead to resolution of the symptoms. Hospitalization is unnecessary unless symptoms are severe or arrhythmias are diagnosed or highly likely.

FOLLOW-UP.   Depending on the etiology of palpitations and the existence of comorbid conditions, the prognosis in patients with palpitations and no underlying cardiac disease generally is favorable, although few studies on this issue are available.

REFERENCES

1.   Diamond TH, Smith R, Myburgh DP. Holter monitoring: A necessity for the evaluation of palpitations. S Afr Med J 1983;63:5–7.

   Symptomatic correlation was achieved in 44% of patients with palpitations referred for Holter monitoring.

2.   Knudson MP. The natural history of palpitations in a family practice. J Fam Pract 1987;24:357–360.

   In a retrospective cohort study of young patients with palpitations, the incidence was less than 1% and there was no increased risk of cardiac morbidity or mortality when compared to a control population.

3. Reid P. Indications for intracardiac electrophysiologic studies in patients with unexplained palpitations. Circulation 1987;75(4 pt 2):III-154–III-160.
    Details electrophysiologic studies most useful for understanding mechanisms involved in paroxysmal supraventricular tachycardia, particularly in patients with underlying cardiac disease.

77 EDEMA

Symptom

STEVEN R. McGEE

EPIDEMIOLOGY.   In one survey of healthy subjects over the age of 65 years, 16% had swelling of the ankles and lower calves that, with firm pressure from an examiner's finger, pitted to a depth of 1 cm or more.

ETIOLOGY.   Swelling of an extremity may result from increased capillary hydrostatic pressure (e.g., congestive heart failure), increased capillary permeability (e.g., inflammation), decreased oncotic pressure (e.g., hypoalbuminemia), reduced lymph removal (lymphedema), or increased amounts of normal tissues (lipedema). Table 77–1 lists the causes of unilateral and bilateral edema. Section 131 (Painful and Swollen Calf) discusses acute unilateral swelling of the lower extremity in further detail.

The ease of pitting reflects the protein content of the edema fluid. Low-protein fluids (hypoalbuminemia, cardiac and venous edema) are of low viscosity and pit easily with local pressure, recovering quickly when the pressure is removed. High-protein fluids (cellulitis edema, lymphedema) are of high viscosity, resist pitting, and once pitted, recover slowly. Leg elevation and diuresis increase the protein content of the edema and make it more firm on examination. All edematous conditions are aggravated by high environmental heat, perhaps because of vasodilation and increased capillary transudation of fluid.

The edema of **chronic venous insufficiency** is worse at the end of the day and is often associated with the sensation of leg heaviness and the findings of superficial venous varicosities, brown pigmentation about the ankle, and in some cases ulceration. Although chronic venous insufficiency is traditionally regarded as a complication of deep venous thrombosis, venograms in these patients show evidence of previous deep venous thrombosis in only one-third, the remainder having isolated incompetent perforator veins.

Lymphedema is painless and firm and, in contrast to venous edema, varies little throughout the day. Squaring of the toes is characteristic, but ulceration

TABLE 77–1. ETIOLOGY OF EDEMA

Bilateral
 Congestive heart failure
 Hepatic cirrhosis
 Nephrotic syndrome
 Acute glomerulonephritis
 Hypoalbuminemia
 Lipedema
 Primary lymphedema
 Medications
  Antihypertensive drugs
   Nifedipine
   Guanethidine
   Prazosin
  Nonsteroidal anti-inflammatory medications

Unilateral
 Acute
  Deep venous thrombosis
  Cellulitis
  Baker's cyst
  Muscle hematoma
 Chronic
  Chronic venous insufficiency
  Primary or secondary lymphedema

is rare unless complicated by trauma or infection. Lymphedema of the lower extremity that begins before age 40 usually results from congenitally abnormal lymphatics (primary lymphedema), may be bilateral, and is much more common in women than men. Lower extremity lymphedema beginning after age 40 is secondary to malignancy or recurrent cellulitis. Secondary lymphedema is unilateral in 95% of cases. When it is secondary to malignancy, prostate cancer is the most common diagnosis in men, lymphoma in women. Lymphedema of the upper extremity is almost always due to breast cancer or the treatment for breast cancer (surgery and radiation therapy).

Lipedema results from increased deposition of fat in the lower extremities, occurs exclusively in obese women, does not pit, and, unlike lymphedema, spares the feet.

CLINICAL APPROACH. The patient interview should determine the distribution of edema, how quickly it developed, and whether there is associated trauma or pain. Edema that develops quickly over days excludes lymphedema and lipedema. Generalized edema that involves the face or sacrum or is associated with abdominal swelling or shortness of breath suggests cardiac, renal, or hepatic disease (anasarca). Severe pain is uncommon in anasarca, lymphedema, and lipedema unless the condition is complicated by infection, ulceration, or thrombosis (see Sections 131 and 134).

Physical examination focusing on the neck veins, chest, abdomen, and pelvis may reveal lymphadenopathy (inflammation, lymphedema), a prostatic or pelvic mass (lymphedema), findings of CHF (elevated jugular venous pressure), or findings of hepatic disease (spider telangiectasia, gynecomastia, palmar erythema). The clinician should determine how easily the edema pits. Routine laboratory tests in patients with bilateral edema include a chemistry profile, complete blood cell (CBC) count, creatinine determination, urinalysis and chest radiography. CT of the abdomen and pelvis is indicated in cases of suspected secondary lymphedema.

MANAGEMENT. General principles in treating edema include (1) elevate the involved extremity, (2) use elastic stockings or custom-made gradient stockings to reduce dependent edema (unless the patient has severe arterial insufficiency), (3) treat the underlying cause (e.g., lymphedema may resolve with treatment of an underlying malignancy), (4) monitor for and promptly treat any cellulitis or ulceration (see Section 134, Leg Ulcers), (5) avoid offending medications if possible (see Table 77–1), and (6) use diuretics (see Section 79, Congestive Heart Failure) when the edema is refractory to more conservative measures. Potential complications of all diuretics include saline depletion, hypokalemia, hyponatremia, and renal insufficiency.

The treatment of generalized edematous disorders (cardiac, renal, or hepatic diseases) includes dietary salt restriction, diuretics, and specific treatments tailored to the underlying disorder (e.g., surgery for valvular heart disease, corticosteroids for some causes of the nephrotic syndrome). Most patients with acute or severe generalized edema are best hospitalized for enforced bed rest (which promotes diuresis) and diagnostic tests.

Cross-references: Eczema (Section 28), Congestive Heart Failure (Section 79), Painful and Swollen Calf (Section 131), Leg Ulcers (Section 134), Proteinuria (Section 183).

REFERENCES

1. Henry JA, Altmann P. Assessment of hypoproteinaemic oedema: A simple physical sign. Br Med J 1978;1:890–891.
   The ease of edema pitting and the rapidity with which the pitting recovers correlate inversely with the serum albumin level.

2. Ruschhaupt WF, Graor RA. Evaluation of the patient with leg edema. Postgrad Med 1985;78:132–139.
   Concise and practical review of unilateral and bilateral swelling.

3. Smith RD, Spittell JA, Schirger A. Secondary lymphedema of the leg: Its characteristics and diagnostic implications. JAMA 1963;185:80–82.
   Clinical features of 80 cases.

78 ANGINA

Problem

DAVID H. HICKAM

EPIDEMIOLOGY/ETIOLOGY. Angina is the syndrome of recurrent chest pain in adults. Classic angina pectoris refers to a characteristic pain that occurs intermittently for a few minutes at a time, is located substernally, radiates to the neck or arms, is described as tight or pressing, is brought on by exertion and relieved by rest, and is severe enough to cause the patient to stop all activities. However, many patients' symptoms lack some of these features, leading to the use of terms such as atypical angina, variant angina, nonanginal chest pain, and noncardiac pain. Angina, particularly in less typical variants, can be caused by any of the etiologies of chest pain (see Section 74, Table 74–1).

Many studies of patients undergoing coronary arteriography have found that patients with classic angina pectoris are more likely to have obstructive disease of the coronary arteries than those with less typical pain. Other risk factors for coronary artery disease (CAD)—male sex, older age, hypertension, hypercholesterolemia, diabetes mellitus, smoking history—increase the likelihood that an individual will have anginal pain and that the pain is caused by CAD.

Studies of patients with angina and negative tests for CAD have found evidence of esophageal motor disorders in half and reflux esophagitis in 10%. However, it is possible that the esophageal disorders were not actually the cause of pain in some of these patients.

SYMPTOMS AND SIGNS. Because the degree to which a patient's pain is typical of angina correlates with the probability that CAD is present, specific criteria should be used to classify pain as typical angina, atypical angina, or nonanginal. The most important criterion is whether the pain is brought on by exertion and relieved by rest. Approximately 80% of patients with exertional chest pain have CAD. Relief of the pain with nitroglycerin also is a helpful characteristic. Pain caused by CAD is usually relieved within 3 minutes. The specificity of this criterion decreases as the time accepted as defining relief is lengthened. Since nitroglycerin relaxes esophageal smooth muscle, esophageal motor disorders should be considered in patients whose pain is relieved by nitroglycerin but who do not have CAD on further evaluation.

Approximately half of patients with the syndrome of atypical angina are found to have CAD on coronary arteriography. Patients should be considered as having atypical angina when there is an inconsistent relationship of the pain to exertion—for example, when a certain level of exercise brings on pain only some of the time, or when mild activities cause the pain but other more strenuous activities do not. It is also appropriate to consider pain atypical angina if it is consistently exertional but other characteristics are atypical, such as a location in the lateral chest, a pleuritic quality, or inconsistent relief achieved with nitroglycerin.

Approximately 20% of patients whose pain was classified as nonanginal have CAD on arteriography studies. Nonanginal chest pain is not exertional, is not relieved by nitroglycerin, is usually located in the lateral chest, and is often aggravated by deep breaths or other movement of the chest.

A clinician's estimate of the probability that a patient's chest pain is caused by CAD should include other patient characteristics. CAD is rare in patients under age 40 unless there are significant risk factors such as a severely elevated cholesterol level or high consumption of cigarettes or cocaine. Patients with a known history of myocardial infarction are more likely to have CAD. The physical examination is of little use, however, because most patients with CAD have no specific physical findings.

The clinician should resist using evidence of other diseases to influence the estimate of the probability of CAD. For example, murmurs suggesting mitral valve prolapse probably are as common in patients with CAD as in those without CAD. Some patients with CAD have chest wall tenderness. Relief of pain by antacids (suggesting reflux esophagitis) does not reliably exclude CAD.

CLINICAL APPROACH.   The reference standard test is coronary arteriography, though rare patients may have ischemia caused by small-vessel obstructions not visible on arteriography. Tests other than arteriography are commonly referred to as noninvasive studies. For all the noninvasive tests, the clinician must estimate the pretest probability of CAD, then use the test result to convert the pretest estimate to a posttest probability. (See Section 12, Principles of Screening.)

The resting ECG is easy to perform, can be interpreted by the average clinician, and should be obtained in all patients except those with a very low pretest probability of CAD. Its greatest value is in detecting Q waves indicative of prior myocardial infarction. If Q waves are absent, the test should be considered positive if there are T wave inversions or ST segment depression of 1 mm or greater. These findings have a sensitivity for CAD of 25% in men and 40% in women, with a specificity of approximately 75%. Thus, the resting ECG is not sensitive enough to exclude CAD in patients with an intermediate pretest probability.

In patients with a high pretest probability of CAD, no diagnostic testing other than the ECG is necessary. If the ECG shows new changes or significant ST segment depressions or elevations, immediate hospitalization should be considered. Otherwise, the patient should be started on medical therapy for CAD pending further evaluation (see below).

The two most commonly used cardiac stress tests are exercise ECG and thallium scintigraphy. Both are based on recordings made before, during, and after the patient undergoes a graded exercise load, usually on a treadmill. On average, the exercise ECG has a sensitivity of 0.70 and a specificity of 0.70 for any CAD. Thallium scintigraphy has a sensitivity of approximately 0.85 and a specificity of approximately 0.80. Thus, the specificity of both tests is such that they have limited value for excluding CAD in patients with a high pretest probability (see Section 89, Exercise Tolerance Testing).

There are two situations in which stress tests are most useful clinically. The first is to help make a diagnosis in patients with an intermediate pretest probability of CAD, such as middle-aged men with atypical angina. A positive result on either exercise ECG and thallium scintigraphy moves the patient's probability to the high range, and a negative result moves the probability to the low range. Because exercise ECG is less expensive and easier to perform than the thallium study, it is preferable for most patients.

The second major clinical indication for stress tests is to help plan management in patients with a high probability of CAD. Some subgroups of these patients may have better long-term outcomes when treated with either coronary bypass surgery or coronary angioplasty. For example, a patient with a single high-grade proximal coronary lesion may be greatly improved by angioplasty. Patients with left main coronary disease, multiple vessel disease, or poor LV function may have improved survival with bypass surgery. If the exercise ECG or thallium study is abnormal, the consulting cardiologist may choose to proceed with arteriography to guide the patient's further treatment.

If CAD has been excluded, tests for esophageal disorders can be considered, though these tests are expensive and uncomfortable for the patient. The only definitive test for reflux esophagitis is endoscopy, and esophageal manometry is necessary to diagnose motor disorders. Barium esophagography is insensitive for motor disorders and lacks specificity for reflux. Thus, the diagnosis of esophageal disease is often based on clinical grounds (atypical chest pain and previous history of peptic disease) rather than on definitive tests.

MANAGEMENT.   Successful reduction of symptoms in CAD is associated with better long-term outcomes in these patients. Three major classes of medications are available to treat symptoms of CAD: nitrates, beta blockers, and calcium channel blockers (Table 78–1). The major pharmacologic action of all three classes is to reduce cardiac workload. While drugs in two of the classes (nitrates and calcium channel blockers) may improve coronary perfusion through dilation of coronary arteries, this probably is a minor effect in patients other than those having coronary artery spasm. Because the pharmacologic effects differ across the three classes, patients often benefit from treatment with more than one medication.

Nearly all patients with CAD should be given sublingual nitroglycerin, which usually brings rapid relief when symptoms occur. It sometimes is useful to instruct the patient to take nitroglycerin prophylactically just before engaging in strenuous activity, though longer acting drugs are generally of greater value for preventing episodes of pain. Any of the three classes can be chosen for initial therapy. Nitrates cause reduced ventricular volume through venous pool-

TABLE 78–1. MEDICATIONS USED TO REDUCE THE FREQUENCY OF ANGINAL CHEST PAIN IN PATIENTS WITH CORONARY ARTERY DISEASE

Generic Name	Brand Name	Starting Dose	Maximal Dose
Sublingual Nitrates[1]			
Nitroglycerin	Nitrostat	0.3 mg PRN	0.8 mg PRN
Topical Nitrates[1]			
Transdermal nitroglycerin	Nitro-Dur	0.2 mg/hr	0.8 mg/hr
	Transderm-Nitro		
Nitroglycerin ointment, 2%	Nitrol	1 inch q.h.s.	6 inches q.h.s.
Oral Nitrates[1]			
Isosorbide dinitrate	Isordil	5 mg q.i.d.	40 mg q.i.d.
	Sorbitrate		
Pentaerythritol tetranitrate	Peritrate	10 mg q.i.d.	60 mg q.i.d.
Erithrityl tetranitrate	Cardilate	10 mg q.i.d.	40 mg q.4h.
Beta Blockers[2]			
Propranolol	Inderal	20 mg q.i.d.	60 mg q.i.d.
Metoprolol	Lopressor	50 mg b.i.d.	100 mg q.i.d.
Atenolol	Tenormin	50 mg q.d.	200 mg q.d.
Nadolol	Corgard	40 mg q.d.	240 mg q.d.
Timolol	Blocadren	10 mg b.i.d.	30 mg b.i.d.
Calcium Channel Blockers[3]			
Nifedipine	Adalat	10 mg t.i.d.	40 mg q.i.d.
	Procardia		
Verapamil	Calan	40 mg t.i.d.	160 mg t.i.d.
	Isoptin		
Diltiazem	Cardizem	30 mg q.i.d.	120 mg q.i.d.

[1]All the nitrate preparations have similar side effects, including headache, hypotension, and tachycardia. Individual patients may tolerate some preparations better than others.

[2]All the beta blockers in this table can cause any of the side effects of this class of medications. The "cardioselective" agents (atenolol and metoprolol) are slightly less prone than the other beta blockers to cause bronchoconstriction, cold extremities, and insulin-mediated hypoglycemia. The "lipophilic" agents (atenolol, nadolol, and timolol) are slightly less prone to cause fatigue and sleep disorders. All of these beta blockers have similar tendencies to cause bradycardia and left ventricular depression. Other beta blockers having intrinsic sympathomimetic activity (acebutolol, carteolol, pindolol) are commonly used to treat hypertension but are not primary agents for the treatment of ischemic heart disease.

[3]The three calcium channel blockers vary in their side effect profiles. Nifedipine is more likely than the other agents to cause headache and hypotension but is less likely to cause problems attributable to bradycardia or left ventricular depression. Verapamil has a greater tendency than nifedipine and diltiazem to cause gastrointestinal symptoms.

ing and are relatively free of side effects. Beta blockers reduce heart rate, ventricular contractility, and blood pressure, making them particularly appropriate in hypertensive patients. They can cause bronchoconstriction and are relatively contraindicated in patients with pulmonary disease. Calcium channel blockers reduce ventricular contractility and peripheral vascular resistance, making them a useful alternative to beta blockers in patients with hypertension.

Medication doses should be increased and additional medications added until the patient has adequate reduction of angina frequency or has achieved maximal hemodynamic effects of the drugs. Doses of beta blockers usually should not be increased if the resting heart rate is less than 60 beats/min or the heart rate with moderate exercise is less than 90 beats/min. Calcium channel blocker doses should not be increased if the systolic blood pressure is less than 100 mm Hg. Nitrates are ineffective at single doses larger than approximately 60 mg for isosorbide and comparable doses for the other agents.

Either calcium channel blockers or nitrates can be used for patients with esophageal motor disorders. Section 97 (Dysphagia and Heartburn) reviews the management of reflux esophagitis.

FOLLOW-UP. Patients with suspected CAD should be seen frequently in the clinic to assess their initial response to treatment. Patients who do not respond to treatment should undergo further diagnostic evaluation. Patients should be instructed to seek care immediately if an episode of pain does not respond to nitroglycerin. If the frequency of a patient's anginal episodes increases while on medical therapy, hospitalization for intensive treatment of unstable angina should be considered.

Cross-references: Chest Pain (Section 74), Essential Hypertension (Section 86), Dysphagia and Heartburn (Section 97).

REFERENCES

1.   Goldman L, Lee TH. Noninvasive tests for diagnosing the presence and extent of coronary artery disease: Exercise electrocardiography, thallium scintigraphy, and radionuclide ventriculography. J Gen Intern Med 1986;1:258–265.
     Good review of noninvasive testing, with strategies for testing in various clinical syndromes.

2.   Katz PO, Dalton CB, Richter JE, et al. Esophageal testing of patients with noncardiac chest pain or dysphagia: Results of three years' experience with 1161 patients. Ann Intern Med 1987;106:593–597.
     Data on prevalence of esophageal disorders and yield of tests for these disorders.

3.   Ladenheim ML, Kotler TS, Pollock BH, et al. Incremental prognostic power of clinical history, exercise electrocardiography and myocardial perfusion scintigraphy in suspected coronary artery disease. Am J Cardiol 1987;59:270–277.
     Useful algorithms for using test results to classify patients' risk of complications of coronary artery disease.

4.   Mark DB, Hlatky MD, Harrell FE, et al. Exercise treadmill score for predicting prognosis in coronary artery disease. Ann Intern Med 1987;106:793–800.
     Additional data on estimating the risk of adverse events in coronary artery disease.

79 CONGESTIVE HEART FAILURE

Problem

STEVEN R. McGEE

EPIDEMIOLOGY. In the United States, the prevalence of congestive heart failure (CHF) is 1%. Although CHF may result from any form of heart disease, major risk factors include hypertension, CAD, rheumatic or congenital heart disease, diabetes mellitus, and older age.

SYMPTOMS AND SIGNS. Table 79–1 lists the symptoms and signs of CHF. Shortness of breath, traditionally regarded as a symptom of left atrial hypertension (pulmonary interstitial edema), may also result from low cardiac output (respiratory muscle fatigue, tachypnea of Cheyne-Stokes respiration), or right atrial hypertension (hydrothorax, ascites).

Early diastolic filling sounds (S_3), if present after 40 years of age, are pathologic and signify rapid diastolic filling, usually from elevated atrial pressures or atrioventricular (AV) valve regurgitation. Additional important physical findings include the following: (1) an abnormal abdominojugular test—elevated jugular venous pressure, produced by midabdominal pressure and sustained longer than 10 seconds—reflects pulmonary wedge pressures greater than 15 mm Hg (in the absence of right ventricular [RV] infarction or isolated RV failure), (2) an apical impulse diameter greater than 3 cm, measured in the left lateral decubitus position, predicts an abnormally elevated left ventricular (LV) end-diastolic volume (sensitivity = 92%, specificity = 75%), and (3) an abnormal Valsalva response (square wave response, absence of phase IV overshoot), detected with a sphygmomanometer, correlates with a depressed ejection fraction and an elevated LV end-diastolic pressure.[3]

TABLE 79–1. CONGESTIVE HEART FAILURE: SYMPTOMS AND SIGNS

Hemodynamics	Symptom	Sign
Low cardiac output	Fatigue, syncope, angina, dyspnea	Cheyne-Stokes respiration, peripheral cyanosis
High right atrial pressure	Edema, abdominal swelling, dyspnea	Elevated central venous pressure, edema, ascites, right ventricular S_3
High left atrial pressure	Dyspnea, orthopnea, paroxysmal nocturnal dyspnea	Lung crackles (more sensitive in acute than chronic CHF), left ventricular S_3

CLINICAL APPROACH.   Characteristic symptoms, signs, and chest radiographic findings (large heart, redistribution of blood flow to upper zones, pleural effusions, pulmonary edema) support the diagnosis of CHF. Ejection fraction, measured by echocardiography or radionuclide ventriculography, remains a valuable prognostic sign but a poor diagnostic test: 20% of patients with abnormally depressed ejection fractions do not have clinical CHF, while 40% of patients with clinical CHF have normal ejection fractions. Explanations for this poor sensitivity include (1) the patient's CHF reflects valvular heart disease, or diastolic instead of systolic dysfunction, or (2) the patient's ejection fraction, normal at rest, decreases during exercise.

The clinician should always attempt to clarify the cause of the patient's cardiomyopathy using the patient interview, physical examination, chest radiography, ECG, and echocardiography, because the specific treatment for many patients depends on a precise diagnosis (e.g., surgery for valvular or pericardial heart disease; control of alcoholism, hypertension, or ischemia for the respective cardiomyopathies; beta blockers or verapamil for diastolic dysfunction).

In patients with unstable symptoms, the clinician should systematically review important precipitating causes (Table 79–2).

MANAGEMENT.   Management goals include reducing symptoms, preventing complications, and improving survival. Most drug treatments for CHF require careful monitoring of blood pressure, serum electrolyte levels, and renal function.

Diuretics.   Diuretics reduce atrial pressures, and therefore symptoms, more rapidly and effectively than any other oral drug available for CHF (Table 79–3). Treatment of patients without diuretics (for example, with vasodilators alone) may result in recurrent pulmonary edema. Long-term treatment with diuretics, in contrast to acute diuresis, may actually enhance cardiac output. Hypokalemia occurs commonly with thiazide and loop diuretics and requires treatment if (1) the potassium level is below 2.9 mEq/liter, (2) hypokalemia is symptomatic, or (3) the patient is taking digoxin. Potential complications of all diuretics include saline depletion, hypotension, and renal insuffiency.

Digoxin.   Digoxin benefits patients with dilated hearts who have an S_3 and poor systolic function. In these patients, serum trough digoxin levels of 1.2 to

TABLE 79–2.   PRECIPITATING CAUSES OF CONGESTIVE HEART FAILURE

Hyperthyroidism
New drug added (beta blocker, nonsteroidal anti-inflammatory drug, alcohol, verapamil, group I antiarrhythmic)
Myocardial ischemia
Noncompliance with diet or medications
Bradyarrhythmia or tachyarrhythmia
Anemia
Renal failure
Fever
Uncontrolled hypertension

TABLE 79–3.   DRUG THERAPY FOR CHF

Drug	Starting Oral Dose	Usual Maintenance Oral Dose	Cost ($)/Day[1]
Thiazide Diuretics			
Hydrochlorthiazide	25 mg q.d.	25–50 mg q.d.	0.03
Metalozone	2.5 mg q.d.	2.5–10 mg q.d.	0.33
Loop Diuretics			
Furosemide	20 mg q.d.	20–160 mg q.d. (b.i.d.)	0.03
K-sparing Diuretics			
Triamterene	100 mg q.d.	100–200 mg q.d.	0.34
Spironolactone	50 mg q.d.	50–200 mg q.d.	0.08
Vasodilators			
Direct-acting			
Hydralazine	25 mg q.8h.	50–100 mg q.6–8h.	0.10
Isosorbide	10 mg q.8h.	20–80 mg q.6–8h.	0.07
dinitrate			
ACE inhibitor			
Captopril	6.25 mg q.8h.	25–50 mg q.8h.	1.56
Enalapril	2.5 mg q.d.	10–20 mg b.i.d.	1.57

[1]Average wholesale price, 1991 *Drug Topics Red Book*, for lower dose under "usual maintenance dose."

1.7 ng/ml result in less dyspnea, increased exercise tolerance, and decreased heart size. Older retrospective studies suggested that digoxin used after myocardial infarction may decrease survival, while more recent studies that controlled for age, ejection fraction, and prior myocardial infarction failed to show adverse effects on survival. Digoxin produces no benefit in patients with normal-sized hearts and normal systolic function (e.g., hypertrophic cardiomyopathy, pericardial diseases). Patients with digoxin toxicity may experience brady- or tachyarrhythmias, confusion, anorexia, nausea, or vomiting. Digoxin blood levels help predict digoxin toxicity, but there is considerable overlap. Decreased renal function, hypokalemia, myocardial disease, and hypothyroidism all predispose patients to digoxin toxicity.

Vasodilator Therapy.   Arterial and venous beds constrict when the cardiac output decreases, presumably to maintain blood pressure and increase preload. In CHF this physiologic response may be maladaptive, because reversal of vasoconstriction by vasodilators (hydralazine + isosorbide [VA cooperative study], enalapril [CONSENSUS study]) not only produces significant improvement in exercise duration, dyspnea, and fatigue but improves 1-year survival by 30%. Captopril also significantly improves symptoms and may decrease mortality. In contrast, hydralazine alone or prasozin alone produce little if any sustained benefit.

Because hydralazine and isosorbide cause more side effects, angiotensin-converting enzyme (ACE) inhibitors are the vasodilators of choice. The initial dose of ACE inhibitors should be small (see Table 79–3); if well tolerated, the dose may be slowly increased every several days, while blood pressure and renal function are monitored. ACE inhibitors may cause significant hypotension, especially in patients who have previously received large doses of diuretics or who have hyponatremia or severe CHF. In these patients, ACE inhibitors are best initiated during a hospitalization; if they are given in the outpatient setting, the clinician should monitor the patient's orthostatic blood pressure frequently after the first dose until the peak effect period has passed (3 hours for captopril, 6 hours for enalapril). Some side effects—hypotension, worsening renal function, and hyperkalemia—occur more often with long-acting agents (e.g., enalapril) and may be minimized by diuretic reduction. Other side effects of ACE inhibitors include dysgeusia, rash, angioedema, and cough.

Vasodilator Therapy versus Digoxin.   It is unclear which drug, digoxin or ACE inhibitor, is optimal second-line therapy after diuretics. Documented vasodilator survival benefit occurs in patients already taking diuretics and digoxin (VA cooperative study and CONSENSUS Study). Vasodilators are more appropriate in patients with mitral regurgitation; digoxin is more appropriate in patients with dilated cardiomyopathy who have hypotension or renal insufficiency induced by ACE inhibitors. In one multicenter trial, patients symptomatic despite diuretics received digoxin, captopril, or placebo: both drugs improved symptoms, captopril to a greater extent but at the expense of more symptomatic hypotension (Captopril-Digoxin Multicenter Research Group[1]).

Other Inotropic Agents.   L-dopa and phosphodiesterase inhibitors (for example amrinore or milrinone) produce sustained symptomatic and hemodynamic improvement. These drugs are still considered experimental, however, because of frequent side effects (nausea with L-dopa, palpitations with milrinone), increased ventricular arrhythmias (milrinone), and a tendency toward increased mortality (amrinore and milrinone).

Ventricular Arrhythmias.   Up to 90% of CHF patients may demonstrate complex ventricular ectopy. **Symptomatic** ventricular tachycardia requires treatment (see Section 84, Chronic Ventricular Arrhythmias). Most authorities do not treat **asymptomatic** ventricular arrhythmias, because (1) evidence that treatment improves survival is lacking and some drugs may actually increase mortality, (2) some antiarrhythmic drugs depress cardiac output and potentially have proarrhythmic effects, and (3) prospective identification of patients at high risk for sudden death is imprecise.

Anticoagulation.   In nonrandomized retrospective studies of patients with dilated cardiomyopathy and normal sinus rhythm, anticoagulation reduced the risk of systemic embolism from 3.5 episodes per 100 patient-years to zero. Without anticoagulation, the lifetime risk of systemic embolism is 18%. If no contraindications exist, many authorities consider anticoagulation. Although echocardiography documents left ventricular mural thrombi in 40% of patients with dilated cardiomyopathy, clinically evident emboli may occur just as frequently when this finding is present as when it is not.

Adverse Reactions to Tricyclic Antidepressants.   Some CHF patients require treatment for depression. Although tricyclic antidepressants possess antiarrhythmic properties and do not affect cardiac output, they may cause severe orthostatic hypotension in CHF patients. This adverse effect may occur with low doses, but it is least problematic with nortryptiline. If preexisting bundle-branch block exists, tricyclic therapy produces second- or third-degree heart block in 25%; these patients require extremely close follow-up by experienced personnel, as well as consideration of alternative antidepressant therapies.

Refractory CHF. Possible reasons include (1) poor absorption of drug (documented in uncontrolled CHF), (2) poor compliance with a low-salt diet, (3) concomitant nonsteroidal anti-inflammatory drug use, (4) renal insufficiency (if the glomerular filtration rate is less than 25 ml/min, thiazide diuretics alone are ineffective), (5) uncontrolled precipitating cause of CHF (see Table 79–2), and (6) the patient's dyspnea is not due to elevated left atrial pressure and therefore should not respond to diuresis (e.g., dyspnea from low cardiac output or chronic obstructive lung disease).

Some patients with refractory CHF benefit from combined loop and thiazide diuretics. Initiation of such therapy may require hospitalization because of the risk of profound hypokalemia, hypotension, and renal insufficiency. Hospitalization of patients with refractory CHF also enforces bed rest (which increases diuresis) and provides the opportunity for parenteral diuretic therapy. For the few patients with severe refractory CHF (ejection fraction < 30%, CHF functional class III or IV despite optimal therapy), cardiac transplantation is the only effective alternative.

FOLLOW-UP.   Major causes of death include progressive CHF (40%) and sudden death (40%). The remaining 20% die of infection, pulmonary embolus, and myocardial infarction, among other causes. Poor prognostic signs include severe symptoms (the 1-year mortality for patients with class IV CHF exceeds 50%), poor ejection fraction, hyponatremia, and ventricular arrhythmias (although arrhythmias predict death from progressive CHF, not sudden death).

REFERENCES

1. Deedwania PC. Angiotensin-converting enzyme inhibitors in congestive heart failure. Arch Intern Med 1990;150:1798–1805.
   Reviews ACE inhibitors: mechanism of action, clinical trials, and safety.

2. Francis GS, Chatterjee K, Prystowsky EN. Should asymptomatic ventricular arrhythmias in patients with congestive heart failure be treated with antiarrhythmic drugs? J Am Coll Cardiol 1988;12:274–283.
   Excellent overview with protagonist's and antagonist's viewpoint. Companion articles in this series review use of digoxin (pp. 265–273) and other inotropic agents (pp. 559–569).

3. Nishimura RA, Tajik AJ. The valsalva maneuver and response revisited. Mayo Clin Proc 1986;61:211–217.
   Utility of Valsalva response in CHF: a normal Valsalva response correlates with an ejection fraction of 69% ± 11%, an absent phase IV overshoot with an ejection fraction of 48% ± 15%, and a square wave response with an ejection fraction of 29% ± 11%. The specificity of the test decreases if the patient is taking beta blockers.

4. Packer M. Therapeutic options in the management of chronic heart failure: Is there a drug of first choice? Circulation 1989;79:198–204.

    Critical review of clinical trials, including diuretics, digoxin, vasodilators, as well as other more controversial forms of therapy.

5. Tsevat J, Eckman MH, McNutt RA, Pauker SG. Warfarin for dilated cardiomyopathy: A bloody tough pill to swallow? Med Decision Making 1989;9:162–169.

    Decision analysis supports chronic anticoagulation, but article concludes that any such recommendation should consider the effects of anticoagulation on the patient's quality of life.

80 AORTIC STENOSIS

Problem

CATHERINE M. OTTO

EPIDEMIOLOGY.   Valvular aortic stenosis is the most common indication for valvular surgery in adults, with over 20,000 aortic valve replacements performed annually in the United States. In addition, many elderly adults have symptoms that may be due to aortic stenosis and have a systolic murmur on examination; in these patients the clinician must exclude severe valvular obstruction.

ETIOLOGY.   In adults, valvular aortic stenosis most often is due to degenerative calcification of a trileaflet valve, with clinical symptoms occurring at age 70 to 80 years. Secondary calcification and fibrosis of a congenital bicuspid valve (occurring in about 1% of the population) results in severe aortic stenosis at age 50 to 60 years. The prevalence of postinflammatory rheumatic aortic stenosis is declining; this condition is always accompanied by rheumatic mitral valve disease.

Valvular aortic stenosis must be distinguished from fixed (membrane or muscular ridge) or dynamic (hypertrophic obstructive cardiomyopathy) subaortic obstruction.

CLINICAL APPROACH.   In the patient with suspected aortic stenosis, the history should determine whether typical symptoms are present: exertional angina, heart failure (dyspnea on exertion is the usual initial symptom), and exertional dizziness or syncope. Physical examination is helpful when the systolic murmur is accompanied by a thrill (grade IV/VI), the carotid upstroke is slow and rising with a reduced systolic impulse, the pulse pressure is reduced, and A_2 is absent (a split S_2 excludes severe aortic stenosis in adults). However, physical examination can be misleading in that most adults with severe aortic stenosis have a softer murmur (grade II/III), and often have a normal carotid upstroke and pulse pressure. The absence of left ventricular (LV) hypertrophy on ECG does not exclude aortic stenosis in adults.

When aortic stenosis is suspected on clinical grounds, further evaluation with two-dimensional and Doppler echocardiography is indicated. Two-dimensional imaging confirms the valvular stenosis, defines the cause of disease, measures any coexisting aortic regurgitation, and excludes subvalvular obstruction. In addition, LV hypertrophy, LV chamber dimensions, and LV systolic function can be assessed. Doppler echocardiography accurately calculates the transaortic pressure gradient and aortic valve orifice area.

Management decisions may be based on echocardiographic findings in most cases. Cardiac catheterization should be employed to evaluate the severity of the stenosis only if the echocardiographic findings are discordant with the clinical impression. Because of the high prevalence (50%) of coexisting coronary disease in patients with aortic stenosis, coronary angiography is indicated prior to aortic valve replacement and may be indicated to define an alternate cause for the patient's symptoms in mild to moderate aortic stenosis.

MANAGEMENT. The prognosis of medically treated severe *symptomatic* valvular aortic stenosis is extremely poor, with a 3-year survival rate of only 25%. Aortic valve replacement can be performed, even in the elderly, with an acceptable operative mortality (10% for patients more than 70 years of age). LV systolic function typically improves after valve replacement (due to afterload reduction). The outcome after percutaneous balloon aortic valvuloplasty has been poor. Thus, the treatment of severe symptomatic aortic stenosis is valve replacement. Coronary bypass grafting can be performed concurrently, if needed, with little increase in the operative risk. In contrast, the prognosis for *asymptomatic* aortic stenosis is no different than that for age-matched controls. Regardless of hemodynamic severity, valve replacement can be deferred until symptoms occur. Medical management in asymptomatic patients should include (1) confirmation of the diagnosis and degree of obstruction with a baseline Doppler echocardiographic study, (2) endocarditis prophylaxis for dental and other procedures, (3) discussion with the patient regarding the eventual need for valve replacement, and (4) counseling the patient to recognize typical symptoms and seek medical attention promptly, since the risk of sudden death is high once symptoms become apparent.

FOLLOW-UP. Symptomatic patients with aortic stenosis need medical follow-up after surgery to monitor anticoagulation (for mechanical prostheses), for endocarditis prophylaxis, and for medical treatment of residual cardiac symptoms. An echocardiogram should be obtained 2 to 3 months following surgery to serve as a baseline should prosthetic valve dysfunction be suspected in the future.

Asymptomatic patients should be followed closely for development of symptoms. The frequency of follow-up echocardiography (every 1–3 years) should be based on the initial severity of disease and on intervening changes in clinical status.

Cross-references: Chest Pain (Section 74), Echocardiography (Section 90), Chronic Anticoagulation (Section 203), Preoperative Cardiovascular Problems (Section 217), Preoperative Infectious Disease Problems (Section 218).

REFERENCES

1.   Judge KW, Otto CM. Doppler echocardiographic evaluation of aortic stenosis. Cardiol Clin 1990;8:203–216.

   Review of the echocardiographic evaluation of aortic stenosis describing methodology and emphasizing limitations.

2.   O'Keefe JH Jr, Shub C, Rettke SR. Risk of noncardiac surgical procedures in patients with aortic stenosis. Mayo Clin Proc 1989;64:400–405.

   Forty-eight patients (mean age 73) with severe aortic stenosis underwent noncardiac surgery with careful diagnostic evaluation and hemodynamic monitoring. There were no intraoperative deaths, although operative morbidity occurred in 9% (transient events in all but one patient).

3.   Otto CM, Pearlman AS. Doppler echocardiography in adults with symptomatic aortic stenosis: Diagnostic utility and cost-effectiveness. Arch Intern Med 1988;148:2553–2560.

   Diagnostic approach to *symptomatic* AS patients: a jet velocity > 4.0 m/sec confirms severe aortic stenosis and need for valve replacement, a velocity < 3.0 m/sec excludes severe aortic stenosis, while a velocity of 3.0 to 4.0 m/sec requires valve area calculation and assessment of coexisting aortic regurgitation.

4.   Pellikka PA, Nishimura RA, Bailey KR, Tajik AJ. The natural history of adults with asymptomatic, hemodynamically significant aortic stenosis. J Am Coll Cardiol 1990;15:1012–1017.

   Asymptomatic AS patients (*n* = 113) with a Doppler jet velocity > 4.0 m/sec had a 2-year actuarial survival of 90%, but only 62% remained symptom free. All three patients with sudden death had symptoms for at least 3 months before death.

5.   Selzer A. Changing aspects of the natural history of valvular aortic stenosis. N Engl J Med 1987;317:91–98.

   Review of natural history of valvular aortic stenosis.

81 MITRAL VALVE PROLAPSE

Problem

ELAINE SACHTER

EPIDEMIOLOGY. Mitral valve prolapse refers to a functional phenomenon and is present when a portion of the mitral valve leaflet(s) crosses the mitral annular plane posterosuperiorly into the left atrium. It is an important cause of isolated mitral regurgitation. The prevalence of mitral valve prolapse is approximately 2.5% to 5.0% of the general population, increases throughout childhood, and peaks in early adulthood. Women are affected twice as often as men. It occurs most commonly as a primary condition, with a greater prevalence among first-degree relatives of affected individuals. The best documented secondary cause, Marfan's syndrome, accounts for only 1 in 500 cases of mitral valve prolapse.

SYMPTOMS AND SIGNS. Mitral valve prolapse is usually an asymptomatic condition. Controlled studies have failed to show an association between mitral valve prolapse and chest pain, anxiety, panic attacks, dyspnea, or syncope. Thoracic bony abnormalities, low body weight, hypotension, and palpitations are associated with mitral valve prolapse but are not sufficiently specific to be useful in the diagnosis.

The auscultatory findings of mitral valve prolapse are midsystolic clicks and/or late systolic apical murmurs that shift timing with changes in body position. Sitting and standing move the click closer to S_1 and prolong the late systolic murmur, while squatting causes the click to move toward S_2 and the murmur to become shorter. Murmurs and clicks can be intermittent in patients with echocardiographic evidence of mitral valve prolapse.

CLINICAL APPROACH. Mitral valve prolapse can be diagnosed from the characteristic auscultatory findings. If the diagnosis is uncertain or if there is concern that mitral regurgitation may be present, echocardiographic confirmation is appropriate (88%–100% sensitivity, 82%–100% specificity).

MANAGEMENT. Asymptomatic patients without mitral regurgitation do not require treatment. Beta blockers have been used empirically in some patients with bothersome palpitations. If severe mitral regurgitation develops, mitral valve replacement is indicated. Patients with mitral valve prolapse and a murmur should receive antibiotic prophylaxis for infective endocarditis. Hypertension should be treated aggressively, since it likely predisposes to chordal rupture and progressive mitral regurgitation in patients with mitral valve prolapse.

FOLLOW-UP. Long-term survival in patients with mitral valve prolapse is not significantly different than in age-matched controls. Appropriate reassur-

233

ance should be given to those in low risk groups and periodic auscultation (every 3–5 years) should be performed to monitor for the development of progressive mitral regurgitation, which occurs in 2% to 4% of unselected patients with mitral valve prolapse. If mitral regurgitation develops, annual follow-up, including auscultation and echocardiography, is indicated.

Complications associated with mitral valve prolapse are concentrated in patients who develop mitral regurgitation. The estimated lifetime risk of needing mitral valve replacement is 4% among men and 1.5% among women with mitral valve prolapse. The absolute risk of infective endocarditis in persons with mitral valve prolapse without a murmur equals that of general population, estimated at 1 in 20,000 adults per year. In patients with mitral valve prolapse and a murmur of mitral regurgitation, the risk is estimated at 1 in 1920 patients per year. The risk of endocarditis associated with mitral valve prolapse is increased threefold in males and fourfold in patients over age 45. Complex arrhythmias are rare in patients with mitral valve prolapse and are more strongly associated with hemodynamically significant mitral regurgitation than with mitral valve prolapse alone. Controversy exists as to whether mitral valve prolapse is an independent risk factor for cerebral ischemia.

Cross-reference: Echocardiography (Section 90).

REFERENCES

1. Devereux RB, Kramer-Fox, Kligfield P. Mitral valve prolapse: Causes, clinical manifestations, and management. Ann Intern Med 1989;111:305–317.
    Overview of etiology, clinical spectrum, and management.

2. Levy D, Savage DD. Prevalence and clinical features of mitral valve prolapse. The Framingham study. Am Heart J 1987;113:1281–1290.
    Discusses epidemiology, symptoms, and auscultatory findings of mitral valve prolapse.

3. MacMahon SW, et al. Mitral valve prolapse and infective endocarditis. Am Heart J 1987;113:1291–1298.
    Discusses the risk of infective endocarditis among subgroups of patients with mitral valve prolapse.

4. Perloff KJ, Child JS. Clinical and epidemiologic issues in mitral valve prolapse: Overview and perspective. Am Heart J 1987;113:1324–1332.
    Reviews diagnostic criteria and clinical features.

82 OTHER VALVULAR DISEASE

Problem

CATHERINE M. OTTO

EPIDEMIOLOGY/ETIOLOGY. **Mitral regurgitation** is the second most common type of valvular disease in adults requiring surgical intervention (aortic stenosis is the most common). Mitral regurgitation may be due to abnormalities of the leaflets themselves (myxomatous mitral valve disease, rheumatic disease, or endocarditis) or of the supporting structures (annular calcification, papillary muscle dysfunction due to myocardial infarction, left ventricular (LV) dilation and systolic dysfunction of any cause). The etiology of **mitral stenosis** is nearly always rheumatic, although an occasional patient may have functional mitral stenosis due to severe degenerative annular and leaflet calcification. The prevalence of rheumatic mitral stenosis has been steadily declining in the past few years as a consequence of the earlier decline in acute rheumatic fever, and rheumatic mitral stenosis now is seen most often in recent immigrants. **Aortic regurgitation** may be due to a congenital bicuspid valve, endocarditis, or aortic root dilation (hypertension, Marfan's syndrome, aortic dissection, annuloaortic ectasia, etc.). **Tricuspid regurgitation** may be due to congenital anomalies (Ebstein's anomaly), endocarditis, rheumatic disease, or carcinoid syndrome, or may be secondary to pulmonary hypertension of any cause. **Tricuspid stenosis** is rare. Hemodynamically significant pulmonic valve disease is uncommon in adults.

CLINICAL APPROACH. The most important methods for detecting valvular heart disease remain a careful history and physical examination. If the physical examination shows a murmur or if the clinical presentation suggests valve disease (a mitral stenosis murmur may be difficult to appreciate on auscultation), echocardiography should be performed. Echocardiography provides definitive information on valve anatomy and dynamics, the cause of valvular disease, the presence and severity of stenosis or regurgitation, compensatory chamber dilation, pulmonary artery pressure, and ventricular function. Cardiac catheterization may be needed to evaluate the degree of CAD but rarely is needed for evaluation of valvular disease per se.

It is important to distinguish between *acute* and *chronic* valvular regurgitation. With acute regurgitation (e.g., mitral regurgitation due to papillary muscle rupture following myocardial infarction or aortic regurgitation due to endocarditis), both compensatory chamber enlargement and the classic physical findings may be absent. A high level of suspicion based on the patient's history and prompt echocardiography are needed to diagnose acute regurgitation.

MANAGEMENT. Medical management includes the appropriate use of diuretics to relieve pulmonary congestion, endocarditis prophylaxis for dental and other procedures, treatment of associated arrhythmias, and careful follow-up. If LV function is normal, digoxin is not needed except for control of the atrial fibrillation rate. In mitral stenosis with atrial fibrillation, chronic anticoagulation with warfarin is indicated to prevent left atrial thrombus formation and systemic embolization. For chronic mitral regurgitation, afterload reduction is beneficial.

In symptomatic patients with severe valvular disease, surgical intervention—valve repair for mitral regurgitation, percutaneous valvuloplasty for stenosis, or valve replacement—is indicated. The timing of valve replacement in asymptomatic patients with chronic valvular regurgitation is controversial insofar as irreversible LV systolic function can occur before symptoms develop.

FOLLOW-UP. Patients with significant valvular regurgitation should be carefully followed with cardiac imaging at 6-month to 1-year intervals (depending on ventricular size and systolic function at entry). Echocardiography is the preferred follow-up method with sequential measurement of LV end-systolic dimension and assessment of LV systolic function. In some settings, resting and exercise radionuclide ventriculography may be useful in patient follow-up. Patients should be referred to a cardiologist when they become symptomatic, for severe regurgitation regardless of LV size and function, for any evidence of deteriorating LV systolic function, or when LV end-systolic dimension exceeds 50 mm.

Cross-references: Dyspnea (Section 19), Echocardiography (Section 90), Chronic Anticoagulation (Section 203), Preoperative Cardiovascular Problems (Section 217), Preoperative Infectious Disease Problems (Section 218).

REFERENCES

1. Biem HJ, Detsky AS, Armstrong PW. Management of asymptomatic chronic aortic regurgitation with left ventricular dysfunction: A decision analysis. J Gen Intern Med 1990;5:394–401.

   Decision analysis (with references to previous literature) of timing of valve replacement in asymptomatic aortic regurgitation, with an accompanying editorial.

2. Cheitlan MD. The timing of surgery in mitral and aortic valve disease. Curr Prob Cardiol 1987;12:69–149.

   Well-referenced review of the diagnosis, natural history, and treatment of valvular disease.

3. Pearlman AS, Otto CM. Quantification of valvular regurgitation. Echocardiography 1987; 4:271–287.

   · Review of Doppler–echocardiographic methods for evaluation of valvular regurgitation.

4. Ross J Jr. Afterload mismatch in aortic and mitral valve disease: Implications for surgical therapy. J Am Coll Cardiol 1985;5:811–826.

   Physiology of left ventricular dysfunction in valvular disease.

5. Stevenson LW, Bellil D, Grover-McKay M, et al. Effects of afterload reduction (diuretics and vasodilators) on LV volumes and mitral regurgitation in severe CHF secondary to ischemic or idiopathic dilated cardiomyopathy. Am J Cardiol 1987;60:654–658.

   Detailed hemodynamic study in a small number of patients illustrating the effects of afterload reduction in mitral regurgitation.

83 ATRIAL FIBRILLATION

Problem

JOYCE E. WIPF

EPIDEMIOLOGY/ETIOLOGY.   Atrial fibrillation, the most common atrial arrhythmia, may be chronic or paroxysmal. The prevalence of atrial fibrillation is 0.4% in adults, increasing with age to 2% to 4% among those over age 60. Paroxysmal atrial fibrillation becomes chronic in about one-third of cases. Although rheumatic mitral valve disease was once the most common cause, coronary artery disease (CAD), hypertension, and congestive heart failure (CHF) now account for over 40% of cases and hyperthyroidism for 15%. Up to 15% of cases of chronic atrial fibrillation occur in otherwise healthy adults with no identifiable risk factors, a condition called "lone" atrial fibrillation. Paroxysmal atrial fibrillation may be precipitated by alcohol ("holiday heart"), stress, caffeine, or intercurrent acute illnesses such as pneumonia or pulmonary embolism.

Atrial fibrillation not only causes immediate hemodynamic effects but increases the potential risk of thromboembolism to the brain and other organs. In comparison with subjects with normal sinus rhythm, the risk of stroke is seventeen times higher for patients with rheumatic heart disease and chronic atrial fibrillation, five times higher for patients with chronic nonrheumatic atrial fibrillation,[2] and two times higher for patients with paroxysmal atrial fibrillation. Carefully defined, lone atrial fibrillation poses a low risk of embolism. Over 20% of patients with atrial fibrillation and a history of stroke will have another embolic event during the first year. The lifetime risk of recurrence is 30% to 75% if not anticoagulated.

SYMPTOMS AND SIGNS.   Atrial fibrillation often produces no symptoms and is discovered incidentally on ECG or by detecting an irregularly irregular pulse on examination. Those with a rapid ventricular rate may experience palpitations, lightheadedness, fatigue, angina, and dyspnea, with hypotension and signs of CHF. Because the atrial contraction contributes approximately 10% of cardiac output, patients with underlying LV dysfunction may become symptomatic even at relatively normal heart rates. Patients with thyrotoxicosis may experience anxiety, restlessness, and diarrhea, although atrial fibrillation without symptoms may be the sole clue to apathetic hyperthyroidism in the elderly. Physical examination focuses on vital signs, thyroid palpation, and evaluation for valvular heart disease and CHF.

CLINICAL APPROACH.   The two major questions in the diagnostic workup of newly noted AF are (1) What is the etiology? and (2) Has the patient had an

237

embolic event? Both help to determine subsequent therapy and the patient's risk of embolism.

Routine laboratory tests are thyroid function tests and echocardiography, which may disclose abnormal heart valves, LV dysfunction, or a cardiac thrombus. Left atrial size does not accurately predict successful cardioversion or maintenance of sinus rhythm. Patients who are acutely symptomatic require hospital admission and evaluation for myocardial ischemia, pulmonary embolism, and pneumonia.

Among patients with acute strokes, 15% to 25% are in atrial fibrillation, and of these, 75% have had an embolism originating from an atrial thrombus. There is no reference standard for determining whether a stroke is cardiogenic, but supporting features include the presence of a cardiac thrombus, infarcts in multiple vascular distributions, the sudden onset of a maximal deficit without prior transient ischemic attacks, and absence of significant atherosclerotic carotid stenoses. Cardiogenic strokes are more likely to be hemorrhagic. To detect carotid stenosis, noninvasive duplex ultrasonography should be performed irrespective of the finding of carotid bruits on examination. Other helpful diagnostic studies include CT of the brain and echocardiography.

MANAGEMENT.   Patients with rapid atrial fibrillation and acute symptoms should be hospitalized for evaluation and treatment in a monitored setting. Patients with acute atrial fibrillation and hemodynamic compromise (angina, hypotension, pulmonary edema) require emergency electrical cardioversion to normal sinus rhythm. No anticoagulation is required for arrhythmias present less than 3 days. If the patient has a rapid ventricular rate but is hemodynamically stable, the physician should lower the rate with antiarrhythmic medications; digoxin is the usual agent of choice unless a preexcitation syndrome (e.g., Wolff-Parkinson-White syndrome) is present. Decisions about cardioversion or antiarrhythmic agents should be made in consultation with a cardiologist if possible. Patients with asymptomatic chronic atrial fibrillation can usually be evaluated as outpatients until they are admitted for cardioversion. Stable patients who are not candidates for cardioversion or anticoagulation may be treated with digoxin alone for rate control.

Because cardioversion carries a 1% to 5% risk of embolism, stable patients with chronic atrial fibrillation should be therapeutically anticoagulated with warfarin (prothrombin time ratio of approximately 1.3–1.7, or International Normalized Ratio [INR] of 2.0–3.0) for 3 weeks prior to the procedure. The usual initial dose of warfarin is 2.5 to 5 mg/day; the prothrombin time should be checked weekly (see Section 203, Chronic Anticoagulation). Once therapeutically anticoagulated, the patient is admitted and chemical cardioversion attempted with a type 1A antiarrhythmic agent such as procainamide or quinidine before electrical cardioversion. Anticoagulation should be continued for 3 to 4 weeks after cardioversion, as embolic events have been documented up to 10 days after the procedure. Patients are more likely to remain in sinus rhythm if the atrial fibrillation had been present for less than 1 year and if they are placed on chronic antiarrhythmic therapy. There is, however, evidence that chronic treatment with quinidine may increase overall mortality. Newer drugs such as amiodarone and flecainide are occasionally used for life-threatening arrhythmias when type 1A agents have failed to control these episodes.

A controversial and complex issue is whether to chronically anticoagulate patients in whom cardioversion fails and who remain in chronic atrial fibrillation. Warfarin anticoagulation reduces embolic risk but is associated with major bleeding complications in 5% to 10% of patients. In patients with acute nonhemorrhagic stroke whose blood pressure is controlled, the risk of converting a nonhemorrhagic to a hemorrhagic stroke by anticoagulation is low. Presently, aspirin is no substitute for warfarin, although preliminary data suggest 375 mg/day of aspirin may reduce the stroke risk in patients under age 75. Absolute and relative contraindications to anticoagulation appear in Section 203.

Patients with chronic atrial fibrillation and valvular heart disease, prosthetic heart valves, or a history of embolism should be anticoagulated. Anticoagulation is also recommended for atrial fibrillation with associated cardiovascular disease in the absence of contraindications (Table 83–1).

FOLLOW-UP. Following successful cardioversion, patients need follow-up within a few weeks to evaluate whether sinus rhythm is maintained, and to monitor antiarrhythmic drug levels and potential side effects of antiarrhythmic therapy. When cardioversion is unsuccessful or if atrial fibrillation recurs, the clinician must decide whether to reattempt cardioversion (if drug levels are subtherapeutic or atrial fibrillation is poorly tolerated) or to initiate chronic anticoagulation. Follow-up of anticoagulated individuals is described in Section

TABLE 83–1. GUIDELINES FOR ANTICOAGULATION IN CHRONIC ATRIAL FIBRILLATION

Anticoagulation Indicated in Atrial Fibrillation
Associated with rheumatic heart disease
History of embolic event
Short-term before and after cardioversion
Prosthetic mitral valve of any type

Anticoagulation Recommended if No Relative Contraindications
Cardiomyopathy with poor LV function
Nonvalvular heart disease
Cardiac thrombus

Unclear Relative Risk and Benefit
Recent onset of atrial fibrillation
Lone atrial fibrillation in the elderly
Thyrotoxicosis and atrial fibrillation
Documented long-standing uncomplicated atrial fibrillation

Anticoagulation not Recommended
Lone atrial fibrillation in patients under 65
Paroxysmal atrial fibrillation without history of embolism

203 (Chronic Anticoagulation). Some 60% to 80% of individuals treated chronically with antiarrhythmic agents will still be in sinus rhythm 1 year after cardioversion. Use of alcohol increases the likelihood of recurrence of atrial fibrillation.

Cross-references: Palpitations (Section 76), Congestive Heart Failure (Section 79), Echocardiography (Section 90), Cerebrovascular Disease (Section 148), Common Thyroid Disorders (Section 156).

REFERENCES

1. Cerebral Embolism Task Force. Cardiogenic brain embolism: The second report of the Cerebral Embolism Task Force. Arch Neurol 1989;146:727–743.
    Discusses etiologies and diagnostic indicators of cardiogenic emboli, and management of atrial fibrillation with embolism.

2. Kannel WB, Abbott RD, Savage DD, McNamara PM. Epidemiologic features of chronic atrial fibrillation: The Framingham Study. N Engl J Med 1982;306:1018–1022.
    Classic epidemiologic study of 5200 residents of Framingham, Massachusetts, followed prospectively for development of cardiovascular disease. The risk of stroke was increased in both valvular and nonvalvular atrial fibrillation.

3. Petersen P, Boysen G, Godtfredsen J, Anderson ED, Andersen B. Placebo-controlled, randomized trial of warfarin and aspirin for prevention of thromboembolic complications in chronic atrial fibrillation. Lancet 1989;1:175–179.
    Two-year prospective trial found that warfarin reduced the risk of stroke in nonvalvular atrial fibrillation to 2% per year; 75 mg aspirin daily and placebo were comparable, with an annual stroke risk of 5.5%.

4. Waldo AL. Clinical evaluation in therapy of patients with atrial fibrillation or flutter. Cardiol Clin 1990;8:479–490.
    Reviews pathophysiology, ECG features, and antiarrhythmic therapy for atrial fibrillation.

5. Wipf JE, Lipsky BA. Atrial fibrillation: Thromboembolic risk and indications for anticoagulation. Arch Intern Med 1990;150:1598–1603.
    Literature review of data on embolic risk of chronic and paroxysmal atrial fibrillation and the hemorrhagic complications of anticoagulation. Article includes algorithms for the management of atrial fibrillation and guidelines for anticoagulation.

84 CHRONIC VENTRICULAR ARRHYTHMIAS

Problem

JEANNE POOLE

EPIDEMIOLOGY/ETIOLOGY. The most dangerous ventricular arrhythmias are ventricular fibrillation and sustained ventricular tachycardia. **Ventricular fibrillation** is a sustained polymorphic disorganized rhythm (rate $\geq$ 300 beats/min) with hemodynamic collapse. Among survivors of out-of-hospital ventricular fibrillation not associated with acute myocardial infarction, the mortality is about 26% at 1 year and 38% at 2 years, with most deaths due to recurrent ventricular fibrillation. Risk factors for recurrent ventricular fibrillation include congestive heart failure (CHF), complex arrhythmias on Holter monitoring, male sex, and previous myocardial infarction. **Sustained ventricular tachycardia** (VT) (rate usually 100–270 beats/min) is defined as VT lasting longer than 30 seconds or requiring intervention because of hemodynamic compromise. Although most patients with ventricular fibrillation and sustained VT have underlying coronary artery disease (CAD), some have dilated cardiomyopathy, hypertrophic cardiomyopathy, valvular heart disease, congenital long QT syndrome, or congenital right ventricular dysplasia.

Nonsustained VT is defined as at least three successive beats of VT that terminate spontaneously in less than 30 seconds. **Ventricular premature contractions** (VPCs) are common and occur in those with heart disease as well as in 40% to 75% of individuals with no evidence of underlying heart disease.

SYMPTOMS AND SIGNS. Symptoms of ventricular arrhythmias range from vague symptoms such as dizziness or light-headedness to palpitations, near-syncope, syncope, or cardiac arrest. The patient's underlying cardiac function and the rate and duration of the tachycardia determine the severity of symptoms. Although most VPCs are asymptomatic, some patients are extremely bothered by the sensation of "skipped" or erratic beats.

Occasional patients present to the outpatient clinic with a stable blood pressure and a wide complex tachycardia (QRS $\geq$ 0.12 sec) on ECG. The physical findings of atrioventricular dissociation (variable intensity of S_1 and intermittent cannon A waves) in these patients support the diagnosis of VT.

CLINICAL APPROACH. Sections 75 and 76 review the approach to syncope and palpitations.

A 12-lead ECG is mandatory in any patient with tachycardia. Specific ECG criteria exist that distinguish VT from supraventricular tachycardia conducted aberrantly.[5]

In patients with documented ventricular arrhythmias, the physician should identify any underlying structural heart disease and determine whether any factors that may provoke arrhythmias are present, such as electrolyte abnormalities (hypokalemia), medications (antiarrhythmics, digoxin) or ongoing myocardial ischemia (chest pain, ECG changes).

The physical examination searches for findings of valvular heart disease, hypertrophic or dilated cardiomyopathy, and CHF.

All patients with ventricular fibrillation and sustained VT should be referred to a cardiologist for consideration of electrophysiologic testing. Coronary angiography is indicated in all patients with ventricular fibrillation or sustained VT, because up to 75% have CAD. Critical coronary lesions should be repaired before electrophysiologic testing is undertaken.

Patients with frequent nonsustained VT should undergo exercise treadmill testing (to identify ischemic heart disease) and echocardiography (to identify valvular heart disease, cardiomyopathy, congenital heart disease, and LV dysfunction).

MANAGEMENT. The decision to treat a patient's ventricular arrhythmias is usually made with consultative help from a cardiologist. The goals of treatment are to improve survival and reduce symptoms. Although recommendations vary widely, several generalizations can be made. First, patients who survive out-of-hospital ventricular fibrillation not associated with acute myocardial infarction should be aggressively treated because they are at high risk for sudden cardiac death. Current approaches include antiarrhythmic drug therapy guided

TABLE 84–1. DRUG PROFILES

Type/Drug	Half-life (hr, Unless Noted)	Major Metabolism	Therapeutic Levels (Trough; μg/ml, Unless Noted)	Oral Maintenance Dose
1A				
Quinidine	3–4	Liver	2–6	200–800 mg q.4–6h.
Procainamide	3	Kidney/liver	4–8	500–2000 mg q.6h.
Disopyramide	5–8	Kidney	2–7	100–300 mg q.6–8h.
1B				
Tocainide	11–22	Kidney/liver	3–11	400–800 mg q.6–12h.
Mexiletine	9–15	Liver	0.8–2.0	200–600 mg q.6–8h.
1C				
Flecainide	10–20	Kidney	200–1000	50–150 mg q.8–12h.
Encainide	3	Liver	10–350 ng/ml	50–100 mg q.8–12h.
Propafenone	6	Liver	70–2000 ng/ml	200–400 mg q.6–8h.
1 (unspecified)				
Moricizine	6–13	Liver	200–1400 ng/ml	200–600 mg q.8h.
3				
Amiodarone	30–45 d	Liver	1.0–2.5	100–300 mg q.24h.
Sotalol	10–28	Kidney	300–3000 ng/ml	80–500 mg q.12–24h.

by electrophysiologic testing and/or implantation of a cardioverter/defibrillator. Implantable devices may provide a survival advantage over antiarrhythmic drug therapy alone. Second, patients who have recurrent symptomatic sustained VT also need aggressive evaluation and therapy. Because antiarrhythmic medications fail in 60% to 70% of patients with this arrhythmia, however, an implantable cardioverter/defibrillator may be necessary. Third, there is no evidence that suppression of VPCs or nonsustained VT prevents sudden cardiac death or improves survival. Although patients with depressed LV function and nonsustained VT or VPCs are at higher risk of sudden death, they also may be more resistant to pharmacologic treatment. Furthermore, recent data from the

TABLE 84–2.   ANTIARRHYTHMIC DRUGS: COMPARISON OF ADVERSE EFFECTS

Drug	CHF?	Proarrhythmic?	Noncardiac Side Effects*	Effect on ECG
Quinidine	±	+ +	+ + nausea, diarrhea, cinchonism, rare hematologic	↑ QRS, ↑ QT
Procainamide	±	+	+ nausea, diarrhea, lupus-like syndrome, rare hematologic	↑ QRS, ↑ QT
Disopyramide	+ + +	+ +	+ + xerostomia, urinary retention	↑ QRS, ↑ QT
Moricizine	±	+	+ nausea, vomiting, tremor, dizziness, urine retention	Mild ↑ PR
Mexiletine	0	0	+ nausea, vomiting, tremor, dizziness	No significant change
Tocainide	+	0	+ + nausea, vomiting, tremor, dizziness	No significant change
Phenytoin	0	0	± nystagmus, slurred speech, ataxia, confusion, dermatitis	No significant change
Encainide	±	+ + + +	± dizziness, visual disturbance, taste perversion, rash, asthenia	↑ PR, ↑ QRS (QT ↑ because of ↑ QRS)
Flecainide	+ +	+ + +	+ dizziness, visual disturbance	↑ PR, ↑ QRS (QT ↑ because of ↑ QRS)
Propafenone	+ +	+ + +	+ nausea, vomiting, metallic taste, dizziness	↑ PR, ↑ QRS (QT ↑ because of ↑ QRS)
Amiodarone	±	±	+ + + + pulmonary toxicity, hyper- and hypothyroidism, nausea, constipation, dermatitis, tremors, ataxia	↑ PR, ↑ QRS, ↑ QT
Beta blockers	+ + +	0	+ + fatigue, depression, insomnia, impotence (side effects are drug variable)	Sinus slowing, possible ↑ PR

*This is not an exhaustive listing of antiarrhythmic drug adverse effects.

Cardiac Arrhythmia Suppression Trial (CAST) suggest that some antiarrhythmics may be proarrhythmic; survivors of myocardial infarction with nonsustained VT and frequent VPCs who were treated with a type 1C antiarrhythmic agent had a threefold increase in sudden cardiac death over those treated with placebo.[2] Until more information is available, only *symptomatic* nonsustained VT or VPCs should be considered for treatment.

Most patients with symptomatic VPCs respond to reassurance. If disabling palpitations persist, beta blocker medications may benefit the patient. Initiation of treatment with any other antiarrhythmic drugs (type 1, type 3) requires hospitalization and continuous ECG monitoring. When choosing an antiarrhythmic drug, the physician should initially use drugs with the least severe side effects, and should document the reason for failure of the drug before proceeding to the next agent. Reasons for failure include intolerable side effects and recurrent arrhythmias despite therapeutic serum levels.

FOLLOW-UP. The physician should be familiar with the appropriate drug levels, dosing schedule, and typical adverse effects of the commonly used antiarrhythmic drugs (Tables 84–1 and 84–2).

When evaluating drug therapy in patients with ventricular fibrillation and sustained VT, Holter monitoring alone does not reliably identify those who will have recurrent disease. Holter monitoring is sometimes used, however, especially in patients with frequent symptomatic nonsustained VT. Because of the extreme natural variation in ventricular ectopy, "successful" antiarrhythmic drug therapy should reduce the number of VPCs per 24 hours by 80% or more and should eliminate complex forms.

Cross-references: Dizziness (Section 20), Syncope (Section 75), Palpitations (Section 76), Congestive Heart Failure (Section 79), Ambulatory Cardiac Monitoring (Section 88).

REFERENCES

1. Adhar GC, Larson LW, Bardy GH, Greene HL. Sustained ventricular arrhythmias: Differences between survivors of cardiac arrest and patients with recurrent sustained ventricular tachycardia. J Am Coll Cardiol 1988;12:159–165.

   The clinical and electrophysiologic features of patients who survive cardiac arrest are distinct from those of patients who present with hemodynamically tolerated, sustained VT.

2. Cardiac Arrhythmia Suppression Trial (CAST) Investigators. Preliminary report: Effect of encainide and flecainide on mortality in a randomized trial of arrhythmia suppression after myocardial infarction. N Engl J Med. 1989;321:406–412.

   In 1725 patients who received the study drug or placebo and were followed over 10 months, patients taking encainide and flecainide had a relative risk of 3.6 for excess deaths over patients in the other groups.

3. Greene HL. Definition of patients at high risk of sudden arrhythmic cardiac death. Clin Cardiol 1988;11:115–116.

   Review article of clinical presentation and evaluation of patients at risk for sudden death.

4. Kennedy HL, Whitlock JA, Sprague MK, Kennedy LJ, Buckingham TA, Goldberg RJ. Long-term follow-up of asymptomatic healthy subjects with frequent and complex ventricular ectopy. N Engl J Med 1985;312:193–197.

Seventy-three asymptomatic patients with frequent and complex ventricular ectopy were followed over 10 years, with an excellent long-term outcome.

5. Wellens HJJ, Bar FWHM, Lie KI. The value of the electrocardiogram in the differential diagnosis of a tachycardia with a widened QRS complex. Am J Med 1978;64:27–33.
    Classic article describing the ECG features helpful in diagnosing wide complex tachycardia.

85 SUPRAVENTRICULAR ARRHYTHMIAS

Problem

JEANNE POOLE

EPIDEMIOLOGY/ETIOLOGY.   Supraventricular tachyarrhythmias are common and affect patients of all ages. Although generally regarded as less serious than ventricular arrhythmias, supraventricular tachyarrhythmias can be dangerous and cause a potentially reversible tachycardia-induced cardiomyopathy, or, in patients with Wolff-Parkinson-White syndrome, rapid atrial fibrillation and sudden death.

Paroxysmal supraventricular tachycardia (PSVT) is a general term for any supraventricular tachycardia that begins and ends abruptly. Eighty to 90% of cases result either from atrioventricular (AV) nodal reentry tachycardias or from reciprocating tachycardias due to an accessory AV bypass pathway. **AV nodal reentry tachycardia** commonly occurs in young, otherwise healthy individuals, often during emotional stress. It accounts for 40% to 70% of all episodes of PSVT. **Reciprocating tachycardia from an accessory AV bypass pathway** accounts for 30% to 50% of PSVT. The direction of conduction of this circus movement tachycardia is referred to as either "orthodromic" (90% of cases, impulse conducts from the atrium to the ventricle through the AV node and back from the ventricle to the atrium through the accessory bypass pathway) or "antidromic" (10%, conducts in the opposite direction). **Wolff-Parkinson-White syndrome** describes patients, some of whom experience reciprocating tachycardias, who have a delta wave on their ECG. Up to 50% of patients with symptomatic Wolff-Parkinson-White syndrome experience atrial fibrillation, a potentially fatal arrhythmia because rapid conduction through the accessory AV pathway may lead to rapid ventricular rates and, in some, ventricular fibrillation.

Atrial fibrillation is discussed in Section 83. **Atrial flutter** may be either paroxysmal or chronic and usually occurs in those with underlying structural heart disease. **Multifocal atrial tachycardia,** defined as a tachycardia with at least three or more different P wave morphologies, develops most often in patients with severe underlying pulmonary, cardiac, or metabolic disease or with digitalis or theophylline toxicity. **Unifocal atrial tachycardia** usually affects patients with underlying heart disease or digitalis toxicity. In contrast to reentrant rhythms, the pulse of an intra-atrial tachycardia slowly increases to its maximal heart rate, and then slowly decreases before the arrhythmia ends. Occasional young patients without underlying heart disease may develop prolonged intra-atrial tachycardia, leading to a tachycardia-induced cardiomyopathy. **Accelerated junctional tachycardia** is seen in critically ill patients, and is usually due to metabolic abnormalities, myocardial infarction, myocarditis, or digoxin or theophylline toxicity.

SYMPTOMS AND SIGNS.   The presence of symptoms, which include palpitations, near syncope and syncope, depend on the patient's left ventricular (LV) function and the duration and rate of the tachycardia. Some patients develop transient polyuria following an episode of supraventricular tachycardia, due to left atrial hypertension and release of atrial natriuretic peptide. The physical examination is generally normal but may reveal structural heart disease.

CLINICAL APPROACH.   Sections 75 and 76 review the approach to palpitations and syncope. The interview should focus on the frequency, duration, and severity of symptoms. In those with palpitations, the physician should inquire about symptoms of hyperthyroidism and pheochromocytoma and about the use of alcohol, caffeine, beta agonists (inhaled or oral), over-the-counter cold medications, and illicit drugs. Arrhythmias in certain patients (e.g., mountain climbers or airline pilots) may be potentially life-threatening and warrant a more aggressive diagnostic approach.

In patients with suspected arrhythmias, the diagnostic goals are (1) to define the nature of the arrhythmia, and (2) to identify any structural heart disease. Because most patients have paroxysmal symptoms, initial attempts to define the arrhythmia utilize ambulatory ECG (Holter) monitoring or arrhythmia event monitoring (see Section 88). Patients should be referred to a cardiologist for consideration of electrophysiologic testing if they have (1) uncontrolled symptomatic tachycardias of unknown diagnosis, despite Holter or event monitoring, (2) tachycardias of known diagnosis but with poor response to therapy (see below), or (3) symptomatic tachycardias and suspected Wolff-Parkinson-White syndrome, i.e., with delta waves on their baseline 12-lead ECG. The evaluation of *asymptomatic* patients found to have delta waves on a routine ECG is controversial.

Routine laboratory tests include thyroid function tests, ECG, chest radiography, and echocardiography. In patients with exercise-induced symptoms, an exercise tolerance test may identify exercise-induced ischemia or arrhythmias (see Section 89). Certain clues from a 12-lead ECG obtained during the tachycardia assist in diagnosis (Table 85–1).

TABLE 85–1.   NARROW QRS COMPLEX (<0.12 SEC) TACHYCARDIA: ECG FEATURES*

Arrhythmia	Atrial Rate	ECG features
Irregularly Irregular		
Atrial fibrillation		No identifiable P waves; rhythm may become regular at rapid rates
Multifocal atrial tachycardia	100–200	Variable P wave morphology; with variable PR and RP intervals
Regular		
Atrial flutter	300	Classic sawtooth atrial deflections (although may be absent); AV conduction usually is 2:1
Unifocal atrial tachycardia	100–250	Single abnormal P wave morphology; usually 1:1 AV conduction, unless digitalis toxicity is present; PR < RP
Accelerated junctional tachycardia	100–250	Retrograde P waves appear immediately prior, within, or just following the QRS complex; PR usually > RP
AV nodal reentry tachycardia	100–280	Retrograde P wave usually hidden in QRS complex
Orthodromic reciprocating tachycardia	100–280	PR > RP

*Any of these rhythms may cause a wide complex tachycardia (QRS > 0.12 sec) if coexistent right or left bundle-branch block is present. Atrial fibrillation in the setting of Wolff-Parkinson-White syndrome produces a rapid irregular wide complex (preexcited) tachycardia.

MANAGEMENT.   Patients who present with a sustained tachycardia should be hospitalized; those with hemodynamic compromise require immediate cardioversion.

Most patients, however, present with paroxysmal arrhythmias. Elimination of caffeine, alcohol, illicit drugs, sympathomimetic medications, and perhaps cigarettes may benefit the patient. Patients with PSVT due to AV nodal or accessory AV pathway reentry may learn to terminate their tachycardia with the Valsalva maneuver. Antiarrhythmic drugs are reserved for patients with documented tachycardias who have frequent distressing palpitations, syncope, or near syncope.

Any of the AV nodal blocking agents (beta blockers, verapamil, or digoxin) are generally safe to administer to unmonitored outpatients, will control the ventricular rate in atrial fibrillation, flutter, or intra-atrial tachycardias, and are the drugs of choice to prevent AV nodal reentrant tachycardia. They should be avoided, however, in patients with accessory AV pathways unless it is known that antidromic conduction does not exist. Digoxin may worsen multifocal atrial tachycardia and is best avoided in this arrhythmia. Although type 1 antiarrhythmic drugs (see Table 84–1) may effectively treat all supraventricular tachycardias, initiation of these drugs requires consultation with a cardiologist, and, especially in those with structural heart disease, hospitalization and continuous ECG monitoring. Some patients with infrequent but prolonged arrhythmias not responsive to the Valsalva maneuver may respond to a single loading dose of procainamide or verapamil (pulsed therapy).

Cross-references: Diagnosis and Management of Drug Abuse (Section 8), Diagnosis and Management of Alcoholism (Section 9), Dizziness (Section 20), Syncope (Section 75), Palpitations (Section 76), Atrial Fibrillation (Section 83), Ambulatory Cardiac Monitoring (Section 88), Common Thyroid Disorders (Section 156).

REFERENCES

1. Bär FW, Brugada P, Dassen WRM, Wellens HJJ. Differential diagnosis of tachycardia with narrow QRS complex (shorter than 0.12 second). Am J Cardiol 1984;54:555–560.
    Using five ECG criteria, a simple algorithm correctly identified 84% of fifty-seven narrow complex tachycardias.

2. Morady F, Scheinman MM, Hess DS. Mechanisms and management of paroxysmal supraventricular tachycardia. Cardiovasc Rev Rep 1981;2:1014–1038.
    Discusses general mechanism, diagnosis, and therapy in an easy-to-read format.

3. Vlay SC. In Viaz SL, Ed. Manual of Cardiac Arrhythmias: A Practical Guide to Clinical Management. Little, Brown, Boston, 1988.
    Comprehensive review of arrhythmias and their treatment.

4. Zipes DP. Cardiac electrophysiology: Promises and contributions. J Am Coll Cardiol 1989;13:1329–1352.
    More detailed discussion of electrophysiologic mechanisms underlying supraventricular and ventricular arrhythmias.

86 ESSENTIAL HYPERTENSION

Problem

JOHN F. STEINER

EPIDEMIOLOGY.   Two aspects of the epidemiology of hypertension have major implications for the clinical diagnosis of the disease. First, about 95% of patients with elevated blood pressure in primary care settings have essential hypertension. Extensive diagnostic workups for secondary hypertension are rarely justified in the absence of characteristic signs or symptoms, onset of disease at the extremes of age, or hypertension refractory to medications. Second, establishing a diagnosis of hypertension requires consistently elevated blood pressure readings over time and in multiple settings, particularly in patients with mild hypertension at screening (<105 mm Hg). Blood pressure readings outside the clinician's office can identify patients who have an exaggerated pressor response to office visits ("white coat" hypertension), while readings over a period of weeks to months can identify patients whose blood pressure elevations are transient.

SYMPTOMS AND SIGNS/CLINICAL APPROACH.   Individuals with hypertension are generally unaware that their blood pressure is elevated. The lack of symptoms complicates diagnosis and treatment, because many individuals seek care or take medications only when they believe their blood pressure is high. The patient's understanding of the causes, symptoms, and treatment of hypertension (his "illness model") should be discussed directly and nonjudgmentally to enhance the therapeutic alliance.

The medical history should focus on a personal or family history of hypertension and its complications, the duration of the hypertension, prior treatment, the reasons for any lapses from treatment, and the presence of other cardiovascular risk factors such as smoking or hyperlipidemia. In addition, the clinician should inquire about symptoms that suggest a cause of secondary hypertension, such as the headaches and palpitations of pheochromocytoma or the hirsutism, myopathy, and menstrual disorders of Cushing's syndrome. During the initial physical examination the physician should (1) use an appropriately sized sphygmomanometer to confirm the presence of hypertension in both arms with the patient supine (or seated) and upright; (2) seek evidence of existing cardiovascular disease (e.g., atherosclerosis or congestive heart failure); and (3) search for evidence of a secondary cause of hypertension (e.g., renal artery bruits, the body habitus of Cushing's syndrome, and blood pressure discrepancies between extremities suggestive of aortic coarctation).

Most hypertensive patients require only limited laboratory testing to screen for cardiovascular risk factors and to establish baseline values for tests to be monitored during treatment.[4] Some of these tests also serve to screen for secondary causes of hypertension, such as unprovoked hypokalemia associated with primary hyperaldosteronism, and elevated creatinine levels in renal parenchymal disease. A reasonable initial evaluation includes an ECG; urinalysis; serum lipids, serum potassium, creatinine, uric acid, hemoglobin, and hematocrit determinations; and a plasma glucose level (preferably fasting).

MANAGEMENT.   In patients with mild hypertension, nonpharmacologic measures should be first-line therapy, particularly for those with diastolic blood pressure below 100 mm Hg.[5] Nonpharmacologic therapy also benefits patients who receive antihypertensive medications and can facilitate subsequent reduction of medications. **Weight reduction** in obese patients is the most consistently effective nonpharmacologic measure, reducing systolic blood pressure by 1 to 4 mm Hg and diastolic blood pressure by 1 to 2 mm Hg per kg of weight loss. **Dietary sodium restriction** to 2 g/day or less induces a substantial fall in blood pressure for "salt-sensitive" hypertensives, but patients who will respond cannot easily be distinguished prospectively from those who will not. Because consumption of more than 2 oz of ethanol a day (2 oz of 100-proof whiskey, 8 oz of wine, or 24 oz of beer) exerts a pressor effect, **reduction or cessation of alcohol use** can obviate or reduce the need for antihypertensive medications. Finally, regular **isometric exercise** can also lower blood pressure independent of its effect on weight, and helps to lower overall cardiovascular risk. Like medications, nonpharmacologic measures pose compliance difficulties and have potential costs and impacts on life-style that should be discussed with the patient.

If the blood pressure remains uncontrolled or if hypertension is moderate or severe (diastolic blood pressure $\geq$ 105 mm Hg), medications are necessary. Most clinical trials of drug therapy have attempted to reduce diastolic blood pressure to below 90 mm Hg, or to achieve at least a 10 mm Hg fall in patients with initial value below 100 mm Hg. In these studies, a long-term reduction in diastolic blood pressure of as little as 5 to 6 mm Hg led to a 42% reduction in strokes and a 14% reduction in coronary heart disease.[2] The merits of more stringent blood pressure control are debated; at present, a target blood pressure of less than 140/90 mm Hg is a reasonable guideline for clinical practice.

The traditional approach to the use of antihypertensive medications has been "stepped care," in which treatment is initiated with a diuretic, supplemented if necessary with a sympatholytic medication (such as a β-adrenergic blocker or a central or peripheral adrenergic inhibitor) and then a peripheral vasodilator. The advent of new drug classes and concerns about the side effects of diuretics have called this management strategy into question. Increasingly, the choice of an initial antihypertensive drug can be individualized on the basis of side effects and costs, since most antihypertensive drugs are effective as single agents in 50% to 60% of patients (Table 86–1). Special characteristics of the patient may also influence drug choices (Table 86–2).

General principles in initiating antihypertensive therapy include the following: (1) Begin treatment at a low dose of a single drug. (2) Minimize the frequency of doses to enhance compliance. (3) Consider drug pharmacokinetics, complications, and potential interactions when choosing medications. (4) Select drugs that potentially benefit the patient's other illnesses (e.g., consider a β-adrenergic blocker in a patient also requiring prophylaxis for migraine). (5) Choose drugs that minimize the costs of treatment.

FOLLOW-UP.   After beginning antihypertensive drugs, patients should be seen at intervals of 2 to 4 weeks until the blood pressure is controlled. Patients should be encouraged to begin monitoring their own blood pressure outside the office. Mercury sphygmomanometers and anaeroid manometers are generally more accurate than digital readout devices and automated machines (such as those in pharmacies and supermarkets), though all home monitoring devices require intermittent calibration to ensure accuracy. The patient should be taught that the pattern of blood pressure readings over time is more important than the results of any single blood pressure determination. Office visits are best spent in counseling about nonpharmacologic management, drug side ef-

Text continued on page 256

TABLE 86–1. USUAL DAILY DOSAGES, SIDE EFFECTS, AND COSTS OF REPRESENTATIVE ANTIHYPERTENSIVE DRUGS

Drug	No. of Doses/Day	Usual Minimum Dose (mg/day)	Usual Maximum Dose (mg/day)	Common Side Effects	Cost*	Other Considerations
Diuretics						
Hydrochlorothiazide	1	12.5	50.0	Hypokalemia, hyperuricemia, hyperglycemia, may worsen lipid profile	1+	Ineffective if creatinine > 2.5–3.0 mg/dl
Furosemide	2	20.0	320.0	Hypokalemia	1+	Useful in chronic renal failure
β-Adrenergic Blockers						
Atenolol	1	25.0	100.0	Bradycardia	3+	Avoid in patients with CHF, claudication; may block gluconeogenesis in diabetics; β_1 selective
Pindolol	1	10.0	60.0		3+	"Intrinsic sympathomimetic activity" attenuates effects on heart rate, lipids
Propranolol	2†	40.0	480.0	Bradycardia, fatigue, insomnia, nightmares	2+	As for atenolol; nonselective for β_1 and β_2 receptors; avoid in patients with bronchospasm

Table continued on following page

TABLE 86–1. USUAL DAILY DOSAGES, SIDE EFFECTS, AND COSTS OF REPRESENTATIVE ANTIHYPERTENSIVE DRUGS *Continued*

Drug	No. of Doses/Day	Usual Minimum Dose (mg/day)	Usual Maximum Dose (mg/day)	Common Side Effects	Cost*	Other Considerations
Adrenergic Inhibitors						
Clonidine	2†	0.1	1.2	Drowsiness, dry mouth, depression	2+	Rapid withdrawal may cause rebound hypertension
Reserpine	1	0.1	0.25	Nasal stuffiness, depression	1+	Least expensive antihypertensive drug
α₁-Adrenergic Blocker						
Prazosin	2	1.0	20.0	Orthostatic hypotension with first dose	3+	
Combined α and β Blocker						
Labetalol	2	200.0	1800.0	Fatigue, dizziness	3+	As for atenolol
Vasodilators						
Hydralazine	2	50.0	300.0	Tachycardia, fluid retention; drug-induced lupus syndrome	1+	Usually used with β blocker
Minoxidil	2	2.5	20.0	Tachycardia, fluid retention, hypertrichosis	2+	Used for refractory hypertension with loop diuretic and β blocker

Calcium Channel Blockers						
Nifedipine	3	30.0	180.0	Tachycardia, fluid retention	4+	Primary mode of action is vasodilation
Slow-release form	1	30.0	180.0		4+	
Diltiazem	3–4	120.0	360.0		4+	Modes of action are reduction in cardiac output and vasodilation; avoid with high-grade AV block, CHF
Slow-release form	2	120.0	360.0		4+	
Verapamil	3–4	120.0	480.0	Constipation	3+	As for diltiazem
Slow-release form	1–2	120.0	480.0		4+	
ACE Inhibitors						
Captopril	2	25.0	300.0	Cough, angioedema, hyperkalemia, renal failure, proteinuria (at high doses)	4+	May reduce proteinuria in diabetics
Enalapril	1	2.5	40.0	As for captopril	4+	As for captopril
Lisinopril	1	5.0	40.0	As for captopril	4+	As for captopril

*Cost estimated from 1990 *Drug Topics Red Book*, using average wholesale price across manufacturers.

†Slow-release forms also available.

TABLE 86–2. CONSIDERATIONS IN CHOOSING ANTIHYPERTENSIVE DRUGS FOR SPECIAL POPULATIONS

Population	Drugs To Consider*	Reasons	Drugs To Avoid*	Reasons
Elderly patients	Thiazides	Demonstrated efficacy (most have low renin), low cost	β-Adrenergic blockers Centrally acting adrenergic inhibitors	Decreased β-adrenergic responsiveness with aging Increased risk of CNS side effects
Black patients	Thiazides	Demonstrated efficacy (most have low renin), low cost	β-Adrenergic blockers ACE inhibitors	Less effective as monotherapy Less effective as monotherapy
Smokers			β-Adrenergic blockers	Less effective
Diabetes	ACE inhibitors	May retard progression of diabetic nephropathy (but may cause hyperkalemia in patients with hyporeninemic hypoaldosteronism)	Thiazides β-Adrenergic blockers	May worsen glucose tolerance (especially if hypokalemic) May impair metabolic response to hypoglycemia
Hyperlipidemia	ACE inhibitors Calcium blockers α₁-Adrenergic blockers	No adverse lipid effects No adverse lipid effects No adverse lipid effects	Thiazides β-Adrenergic blockers without sympathomimetic activity	May raise total cholesterol and LDL, lower HDL May raise VLDL and lower HDL

Condition	Preferred drugs	Comments	Drugs to avoid	Comments
Congestive heart failure	ACE inhibitors	Efficacy for both CHF and hypertension	β-Adrenergic blockers; Verapamil, diltiazem	Negative inotropic effect; Negative inotropic effect
Renal failure	Furosemide; ACE inhibitors	Promotes sodium excretion; May slow progression of disease	Thiazides	Ineffective if serum creatinine > 2.5–3.0 mg/dl
Coronary artery disease	β-Adrenergic blockers; Calcium blockers	Also treat angina pectoris, prevent reinfarction after myocardial infarction (MI), may prevent initial MI; Also treat angina pectoris	Thiazides	May worsen lipids; hypokalemia may provoke arrhythmias
Benign prostatic hypertrophy	α₁-Adrenergic blockers; Methyldopa	May improve bladder emptying; Proven effectiveness and safety	Thiazides; Loop diuretics; ACE inhibitors	May worsen frequency and nocturia; Possible teratogenesis
Pregnancy	Hydralazine; β-Adrenergic blockers	Proven effectiveness and safety; Also effective and appear safe	Calcium blockers	Inhibit uterine contractions at term

*Few of these recommendations are absolute. Individual patients vary in their response to any drug.

fects, and compliance. If the patient's blood pressure is still above the target range, the dose of the initial drug can be gradually increased. Most medications reach a plateau of effectiveness in the middle of the recommended dosage range; maximal doses often confer little additional benefit but magnify side effects.

If the blood pressure remains elevated despite reasonable doses of a single antihypertensive drug, the clinician must decide whether the failure to attain blood pressure control is due to noncompliance, inadequate dosage, or true drug resistance. Approximately 50% to 80% of patients with uncontrolled hypertension are not compliant with medication regimens. Strategies for assessing and treating noncompliance are discussed in Section 4. If the patient is compliant, the physician should consider switching to an antihypertensive drug with a different mechanism of action. If monotherapy with a range of drugs is unsuccessful, moderate doses of drugs with complementary mechanisms of action should be added to the treatment regimen. In the rare patient for whom multidrug therapy is ineffective despite good compliance, problems with measurement of blood pressure ("white coat" hypertension or "pseudohypertension" due to sclerotic, poorly compressible brachial arteries), drug-drug interactions (e.g., with oral contraceptives), failure to adequately reduce intravascular volume, and secondary causes of hypertension must be considered.[3]

After the patient attains normal blood pressure, office visits can become less frequent. Some patients benefit from regular reevaluation and counseling to maintain adherence, others are able to manage their medications, monitor their own blood pressure, and visit their physician infrequently. Ongoing home monitoring of blood pressure should be encouraged, to enlist the patient as a participant in his own care and to detect discrepancies between home and office blood pressure readings. The timing of laboratory monitoring is also a matter of judgment. For drugs such as diuretics and angiotensin-converting enzyme (ACE) inhibitors, which have potentially serious metabolic effects, serum electrolytes should be repeated after the first month of therapy. After the patient attains a stable treatment regimen, laboratory tests need to be monitored as infrequently as once a year.

After the blood pressure has been under good control for a year or more, consideration should be given to a trial of treatment reduction. Few patients in whom hypertension is properly diagnosed are able to stop medications permanently, but many can reduce drug dosages for a prolonged period. Such "stepdown" of antihypertensive medications is particularly likely to be successful in patients with blood pressure lower than the usual target range and in those who have successfully instituted nonpharmacologic measures of blood pressure control.

HYPERTENSIVE CRISES. Patients with a diastolic blood pressure above 120 to 130 mm Hg are at substantially increased short-term risk of complications and must be treated immediately. If the patient manifests end-organ disease of the CNS (encephalopathy, focal neurologic deficits), cardiovascular system (angina pectoris, myocardial infarction, pulmonary edema, aortic dissection), renal deterioration, or eclampsia in pregnancy, prompt hospital admission and the use of parenteral antihypertensive agents is necessary.[1] If blood pressure elevations are extreme but end-organ disease is absent, treatment can be promptly instituted in the outpatient department with oral or sublingual medications. The goal of immediate therapy is to produce a *gradual* reduction in blood pressure to a target diastolic blood pressure of 100 to 110 mm Hg; more rapid lowering of the blood pressure may lead to hypoperfusion of end-organs because of changes in autoregulation of blood flow. The drugs most commonly used to treat hypertensive "urgencies" in primary care are clonidine and nifedipine. Oral clonidine loading can be accomplished with an initial dose of 0.1 to 0.2 mg orally, followed by repeated doses of 0.05 to 0.1 mg every hour until the blood pressure reaches the target range or a total of 0.6 to 0.7 mg has been given. Nifedipine can be administered either by mouth or sublingually, with an initial dose of 10 mg, repeated once if necessary. Patients should be observed for several hours after either mode of therapy to ensure that the blood pressure does not fall excessively. When the blood pressure is stable, patients should leave the clinic with a prescription for medications and should receive frequent follow-up, as often as daily, to assure that the blood pressure is coming under control.

Cross-references: Compliance (Section 4), Periodic Health Assessment (Section 7), Diagnosis and Management of Alcoholism (Section 9), Obesity (Section 15), Assessment of Physical Activity (Section 72), Hypertension Screening (Section 73), Congestive Heart Failure (Section 79).

REFERENCES

1. Calhoun DA, Oparil S. Treatment of hypertensive crisis. N Engl J Med 1990;323:1177–1183.
    The most recent review of practical strategies for managing hypertensive urgencies or emergencies and their complications.

2. Collins R, Peto R, MacMahon S, Hebert P, et al. Blood pressure, stroke, and coronary heart disease. Lancet 1990;2:827–838.
    A meta-analysis of the fourteen randomized clinical trials that assess cardiovascular outcomes of therapy for hypertension.

3. Gifford RW. An algorithm for the management of resistant hypertension. Hypertension 1988;11(suppl II):II-101–II-105.
    A sequential method for evaluating patients whose blood pressure appears refractory to three-drug antihypertensive therapy.

4. 1988 Joint National Committee. The 1988 report of the Joint National Committee on Detection, Evaluation, and Treatment of High Blood Pressure. Arch Intern Med 1988; 148:1023–1038.
    The report of a consensus panel on hypertension management. Emphasizes a practical approach for ambulatory care.

5. Subcommittee on Nonpharmacological Therapy of the 1984 Joint National Committee on Detection, Evaluation, and Treatment of High Blood Pressure. Nonpharmacological approaches to the control of high blood pressure. Hypertension 1986;8:444–467.
    Reviews the evidence for a wide variety of approaches to nonpharmacologic management of hypertension. Alhough they advocate only weight loss, sodium restriction, and reduction of alcohol consumption, more recent studies have strengthened the evidence for the role of isometric exercise in hypertension treatment.

87 RADIONUCLIDE ASSESSMENT OF CARDIAC FUNCTION

Procedure

MANUEL CERQUEIRA

INDICATIONS/CONTRAINDICATIONS.   The presence and extent of coronary artery disease (CAD) can be evaluated by radionuclide methods using exercise or pharmacologic stress thallium 201 imaging or exercise radionuclide angiography. These studies are indicated in the same clinical situations in which conventional exercise tolerance testing has been useful: (1) in the diagnosis of patients with chest pain and a moderate probability of CAD, (2) in the prognosis of patients with known CAD, including acute myocardial infarction, and (3) in preoperative risk assessment. Radionuclide methods are superior to conventional exercise tolerance testing for the following patient groups: (1) those with abnormal baseline ECGs, (2) those unable to exercise owing to stroke, spinal cord injury, amputation, severe arthritis, peripheral vascular disease, or chronic obstructive pulmonary disease, and (3) for assessing the significance of known coronary artery lesions.

Contraindications to exercise evaluation by radionuclide methods are similar to those for conventional exercise tolerance testing. Contraindications to pharmacologic stress evaluation using intravenous dipyridamole or adenosine include the above plus a history of asthma and the concurrent use of methylxanthines or dipyridamole.

RATIONALE.   *Diagnosis of Coronary Artery Disease.*   Thallium 201 is a radioactive material that is concentrated by myocytes in direct proportion to blood flow. When thallium is injected during exercise or pharmacologic stress, images obtained with a gamma camera show normal myocardium as areas of increased concentration and display ischemic (areas distal to >50% stenosis) or infarcted myocardium as areas of diminished or absent activity. Over 3 to 4 hours, the thallium distribution decreases in normal myocardium, increases in ischemic myocardium, and is never concentrated in infarcted myocardium. Repeat imaging, therefore, separates ischemic from infarcted myocardium.

Exercise radionuclide angiography measures ejection fraction at rest and at peak bicycle exercise. Normal hearts increase ejection fraction by 5% or more with maximal exercise, but in the presence of coronary stenosis the ejection fraction may drop or fail to increase appropriately.

Both techniques are more expensive than conventional exercise tolerance testing, but offer improved sensitivity (85% to 96% with thallium tomography and 85% with exercise radionuclide angiography) and comparable or slightly lower specificity. Patients with a normal thallium study have a very low adverse cardiac event rate over 5 years of follow-up. As with conventional exercise stress testing, it is not recommended that asymptomatic patients undergo evaluation, owing to the low specificity in such populations. In patients capable of maximal exercise and with normal resting ECGs, exercise tolerance testing is preferable because of lower cost and comparable accuracy.

Assessing the Significance of Known Coronary Artery Disease. In patients with known CAD, radionuclide evaluation provides prognostic information and is useful for management. In patients with an acute myocardial infarction and no recurrence of chest pain or CHF, predischarge low-level exercise or pharmacologic stress imaging is more accurate than coronary arteriography or a low-level exercise tolerance test in predicting the occurrence at 1 year of ischemic events and death. In patients with multivessel CAD being evaluated for percutaneous transluminal coronary angioplasty, thallium imaging identifies the critical lesion and is also useful in evaluating restenosis.

Preoperative Risk Assessment. In patients undergoing elective surgery, exercise or dipyridamole ^{201}Tl imaging accurately stratifies the risk for intra- and postoperative cardiac events. Patients should first be screened for the presence of risk factors and symptoms of CAD or ventricular dysfunction. Low-risk patients may proceed to surgery without further evaluation, high-risk patients may benefit from invasive evaluation, and intermediate-risk patients may benefit from radionuclide evaluation. Patients with strongly positive radionuclide studies are at high risk for adverse events, and invasive evaluation should be considered.

METHODS. For both radionuclide studies, an intravenous catheter is required and the blood pressure and ECG are monitored. Thallium studies are performed with upright treadmill exercise or in the supine position for dipyridamole or adenosine infusions. After injection of thallium at peak exercise or peak pharmacologic effect, 30-minute images are taken immediately and 4 hours later. Exercise radionuclide angiography is performed by labeling the patient's red blood cells with technetium, and measuring the ejection fraction at rest and during peak bicycle exercise in the supine or upright position.

Cross-references: Chest Pain (Section 74), Angina (Section 78), Exercise Tolerance Testing (Section 89), Preoperative Cardiovascular Problems (Section 217).

REFERENCES

1. American College of Cardiology/American Heart Association. Guidelines for Clinical Use of Cardiac Radionuclide Imaging, December 1986. A report of the American College of Cardiology/American Heart Association Task Force on Assessment of Cardiovascular Procedures (Subcommittee on Nuclear Imaging). Circulation 1986;74:1469A–1482A.
   Although some may disagree with the classifications, these recommendations provide an excellent framework for evaluating the clinical use of these techniques. Indications are ranked as class I (frequently

indicated and often providing important clinical information) through class IV (not recommended as a diagnostic technique).

2. Eagle K, Coley C, Newell J, et al. Combining clinical and thallium data optimizes preoperative assessment of cardiac risk before major vascular surgery. Ann Intern Med 1989; 110:859–866.
    Systematic approach using clinical and thallium information for preoperative risk evaluation.

3. Gibbons R, Zinsmeister A, Miller T, Clements I. Supine exercise electrocardiograph compared with exercise radionuclide angiography in noninvasive identification of severe coronary artery disease. Ann Intern Med 1990;112:743–749.
    A comparison between conventional exercise ECG and exercise radionuclide angiography for identifying severe CAD.

4. Gibson R, Watson D, Craddock G, et al. Prediction of cardiac events after uncomplicated myocardial infarction: A prospective study comparing predischarge exercise thallium-201 scintigraphy and coronary angiography. Circulation 1983;68:321–336.
    Large trial examining multiple invasive and noninvasive strategies for evaluation of patients after myocardial infarction.

5. Kotler T, Diamond G. Exercise thallium-201 scintigraphy in the diagnosis and prognosis of coronary artery disease. Ann Intern Med 1990;113:684–702.
    Extensive review of early exercise tolerance testing studies using thallium for detecting CAD, and an accompanying American College of Physicians position paper.

88 AMBULATORY CARDIAC MONITORING

Procedure

MANUEL J. ARBO
WISHWA N. KAPOOR

INDICATIONS.   Common reasons for ambulatory cardiac monitoring include the following:

1. *Evaluation of unexplained symptoms.* ECG monitoring is often used in the evaluation of syncope, presyncope, dizziness, and palpitations when a cause of these symptoms cannot be determined from initial clinical information or baseline laboratory tests. Less commonly, it is used to evaluate chest pain or suspected silent coronary ischemia. Rarely, this test has been used in patients with episodes of sudden dyspnea or fatigue when paroxysmal arrhythmias are suspected clinically.

2. *Determining prognosis.* In patients with myocardial infarction, hypertrophic cardiomyopathy, or other conditions, although the use of the test for this purpose is not well supported (see Rationale).

3. *To guide antiarrhythmic therapy.*

4. *Miscellaneous.* Other rare indications include sleep apnea (to look for marked bradycardia during episodes of apnea), pacemaker follow-up, evaluation of chest pain when a patient cannot undergo exercise stress testing, and for the diagnosis of visceral diabetic neuropathy (to look for RR variability).

RATIONALE.   *Evaluation of Unexplained Symptoms.*   Ascribing episodic unexplained symptoms to arrhythmias is often difficult, because most patients have no symptoms during monitoring. Furthermore some arrhythmias, including nonsustained VT and sinus pauses, are occasionally reported in asymptomatic individuals. Because there is no reference standard with which to compare the performance of ambulatory monitoring for unexplained symptoms, it is impossible to calculate the sensitivity, specificity, or predictive values. Nonetheless, the yield of ambulatory monitoring is relatively low. Section 75 reviews the diagnostic value of monitoring in patients with syncope.

In patients with coronary disease, ST segment changes may indicate episodes of ischemia, but false-positive and false-negative results are frequent. Because the assessment of ST segment changes with ambulatory ECG is still in the early stages of development, routine use is not recommended for the diagnosis of coronary artery disease (CAD), determination of its prognosis, or monitoring of therapy.

Determination of Prognosis.   MYOCARDIAL INFARCTION.   The findings of ventricular trichycardia (VT) and frequent (>10/hr) or complex ventricular ectopy are associated with increased total mortality, sudden death, and cardiac mortality in patients with recent myocardial infarction. This increased risk, however, can be predicted from other variables (cardiomegaly, ejection fraction, extent of myocardial necrosis, ST segment depression, prior myocardial infarction, exercise testing). Moreover, studies are not available to show that treatment of these arrhythmias has a favorable or negative impact on outcome. Therefore, routine ambulatory monitoring is not recommended in asymptomatic survivors of myocardial infarction.

HYPERTROPHIC CARDIOMYOPATHY.   VT is reported in up to 25% of patients with hypertrophic cardiomyopathy. In small studies, nonsustained VT was a predictor of sudden death. However, the routine use of this test in patients with hypertrophic cardiomyopathy is not established, and studies are not available to show that therapy may alter outcome.

OTHER CONDITIONS.   In patients with known CAD (but not acute myocardial infarction), congestive heart failure (CHF), or chronic obstructive lung disease, ventricular arrhythmias have not generally been shown to be an independent predictor of mortality or sudden death. Thus, there is no evidence to support the routine use of ambulatory monitoring in these settings.

To Guide Antiarrhythmic Therapy.   The ability of antiarrhythmic drugs to suppress ventricular ectopy and supraventricular arrhythmias has been well documented by continuous ECG monitoring. *Symptomatic* patients with ventricular or supraventricular arrhythmias can be followed with ambulatory monitoring to determine adequate suppression of arrhythmias and adjust treatment. Because of marked spontaneous variability and the absence of a reference standard, it is difficult to define "adequate suppression of arrhythmia." Most authors recommend at least 80% to 90% decrease in the frequency of arrhythmia compared to baseline. Clinical trials have not shown an improved outcome for *asymptomatic* patients given antiarrhythmic therapy for ventricular ectopy, and one study has shown a worse outcome with encainide or flecainide (see Section 84).

An alternative mode of management of tachyarrhythmias is the use of electrophysiologic studies. However, because arrhythmias in up to 50% of patients with spontaneous ventricular tachyarrhythmias are not inducible during ventricular stimulation, and because no conclusive evidence has shown an improved outcome with electrophysiologic studies as compared to ambulatory monitoring, using ambulatory monitoring as a guide to antiarrhythmic therapy is currently an acceptable alternative.

METHODS. The traditional system uses a battery-powered tape recorder to record a two-lead ECG continuously over a 24- to 48-hour period. Only bathing and swimming are restricted during the recording period. The patient is instructed to keep a diary of symptoms to determine which if any correlate with arrhythmias. The recorded information is analyzed by a computer comparing each QRST with a series of templates already classified and determined to be either normal, aberrant supraventricular or ventricular. All questionable signals are analyzed by an operator to eliminate artifacts. Other types of recorders include the patient-activated monitor, which is useful when symptoms are recurrent but infrequent. Some devices have a memory loop (loop recorders) that allows the patient to record the cardiac rhythm after symptoms have occurred. These monitors can be worn continuously for prolonged periods (up to several months). The major advantage of an intermittent loop recorder is that after being activated it records the rhythm from the previous 4 minutes as well as the subsequent 60 seconds. This stored information can then be transmitted by telephone to a central station for analysis. Small studies suggest that this test may provide symptomatic correlation in a subset of patients with recurrent unexplained symptoms (syncope, presyncope, and palpitation). Currently, loop monitoring is complementary to Holter monitoring and has not eliminated the need for initial Holter monitoring for the evaluation of unexplained symptoms.

COST. The cost for standard Holter monitoring ranges from $250 to $350 per 24 hours. The charges for cardiac loop ECG recorders are similar, with the major advantage of increasing the observational period to several weeks. There are no studies on the cost-effectiveness of cardiac monitoring.

Cross-references: Dizziness (Section 20), Syncope (Section 75), Palpitations (Section 76), Chronic Ventricular Arrhythmias (Section 84), Supraventricular Arrhythmias (Section 85).

REFERENCES

1. American College of Physicians. Ambulatory ECG (Holter) monitoring: Position paper. Ann Intern Med 1990;113:77–79.

Review of recommendations by the American College of Physicians for use of ambulatory Holter monitoring.

2. DiMarco JP, Philbrick JT. Use of ambulatory electrocardiographic (Holter) monitoring. Ann Intern Med 1990;113:53–68.
    Most recent review of efficacy of ECG monitoring and guidelines for its use in clinical practice.

3. Fisch C, DeSanctis RW, Dodge HT, Reeves TJ, Weinberg SL. Guidelines for ambulatory electrocardiography. J Am Coll Cardiol 1989;13:249–258.
    Report of the American College of Cardiology and American Heart Association Task Force on Ambulatory ECG Monitoring.

89 EXERCISE TOLERANCE TESTING

Procedure

STEVEN R. McGEE

INDICATIONS/CONTRAINDICATIONS. Exercise testing adds useful information in three common clinical settings: (1) in the diagnosis of chest pain in patients with an intermediate pretest probability of coronary artery disease, (2) in evaluating the prognosis of patients with known CAD, and (3) in predicting future coronary events after uncomplicated myocardial infarction. Less frequent indications include the evaluation of pulmonary disease and exercise-induced arrhythmias.

Contraindications include (1) acute myocardial infarction in the previous 10 to 14 days, (2) unstable angina, (3) severe aortic stenosis (exercise-induced vasodilation causes syncope), (4) uncompensated CHF, (5) acute systemic illness, (6) uncontrolled hypertension, and (7) uncontrolled significant cardiac arrhythmias.

RATIONALE. *Diagnosis of Coronary Artery Disease.* Abnormal exercise test ST responses (>1 mm horizontal or downsloping depression) predict anatomic coronary artery disease (CAD) with a sensitivity of 50% to 70% and a specificity of 90%. Table 89–1 lists causes of false-positive and false-negative results. The physician should address the patient's age, quality of chest pain, and risk factors to determine the pretest likelihood of CAD. Diagnostic exercise testing benefits those patients with an *intermediate* pretest probability (40% to 60%) (Table 89–2). Most patients with a *high* pretest likelihood of CAD and negative test results actually have CAD (false negative); most with a *low* pretest likelihood and positive results do not have disease (false positive). Easy-to-use nomograms simplify these calculations.[4]

TABLE 89–1.   CAUSES OF FALSE-POSITIVE AND FALSE-NEGATIVE EXERCISE TESTS

False-positive Test Results
Digoxin
LV hypertrophy
Left bundle-branch block
Preexcitation syndromes
Hyperventilation

False-negative Test Results
Antianginal medication
Single-vessel disease
Test limited by noncardiac symptoms (claudication, fatigue)

Exercise thallium scintigraphy, with its higher sensitivity (80%), is preferable when the physician anticipates either false-positive results on conventional exercise testing (see Table 89–1) or poor patient effort.

Prognosis in Coronary Artery Disease.   Three variables predict prognosis: the duration of exercise (testing stopped early because of abnormal findings signifies higher risk), the presence of angina during testing, and an abnormal ST response. Simple arithmetic scores identify patients at high, moderate, and low risk, who have respective 5-year myocardial infarction–free survivals of 63%, 86%, and 93% with medical treatment.[2] Exercise-induced hypotension in the absence of obstructive cardiomyopathy or valvular heart disease is highly specific for left main or triple-vessel disease (its sensitivity, however, is less than 20%). Exercise-induced premature beats add little independent information. In low-risk patients, medical treatment may be safely continued, because survival benefit with surgery is difficult to demonstrate. Higher risk patients are most likely to benefit from cardiac catheterization, which may further define those who will benefit from revascularization or angioplasty.

Prognosis After Myocardial Infarction.   Two to three weeks after an uncomplicated myocardial infarction, low-level exercise testing stratifies patients into low- and high-risk groups. Exercise testing is not appropriate when patients experience early recurrent angina or severe pump failure, because the risk of

TABLE 89–2.   POSTTEST LIKELIHOOD OF CORONARY ARTERY DISEASE

Patient	Pretest Likelihood	Posttest Likelihood if Test Is:	
		Positive	*Negative*
45-year-old woman with nonanginal chest pain	0.05 (low)	0.24	0.02
50-year-old man with atypical angina	0.50 (intermediate)	0.86	0.31
60-year-old man with typical angina	0.90 (high)	0.98	0.80

future cardiac events in these patients is already high. Of the remaining 80% who may safely undergo exercise testing, two-thirds have normal results and a subsequent 1-year mortality of 2.6%. Medical therapy is appropriate for these low-risk patients. The one-third of patients with abnormal results (ST changes, poor exercise duration, or angina) have a 1-year mortality of 20% and account for 80% of posthospitalization deaths. Cardiac catheterization in this high-risk group may identify disease amenable to angioplasty or bypass surgery. Exercise-induced hypotension in the first few weeks after myocardial infarction is a nonspecific, self-limited finding and does not signify severe myocardial ischemia, as it does in those without recent infarction.

Asymptomatic Patients. Exercise testing in asymptomatic patients is inappropriate for two reasons: (1) even though positive test results (abnormal ST change) increase the asymptomatic patient's risk for future coronary events (death, myocardial infarction, angina) fivefold, the overwhelming majority of positive results are false positive because of a very low pretest probability of disease (see Table 89–2), and (2) the initial cardiac event during follow-up is usually angina (potentially reversible), and not myocardial infarction or sudden death.

METHODS. Patients progressively increase the exercise workload at regularly timed intervals, or stages, while the physician monitors the patient's symptoms, signs, and physiologic responses. In treadmill testing, the most popular form of exercise testing, either treadmill speed or grade (or both) is increased at each stage. Exercise testing after myocardial infarction employs modified protocols, which change workload more gradually.

Exercise testing begins after informed consent, history, physical examination, and resting ECG. During testing the physician watches for end points listed in Table 89–3. Low-level modified protocols usually include heart rate as an end point (determined to be 70% to 75% maximal heart rate, or approximately 120–130 beats/min).

COST/COMPLICATIONS. The risk of death, which usually occurs because of acute myocardial infarction or arrhythmia, is 0.5 per 10,000 during exercise

TABLE 89–3. REASONS TO TERMINATE EXERCISE TESTING

Symptoms
Progressive angina
Extreme fatigue or dyspnea

Signs
Fall in systolic blood pressure
Confusion, staggering gait
Pallor, clammy skin

ECG Criteria
Arrhythmia (frequent ventricular salvos, ventricular tachycardia, heart block, supraventricular tachycardia)
Excessive ST change (criteria vary, usually > 3 mm ST depression or > 2 mm ST elevation)

testing. Although this is extremely low, resuscitation equipment and skills must be nearby. The cost of treadmill exercise testing is $268.00 (based on 1991 University of Washington hospital and professional fees).

Cross-references: Prescription of Physical Activity (Section 72), Chest Pain (Section 74), Angina (Section 78), Radionuclide Assessment of Cardiac Function (Section 87).

REFERENCES

1. DeBusk RF. Specialized testing after recent acute myocardial infarction. Ann Intern Med 1989;110:470–481.

    Excellent review, with accompanying American College of Physicians position paper, which compares role of exercise testing, radionuclide testing, Holter monitoring, and echocardiography after myocardial infarction.

2. Mark DB, Hlatky MA, Harrel FE, Lee KL, Califf RM, et al. Exercise treadmill score for predicting prognosis in coronary artery disease. Ann Intern Med 1987;106:793–800.

    Discusses derivation and testing of an arithmetic treadmill score that adds prognostic information independent from coronary anatomy and left ventricular function.

3. McHenry PL, O'Donnell J, Morris SN, Jordan JJ. The abnormal exercise electrocardiogram in apparently healthy men: A predictor of angina pectoris as an initial coronary event during long-term follow-up. Circulation 1984;70:547–551.

    Among 916 asymptomatic Indiana State patrolmen, 34% with ST changes during exercise testing developed a cardiac event (angina, infarction or sudden death) during a mean 12 years of follow-up, compared to 5% of those with negative test results (i.e., although ETT identified increased risk, most positive results were false negative).

4. Patterson RE, Eng C, Horowitz SF. Practical diagnosis of coronary artery disease: A Bayes' theorem nomogram to correlate clinical data with noninvasive exercise tests. Am J Cardiol 1984;53:252–256.

    Nomograms that incorporate patient's age, sex, risk factors, and treadmill and thallium testing results define the posttest likelihood of anatomic CAD.

5. Schlant RC, Blomqvist CG, Brandenburg RO, DeBusk R, Ellestad MH, et al. Guidelines for exercise testing. J Am Coll Cardiol 1986;8:725–738.

    Recommendations for exercise testing, prepared by the American College of Cardiology/American Heart Association task force.

90 ECHOCARDIOGRAPHY

Procedure

CATHERINE M. OTTO

INDICATIONS. Echocardiography is useful for evaluating a broad range of cardiac diseases (Table 90–1). Echocardiography is *not* routinely indicated in the evaluation of supraventricular arrhythmia or to search for a source of embolism unless the history or physical examination suggests the possibility of structural heart disease.

Transesophageal echocardiography (TEE) is a relatively new procedure, and indications for its use have not been fully defined. TEE should be considered for evaluation of prosthetic valve dysfunction, endocarditis, paravalvular abscess, left atrial thrombus, complex congenital heart disease, aortic dissection, and in other situations when transthoracic images are nondiagnostic.

RATIONALE. Echocardiography uses ultrasound waves (nonionizing radiation) to generate two-dimensional images of cardiac structures in motion and to display intracardiac blood flow information in a variety of formats. Echocardiography has no known adverse effects, is noninvasive (except for TEE), is portable, and can be performed quickly and repeatedly.

METHODS. Standard echocardiographic data are obtained with the ultrasound transducer placed on the patient's chest using a water-soluble acoustic coupling gel. Because ultrasound waves do not transmit well through air or bone, the major limitation to echocardiography is suboptimal data quality in some patients owing to poor tissue penetration. TEE provides superior images of posterior cardiac structures owing to the absence of interposing lung (containing air) and the decreased distance of cardiac structures from the ultrasound transducer.

Two-dimensional echocardiography (2DE) provides detailed tomographic cardiac images in a dynamic (real-time) format that allows assessment of both normal anatomy (ventricular endocardial motion and wall thickening, valve anatomy and motion), and abnormal intracardiac structures (e.g., tumor, vegetation, thrombus). These images also provide accurate measurements of wall thickness, chamber dimensions, and great vessel diameters, and allow calculation of left ventricular (LV) volumes, LV mass, and ejection fraction. Not all laboratories quantitate LV systolic function by 2DE because of the laborious task of tracing endocardial borders, but as automated methods become available, this will become routine. When carefully measured, echocardiographic, angiographic, and radionuclide procedures are equally accurate. In general, echocardiography is the procedure of choice, even if only a qualitative estimate

267

TABLE 90–1. INDICATIONS FOR ECHOCARDIOGRAPHY

Clinical Problem	Information Obtainable by Echocardiography	Limitations	Alternative Diagnostic Tests
Valvular Disease	Valve anatomy, etiology of disease Transvalvular pressure gradients and valve areas Regurgitant severity PA pressures Compensatory chamber enlargement Ventricular function	Possible underestimation of stenosis severity Prosthetic valve dysfunction may require TEE	If echocardiographic data are of good quality, cardiac catheterization is rarely needed
Pericardial Disease	Presence, size, distribution of effusion Evidence of tamponade physiology Possible evidence of pericardial constriction (difficult diagnosis)	Not all patients with acute pericarditis have an effusion The diagnosis of tamponade requires correlation with clinical findings	Echocardiography is the most sensitive method for diagnosing effusion Cardiac catheterization and CT (pericardial thickness) may be needed to diagnose constriction
Cardiomyopathy	Chamber sizes, wall thickness LV systolic function Outflow obstruction in hypertrophic cardiomyopathy PA pressures LV thrombus RV systolic function Associated valve dysfunction (e.g., mitral regurgitation)		Coronary angiography if indicated Radionuclide or contrast angiography measures LV ejection fraction but does not provide assessment of valve function, thickness, etc.
Ischemic Heart Disease Acute myocardial infarction	Bedside evaluation of global and segmental LV function Extent of myocardium at risk Complications: acute mitral regurgitation or VSD, pericarditis, LV thrombus, aneurysm, RV infarct	Direct visualization of coronary anatomy is not feasible	Coronary angiography

268

TABLE 90–1. INDICATIONS FOR ECHOCARDIOGRAPHY *Continued*

Clinical Problem	Information Obtainable by Echocardiography	Limitations	Alternative Diagnostic Tests
Angina	LV systolic function Resting wall motion abnormalities Exercise echocardiographic testing for reversible ischemia	Wall motion may be normal at rest despite severe coronary disease	Exercise testing with thallium imaging Coronary angiography Radionuclide ventriculography
Cardiac Masses LV thrombus	High sensitivity (95%) and specificity (86%) for detection of LV thrombus	Technical artifacts can be misleading	LV thrombus may be suspected on radionuclide or contrast angiography, but is often missed
LA thrombus	Transthoracic echo has a low sensitivity (33%–50%) for diagnosis of LA thrombus, although specificity is high (99%–100%)	TEE is needed to detect LA thrombus reliably	
Cardiac tumors	Size, location, physiologic consequences of tumor mass		CT with cardiac gating, MRI
Endocarditis	Detection of vegetations Evaluation of valve regurgitation Chamber sizes LV systolic function	Detection of paravalvular abscess often requires TEE Endocarditis cannot be excluded by echocardiography Vegetations may persist long after the acute episode	Blood cultures and clinical exam form the basis for diagnosis of endocarditis
Aortic Dissection	Aortic root, arch, and descending thoracic aortic size Imaging of dissection flap Detection of severity and mechanism of aortic regurgitation Detection of pericardial effusion	Often requires TEE Images of ascending aorta may be suboptimal Cannot assess distal vascular beds	Aortography, CT, MRI
Congenital Heart Disease	Detection and assessment of anatomic abnormalities Quantitation of physiologic abnormalities Chamber enlargement Ventricular function		Echocardiography is the initial diagnostic test of choice for congenital heart disease Cardiac catheterization by an experienced operator may be needed

of LV function is reported, because of the additional clinically relevant information obtained with this technique. In some specific situations, for example if sequential numerical ejection fractions are needed, then a radionuclide study may be appropriate.

A Doppler examination typically includes three different modalities—pulsed, continuous wave, and color flow imaging Doppler. Pulsed Doppler accurately measures blood flow velocity at specific intracardiac sites and is useful for evaluation of LV diastolic filling and systolic ejection dynamics, for calculation of stroke volume, and for determination of the pulmonary-to-systemic shunt ratio. Continuous wave Doppler accurately measures high velocities and is useful in determining pressure gradients across stenotic valves, pulmonary artery systolic pressure (based on the tricuspid regurgitant jet velocity), and intracardiac hemodynamics in patients with aortic or mitral regurgitation. Color flow Doppler displays mean velocity information superimposed on the two-dimensional image in a real-time format, and is most useful for detecting intracardiac shunts and for evaluating valvular regurgitation.

COST/COMPLICATIONS.   There are no known adverse effects of standard transthoracic echocardiography. The risk of TEE is low, with potential complications similar to those of upper endoscopy, including infection (endocarditis prophylaxis is given), bleeding, aspiration (patients are fasting), and rarely, esophageal perforation (a careful swallowing history is taken and a barium swallow or screening upper endoscopy is performed if indicated). The cost of echocardiography is lower than alternative cardiac imaging procedures. Costs vary geographically and with the extent of the procedure performed, but total costs (procedure and professional fees) for a comprehensive 2DE and Doppler study range from $500 to $1000.

Cross-references: Congestive Heart Failure (Section 79), Aortic Stenosis (Section 80), Mitral Valve Prolapse (Section 81), Other Valvular Disease (Section 82).

REFERENCES

1. Felner JM. Echocardiography. In Hurst JW, Schlant RC, et al, Eds. The Heart, 7th ed. McGraw-Hill, N.Y., 1990, pp. 1990–2034.
    Comprehensive review of M-mode and two-dimensional echocardiography.

2. Fisher EA, Goldman ME. Transesophageal echocardiography: A new view of the heart. Ann Intern Med 1990;113:91–93.
    Editorial summarizing techniques and indications for transesophageal echocardiography; 20 references.

3. Pearlman AS. The use of Doppler in the evaluation of cardiac disorders and function. In Hurst JW, Schlant RC, et al, Eds. The Heart, 7th ed. McGraw-Hill, N.Y., 1990, pp. 2039–2062.
    Comprehensive and readable review of Doppler echocardiography.

4. Popp RL. Echocardiography. N Engl J Med 1990;323:101–109, 165–172.
    Brief review of indications for and principles of echocardiography; more than 150 references.

GASTROINTESTINAL DISORDERS

91 COLORECTAL CANCER SCREENING

Screening

STEPHAN D. FIHN

EPIDEMIOLOGY. Colorectal cancer is the second most common cancer in the United States, causing 61,000 deaths annually. There are 150,000 new cases diagnosed each year. The mean age at diagnosis is 69. Well-established risk factors include a family history of colorectal cancer or familial polyposis, prior colorectal, endometrial, breast, or ovarian cancer, adenomatous polyps, and long-standing ulcerative colitis.

RATIONALE. Colorectal cancer is a significant cause of pain and suffering as well as death. Although early cancers are amenable to surgical extirpation, most cancers are detected at a late stage for which therapy is unsatisfactory. Many, if not most, cancers are thought to arise from polyps that have a long preclinical phase. Thus, in many respects, colorectal cancer would seem to be an ideal candidate for screening. Unfortunately, all of the currently available screening tests have serious deficiencies, and none has been shown to improve mortality or lessen morbidity.

Less than 10% of cancers occur within 8 cm of the anal verge, making digital examination exceedingly insensitive. Testing for fecal occult blood is widely practiced but produces both false-positive and false-negative results (Table 91–1). Results from uncontrolled trials suggest the sensitivity can be as high as 75%. When performed in mass screening programs involving persons over 50 years of age, 1% to 2% of participants are found to have at least one positive slide, and the predictive value of a positive test is 5% to 10% for cancer. Thus, 90% to 95% of those with positive tests will undergo expensive and uncomfortable examinations of the colon for no benefit. If detection of adenomatous polyps is included, the predictive value of a positive test is 30%. However,

271

TABLE 91–1.   CAUSES OF FALSE-POSITIVE AND FALSE-NEGATIVE TESTS FOR FECAL OCCULT BLOOD

False-Positive Tests	False-Negative Tests
Meat in diet	Vitamin C in diet
Iron supplements	Failure to process slides promptly
Diverticulosis with bleeding	Failure to properly prepare slides or use
Minor anorectal problems (hemorrhoids,	of outdated slides
fissures, proctitis)	Testing dry stool
Peroxidases in skins of fruits (cherries)	Lesion that bleeds intermittently or
and vegetables (tomatoes)	not at all
Upper gastrointestinal bleeding due to	
gastritis or peptic ulcer disease	

since 10% to 33% of older adults are found to have adenomas at autopsy, only a fraction of such lesions can be assumed to progress to clinically significant malignancies. To date, no adequately designed trial has demonstrated a benefit from mass screening for fecal occult blood among asymptomatic individuals.

The sensitivity of sigmoidoscopy is directly related to the length of instrument. Modern 35-cm (short bundle) sigmoidoscopes disclose 30% to 40% of cancers, while longer 60-cm instruments disclose 50% to 60%. During the examination polyps are also removed. It has been postulated that such prophylactic polypectomies prevent the development of cancer. To date, however, no prospective trial has shown that the mortality or morbidity among asymptomatic individuals is improved by routine screening with sigmoidoscopy. Many patients find this procedure unpleasant, uncomfortable, and costly. A single examination costs $100 to $200. Moreover, there is a very small risk of colonic perforation or bleeding following biopsy.

ACTION.   As a result of the lack of well-controlled studies, intense controversy surrounds the issue of colorectal cancer screening. Several professional organizations, including the American Cancer Society, recommend annual digital rectal examinations commencing at age 40 and annual fecal occult blood testing along with sigmoidoscopy every 3 to 5 years after age 49. Other experts have advised against mass screening and advocate periodic testing with occult blood testing or sigmoidoscopy for high-risk individuals. A recent report from the U.S. Preventive Services Task Force states that there is insufficient evidence for or against screening of asymptomatic patients. At present a prudent approach is to offer screening to patients over 50 years of age who have one or more risk factors. All patients to whom screening is offered should be carefully advised of the potential costs, risks, and benefits.

Cross-reference: Periodic Health Assessment (Section 7).

REFERENCES

1.   Clayman CB. Mass screening for colorectal cancer: Are we ready yet? JAMA 1989;261:609.
Editorial calculating that routine mass screening with fecal occult blood testing and sigmoidoscopy would cost the nation $1 billion annually, with uncertain benefits.

2. Eddy DM. Screening for colorectal cancer. Ann Intern Med 1990;113:373–384.

    Reviews current data related to screening and uses them in a sophisticated mathematical model to compare screening strategies.

3. Frame PS. Screening flexible sigmoidoscopy: Is it worthwhile? An opposing view. J Fam Pract 1987;25:604–607.

    To adhere to American Cancer Society recommendations, a typical family physician with 1000 patients over age 50 would have to perform five sigmoidoscopies daily for initial screening and two per day thereafter.

4. Knight KK, Fielding JE, Battista RN. Occult blood screening for colorectal cancer. JAMA 1989;261:587–593.

5. Selby JV, Friedman GD. Sigmoidoscopy in the periodic health examination of asymptomatic adults. JAMA 1989;261:595–601.

    Two thoughtful background papers for the U.S. Preventive Services Task Force reviewing the pros and cons of screening.

92 DIARRHEA

Symptom

JOHN S. HALSEY

EPIDEMIOLOGY.   Diarrhea is second only to the common cold as a symptom of illness in the United States. Adults usually experience one diarrheal illness per year, which on average lasts 36 to 48 hours. Although diarrheal illnesses limit activities in 50% of cases, only a minority of symptomatic individuals consult a physician.

Patients usually describe diarrhea as an increase in stool frequency, volume, or fluidity. It is often accompanied by urgency, discomfort, and/or fecal incontinence. Objectively, diarrhea is defined as a stool weight exceeding 200 g per 24 hours. Diarrhea is considered acute if it lasts less than 3 weeks and chronic if it lasts longer than 3 weeks.

ETIOLOGY.   Diarrhea may result from increased intestinal fluid secretion, decreased fluid absorption, or altered bowel motility. The normal adult small intestine absorbs about 80% of the 1 to 2 liters of ingested fluid and 8 liters of secreted fluid received per day. Ninety percent of the remaining 2 liters is absorbed in the large bowel, leaving 200 ml to be expelled as stool. Mechanisms that disturb this process produce diarrhea.

Invasive organisms induce dysentery by mucosal inflammation, resulting in blood, leukocytes, and mucus in the stool. In the United States, *Campylobac-*

ter jejuni, Salmonella spp., and *Shigella* spp. are the most common causes of the acute dysenteries (Table 92–1). Noninvasive organisms cause watery diarrhea that is free of blood and leukocytes. Rotavirus is the most common cause of watery diarrhea in children and in their adult contacts. Norwalk and similar viruses cause community outbreaks. Most travelers' diarrheas are caused by enterotoxigenic *Escherichia coli.*

Medications cause both acute and chronic diarrhea (Table 92–2). Fecal impaction, radiation therapy, and nonenteric pelvic inflammation may also cause acute diarrhea.

The most common causes of chronic diarrhea are listed in Table 92–3.

CLINICAL APPROACH.   In addition to previous surgeries, current medications, and recent travel, the clinician should determine (1) the approximate daily stool volume (large or small), (2) the duration of the diarrhea, (3) whether the stool is bloody, and (4) whether there are systemic findings such as fever, weight loss, or intravascular volume depletion. Figure 92–1 presents a general approach to diarrhea, though the initial approach for some patients may not

TABLE 92–1.   PATHOGENS CAUSING ACUTE DIARRHEA

Cause and Site	Features	Examples
Viral Infection	Noninvasive	Rotavirus Norwalk virus Enteric adenovirus
Bacterial Infection Small bowel	Noninvasive	*Vibrio cholerae* Toxigenic *E. coli*
	Invasive	*Yersinia enterocolitica* *Mycobacterium tuberculosis*
Large bowel	Noninvasive, but toxin may cause inflammation	*Clostridium difficile* *Vibrio parahaemolyticus*
	Invasive	*Salmonella* spp. *Shigella* spp. *Campylobacter* Invasive *E. coli*
Rectum	Invasive	*Chlamydia trachomatis* *Neisseria gonorrhoeae*
Parasitic Infection Small bowel	Noninvasive	*Giardia lamblia* *Cryptosporidium*
Large bowel	Invasive	*Entamoeba histolytica*
Toxin Ingestion ("Food poisoning")	Noninvasive	*Staphylococcus aureus* *Bacillus cereus* *Clostridium perfringens* *Clostridium botulinum*

TABLE 92–2.   SELECTED DRUGS CAUSING ACUTE OR CHRONIC DIARRHEA

Alcohol
Antibiotics
Bile salts
Colchicine
Digitalis
Lactulose
Laxatives
Mg^{2+}-containing antacids
Nonsteroidal anti-inflammatory drugs
Prostaglandins
Quinidine
Sorbitol (some foods)
Theophylline

TABLE 92–3.   ETIOLOGY OF CHRONIC DIARRHEA

Etiology	Examples
Infection	*Giardia lamblia* *Clostridium difficile* *Entamoeba histolytica* *Cryptosporidium* *Isospora belli* *Mycobacterium tuberculosis*
Inflammation	Ulcerative colitis Crohn's disease Ischemic colitis/enteritis Solitary rectal ulcer Collagenous colitis Microscopic colitis
Drugs	See Table 92–2
Malabsorption	Short bowel syndrome Ileal resection Enteric fistula Radiation enteritis Bacterial overgrowth Disaccharidase deficiency Pancreatic insufficiency
Endocrine	Diabetes mellitus Hyperthyroidism Hypothyroidism Zollinger-Ellison syndrome Carcinoid
Motility disorders	Irritable bowel syndrome Postvagotomy syndrome Postgastrectomy syndromes Fecal impaction Narcotic bowel

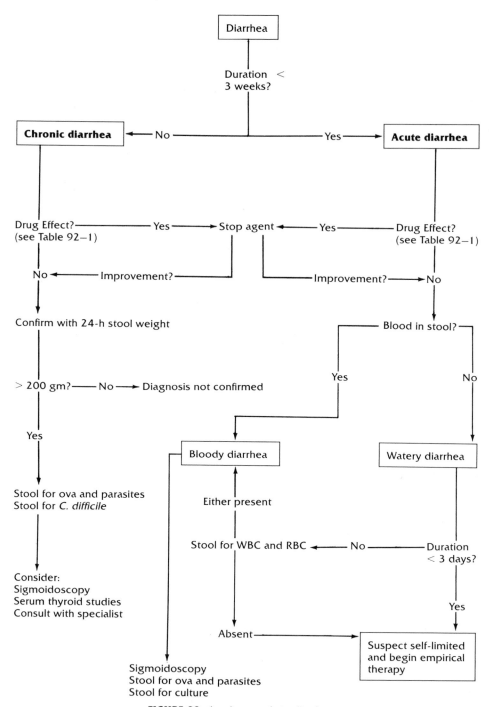

FIGURE 92–1. Approach to diarrhea.

TABLE 92–4.   NONPRESCRIPTION ANTIDIARRHEAL AGENTS

Agent	Action	Dose	Cost ($)[1]
Bismuth subsalicylate (Peptobismol)	Antisecretory	30 ml or 2 tabs q.30 min. × 8 doses	1.94 for 120 ml 4.82 for 24 tabs
Loperamide (Imodium A-D)	Delayed motility	2 tab stat; then 1 after each unformed stool (≤8/day)	4.94 for 12 caplets
Kaolin (Kaopectate)	Absorbent	60 ml stat; then repeat after each unformed stool	1.33 for 90 ml

[1]Average wholesale price, 1991 *Drug Topics Red Book.*

include all the recommended tests. Failure to respond to initial therapy should prompt a more thorough reevaluation.

MANAGEMENT.   Most adults with acute, nonspecific diarrhea are treated in the ambulatory setting with dietary modification and nonprescription drugs. Adequate hydration is important. Patients should avoid their usual diet (including milk products) and substitute 2 to 3 liters per day of liquids containing sugar and electrolytes, such as uncaffeinated soft drinks, broths, gelatins, and Gatorade. The World Health Organization rehydration formula is available in

TABLE 92–5.   ANTIMICROBIAL THERAPY FOR SELECTED ENTERIC PATHOGENS

Pathogen	Medication	Cost ($)[1]
Campylobacter jejuni[2]	Erythromycin, 250 mg PO q.i.d. × 5 d	4.00
	or	
	Ciprofloxacin, 500 mg b.i.d. × 3–5 d	25.50
Clostridium difficile	Metronidazole, 250 mg PO q.i.d. × 7 d	1.12
	or	
	Vancomycin, 125 mg PO q.i.d. × 10 d	189.20
Escherichia coli (invasive)	Trimethoprim-sulfamethoxazole, 160 mg/800 mg PO b.i.d. × 5 d	1.20
Salmonella spp.	Symptomatic treatment	—
Salmonella typhi	Trimethoprim-sulfamethoxazole, 160 mg/800 mg PO b.i.d. × 5 d	1.20
	or	
	Ampicillin, 1.6 g IV q.4h. × 10–14 d	160.00
Shigella spp.	Trimethoprim-sulfamethoxazole, 160 mg/800 mg PO b.i.d. × 5 d	1.20
	or	
	Ciprofloxacin, 500 mg PO b.i.d. × 3–5 d	25.50
01 *Vibrio cholera*	Tetracycline, 250 mg PO q.i.d. × 5 d	0.80
Yersinia enterocolitica	Tetracycline, 250 mg PO q.i.d. × 7 d	1.12
Giardia lamblia	Metronidazole, 250 mg PO t.i.d. × 7 d	0.84
	or	
	Quinacrine, 100 mg PO t.i.d. × 5 d	4.05
Entamoeba histolytica	Metronidazole, 750 mg PO t.i.d. × 7 d, followed by Iodoquinol, 650 mg PO t.i.d. × 20 d	19.92

[1]Average wholesale price, 1991 *Drug Topics Red Book,* generic if available.
[2]Therapy for *Campylobacter* may not change duration of symptoms.

packets to be mixed with water. Homemade solutions created by mixing half a teaspoon of salt (3.5 g) and 8 teaspoons of sugar (40 g) in 1 liter of water are often prescribed when other regimens are unavailable, but they are inferior because they lack potassium and base. When diarrhea has subsided, the patient may begin eating simple foods such as cooked cereals, rice, bread, and baked potatoes, advancing the diet as symptoms allow.

Useful nonprescription drugs for diarrhea are listed in Table 92–4 and recommended treatment for specific enteric pathogens in Table 92–5. Therapy for chronic diarrhea must be based on the specific diagnosis.

Cross-reference: Inflammatory Bowel Disease (Section 98).

REFERENCES

1. Brownlee HJ, Ed. Symposium on Management of Acute Nonspecific Diarrhea. Am J Med 1990;88(6A):1S–37S.

    A series of review papers emphasizing various therapeutic approaches to symptomatic control as well as definitive treatment. Special attention is given to outpatient and self-treatment.

2. DuBois D, Binder L, Nelson B. Usefulness of the stool Wright's stain in the emergency department. J Emerg Med 1988;6:483–486.

    Estimates the utility of fecal leukocytes in predicting bacterial pathogens: the predictive value of a positive test is 61%, the predictive value of a negative test is 94%.

3. Fine KD, Krejs GJ, Fordtran JS. Diarrhea. In Sleisenger MH, Fortran JS, Eds. Gastrointestinal Disease, 4th ed. W.B. Saunders, Philadelphia, 1989, pp. 290–317.

    A comprehensive chapter that approaches diarrhea from a pathophysiologic viewpoint.

93 JAUNDICE

Symptom

JOHN S. HALSEY

EPIDEMIOLOGY.   Jaundice occurs when serum bilirubin exceeds about 2.5 mg/dl. In the United States, acute viral hepatitis accounts for 75% of cases in patients younger than 30 years, whereas common bile duct obstruction from gallstones or pancreatic cancer accounts for 50% of cases in people older than 60 years.

ETIOLOGY.   Jaundice may be caused by increased bilirubin production (e.g., hemolysis), decreased bilirubin conjugation (e.g., Gilbert's syndrome), or decreased bilirubin excretion (e.g., intrahepatic or extrahepatic cholestasis) (Table 93–1).

CLINICAL APPROACH. The patient interview should focus on risk factors for biliary obstruction, which include prior episodes of jaundice, previous biliary surgery, known malignancies, and the presence of gallstones. The patient should be asked about risk factors for hepatitis, including alcohol use, recent exposure to viral hepatitis, raw shellfish ingestion, travel, occupational or recreational exposure to hepatotoxins, homosexual activity, and intravenous (IV) drug use. Important associated symptoms include fever, easy bruising, pale stools, dark urine, or confusion.

On physical examination, the clinician should search for signs of weight loss and confirm scleral icterus to avoid confusion with the yellow hue produced by carotenemia. Mild degrees of icterus may be detectable only in the peripheral sclera. Abdominal examination should begin with visual inspection for distorted contours caused by underlying masses or ascites and for prominent superficial veins arranged radially about the umbilicus, indicating portal hypertension. Other important findings include hepatomegaly (e.g., cholestatic disorders), splenomegaly (e.g., portal hypertension), ascites, abdominal masses, or a nontender dilated gallbladder (suggesting malignant extrahepatic obstruction). Spider angiomas, palmar erythema, lack of axillary or pectoral hair, and Dupuytren's contracture may indicate chronic liver disease.

The clinician should focus on potentially treatable causes while minimizing expensive and invasive tests. Using just the patient interview, physical examination, and routine liver chemistries, experienced clinicians correctly classify the liver disease 85% of the time as hemolytic, hepatocellular, or extrahepatic cholestasis. Initial diagnostic testing should focus on identifying extrahepatic biliary obstruction, which requires urgent intervention. Figure 93–1 presents one logical approach.

A low hemoglobin suggests increased bilirubin production from hemolysis or hematoma; an elevated white blood cell (WBC) count suggests an inflammatory

TABLE 93–1.   ETIOLOGY OF HYPERBILIRUBINEMIA

Unconjugated Bilirubin	Conjugated Bilirubin
Increased Production	*Intrahepatic Cholestasis*
Hemolytic anemia	Hepatocellular disease (e.g., cirrhosis, viral hepatitis)
Ineffective erythropoiesis	Infiltrative disease (e.g., lymphoma, metastatic cancer)
Transfusion	Drugs and hormones
Hematoma	Pregnancy
	Sepsis
Decreased Conjugation	
Gilbert's syndrome	*Extrahepatic Cholestasis*
Crigler-Najjar syndrome	Biliary stricture
Drugs	Choledocholithiasis
	Tumors
	Pancreatic disease

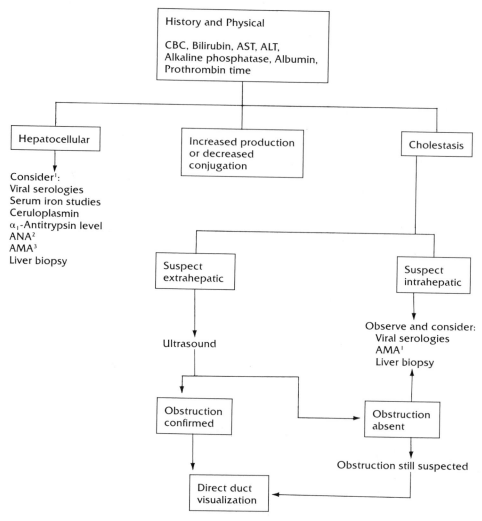

[1]Not all tests appropriate in all patients; see text.
[2]Antinuclear antibody.
[3]Antimitochondrial antibody.

FIGURE 93–1. Clinical approach to the jaundiced patient.

or viral illness. Partitioning of serum bilirubin into direct and indirect fractions is helpful only when the total bilirubin is less than 5 to 6 mg/dl. Pure unconjugated hyperbilirubinemia seldom exceeds 5 mg/dl. Aspartate aminotransferase (AST), also known as glutamic-oxaloacetic transaminase (SGOT), and alanine aminotransferase (ALT), also known as glutamic-pyruvic transaminase (SGPT), are sensitive indicators of liver cell injury. In a jaundiced patient, values exceeding 300 to 400 mg/dl usually indicate acute hepatocellular disease, especially when associated with a normal or minimally elevated alkaline phosphatase level. Levels exceeding 1000 mg/dl are seen in acute viral hepatitis, acute toxin- or drug-induced injury, and congestive heart failure. Levels below 300 mg/dl are nonspecific.

The AST/ALT ratio is useful only in recognizing liver disease due to alcohol. In patients whose ALT level is less than 300 mg/dl, alcoholic liver disease is probable if the AST/ALT ratio is greater than 2, and highly probable if it is greater than 3. A markedly elevated alkaline phosphatase level with modestly elevated transaminase levels is typical of mechanical obstruction and intrahepatic cholestasis. Elevated 5′-nucleotidase and γ-glutamyltranspeptidase (GGT) levels are used to confirm the hepatic source for the elevated alkaline phosphatase.

Although not specific for liver disease, a reduced serum albumin level and prolonged prothrombin time suggest reduced hepatocellular synthetic ability. A prolonged prothrombin time may also occur in obstructive jaundice due to malabsorption of vitamin K. Administration of vitamin K (10 mg subcutaneously) will normalize the prothrombin time within 24 hours in patients with normal hepatocellular function. If the initial evaluation indicates hepatocellular disease and there is no history of drug or toxin exposure and viral serologies are negative, it may be useful to obtain serum iron studies (to rule out hemochromatosis), ceruloplasmin (to rule out Wilson's disease), or α_1-antitrypsin assay (to rule out α_1-antitrypsin deficiency). If all of these investigations are negative and liver chemistry abnormalities persist for more than 6 months, a liver biopsy should be performed.

When liver chemistries suggest cholestasis but intrahepatic cholestasis is unlikely, patients should undergo abdominal ultrasound (US) to exclude extrahepatic obstruction. A technically adequate ultrasound study detects both dilation of the intrahepatic or extrahepatic bile ducts (sensitivity, 90%–95%) and pancreatic masses. The sensitivity and specificity of abdominal computed tomography (CT) are similar to that of ultrasound, but because of the ionizing radiation exposure, greater expense, and frequent need for contrast agents, CT should be reserved for patients with equivocal findings on ultrasound. If US confirms obstruction or if clinical suspicion of ductal obstruction remains strong despite a normal ultrasound study, direct ductal visualization by endoscopic retrograde or percutaneous transhepatic cholangiography is indicated.

If ultrasound fails to demonstrate extrahepatic obstruction, the patient should be closely observed while all potentially offending agents are withheld. Further testing may include viral serologies or antimitochondrial antibody assay (for primary biliary cirrhosis). Liver biopsy should be performed if abnormalities persist without a specific diagnosis.

When the initial clinical evaluation indicates increased bilirubin production or decreased conjugation, a workup for hemolysis is warranted. Further evaluation of the liver is unnecessary.

MANAGEMENT.   Jaundice per se is harmless and therapy is directed toward the underlying disease. Disabling pruritus, however, may require symptomatic relief. Oral antihistamines can be used initially, followed by the binding resin cholestyramine (4 g t.i.d. with juice), which is effective as long as bile acids pass the obstruction and enter the small bowel. Because cholestyramine may further hinder absorption of fat-soluble vitamins, oral or parenteral supplementation with vitamins A, D, and K may be necessary.

Cross-references: Diagnosis and Management of Alcoholism (Section 9), Abdominal Pain (Section 95), Biliary Tract Disease (Section 99), Cirrhosis and Chronic Liver Failure (Section 100), Viral Hepatitis (Section 101), Anemia (Section 201).

REFERENCES

1. Frank BB, et al. Clinical evaluation of jaundice. JAMA 1989;262:3031–3034.
    Guide to the utility of various approaches to patient evaluation, based on reported sensitivity and predictive value of available procedures.

2. McKenna JP, Moskovitz M, Cox JL. Abnormal liver function tests in asymptomatic patients. Am Fam Physician 1989;39:117–126.

3. Van Ness MM, Diehl AM. Is liver biopsy useful in the evaluation of patients with chronically elevated liver enzymes? Ann Intern Med 1989;111:473–478.
    A recent study confirming the utility of liver biopsy in cases remaining undiagnosed after appropriate laboratory and imaging studies.

94 CONSTIPATION

Symptom

SHOBA KRISHNAMURTHY

EPIDEMIOLOGY.   Constipation is one of the most common chronic digestive complaints, affecting 1 in every 50 persons. Although there is no universally accepted or precise definition of this complaint, one objective definition is passage of less than three stools per week. Subjective definitions (small or hard stools, difficult passage of stools, or a feeling of incomplete evacuation) are difficult to quantify or assess. Recent analysis suggests a prevalence of 1% to 2%, with 2.5 million physician visits per year for constipation. It is more common in people over 65 years of age and in women, and affects nonwhites more than whites.

ETIOLOGY.   It is widely believed that inadequate intake of dietary fiber is a common cause of constipation, despite the lack of evidence that constipated individuals consume less fiber. Constipation can be caused by gastrointestinal disorders (primarily colonic and anorectal disorders), drugs, and metabolic, endocrine, and neurologic disorders (Table 94–1). Although inactivity and suppression of the urge to defecate are often considered causes of constipation, these factors have not been adequately studied.

Irritable bowel syndrome is the most common gastrointestinal disorder associated with constipation. The onset is usually before age 35, and affected women outnumber men 2 to 1. This syndrome, which is characterized by disordered intestinal motility, causes abdominal pain, passage of small, hard stools, bloating, and a sense of incomplete evacuation. In 50% of cases, symptoms are induced by stress and associated with abnormal psychological features such as depression, anxiety, and somatization. The diagnosis depends on a long duration of symptoms beginning at a young age, the absence of weight loss, nocturnal abdominal pain and hematochezia, and the lack of laboratory or radiologic abnormalities. **Diverticular disease** is present in 50% of patients over 60 years of age, with symptoms similar to those of irritable bowel syndrome. Diverticulitis and stricture formation can cause or exacerbate constipation.

Colonic carcinoma must be considered in any patient over 40 years with a history of recent constipation. Associated hematochezia, weight loss, a personal history of colonic polyps and ulcerative colitis, and a family history of colonic cancer or familial polyposis support this diagnosis. **Hirschsprung's disease** is an uncommon disorder (1 in 5000 live births) caused by the absence of ganglion cells along a variable length of the distal colon. This diagnosis should be considered in patients with a history of constipation from birth or infancy. **Neuromuscular disorders** affecting either the colonic smooth muscle or the colonic myenteric plexus can cause severe constipation and prolonged colonic transit that responds poorly to laxatives.

Of the metabolic disorders, **diabetes** commonly causes constipation, and affects 80% to 90% of patients with autonomic and peripheral neuropathy and 30% of patients without neuropathy. Among the endocrine disorders, **hypothyroidism** is the most common cause of constipation. It is sometimes associated with a megacolon (an enlarged and dilated colon on abdominal radiographs). Constipation may be the only symptom of hypothyroidism.

Constipation is commonly present with neurologic disorders. Megacolon is present in 10% of patients with **Parkinson's disease,** though constipation is more common. Antiparkinson medications may also cause constipation. About 40% of patients with **multiple sclerosis** complain of constipation.

CLINICAL APPROACH.   The patient interview should focus on the exact nature of the patient's complaint, including a detailed account of drug intake and

TABLE 94–1.   CAUSES OF CONSTIPATION

Medications

Analgesics/opiates*
Antacids (calcium and aluminum)
Anticholinergics*
Anticonvulsants
Antidepressants*
Antihypertensives
Antiparkinson agents

Iron
Heavy metal poisoning
   (lead, mercury, arsenic)
Calcium channel blockers*
Sucralfate
Barium sulfate

Metabolic Disorders

Diabetes*
Porphyria
Amyloidosis

Uremia
Hypokalemia
Hypercalcemia

Endocrine Disorders

Panhypopituitarism
Hypothyroidism*
Pheochromocytoma

Pregnancy
Glucagonoma

Gastrointestinal Disorders

Colonic obstruction
   Extraluminal (tumors, chronic volvulus, hernias)
   Luminal (tumors*, benign strictures)
Abnormalities of colonic motor function
   Irritable bowel syndrome*
   Diverticular disease*
Pseudo-obstruction
   Disorder of intestinal muscle (scleroderma, hollow visceral myopathy)
   Disorders of myenteric nerves (visceral neuropathy, paraneoplastic neuropathy, Chagas'
      disease, neuronal intestinal dysplasia, Hirschsprung's disease)
Rectal disorders
   Rectocele
   Intussusception
   Prolapse
   Rectosphincteric dyssynergia
Anal problems
   Stenosis
   Fissures

Neurologic Disorders

Brain
   Parkinson's disease
   Tumors
   Cerebrovascular accidents*
Other
   Trauma to nervi erigentes and lumbosacral cord
   Cauda equina tumor
   Meningocele
   Autonomic insufficiency
   Tabes dorsalis
   Multiple sclerosis

*Most common causes.

symptoms of metabolic, endocrine, and neurologic disease. A careful physical examination of the gastrointestinal and neurologic systems is mandatory. Anorectal and perineal examination should include a search for perineal disease, rectal prolapse, and anal fissure. A digital rectal examination may detect a rectal mass, tenderness of a fissure, or anal stenosis.

Routine laboratory tests include a complete blood cell (CBC) count, fecal occult blood test, thyroid function tests, and blood urea nitrogen, serum calcium, electrolyte, and fasting blood glucose determinations. Patients with recent onset of symptoms or especially severe symptoms should undergo sigmoidoscopy and barium enema examination to look for colorectal neoplasms, strictures, diverticula, megacolon, or a narrowed distal segment with dilated proximal colon (suggesting Hirschsprung's disease).

If the above evaluation is entirely normal, the patient should be started on a high-fiber diet (20–30 g of fiber per day, generally in the form of 1 cup of All-Bran cereal or 1–2 tbsp of psyllium) for 30 days. If constipation resolves, no further workup is required. In patients with persistent constipation who complain primarily of infrequent defecation, a colonic transit study on a high-fiber diet is indicated. Although many transit studies are described, it is most simply done by having the patient ingest 20 radiopaque markers (5-mm pieces cut from a No. 16 French nasogastric tube or commercially available markers) which are taken on day 0, a day after the patient has had a bowel movement. Plain abdominal radiographs are obtained on days 5 and 7. Normal subjects pass 80% of markers by day 5 and 100% by day 7. The patient should avoid laxatives or enemas during the test. This is an excellent way of objectively confirming prolonged colonic transit time. An abnormal test suggests a neuromuscular disorder ("colonic inertia"). These patients are best referred to a gastroenterologist for further evaluation and management. Anorectal manometry and rectal biopsy are necessary to exclude Hirschsprung's disease.

In the patient with persistent constipation who complains of difficulty with defecation, anorectal manometry and defecography may be helpful. Defecography (evacuation of thick barium paste monitored by fluoroscopy and videotape while the patient sits on a translucent commode) may be used to demonstrate a rectocele and internal rectal intussusception. This test, however, needs further study. Anorectal manometry and electromyography may be helpful in demonstrating rectosphinceteric dyssynergia (paradoxical contraction of the puborectalis muscle on attempted defecation).

MANAGEMENT.   Although appropriate treatment of constipation depends on the underlying cause, there are several important principles: (1) An increase in fiber intake to 20 to 30 g/day in the form of dietary fiber or supplemental fiber (psyllium, calcium polycarbophil, or cellulose) benefits most patients. Of the dietary fibers, wheat bran is most effective in increasing stool weight, followed by fruits and vegetables, oats, mucilage, corn, cellulose, soya, and pectin. (2) Routine use of laxatives over long periods should be discouraged. (3) Biofeedback has been reported to be helpful in patients with rectosphincteric dyssynergia. (4) Surgical treatment is useful in (a) Hirschsprung's disease, (b) selected patients with "colonic inertia," and (c) occasionally in patients with large rectoceles, prolapse, and rectal intussusception. Habit training (i.e., having a scheduled time each day for bowel movements, usually after a meal) and contingency management (i.e., using a cleansing enema if defecation does not occur after 2 days) have been used in the management of constipation in children but have not been adequately studied in adults.

Cross-references: Colorectal Cancer Screening (Section 91), Abdominal Pain (Section 95), Multiple Sclerosis (Section 143), Parkinsonism (Section 147), Common Thyroid Disorders (Section 156).

REFERENCES

1. Devroede G. Constipation. In Sleisinger MH, Fordthan JS, Eds. Gastrointestinal Disease: Pathophysiology, Diagnosis and Management. W.B. Saunders, Philadelphia, 1989, pp. 331–368.
    A detailed review.

2. Johanson JF, Sonnenberg A, Koch TR. Clinical epidemiology of chronic constipation. J Clin Gastroenterol 1989;11:525–536.
    An analysis of various national surveys.

3. Wald A. Approach to the patient with constipation. In Yamada T, Ed. Textbook of Gastroenterology. J.B. Lippincott, Philadelphia, 1991, pp. 779–795.
    A comprehensive, practical review.

4. Wald A, Hinds JP, Caruana BJ. Psychological and physiological characteristics of patients with severe idiopathic constipation. Gastroenterology 1989;97:932–937.
    Patients with severe, idiopathic constipation could be divided into two major groups on the basis of transit studies, with different implications for therapy and prognosis.

95 ABDOMINAL PAIN

Symptom

TIMOTHY E. LITTLE

EPIDEMIOLOGY.   Acute abdominal pain of less than 1 week's duration is responsible for 5% of emergency room visits. Recurrent abdominal pain without an identifiable cause affects 3% to 15% of the U.S. population and accounts for 40% of patients seen in many gastrointestinal specialty practices.

ETIOLOGY.   *Acute Abdominal Pain.*   Table 95–1 lists the important causes of acute abdominal pain. The most common cause, "nonspecific abdominal pain,"

TABLE 95–1. CAUSES OF ACUTE ABDOMINAL PAIN

Diagnosis	% of Cases
Nonspecific abdominal pain	40–45
Appendicitis	6–24
Biliary pain	>10
Acute cholecystitis	7–9
Gastroenteritis	7
Small bowel obstruction	2–4
Renal colic	2–8
Perforated peptic ulcer	3
Acute pancreatitis	1–2
Acute diverticulitis	1–2
Acute salpingitis	2
Ectopic pregnancy	0.2
Aortic rupture	<2
Acute mesenteric ischemia	<2

refers to acute abdominal pain that remains undiagnosed after the initial evaluation but is not believed to represent surgical disease; follow-up may reveal an organic or functional cause. It affects women more than men (2:1 ratio) and usually occurs in younger patients (<30 years, 60% of cases). In the elderly, cholecystitis is the most frequent cause of acute abdominal pain. Appendicitis affects all age groups, with a peak incidence between the ages of 10 and 20 years, and is the most common missed diagnosis in patients with abdominal pain.

Several nonsurgical diseases may cause acute abdominal pain, including vasculitis, splenic infarction, renal infarction, sickle cell crisis, and infectious colitides.

Chronic Abdominal Pain.   The irritable bowel syndrome is the most common cause of chronic abdominal pain. The pain is gradual in onset with an undulating continuous pattern, is located in periumbilical or hypogastric areas, and may be so severe as to lead to emesis. The pain usually decreases with defecation or is associated with a change in frequency or consistency of stool. Patients may experience gaseous distention, bloating, or intermittent constipation. Although the etiology of irritable bowel syndrome is unclear, gut motility is usually abnormal and the perception of pain from luminal gut distention is increased. Despite traditional teachings, many patients with irritable bowel syndrome do not have major psychiatric disorders.

Other common causes of chronic abdominal pain include chronic pancreatitis, depression, visceral cancer pain, abdominal wall neuromuscular pain, the pain of benign organomegaly, chronic peptic disease, subacute presentations of contained perforations in the elderly, endometriosis, and subclinical Crohn's disease.

Chronic intractable (or idiopathic) abdominal pain refers to the relatively continuous pain over months seen in patients without identifiable disease or features of irritable bowel syndrome. Women are more commonly affected (70%), bowel movements may be normal, the pain may be incapacitating, and psychiatric illness is common. Risk factors include abdominal pain that begins in childhood or adolescence, a history of sexual abuse, a history of nondefinitive pelvic or abdominal surgery, other organ system chronic pain syndromes, and DSM-III-R criteria for somatoform disorders.

CLINICAL APPROACH.   *Acute Abdominal Pain.*   Acute abdominal pain represents surgical disease until proven otherwise. Systematic evaluation using the patient interview and serial abdominal examinations leads to the correct diagnosis in 70% to 90% of cases. The chart shown in Figure 95–1 lists important historical, physical examination, and laboratory data to collect during the initial evaluation. The location of perceived pain, the location of tenderness on examination, and the evolution of the abdominal examination are especially important. Nonspecific abdominal pain, in contrast to most surgical diseases, tends to diminish with time.

Common causes of **midepigastric pain** are biliary pain (biliary colic, cholecystitis, cholangitis), peptic pain, acute pancreatitis, and early appendicitis. *Biliary pain* gradually appears in the midline or just to the right of midline, may radiate into the subscapular area or back, is continuous (not "colicky"), and is not necessarily related to meals (see Section 99, Biliary Tract Disease). Biliary pain may gradually resolve without systemic signs over 1 or 2 hours or progress to frank cholecystitis, with tenderness and a vague mass in the right upper quadrant. Cholangitis is accompanied by fever, tachycardia, and percussion tenderness over the liver. *Peptic pain* is often burning in quality, is well localized to the midepigastrium, and may temporarily resolve with antacids or have a clear association with eating (see Section 96, Dyspepsia). Epigastric pain that rapidly becomes generalized or spreads to the right lower quadrant suggests peptic perforation. *Acute pancreatitis* usually causes a continuous boring epigastric pain that may radiate to the flanks or back and is accompanied by vomiting. Dehydration and fever are typical in severe cases, and elevated serum amylase levels confirm the diagnosis. Although appendicitis may occasionally cause epigastric pain, right lower quadrant findings appear within several hours in 70% to 85% of patients.

Right upper quadrant pain usually results from biliary disease (see above), duodenal ulcer disease, hepatitis, ascending appendicitis, or primary renal disease. *Acute hepatitis* usually causes mild pain with a diffusely tender liver on examination. The serum AST (SGOT) and ALT (SGPT) levels are markedly elevated in most patients with hepatitis, except those with alcoholic hepatitis (see Section 93, Jaundice). *Pyelonephritis* and *hydronephrosis* are usually evident after urinalysis and renal ultrasound, respectively. *Retrocecal appendicitis* should be considered when ultrasound in a patient with suspected cholecystitis does not confirm the presence of gallstones.

Isolated **left upper quadrant pain** may result from splenic infarction, splenic hemorrhage, or left kidney inflammation, infarction, or obstruction. Computed tomography may clarify confusing cases.

Sex:

Age:

Pain (indicate on a drawing the location of maximal pain):

Aggravating factors: Pain character at onset:

Mitigating factors: Areas of pain radiation:

Duration: Severity:

Quality of pain:

Nausea/vomiting: Female:

Appetite: Periods:

Bowels: Vaginal discharge:

Micturition: Pregnancy risk:

Past medical history:

Previous similar pain:

Previous abdominal surgery:

Prior serious illness:

Immune status (e.g., systemic steroids, HIV infection):

Drugs:

Exam:

Color: Guarding:

Mood: Rigidity:

Vital signs: Swellings:

Movement: Bowel sounds:

Scars: Rectal examination:

Distention: Vaginal examination:

Rebound:

Laboratory:

WBC: X-ray:

Urine: Amylase:

FIGURE 95—1.   Chart for evaluation of acute abdominal pain.

Acute **right lower quadrant pain** strongly suggests appendicitis. Approximately 85% of patients with *appendicitis* have fever (usually $< 38°C$) and 86% have leukocytosis (10–20,000/mm^3). In women, ectopic pregnancy, salpingitis, and ruptured ovarian cysts should be considered (see Sections 163 and 168). Salpingitis is the most commonly missed diagnosis leading to unnecessary laparotomy in the general population. Ileal-colonic Crohn's disease may occasionally cause right lower quadrant pain but usually is associated with diarrhea, weight loss, or fatigue (see Section 98, Inflammatory Bowel Disease).

Periumbilical pain should suggest diseases that cause dilation, inflammation, or ischemia of the small bowel and appendix. *Small bowel pain* is usually spasmodic (but may be relatively constant) and increases slowly in intensity. Risk factors for small bowel obstruction include prior abdominal surgery, inflammatory bowel disease, gallstones, and a history of foreign body ingestion. Vomiting is usually prominent and bowel sounds are present but abnormal in quality. The clinician should carefully inspect the patient for hernias. Radiographs taken during early obstruction may not reveal the characteristic dilated loops of bowel. *Small bowel ischemia* should always be considered when continuous periumbilical pain occurs in the elderly or in those at risk of thromboembolic disease. Because physical examination and laboratory findings may be normal in early intestinal ischemia, surgical consultation should be considered in these patients.

Hypogastric pain usually represents pelvic disease, disease of the urinary bladder, colonic disease, or appendicitis. A distended bladder may be evident on abdominal palpation or percussion. Fever and leukocytosis in an elderly patient suggest diverticular disease (see Section 102, Diverticulitis). Other causes of hypogastric pain are constipation with or without stercoral ulceration (see Section 94, Constipation), discrete attacks of irritable bowel syndrome, and ulcerative, ischemic, or infectious colitis (associated with diarrhea and microscopic blood in the stool).

Left lower quadrant pain suggests diverticulitis, distal colonic neoplasia, or inflammation. Gynecologic causes must be considered in women (see Sections 163 and 168).

DIAGNOSIS BY PATTERN OF RADIATION. Flank or abdominal pain radiating to the vulva or testicle occurs commonly in ureteral colic and aortic rupture or leakage. The pain of aortic rupture is acute or subacute, relatively continuous, and sometimes (but not always) associated with hypotension, anemia, and an abdominal mass.

Pain radiating into the mid-back usually reflects disease in the retroperitoneum (i.e., the duodenum, pancreas, aorta, and kidneys).

Chronic Abdominal Pain. The clinical approach to chronic abdominal pain depends on the duration of symptoms and the presence of objective signs. Extensive diagnostic evaluation of pain syndromes that have recurred for decades or since adolescence is rarely productive. The approach to these patients should include careful history (including dietary, psychiatric, social, and surgical histories), physical examination, some laboratory tests (liver blood tests, amylase, CBC, urinalysis), and, most important, careful, regular follow-up.

Even the most severe abdominal pain of irritable bowel syndrome or chronic intractable abdominal pain is not associated with persistent anorexia, weight loss, or diarrhea that wakes the patient or exceeds 300 g/day. Patients with chronic abdominal pain and associated anorexia or weight loss should be evaluated for gastrointestinal malignancy, depression, and chronic intra-abdominal inflammation, including inflammatory bowel disease. Patients with vague abdominal pain and weight loss but with a good appetite should be referred to a gastroenterologist for evaluation of possible malabsorption.

Elderly patients with chronic abdominal pain should be referred to a gastroenterologist if the diagnosis is not obvious. Most will have organic disease.

MANAGEMENT. *Acute Abdominal Pain.* Patients with suspected appendicitis, cholecystitis, bowel obstruction, or other suspected surgical conditions should be seen promptly by a surgeon. Hospital admission should be also considered for patients with new undiagnosed abdominal pain if (1) the pain shows no signs of relenting, (2) vital signs are abnormal, (3) appendicitis cannot be reliably excluded, or (4) the patient is elderly. In patients with nonspecific acute abdominal pain, follow-up in 24 to 48 hours often reveals significant organic disease.

Chronic Abdominal Pain. The clinician should acknowledge the pain of irritable bowel syndrome and reassure patients that medical support will be provided. Management focuses on educating the patient,[4] involving the patient in treatment plans, and advising the patient to be watchful for life events or foods that seem to precipitate symptoms (although in many cases no specific event is found). Careful trials with many different pharmacologic agents have not conclusively shown benefit for any specific agents,[3] in part because of a strong placebo response. Antimuscarinics such as dicyclomine, 10 mg PO at the first suggestion of the onset of a pain attack, may abort pain progression in selected patients.[2] Psyllium seed, two tablespoons in juice or water twice daily, is helpful in some patients, but trials of bulking agents overall have been contradictory. Narcotics have no role in the treatment of this disorder.

Many patients with chronic intractable abdominal pain are profoundly disabled. Although management is similar to that for irritable bowel syndrome, clinicians should tell patients to expect setbacks, simultaneously reassuring them that support will be provided. The goal of therapy is to improve the patient's function rather than to cure the patient of pain. These patients may benefit from early referral to a multispecialty pain clinic that includes psychiatric consultation. Family counseling, physical therapy, and exercise programs may also be beneficial. Patients with chronic intractable abdominal pain tolerate drugs poorly. Antidepressants have not been adequately investigated in this disorder but may be of some benefit in selected patients. Although narcotics are contraindicated, most patients use these agents at some time during their course.

Cross-references: Chronic Pain Syndrome (Section 13), Jaundice (Section 93), Constipation (Section 94), Dyspepsia (Section 96), Inflammatory Bowel Disease (Section 98), Biliary Tract Disease (Section 99), Diverticulitis (Section 102), Peptic Ulcer Disease (Section 103), Sigmoidoscopy and Colonoscopy (Section 105), Upper Gastrointestinal Endoscopy (Section 106), Diabetes Mellitus (Section 157), Pelvic Pain in Women (Section 163), Pelvic Inflammatory Disease (Section 168), Nephrolithiasis (Section 176), Urinary Tract Infections in Women (Section 177), Somatization (Section 191).

REFERENCES

1. de Dombal FT. Acute abdominal pain: An O.M.G.E. survey. Scand J Gastroenterol 1979;56(suppl 14):29–43.
    Multinational standardized data collection survey of 6097 patients admitted for abdominal pain, with outcome results.

2. Freidman G. Treatment of the irritable syndrome. Gastroenterol Clin North Am 1991; 20:325–334.
    A balanced discussion of therapy for irritable bowel syndrome.

3. Klein KB. Controlled treatment trials in the irritable bowel syndrome: A critique. Gastroenterology 1988;95:232–241.
    No single study offered convincing evidence that any therapy is effective in treating IBS.

4. Shimberg EF. Relief from IBS: Irritable Bowel Syndrome. Ballantine Books, New York, 1991.
    A useful lay monograph that provides education and validation for the patient.

5. Silen W. Cope's Early Diagnosis of the Acute Abdomen, 15th ed. Oxford University Press, New York, 1979.
    Classic treatise on abdominal pain syndromes, with remarkable and timely observations on clinical diagnosis. Abdominal presentations with sparse clinical signs are not addressed in depth.

96 DYSPEPSIA

Symptom

STEVEN R. McGEE

EPIDEMIOLOGY.   Although definitions vary, dyspepsia usually refers to chronic or recurrent upper abdominal discomfort not related to exertion and not associated with jaundice, bleeding, or dysphagia. Point prevalence rates for dyspepsia approach 30%, although only 25% of affected patients seek medical attention.

ETIOLOGY.   Among general practice patients with dyspepsia, esophagogastroduodenoscopy (EGD) reveals duodenal ulcer in 12% to 25%, gastric ulcer in 2% to 13%, esophagitis in 3% to 5%, and gastric cancer in 0.05% to 1.8%. "Non-ulcer dyspepsia" is diagnosed when EGD demonstrates either normal findings or gastritis. Some patients with non-ulcer dyspepsia experience classic reflux esophagitis symptoms and benefit from antireflux therapy despite normal findings on EGD. Others may describe biliary pain, which usually appears suddenly in the right hypochondrium or epigastrium, is severe and constant, and fades gradually over hours. Medications such as potassium chloride, antibiotics, or nonsteroidal anti-inflammatory agents may provoke dyspepsia.

The etiology of most cases of non-ulcer dyspepsia remains unknown. Proposed mechanisms include gastric acid hypersecretion, motility disorders, and *Helicobacter pylori* (formerly *Campylobacter pylori*) gastritis. Acid hypersecretion probably plays a minor role, because placebo-controlled trials of antacids or cimetidine show little benefit. *H. pylori* is recovered from the stomachs of as many as 70% of patients with non-ulcer dyspepsia and does correlate with histologic type B gastritis, but successful treatment of the bacterium does not significantly change symptoms. Furthermore, there is no correlation between the severity of histologic gastritis and symptoms, and *H. pylori* is found in 50% of elderly asymptomatic subjects. Motility disturbances may play a role, especially when dyspepsia refers to nonpeptic symptoms such as bloating, nausea, distention, or early satiety. In these patients, manometric studies frequently document abnormalities (especially antral hypomotility), irritable bowel symptoms are frequent, and promotility drugs such as domperidone, metoclopramide, and cispralide are effective in double-blind placebo trials.

CLINICAL APPROACH/MANAGEMENT.   Nocturnal pain and pain *relieved* by food, milk, or antacids favors peptic ulcer disease; pain *provoked* by meals and pain insufficient to influence daily activities favors non-ulcer dyspepsia. No symptom, however, reliably distinguishes non-ulcer dyspepsia from ulcer disease or gastric cancer. Epigastric tenderness, though reproducible, occurs just as often in non-ulcer dyspepsia as in other causes. All causes of dyspepsia may produce weight loss.

The physical examination should search for complications of peptic ulcer disease and gastric cancer. Patients with weight loss, abdominal masses, gastrointestinal bleeding, obstruction, or jaundice should undergo prompt diagnostic evaluation. Patients without such complications should avoid potentially offending agents (nonsteroidal anti-inflammatory drugs, alcohol, cigarettes) and begin empirical therapy with antacids, H_2 antagonists, or sucralfate. Patients who do not respond to 7 to 10 days of empirical therapy, who have persistent symptoms at the end of 8 weeks of therapy, or who have recurrent symptoms after withdrawal of therapy should undergo diagnostic evaluation. An upper gastrointestinal series, though more accessible and less expensive than EGD, misses some gastric lesions, especially when the patient has had prior gastric surgery or ulcer disease. Most authorities prefer EGD over an upper gastrointestinal series because EGD is more accurate and allows biopsy of suspicious lesions (see Section 106).

This approach, which emphasizes empirical treatment for no more than 8 weeks, is based on the following rationale: (1) the diagnostic screening of all dyspepsia patients is too expensive, (2) the treatment for all organic causes of dyspepsia, except gastric cancer, is the same (antacid therapy), (3) gastric cancer is rare in general practice (<1%), (4) refractory ulcers and gastric cancer, if symptomatically improved on empirical therapy, will recrudesce after withdrawal of therapy, and (5) there is no evidence demonstrating increased complications from an 8-week diagnostic delay.

FOLLOW-UP. Approximately 70% of peptic ulcers respond to 8 weeks of empirical therapy. Between 50% and 80% of ulcer patients experience recurrences within 12 months of cessation of therapy. In non-ulcer dyspepsia patients, symptoms improve over several years in 75% and the risk of subsequent peptic ulcer disease is low.

Cross-references: Diagnosis and Management of Alcoholism (Section 9), Smoking Cessation (Section 11), Abdominal Pain (Section 95), Peptic Ulcer Disease (Section 103), Upper Gastrointestinal Endoscopy (Section 106).

REFERENCES

1. Dobrilla G, Comberlato M, Steele A, Vallaperta P. Drug treatment of functional dyspepsia: A meta-analysis of randomized controlled clinical trials. J Clin Gastroenterol 1989;11:169–177.
    Reviews many non-ulcer dyspepsia drug trials. The placebo effect is strong, and promotility drugs are most effective.

2. Kahn KL, Greenfield S. The efficacy of endoscopy in the evaluation of dyspepsia: A review of the literature and development of a sound strategy. J Clin Gastroenterol 1986;8:346–358.
    Excellent review of the literature by authors of American College of Physicians position paper (Ann Intern Med 1985;102:266–269).

3. Nyren O, Adami H, Bates S, Bergström R, Gustavsson S, Lööf L, Nyberg A. Absence of therapeutic benefit from antacids or cimetidine in non-ulcer dyspepsia. N Engl J Med 1986;314:339–343.
    Patients with non-ulcer dyspepsia defined by endoscopy experienced peptic symptoms such as epigastric pain and heartburn.

4. Talley N, Phillips S. Non-ulcer dyspepsia: Potential causes and pathophysiology. Ann Intern Med 1988;108:865–879.
    Encyclopedic overview of pathogenesis of non-ulcer dyspepsia.

5. Zell S, Budhraja M. An approach to dyspepsia in the ambulatory care setting: Evaluation based on risk stratification. J Gen Intern Med 1989;4:144–150.
    Stratifies risk more thoroughly and advocates less aggressive approach in the lowest risk patients in whom antacid therapy fails.

97 DYSPHAGIA AND HEARTBURN

Symptom

STEVEN R. McGEE

DYSPHAGIA

EPIDEMIOLOGY. Dysphagia, defined as difficulty swallowing, accounts for about 10% of referrals for barium esophagography or upper endoscopy.

ETIOLOGY. Table 97–1 lists the important causes of dysphagia, which are traditionally divided into disorders occurring above the cricopharyngeal muscle in the mouth or pharynx (oropharyngeal dysphagia) and those occurring below the cricopharyngeal muscle in the esophagus (esophageal dysphagia).

CLINICAL APPROACH. Dysphagia is always associated with the act of swallowing. The **globus** sensation, in contrast, is a constant tightness or lump in the middle of the throat that is sometimes relieved by swallowing. In some patients, globus results from reflux esophagitis. **Odynophagia,** or painful swallowing, usually reflects infectious esophagitis (*Candida,* herpesvirus, cytomegalovirus [CMV]), or severe reflux, caustic (lye ingestion), or pill-induced esophagitis.

Although acute dysphagia requires urgent evaluation, chronic dysphagia is commonly evaluated in the outpatient clinic. The patient interview should initially distinguish oropharyngeal from esophageal dysphagia. Patients with oropharyngeal dysphagia have difficulty initiating a swallow (especially of liquids or dry solids such as biscuits), may experience immediate coughing or nasopharyngeal regurgitation with liquid swallows, and usually exhibit other symptoms of neuromuscular disease. Esophageal dysphagia lacks these features; instead, soon after initiation of the swallow, the bolus "sticks."

In patients with esophageal dysphagia, the history helps distinguish obstructive from motility disorders. Patients with obstructive causes have more trouble with solid boluses than liquid, are not affected by the temperature of the food, and usually regurgitate the food after bolus impaction. Those with motility disorders, in contrast, have equal difficulty with solids and liquids, may have more trouble with cold liquids, and, after bolus impaction, can usually eventually swallow the food by maneuvers such as swallowing more liquids or hyperextending the neck.

Dysphagia from esophageal rings is intermittent, with months between episodes; that from strictures progresses gradually over months; and that from cancer progresses over weeks, with associated weight loss. Achalasia leads to continuous dysphagia without heartburn, scleroderma leads to continuous dysphagia with heartburn, and diffuse esophageal spasm leads to intermittent dysphagia with chest pain.

295

TABLE 97–1.   ETIOLOGY OF DYSPHAGIA

Oropharyngeal Dysphagia (above the cricopharyngeal muscle)
Neuromuscular disease
  Central nervous system*
    CNS depression from any cause
    Stroke
    Parkinson's disease
    Multiple sclerosis
    Amyotrophic lateral sclerosis
  Peripheral nervous system
    Guillain-Barré syndrome
    Poliomyelitis
  Neuromuscular junction
    Botulism
    Myasthenia gravis
  Myopathies
    Polymyositis/dermatomyositis
    Muscular dystrophy

Obstructive disease
  Zenker's diverticulum
  Cancer

Esophageal Dysphagia (below the cricopharyngeal muscle)
Neuromuscular (motility) disorders
  Achalasia*
  Scleroderma
  Diffuse esophageal spasm
  Nonspecific motility disorders*

Obstructive disease
  Intrinsic
    Peptic stricture*
    Cancer*
    Schatzki ring*
    Webs
  Extrinsic—mediastinal blood vessels or tumors

*Most common causes.

Although the patient interview accurately defines the cause of dysphagia in 80% of cases, the patient's opinion of the site of a lesion, demonstrated with a finger pointed on the chest, is often inaccurate.[2]

A barium esophagram reliably identifies strictures, esophageal cancers, and, if a marshmallow is swallowed during the test, esophageal rings. Because it better evaluates the pharynx and upper esophagus, esophagography should always precede endoscopy. Endoscopy is indicated when esophagrams demonstrate an abnormality, because most require biopsy, and in patients with persistent symptoms and normal esophagrams, although the yield may be low.[1] Patients with persistent unexplained dysphagia or whose esophagrams suggest motility disorders should be referred for manometry.

MANAGEMENT.   An experienced speech pathologist best determines the safety of swallowing in patients with oropharyngeal dysphagia. In general, patients should be alert, be able to elevate the larynx with a dry swallow and sit up for 20 minutes after a meal, and have a clear voice and good cough. Severe cases may require a temporary nasogastric tube or feeding gastrostomy (placed percutaneously by endoscopy). Tracheostomy is best avoided because it may actually promote rather than prevent aspiration.

Gastroenterologists manage esophageal rings, strictures, and achalasia with esophageal dilation. Inoperable esophageal cancer may require placement of an esophageal stent.

HEARTBURN AND REFLUX ESOPHAGITIS

EPIDEMIOLOGY.   Heartburn, a symptom of reflux esophagitis, is a substernal burning sensation that radiates toward the mouth, decreases with antacids, and is provoked by bending over, lying down, heavy lifting, and ingestion of particular foods (alcohol, spicy foods, chocolate). In one survey of hospital workers, heartburn occurred daily in 7% and at least monthly in 36%. Other than during pregnancy, when 25% have daily heartburn, there is no age or sex predilection.

SIGNS AND SYMPTOMS.   Other symptoms that may be associated with reflux esophagitis include acid regurgitation (effortless appearance of bitter fluid in mouth without nausea), water brash (nonbitter fluid in mouth, from excess salivary fluid production), retrosternal chest pain, hiccoughs, nocturnal asthma, dysphagia (even without stricture), and hoarseness.

The correlation between the severity of heartburn and the endoscopic grade of esophagitis is poor. In endoscopic surveys of patients with heartburn, about 50% have reflux esophagitis, 35% have normal findings, and 15% have peptic ulcer disease. Cancer is rare (<1%).

CLINICAL APPROACH.   As with dyspepsia, patients with classic heartburn and no complications should receive empirical treatment for reflux esophagitis without further testing (see Section 96, Dyspepsia). Early diagnostic evaluation is indicated when (1) complications are present, such as dysphagia, severe nausea and vomiting, weight loss, or gastrointestinal bleeding, (2) the patient fails to respond to empirical therapy, or (3) the heartburn worsens with exercise, which suggests angina.

Barium radiography is less expensive and more accessible to general practitioners than endoscopy, and accurately demonstrates esophageal strictures and peptic ulcer disease. Endoscopy is preferred in those with persistent symptoms, however, because it has superior diagnostic sensitivity for esophagitis and is the only test that identifies Barrett's esophagus, a precursor of esophageal adenocarcinoma found in 0 to 20% of endoscopic examinations undertaken for persistent heartburn.

TABLE 97–2.   THERAPY FOR REFLUX ESOPHAGITIS

Drug	Dose	Cost ($), per Day[1]
Cimetidine	300 mg PO q.i.d.	2.84
Ranitidine	150 mg PO b.i.d.	2.80
Famotidine	20 mg PO b.i.d.	2.42
Omeprazole	20 mg PO q.d.	3.21

[1]Average wholesale price, 1991 *Drug Topics Red Book.*

MANAGEMENT.   In controlled trials, elevation of the head of the bed and the use of H_2 receptor antagonists or omeprazole effectively reduce heartburn and heal esophagitis. Omeprazole is superior to H_2 receptor antagonists, although its long-term safety is unknown.

All patients should elevate the head of the bed, avoid troublesome foods, stop smoking, limit alcohol, and use antacids as needed. This conservative approach alone is effective in mild cases and is the backbone of all more aggressive therapies. Patients with more severe cases should additionally receive H_2 receptor antagonists (Table 97–2). Patients with refractory symptoms, who require referral for endoscopy, may benefit from omeprazole.

FOLLOW-UP.   In most patients, symptoms dramatically improve during the first 2 weeks of therapy. Therapy should continue for a total of 6 to 8 weeks, after which it is withdrawn. Although some patients relapse (up to 50% of those with severe disease), many experience no further symptoms. Anti-ulcer maintenance doses of H_2 receptor antagonists (see Section 103, Peptic Ulcer Disease) may be less effective in reflux esophagitis.

Complications of reflux esophagitis include esophageal stricture, Barrett's esophagus, and, rarely, gastrointestinal bleeding. Although antireflux therapy improves the symptoms of those with Barrett's esophagus, there is no evidence that Barrett's epithelium regresses or that the risk of cancer is reduced. Endoscopic surveillance is recommended for most patients with Barrett's esophagus, but the exact timing is controversial.

Cross-references: Diagnosis and Management of Alcoholism (Section 9), Smoking Cessation (Section 11), Chest Pain (Section 74), Dyspepsia (Section 96), Peptic Ulcer Disease (Section 103), Upper Gastrointestinal Endoscopy (Section 106).

REFERENCES

1. DiPalma JA, Prechter GC, Brady CE. X-ray-negative dysphagia: Is endoscopy necessary? J Clin Gastroenterol 1984;6:409–411.

   In 195 patients with dysphagia and prior normal barium esophagograms, endoscopy revealed normal findings in 66%, esophagitis in 27%, and miscellaneous lesions (stricture, rings, candidiasis, among others) in 7%. In no patient was cancer identified.

2. Edwards DAW. Discriminatory value of symptoms in the differential diagnosis of dysphagia. Clin Gastroenterol 1976;5:49–57.

Overview of the importance of the patient interview, based on evaluation of more than 1200 cases of dysphagia (see also J R Coll Phys 1975;9:257–263).

3. Kitchin LI, Castell DO. Rationale and efficacy of conservative therapy for gastroesophageal reflux disease. Arch Intern Med 1991;151:448–454.
    Reviews evidence supporting conservative antireflux treatments: head of bed elevation, selective food and medicine avoidance, smoking cessation, and antacids.

4. Koelz HR. Treatment of reflux esophagitis with H2-blockers, antacids and prokinetic drugs. Scand J Gastroenterol Suppl 1989;156:25–36.
    Critical review of randomized clinical trials.

5. Wesdorp ICE. Reflux oesophagitis: A review. Postgrad Med J 1986;62 (suppl 2):43–55.
    Excellent review of pathogenesis, clinical approach, and management.

98 INFLAMMATORY BOWEL DISEASE

Problem

EDWARD J. BOYKO

EPIDEMIOLOGY.   Inflammatory bowel disease (IBD) refers to three chronic gastrointestinal diseases of unknown etiology—ulcerative colitis, ulcerative proctitis, and Crohn's disease—which afflict about 1 in every 1000 persons in the United States. These diseases share a peak incidence between ages 20 and 40 years, have no clear sex predominance, and occur with a higher incidence in caucasians, Jews, and possibly residents of developed countries. Smoking may increase the risk for Crohn's disease but decrease the risk for ulcerative colitis. There is little evidence that stress and psychiatric disorders cause these diseases.

SYMPTOMS AND SIGNS.   The most common presentation of ulcerative colitis or ulcerative proctitis is bloody diarrhea. Other presenting features include fever, weight loss, or extraintestinal manifestations, including large joint arthritis, ankylosing spondylitis, erythema nodosum, pyoderma gangrenosum, iritis, thromboembolic events, and several hepatobiliary disorders.

About one-half of patients with Crohn's disease have colonic involvement and present with bloody diarrhea. Small bowel disease (about 40% of patients) leads to chronic diarrhea, weight loss, or fever. Because Crohn's disease may affect any part of the gastrointestinal tract from mouth to anus, initial symptoms may include dysphagia, oral complaints, or gastric outlet obstruction. The extraintestinal events seen in ulcerative colitis also occur with Crohn's disease except that ankylosing spondylitis and thromboembolic events are less frequent.

Several clinical features distinguish ulcerative colitis from Crohn's disease. Ulcerative colitis spares the small intestine and, in contrast to Crohn's disease, rarely causes malabsorption, bowel obstruction, or intestinal fistulas. The transmural Crohn's disease process may produce fistulas with other loops of bowel or adjoining organs such as bladder, vagina, or skin. Severe perirectal fissure, fistulas, or abscess are much more common in Crohn's disease than ulcerative colitis.

CLINICAL APPROACH.   Most patients will present with diarrhea (see Section 92). If fecal leukocytes and diarrhea persist beyond 6 weeks without an identifiable pathogen, the diagnosis of IBD is possible, and sigmoidoscopic examination should be performed. Friable, erythematous mucosa extending proximally from the rectum without interruption suggests the diagnosis of ulcerative colitis. If normal mucosa appears above the abnormal mucosa, the patient probably has ulcerative proctitis. Areas of erythema, friability, or ulceration separated by normal mucosa suggest Crohn's disease. Normal rectal mucosa excludes active ulcerative colitis but should lead to further investigation for Crohn's disease, including colonoscopy or air contrast barium enema, and an upper gastrointestinal series with small bowel follow-through (to examine the terminal ileum).

Because the initial symptoms of IBD may appear identical to those of self-limited infectious diarrhea, and because misdiagnosis of chronic disease may inflict psychological damage on patients, the clinician should refrain from diagnosing IBD until duration criteria for disease are satisfied. Although 6 weeks of diarrhea establishes the diagnosis of IBD in clinical studies, self-limited diarrhea without an identifiable pathogen may persist longer than 6 weeks, as has been reported in recent Third World travelers or in community outbreaks of chronic diarrhea linked to untreated water or unpasteurized milk. Diagnostic restraint in these settings is advised.

MANAGEMENT.   A gastroenterologist should see all patients with IBD soon after diagnosis to confirm the diagnosis, measure the extent of disease, and help plan therapy. Although primary care physicians may manage quiescent and mild disease, moderate to severe symptoms usually require continuing care by a gastroenterologist.

Mild ulcerative proctitis usually responds to hydrocortisone enemas (100 mg/ 60 ml) at bedtime for 2 to 3 weeks, followed by an every other night taper for 2 to 3 weeks. Further treatment is unnecessary for patients who respond rapidly and completely.

Patients with relapsing ulcerative proctitis or more extensive ulcerative colitis but mild symptoms should in addition receive sulfasalazine, 2 to 4 g/day in divided doses. 5-Aminosalicylic acid in an enema or rectal suppository preparation is now available to treat distal ulcerative proctitis in patients who are intolerant of sulfasalazine or hydrocortisone enemas. More severe symptoms, such as fever, weight loss, and six to eight stools per day, necessitate predni-sone, 40 mg/day for 2 to 4 weeks, followed by a slow taper. Very ill patients with ulcerative colitis require hospitalization for intensive treatment, including bowel rest and observation for the development of toxic megacolon. Anticho-linergic agents increase the risk of this life-threatening condition and are con-traindicated. Colectomy cures severe ulcerative colitis refractory to medical treatment. After resolution of acute symptoms, sulfasalazine, 2 to 4 g/day, re-duces the relapse rate. Immunosuppressive agents have not been conclusively shown to effectively treat either ulcerative colitis or Crohn's disease.

Fewer treatment options exist for Crohn's disease. Sulfasalazine, 2 to 4 g/day, effectively treats colonic Crohn's disease. Metronidazole, 20 mg/kg in divided doses, is an alternative treatment, particularly if severe perirectal dis-ease is present. Sulfasalazine does not consistently benefit Crohn's disease of the small bowel. Severe disease activity requires prednisone treatment as de-scribed above, and hospitalization if severe diarrhea (more than six to eight stools per day), brisk intestinal bleeding, bowel obstruction, signs of abdominal abscess/fistulas, or other serious condition is present. Disease unresponsive to medical therapy can be managed surgically, but recurrences are frequent. Sul-fasalazine does not reduce the relapse rate of Crohn's disease.

FOLLOW-UP.   Ulcerative proctitis progresses to pancolitis in 5% to 10% of cases after 10 years. The disease is usually more severe in the first 5 years and often "burns out" after 10 to 15 years. The risk of colon cancer is slightly higher in ulcerative proctitis and left-sided ulcerative colitis, especially if dis-ease began before age 30 years. Because pancolitis results in a 40% cumulative incidence of colon cancer after a disease duration of 35 years, patients with long-standing, extensive disease should probably be screened for colon cancer with colonoscopy and biopsy.

Crohn's disease of the small bowel leads to surgical resection in 50% of pa-tients; recurrences occur in about 40%. Colonic Crohn's disease probably in-creases the risk of acquiring colorectal carcinoma, but not to the same degree as ulcerative colitis. It is not clear whether cancer surveillance is warranted.

Cross-references: Colorectal Cancer Screening (Section 91), Diarrhea (Sec-tion 92), Abdominal Pain (Section 95), Sigmoidoscopy and Colonoscopy (Section 105), General Approach to Arthritic Symptoms (Section 107).

REFERENCES

1. Ekbom A, Helmick C, Zack M, Adami HO. Ulcerative colitis and colorectal cancer: A population based study. N Engl J Med 1990;323:1228–1233.
    The largest and most methodologically sound study of colorectal cancer risk and ulcerative colitis per-formed to date.

2. Kirsner JB, Shorter RG. Inflammatory Bowel Disease, 3rd ed. Lea & Febiger, Philadelphia, 1988.
    A comprehensive and up-to-date textbook covering all aspects of inflammatory bowel disease, includ-ing epidemiology, etiology, clinical course, medical and surgical treatment, and psychosocial issues.

3. Peppercorn MA. Advances in drug therapy for inflammatory bowel disease. Ann Intern Med 1990;112:50–60.

Treatments for inflammatory bowel disease changed very little from the 1940s until very recently. This article reviews the efficacy of old and new treatments for these chronic disorders.

99 BILIARY TRACT DISEASE

Problem

ANDREW K. DIEHL

EPIDEMIOLOGY.   Gallstones occur in 5% to 15% of white women under age 50 and in 25% of older women. For men, prevalences range from 4% to 10% for those less than 50 years old and 10% to 15% thereafter. Hispanics of Mexican origin have rates approximately twice those of other whites, but blacks have a lower prevalence. Almost 90% of gallstone patients have cholesterol or mixed composition stones, with the remainder having pigment stones. The most important risk factors are advancing age and female sex. Obesity, upper body fat distribution, childbearing, parental history of stones, diabetes, exogenous estrogens, and rapid weight loss increase the risk of gallstone development. Moderate alcohol intake is associated with a lower risk. The role of diet in gallstone formation is unsettled.

Choledocholithiasis occurs most commonly in older patients with gallbladder stones. Gallbladder cancer is strongly associated with gallstones. Patients with gallstones 30 mm in diameter or larger have a tenfold risk of cancer.

SYMPTOMS AND SIGNS.   Half of patients with gallstones are unaware of their presence. The symptom most closely linked to stones is severe epigastric or right upper quadrant pain (biliary colic), which characteristically persists 30 minutes to several hours before resolving gradually over 24 hours. It is usually steady in intensity (rather than fluctuating), and radiates to the upper back in a minority of patients. The pain may follow meals, most typically after more than 1 hour, and is often accompanied by nausea. However, fatty food intolerance, bloating, belching, and heartburn are no more common in those with gallstones than in normal subjects. Physical examination during a pain attack may reveal local abdominal tenderness. Those with lower abdominal symptoms or signs are significantly less likely to have gallstones.

Acute cholecystitis is defined by prolonged biliary pain accompanied by fever, leukocytosis, or guarding on physical examination. Vomiting is commonly reported. Those with choledocholithiasis may also develop jaundice. Gall-stones are a common cause of acute pancreatitis. Stones may also erode into the small intestine, resulting in fistula formation and gallstone ileus. Gallbladder cancer presents insidiously with abdominal pain, weight loss, and jaundice.

The symptoms and signs of biliary tract disease are nonspecific, and it is hazardous to base a diagnosis on the clinical assessment alone. Imaging studies are required to confirm the diagnosis.

CLINICAL APPROACH.   Patients whose presentation suggests biliary tract disease should first undergo gallbladder ultrasound. This study, which requires that the patient be fasting, has a sensitivity for gallstones of 90% to 95% and a specificity of 94% to 98%. Stones as small as 3 mm in diameter can be detected. Oral cholecystography has comparable sensitivity and specificity but requires more time and patient preparation and yields many more inconclusive results. Plain abdominal radiographs occasionally suggest pigment stones but rarely establish a diagnosis. Liver chemistry tests are of no value in distinguishing gallstone-related conditions from other diagnoses.

Patients with severe abdominal pain and fever may have acute cholecystitis. Physical examination may reveal guarding in the right upper quadrant and Murphy's sign (tenderness in the area of the gallbladder that halts the patient's inspiration, found in 27%). Leukocytosis is often observed. Ultrasound can demonstrate gallstones and gallbladder wall thickening, as well as the "sonographic Murphy's sign" (tenderness over the gallbladder elicited by the ultrasonic transducer). Indeterminate evaluations should be followed by technetium-99m iminodiacetic acid scans (e.g., DISIDA), which have a sensitivity of 95% to 97% and a specificity of 90% to 97% for acute cholecystitis.

Patients thought to have common duct stones generally should undergo endoscopic retrograde cholangiopancreatography (ERCP) or percutaneous transhepatic cholangiography (PTC), as ultrasound is insensitive in this situation. Gallbladder cancer can be detected by ultrasound, but only in late stages, when it is incurable. However, patients with calcification of the gallbladder wall on plain radiography ("porcelain gallbladder") are at increased risk for cancer.

Oral cholecystography is required before consideration of most nonsurgical treatments because it provides more accurate information on physiologic function, stone number, and stone dimensions than does ultrasound.

MANAGEMENT.   Patients found to have asymptomatic gallstones may be observed, as less than half will develop clear symptoms within 20 years of diagnosis, and even fewer will present with complications. Gallstone patients with diabetes should be considered for treatment even in the absence of symptoms, although close observation is an acceptable alternative. Patients with definite symptoms should be treated, as their risks for further symptoms and complications outweigh the risks of surgery. Cholecystectomy remains the treatment of choice because of its high success rate and low mortality. It is likely that the recently introduced laparoscopic approach will become the standard because of its lower morbidity.

Nonsurgical approaches, although disappointing, are indicated for symptomatic patients at high risk for surgery. Oral dissolution therapy with ursodiol can be attempted for those with radiolucent stones less than 20 mm in diameter, but complete dissolution occurs in only 20% to 30% within 2 years. Gallstone lithotripsy is most successful in those with a solitary radiolucent stone less than 20 mm in diameter but complete dissolution occurs in only 35% after 6 months. Percutaneous gallbladder lavage with methyl *tert*-butyl ether is still experimental. Both lithotripsy and ether treatments require subsequent treatment with ursodiol until dissolution of the stones is complete. Nonsurgical treatments are indicated for symptomatic patients who are at high risk for surgery.

FOLLOW-UP.   Patients who have successfully undergone cholecystectomy do not require long-term follow-up and may eat a normal diet. After nonsurgical treatments, gallstones recur at a rate of 10% annually, less often in those with small solitary stones. Although ursodiol or aspirin may prevent recurrent stones in such patients, most recurrences will respond to repeat dissolution therapy.

Cross-references: Jaundice (Section 93), Abdominal Pain (Section 95).

REFERENCES

1. Diehl AK. Epidemiology and natural history of gallstones. Gastroenterol Clin North Am 1991;20:1–19.
    Comprehensive review of prevalence, risk factors, time trends, and possibilities for preventive interventions.

2. Diehl AK, Sugarek NJ, Todd KH. Clinical evaluation for gallstone disease: Usefulness of symptoms and signs in diagnosis. Am J Med 1990;89:29–33.
    Prospective study comparing symptoms and signs in patients found to have gallstones with those in contemporaneous patients found to be gallstone-free.

3. Marton KI, Doubilet P. How to image the gallbladder in suspected cholecystitis. Ann Intern Med 1988;109:722–729.
    Comprehensive and critical review of available diagnostic tests for gallbladder disease.

4. Way LW. Changing therapy for gallstone disease. N Engl J Med 1990;323:1273–1274.
    Editorial accompanying paper reporting the disappointing results of gallstone lithotripsy; reviews the present options for gallstone treatment, including laparoscopic cholecystectomy.

100 CIRRHOSIS AND CHRONIC LIVER FAILURE

Problem

JOHN S. HALSEY

EPIDEMIOLOGY. Cirrhosis may result from many different chronic liver diseases that destroy liver parenchyma and replace it with scars and nodules. In the United States, alcohol toxicity and viral hepatitis are the most common causes.

SYMPTOMS AND SIGNS. Fatigue is often the major complaint in uncomplicated cirrhosis. Physical examination may reveal an enlarged firm liver, although a nonpalpable shrunken and hard liver is common late in the disease. Palmar erythema, Dupuytren's contracture, spider angiomas, lack of axillary or pectoral hair, and signs of portal hypertension (e.g., splenomegaly, ascites, and prominent superficial veins of the abdominal wall) may be present. Somnolence, defiant behavior, or mild confusion suggest early encephalopathy.

CLINICAL APPROACH. The clinician should always attempt to identify the specific cause, because specific therapy is available for several of the diseases that produce cirrhosis. Section 93 reviews the diagnostic approach to patients with abnormal liver function tests.

MANAGEMENT. With appropriate management, patients with cirrhosis remain comfortable and active for prolonged periods. The cardinal objective is to prevent further liver injury. Patients with alcohol-related cirrhosis who stop drinking have a significantly better 5-year survival rate than those who continue to drink. Toxin- or drug-induced cirrhosis also may improve after removal of the offending agent. In all cases, adequate caloric intake of 2000 to 3000 kcal/day should be maintained, potentially hepatotoxic agents should be avoided, and the use of tranquilizers and sedatives should be minimized. The patient should be carefully monitored for early signs of complications (e.g., encephalopathy, spontaneous bacterial peritonitis, gastrointestinal bleeding, ascites). Often, daily home monitoring by family members will give warning of impending deterioration.

Patients with new-onset **ascites** should undergo diagnostic ultrasound (to confirm ascites, identify hepatic masses, and detect portal vein thrombosis) and abdominocentesis (to exclude infection or malignancy). Treatment of ascites is indicated only when it causes patient discomfort or affects respiratory mechanics. Initial management should include withdrawal of offending agents (e.g., alcohol) and adequate dietary protein intake. If these measures are insufficient, the clinician should prescribe a 1 to 2 g sodium diet while monitoring serum

305

sodium and potassium levels and restricting water intake to 1.5 liters/day if hyponatremia ensues.

If ascites persists despite adequate sodium restriction, diuretic therapy may be initiated, beginning with spironolactone (50 mg PO b.i.d.). Its onset of action may be delayed for 2 to 3 days, with maximum diuresis sometimes not observed for 2 to 3 weeks. Spironolactone should be increased until the urinary sodium concentration is twice the urinary potassium concentration. Furosemide provides additional diuresis, but at the risk of volume depletion and hepatorenal syndrome. Patients without edema should lose no more than 1 pound per day. All patients require frequent monitoring of postural blood pressure, weight, and serum electrolytes. Responsible patients may learn to direct their own diuretic schedule by monitoring their weight daily at home.

Ascites that is refractory to dietary and diuretic therapy may respond to repeated large volume paracentesis performed in the clinic. Peritoneovenous shunts, once popular, have not been shown to improve survival when compared with conventional therapy; they also increase the risks of infection and coagulopathy.

Spontaneous bacterial peritonitis, which occurs in roughly 10% of patients, should be considered whenever a patient with cirrhosis deteriorates unexplainably (e.g., worsening encephalopathy, increased liver failure, fever, or abdominal pain). Diagnostic abdominocentesis demonstrating over 250 polymorphonuclear leukocytes/mm^3 should be considered positive and prompt hospital admission for administration of parenteral antibiotics.

Portosystemic encephalopathy is a reversible metabolic cerebral dysfunction that results from inability of the liver to remove various neurotoxins or to synthesize certain protective substances. Encephalopathy is often precipitated by gastrointestinal bleeding, fever, infection, increased dietary protein intake, diuresis-related hyponatremia or hypokalemia, or injudicious use of sedatives.

Therapy for encephalopathy includes limiting dietary protein to less than 50 g/day, maintaining standard caloric intake with fat and carbohydrate, and giving the nonabsorbable disaccharide lactulose. The dose of lactulose prescribed should induce two or three loose bowel movements per day (usually 60–120 mg/day), though patient compliance often improves if patients are allowed to choose their own dose based on stool frequency and mental status. Neomycin (2–6 g PO q.d.) is a second-line agent, owing to concerns about renal and neurotoxicity.

Clinically significant **upper gastrointestinal hemorrhage** requires endoscopy. In about 60% of patients, the source of acute bleeding is esophageal varices, with other sources (e.g., peptic ulcer disease, Mallory-Weiss tear) accounting for the remaining 40%. Direct injection of a sclerosing agent into the varices is often effective for the immediate control of variceal bleeding and may be repeated periodically to prevent recurrent bleeding. Varices that have not bled do not require sclerotherapy. Treatment with propranolol, in a dose sufficient to reduce the resting pulse about 25%, appears to decrease bleeding episodes and fatal hemorrhage, although the survival benefit is meager.[2]

Orthotopic liver transplantation is an option in patients with irreversible chronic liver disease, especially those with primary biliary cirrhosis, sclerosing cholangitis, toxin-induced injury, and some patients with chronic viral hepatitis. Ideally, candidates should be evaluated at a transplant center before they become seriously ill.

Cross-references: Diagnosis and Management of Alcoholism (Section 9), Upper Gastrointestinal Endoscopy (Section 106).

REFERENCES

1. Kellerman PS, Linas SL. Large volume paracentesis of ascites. Ann Intern Med 1990;112:889–891.
   Editorial summarizing current thought on the subject.

2. Poynard T, Calès P, Pasta L, Ideo G, Pascal JP, et al. Beta-adrenergic-antagonist drugs in the prevention of gastrointestinal bleeding in patients with cirrhosis and esophageal varices: An analysis of data and prognostic factors in 589 patients from four randomized clinical trials. N Engl J Med 1991;324:1532–1538.
   Propranolol and nadolol effectively prevented first bleeding and reduced the mortality from gastrointestinal bleeding, independent of the cause and severity of cirrhosis.

3. Stanley MM, et al. Peritoneovenous shunting as compared with medical treatment in patients with alcoholic cirrhosis and massive ascites. N Engl J Med 1989;321:1632–1638.
   Report of a Veterans Administration cooperative study.

101 VIRAL HEPATITIS

Problem

JOHN S. HALSEY

EPIDEMIOLOGY/ETIOLOGY.   Viral hepatitis is a systemic illness that causes hepatic inflammation and hepatic cell necrosis. Besides the hepatitis viruses listed in Table 101–1, other less common causes are Epstein-Barr virus, CMV, and herpesvirus.

In the United States, hepatitis A virus (HAV) accounts for about 25% of clinically apparent cases of acute viral hepatitis and a larger number of subclinical infections. By age 50, 70% of U.S. adults have contracted hepatitis A and are immune.

Groups at risk for hepatitis B and hepatitis delta infection are IV drug abusers, hemophiliacs, hemodialysis patients, and homosexual men. Because the

TABLE 101–1. CLINICAL FEATURES OF VIRAL HEPATITIS INFECTION

	Hepatitis A Virus	Hepatitis B Virus	Hepatitis Delta Virus	Hepatitis C Virus	Enteric Non-A, Non-B Hepatitis
Genome	RNA	DNA	RNA	RNA	Unknown
Mean incubation time	25 days	75 days	35 days	50 days	27 days
Transmission mode	Fecal-oral, sexual	Parenteral, sexual	Parenteral in U.S., sexual	Parenteral	Fecal-oral
Acute mortality	0.1%–0.2%	0.2%–1.0%	1%–20%	0.2%–1.0%	1%–2%
Risk of chronicity	None	1%–10%	1%–80%	50%	None
Risk of hepatocellular carcinoma	No	Yes	Unknown	Yes	No

hepatitis delta virus requires the presence of hepatitis B virus (HBV) to replicate, it occurs only as a coinfection with acute HBV hepatitis or as a superinfection in chronic carriers of HBV.

In the United States, hepatitis C accounts for 40% to 50% of hepatitis in IV drug abusers and 80% to 90% of cases of posttransfusion hepatitis.

Enteric non-A, non-B hepatitis (tentatively termed hepatitis E) is epidemically transmitted by the fecal-oral route. Although the specific virus has not been identified, accumulating evidence suggests an RNA virus similar to HAV. Pregnant individuals with enteric non-A, non-B hepatitis are at risk for a fulminant course and death.

SYMPTOMS AND SIGNS. The course of acute viral hepatitis varies from an asymptomatic disorder to fulminant hepatic necrosis and death. Patients classically present with acute malaise, fever, anorexia, and nausea, soon followed by poorly localized or right upper quadrant abdominal discomfort. Jaundice, itching, dark-colored urine, and light-colored stools declare the icteric phase. Systemic symptoms may already be improving by the time jaundice appears.

Table 101–1 lists the other important clinical features. Fulminant hepatitis is unusual in HAV infection; even when it occurs, complete recovery is common. HBV infection is subclinical in two-thirds of cases. Some patients with HBV infection have findings due to circulating antigen-antibody complexes (rash, neuralgia, arthralgia, arthritis, and vasculitis) before jaundice appears. Although acute HBV infection usually completely resolves, about 10% of patients will develop chronic hepatitis or the asymptomatic carrier state. Some 10% to 30% of individuals with chronic HBV infection eventually develop cirrhosis. Both chronic HBV infection and the asymptomatic carrier state increase the risk of hepatocellular carcinoma.

In general, acute hepatitis delta infection causes a more severe illness than other hepatitis viruses. Chronic infection develops in 5% of patients who are infected simultaneously with hepatitis delta virus and HBV, and in most chronic HBV carriers following superinfection of hepatitis delta. Eighty percent of those with chronic hepatitis delta infection eventually develop cirrhosis.

Acute hepatitis C infection is usually anicteric and rarely fulminant, but at least 50% of patients develop chronic hepatitis. Cirrhosis eventually occurs in 20%.

CLINICAL APPROACH. Symptoms and signs are not specific for a viral etiology or a particular virus; serologic evaluation is required to make these distinctions (Table 101–2). The patient's history, which focuses on previous travel, parenteral drug abuse, known exposure, or other risk factors, should guide the choice of studies. As many as 10% of individuals with acute HBV infection have a negative hepatitis B surface antigen (HBsAg) and negative IgM anti-HBs serology ("window" between the clearance of HBsAg and appearance of anti-HBs antibody), but positive IgM anti-hepatitis B core (HBc) assays.

HCV infection is confirmed by demonstrating the presence of antibody to an antigenic component of HCV. Unlike HAV, this antibody does not confer im-

TABLE 101–2. SEROLOGIC PATTERNS IN ACUTE VIRAL HEPATITIS

Anti-HAV Total	Anti-HAV IgM¹	HBsAG	Anti-HBc Total	Anti-HBc IgM	Anti-HBs	Anti-HD	Interpretation
+	+	–	–	–	–	–	Acute hepatitis A
–	–	+	+	+	–	–	Acute hepatitis B
+	–	+	+	+	–	–	Acute hepatitis B, prior hepatitis A
+	+	–	+	–	+	–	Acute hepatitis A, prior hepatitis B
–	–	–	+	–	+	–	Prior hepatitis B
–	–	+	+	–	–	–	Chronic hepatitis B
–	–	+	+	–	–	+	Hepatitis delta superinfection (chronic HBV, acute delta)
–	–	+	+	+	–	+	Acute hepatitis B and delta coinfection (acute HBV and acute delta)
–	–	–	–	–	+	–	Hepatitis B immunization

¹Persists 3–6 months after acute infection.

munity and may in fact be present only during active viral replication. Because serologic conversion occurs approximately 5 months after onset of the infection, testing during the acute phase often produces false-negative results. A positive assay does not differentiate between chronic and acute disease.

No specific serologic assay is available for epidemic non-A, non-B hepatitis.

The differential diagnosis of acute hepatitis includes drug reactions, alcohol use, and ischemic liver injury (see Section 93, Jaundice). Confusing cases may require consultation with a gastroenterologist.

MANAGEMENT. There is no definitive therapy for acute viral hepatitis. The initial management is supportive, usually occurring in the outpatient setting. Patients should receive good nutrition without protein restriction and should avoid alcohol and other hepatotoxins. Strict bed rest is unnecessary, though patients may choose to limit their activity based on their symptoms. Nausea and vomiting may respond to prochlorperazine (5–10 mg PO t.i.d. or q.i.d.), but the clinician should be alert for the potential of drug-induced cholestasis. Pruritus may respond to antihistamines or cholestyramine (see Section 93, Jaundice). Abdominal pain from stretching of the hepatic capsule may require narcotic analgesia, using the minimal dose to avoid portal-systemic encephalopathy.

Fulminant viral hepatitis occurs rarely but is associated with a mortality of 70% to 80%. Altered mentation is the initial sign and its appearance requires immediate attention by physicians experienced in managing fulminant hepatic failure. Orthotopic liver transplantation may be lifesaving.

FOLLOW-UP. Patients with acute HAV infection need no specific follow-up after their symptoms resolve. Follow-up of patients with acute hepatitis B, C, or delta virus infection is mandatory, owing to the possibility of chronicity following the initial infection. Patients with any of these acute infections should be seen at 1- to 2-month intervals during the first 6 months to document that the serum transaminase levels return to normal. In patients with HBV infection, clinicians should monitor serial HBsAg and anti-HBsAg titers until anti-HBsAg antibody is present. Persistence of symptoms, prolonged elevations of HBsAg, serum transaminases, or bilirubin, or an elevated prothrombin time are all indications for referral to a specialist.

Cross-references: Diagnosis and Management of Drug Abuse (Section 8), Jaundice (Section 93), Abdominal Pain (Section 95), Cirrhosis and Chronic Liver Failure (Section 100).

REFERENCES

1. Centers for Disease Control. Protection against viral hepatitis. MMWR 1990;39(S-2):1–26.
   Recommendations for protection against viral hepatitis. Reviews the use of hepatitis B vaccine, hepatitis B immune globulin, and gamma-globulin.

2. Hollinger FB. Serologic evaluation of viral hepatitis. Hosp Pract 1987;22(2):101–114.
   Step-by-step details, including an algorithm.

3. Hoofnagle JH. Type D (delta) hepatitis. JAMA 1990;261:1321–1325.
    Comprehensive review from grand rounds at the Clinical Center of the National Institutes of Health.
4. Zuckerman AJ, Ed. Viral hepatitis. Br Med Bull 1990;46:301–564.
    A series of expert reviews.

102 DIVERTICULITIS

Problem

ROBERT G. HOLMAN
HUBERT N. RADKE

EPIDEMIOLOGY.   Diverticulitis results from obstruction and inflammation of a colonic diverticulum. Most colonic diverticula develop as people age; in the United States, 50% to 67% of people have diverticula by 80 years of age. Ninety-five percent of patients with diverticulosis have involvement of the sigmoid colon either alone or as part of a more diffuse process. About 20% to 30% of people with diverticula develop diverticulitis during their lifetime.

SYMPTOMS AND SIGNS.   Initial symptoms may be mild and nonspecific and include abdominal pain, chronic constipation, or, less frequently, diarrhea. Progressive signs of localized peritonitis such as left lower quadrant abdominal pain, tenderness, guarding, and mass may develop. Fever and/or leukocytosis occur in only two-thirds of patients. Extension of the infection (chronic inflammatory process) to pericolic tissues produces a variety of complications that include diffuse peritonitis after free perforation, abscess formation, obstruction, and fistula formation between the colon and the bladder, other segments of bowel, skin, or uterus. Sepsis with multiple organ failure, abdominal distention, pyuria, or pneumaturia may appear in severe episodes. Gross colonic bleeding is not a common complication of diverticulitis and occurs much more often in patients with diverticula that are not inflamed.

CLINICAL APPROACH.   After examination of the chest, abdomen, pelvis, and rectum, routine laboratory studies should include a WBC count, urinalysis, and abdominal and upright chest radiography (upright position to detect pneumoperitoneum). Radiography may be omitted when the history, physical examination, and laboratory data suggest only mild inflammation. The differential diagnosis, depending on the severity of the patient's symptoms, includes acute constipation, urinary tract infection, colon cancer, inflammatory bowel disease, ischemic colitis, and hollow viscus perforation. Barium enema is useful for detecting mucosal disease, inflammatory bowel disease, cancer, ischemia, and luminal distortion (obstruction), while computed tomography (CT) better defines extraluminal extension of disease. Because neither study is clearly superior, the choice is usually based on the resources available. Barium enema examination is contraindicated if a free or poorly contained perforation is likely. Ultrasound may be helpful but is extremely operator dependent and its precise role is yet to be defined. Endoscopy has little utility.

The recommended evaluation depends on whether the patient's symptoms and signs reflect mild, moderate, or severe diverticulitis. In **mild** cases, left lower quadrant pain, mild tenderness, and a change in bowel habits are the only findings. There are no peritoneal signs (e.g., guarding, rebound tenderness) and no signs of systemic response (e.g., fever, leukocytosis). In these patients, definitive radiologic diagnosis (barium enema examination or abdominal CT) is not urgent but should be performed within 1 to 2 weeks to document the presence of diverticulitis and to exclude other diseases from the differential diagnosis such as carcinoma. Tests delayed beyond this period may fail to reveal the characteristic abnormalities of diverticulitis. In **moderate** cases, patients have significant abdominal pain and tenderness with varying degrees of fever and leukocytosis; surgical consultation should be obtained to assist in initial assessment and planning of the appropriate timing of radiologic evaluation. In **severe** cases, the symptoms and signs suggest complicated disease; findings include peritoneal signs, mass, intestinal obstruction, sepsis, pyuria, and pneumaturia. Hospital admission and early surgical consultation are imperative. Because they have a very high complication rate, men less than 45 years old, diabetics and immunocompromised patients require an aggressive approach with early surgical consultation.

MANAGEMENT. In mild cases, therapy includes oral fiber supplementation (a low-fiber diet is thought to be important in the development of diverticulosis and diverticulitis) and mild analgesics such as acetaminophen or ibuprofen (narcotics, especially morphine, are contraindicated). Antibiotics to cover both aerobic and anaerobic gram-negative enteric pathogens are often prescribed, although no available data support their use in mild diverticulitis (in contrast to the good evidence for antibiotic use in moderate and severe diverticulitis) (Table 102–1). If the patient is reliable and can be followed closely, outpatient therapy is satisfactory in mild cases.

All patients with moderate and severe disease require hospital admission for observation, surgical consultation, bowel rest, parenteral antibiotics, and hydration. Because no immediately available and simple diagnostic test exists that reliably confirms diverticulitis and excludes other life-threatening diseases in the differential diagnosis, in-patient observation is important. Severe cases may additionally require intensive monitoring and early consideration of surgical or percutaneous treatment of infection. When possible, it is preferable to

TABLE 102–1. ANTIBIOTIC THERAPY FOR DIVERTICULITIS[1]

Diverticulitis Severity	Antimicrobial Agent	Administration	Cost ($)[2]
Mild	Clindamycin	300 mg PO q.8h. × 7–10 d	57.60
	+	+	
	TMP-SMX (DS)[3]	1 tab PO q.12h. × 7–10 d	6.00
	or	or	
	Metronidazole	500 mg PO q.6–8h. × 7–10 d	4.00
	+	+	
	Cefaclor	250 mg PO q.8h. × 7–10 d	48.30
Moderate or Severe	Inpatient parenteral antibiotics to cover aerobic gram-negative rods and anaerobes		

[1]The choice of therapy in any individual patient must be guided by specific clinical factors. There are no data supporting or refuting the use of antibiotics in mild diverticulitis.
[2]Average wholesale price, 1991 *Drug Topics Red Book* (for 10 days).
[3]TMP-SMX (DS) = trimethoprim-sulfamethoxazole, double strength.

initially stabilize the patient and perform colonic resection days to weeks after the acute episode to avoid a temporary colostomy.

FOLLOW-UP. Diverticulitis is usually self-limited and results in complete recovery. Although dietary fiber therapy is often prescribed to maintain one or more soft, bulky stools per day, data supporting a decreased incidence of diverticulitis are lacking (other than the epidemiologic data that associate diverticuli with cultures eating low-fiber food).

Only 25% of patients will have a second attack of diverticulitis. Moderate or severe diverticulitis that is recurrent or that occurs in men under 45 years of age, diabetics, or patients with immunodeficiencies is an indication for colonic resection because of the high complication and recurrence rates in these groups.

Cross-references: Constipation (Section 94), Abdominal Pain (Section 95).

REFERENCES

1. Hackford AW, Veidenheimer MC. Diverticular disease of the colon: Current concepts and management. Surg Clin North Am 1985;65:347–363.
   A review of diverticular disease, including diverticulitis, with particular emphasis on surgical indications and options.

2. Pohlman T. Diverticulitis. Gastroenterol Clin North Am 1988;17:357–385.
   Emphasizes the complications and medical treatment of diverticulitis.

3. Rodkey GV, Welch CE. Changing patterns in the surgical treatment of diverticular disease. Ann Surg 1984;200:466–478.
   Discusses changing epidemiology of diverticulitis requiring hospitalization, compares various surgical options for treatment, and describes indications for surgery.

4. Smith TR, Cho KC, Morehouse HT, Kratka PS. Comparison of computed tomography and contrast enema evaluation of diverticulitis. Dis Colon Rectum 1990;33:1–6.
   Authors favored barium enema; other studies (cited in references) favored computed tomography. Differences may be largely based on the local availability and quality of the examination.

103 PEPTIC ULCER DISEASE

Problem

MICHAEL B. KIMMEY

EPIDEMIOLOGY. The lifetime prevalence of peptic ulcer is approximately 10%; at any one time between 1% and 2% of adults have an ulcer. Although ulcer disease used to be more frequent in men, and duodenal ulcers more common than gastric ulcers, the prevalence of gastric and duodenal ulcers is now approximately equal, with little sex difference. The most important risk factors are cigarette smoking and the consumption of nonsteroidal anti-inflammatory drugs (NSAIDs). Glucocorticoid therapy may increase the risk of gastric ulcer development slightly. Increased use of NSAIDs among the elderly has led to more ulcers and ulcer complications. Although *Helicobacter pylori* has been associated with both gastric and duodenal ulcers, whether this organism is truly causative is unknown.

SYMPTOMS AND SIGNS. Although many patients are asymptomatic, the cardinal symptom of ulcer disease is epigastric pain. Duodenal ulcer pain typically occurs 1 to 2 hours after a meal and during the night, and is relieved by antacids or food. Gastric ulcer pain is also felt in the epigastrium but is less clearly related to meals and is not always relieved by antacids. Ulcers associated with NSAID consumption are frequently painless. Although some patients with ulcers have nausea and vomiting, this may reflect the complication of gastric outlet obstruction. Epigastric tenderness has no predictive value for the diagnosis of peptic ulcer.

CLINICAL APPROACH. The clinician must first determine whether the patient has an ulcer complication, such as gastric outlet obstruction, acute or chronic GI bleeding, weight loss, or unusually severe or prolonged pain. Patients with suspected complications from ulcers should undergo immediate diagnostic evaluation with either upper GI radiography or upper endoscopy. If no complications are present, an empiric 2-week trial of oral H_2 receptor antagonist therapy is indicated. If the pain completely resolves within 2 weeks and there are no other signs of complications, a 6-week course of these drugs is appropriate; further diagnostic workup is unnecessary. If ulcer pain does not resolve after 2 weeks of H_2 receptor antagonist therapy, diagnostic tests are indicated (see Section 96, Dyspepsia).

The decision whether to perform upper GI radiography or upper endoscopy to diagnose an ulcer should be individualized. An upper GI series costs about half as much as upper endoscopy and is more readily available to the primary care physician. The sensitivity of endoscopy in detecting superficial ulcers is greater than that of upper GI radiography. However, high-quality air contrast barium radiographs reveal over 90% of chronic gastric and duodenal ulcers. Endoscopy is preferred in patients with GI bleeding, because barium will confound further attempts at endoscopic or angiographic therapy. If an upper GI series demonstrates a gastric ulcer with radiographic signs suspicious for malignancy, the patient should be referred for endoscopy and biopsy. Endoscopy is also preferred in patients who have a history of ulcers or prior gastric surgery.

A serum gastrin level is a good screening test for the presence of gastrinoma, a neoplastic condition that results in acid hypersecretion. The gastrin level should be checked when duodenal ulcers are multiple, are recurrent, are found distal to the duodenal bulb, recur after ulcer surgery, or resist standard treatment.

MANAGEMENT. The advent of specific drug therapy that promotes ulcer healing has limited the roles for diet, life-style changes, and surgery in management. There is little evidence that specific dietary components, including caffeinated beverages, dairy products, and fiber, affect ulcer healing.

Even with anti-ulcer medications, cigarette smoking impairs ulcer healing. Smoking also favors an earlier recurrence after the ulcer has healed and anti-ulcer therapy is stopped. Even if smoking cannot be stopped, reducing cigarette consumption to less than ten cigarettes per day will benefit ulcer healing. Because NSAIDs impair healing of gastric but not duodenal ulcers, they should be stopped if possible during treatment of gastric ulcers.

Most gastric and duodenal ulcers respond to either antacids or H_2 receptor antagonists. H_2 receptor antagonists are favored over antacids because they can be given once a day with fewer side effects. The choice among the various H_2 receptor antagonists depends primarily on cost, because they are all equally efficacious and have similar side effects (Table 103–1). One exception is pa-

TABLE 103–1. STANDARD ANTI-ULCER REGIMENS

Drug	Regimen	Cost ($) per Day[1]	Cost ($) per 6 Weeks[1]
Mylanta II	30 ml q.i.d.	2.31	97.02
Maalox	30 ml q.i.d.	1.37	57.54
Riopan	30 ml q.i.d.	1.22	51.24
Cimetidine	800 mg h.s.	2.40	100.80
	400 mg b.i.d.	2.40	100.80
Ranitidine	300 mg h.s.	2.80	117.60
	150 mg b.i.d.	2.80	117.60
Nizatidine	300 mg h.s.	2.14	89.88
	150 mg b.i.d.	2.14	89.88
Famotidine	40 mg h.s.	2.44	102.48
	20 mg b.i.d.	2.44	102.48
Sucralfate	1 g q.i.d.	2.32	97.44
Misoprostol	200 µg q.i.d.	2.40	100.80
Omeprazole	20 mg q.d.	3.21	134.82

[1]Average wholesale price, 1991 *Drug Topics Red Book.*

tients who are also taking theophylline, warfarin, or phenytoin; famotidine is then preferred over other H_2 receptor antagonists because it is less likely to inhibit hepatic drug metabolism.

Patients with duodenal ulcers may be treated with a single dose of an H_2 receptor antagonist at bedtime. Because gastric ulcers are more difficult to heal, twice daily therapy with the H_2 receptor blockers may offer a slight therapeutic advantage. Sucralfate is as effective as H_2 receptor antagonists in treating duodenal ulcers but is less effective in treating gastric ulcers. Although misoprostol may heal gastric ulcers when NSAIDs are continued, significant diarrhea and abdominal cramping has limited its clinical usefulness. Omeprazole is useful for treating refractory ulcers and for treating gastric ulcers when NSAIDs must be continued, but has the disadvantages of being more expensive and relatively new with unknown long-term side effects. Sucralfate is not effective in healing gastric ulcers when NSAIDs are continued.

FOLLOW-UP.   Pain in most patients resolves within 1 week of beginning therapy with antacids or H_2 receptor antagonists. Nevertheless, these treatments should be continued for a total of 6 to 8 weeks to assure ulcer healing. Patients with duodenal ulcers need no documentation of ulcer healing. Patients with gastric ulcers should have follow-up endoscopic documentation of healing after 8 weeks of therapy, because of the 3% risk of gastric cancer masquerading as a benign gastric ulcer.

Candidates for maintenance therapy to prevent ulcer recurrence include patients with complications such as hemorrhage or perforation, those with more than two recurrences per year, cigarette smokers, and those with significant medical illnesses such that an ulcer recurrence or complication might be life-threatening. The best studied agents for maintenance therapy are the H_2 receptor antagonists, given as half the acute healing dose at night (cimetidine, 400 mg; ranitidine, 150 mg; nizatidine, 150 mg; famotidine, 20 mg). The optimum duration of maintenance therapy is unknown and should be individualized; some high-risk patients may need lifelong treatment.

Patients with ulcer complications such as upper GI hemorrhage or perforation should be hospitalized. Perforation is managed surgically by oversewing the ulcer. Hemorrhage can usually be managed with endoscopic injection or coagulation therapy. Although infrequently necessary, some patients with intractable pain, failed healing, or gastric outlet obstruction may require surgical treatment with selective vagotomy or gastric resection.

Cross-references: Smoking Cessation (Section 11), Abdominal Pain (Section 95), Dyspepsia (Section 96), Upper Gastrointestinal Endoscopy (Section 106).

REFERENCES

1. Feldman M, Burton ME. Histamine2-receptor antagonists: Standard therapy for acid-peptic diseases. N Engl J Med 1990;323:1672–1680, 1749–1755.
    Comprehensive review of the H_2 receptor antagonists.

2. Freston JW. Overview of medical therapy of peptic ulcer disease. In Hunt RH, Ed. Peptic Ulcer Disease. Gastroenterol Clin North Am 1990;19:121–140.

    Comprehensive review of the medical treatment of ulcer disease.

3. Peterson WL. *Helicobacter pylori* and peptic ulcer disease. N Engl J Med 1991;324:1043–1048.

    This spiral-shaped bacterium causes gastritis and may contribute to the pathogenesis of ulcer disease and ulcer recurrence, but is not the sole cause of ulcers.

4. Walan A, Bodey JP, Classen M, et al. Effects of omeprazole and ranitidine on ulcer healing and relapse rates in patients with benign gastric ulcer. N Engl J Med 1989;320:69–75.

    Omeprazole heals gastric ulcers more rapidly than ranitidine, even when NSAIDs are continued during treatment.

104 HEMORRHOIDS AND FISSURES

Problem

STEVEN R. McGEE

EPIDEMIOLOGY.   In the United States, the prevalence of hemorrhoids is 4.4%, though only one-third of affected patients seek medical attention. Hemorrhoids affect whites more than blacks, are rare below the age of 20 years, have a peak incidence between ages 45 and 65 years, and diminish in frequency after age 65 years. Despite traditional teachings, hemorrhoids are not more prevalent in patients with portal hypertension.

Anal fissures, common in middle-aged patients, are the most common cause of anal pain.

SYMPTOMS AND SIGNS.   **Hemorrhoids** consist of anatomically normal vascular anal cushions, oriented in the left lateral, right anterior, and right posterior position, that have lost their fibromuscular support and become trapped by the anal sphincter in the prolapsed position. Common symptoms include bright red bleeding after defecation (85%–90%), prolapse (40%–60%), anal discomfort (15%–50%), and pruritus (20%–50%). Severe pain is uncommon and suggests thrombosed external hemorrhoids, which appear as tender blue swellings at the anal verge and usually occur after strenuous effort such as heavy lifting. Hemorrhoids are traditionally classified both by stage (stage 1, no prolapse; stage 2, prolapse reducing spontaneously; stage 3, prolapse requiring manual reduction; stage 4, irreducible prolapse) and whether they are external or internal (depending on whether the involved tissue is below or above the dentate line). This classification has limited value, however, because most symptomatic hemorrhoids involve both internal and external tissues and move between different stages over hours or days.

Fissures cause acute severe anal pain, sometimes accompanied by bright red blood, immediately after passage of hard stool or, less commonly, after explosive diarrhea. Pain from fissures, in contrast to pain from other common causes of anal pain (thrombosed external hemorrhoid and perirectal abscess), decreases between bowel movements. All fissures are visible during examination as tears in the anal mucosa located below the dentate line in the posterior (90% women, 98% men) or anterior midline. Fissures that are not anterior or posterior should suggest Crohn's disease, syphilis, or tuberculosis.

CLINICAL APPROACH.   Most patients with anal discomfort or bleeding believe they have hemorrhoids, although the differential diagnosis includes tumors, inflammatory bowel disease, and infections (herpes, syphilis, gonorrhea, chlamydia, perirectal abscess). The patient interview should identify risk factors for trauma and infection (e.g., anal intercourse), any self-prescribed medications (some nonprescription anesthetics cause contact dermatitis), and any family history of Crohn's disease, ulcerative colitis, polyps, or cancer. No symptom, however, reliably distinguishes hemorrhoids from cancer; even bright red blood on top of the stool, the traditional symptom of hemorrhoids, may be the result of cancer.

The recommended minimal clinical approach in all patients with perirectal bleeding or discomfort is digital rectal examination and rigid sigmoidoscopy. In addition, the following groups of patients with perirectal symptoms should undergo examination of the entire colon (double contrast barium enema examination or colonoscopy): (1) patients older than 40 years, (2) patients with hemorrhoids identified but no response to conservative treatment, (3) patients with a family history of cancer, polyps, or inflammatory bowel disease, and (4) patients in whom rigid sigmoidoscopy discloses blood in the stool above the sigmoidoscope. In one study of elderly men with hematochezia and in whom hemorrhoids were identified during anoscopy, other important lesions were identified during colonoscopy in 35% (e.g., carcinomatous polyps, villous adenoma, tubular adenoma).

In contrast, the physical examination does differentiate among the causes of *severe* anal pain. Fissures are always visible on examination. Thrombosed hemorrhoids appear as tender firm blue swellings. If a fissure or thrombosed hemorrhoids are not present and there is tenderness in the perirectal tissues, the clinician should consider the diagnosis of perirectal abscess. In these settings, digital rectal examination and anoscopy are unnecessarily painful and best postponed. Patients with suspected perirectal abscesses should be referred to a surgeon for consideration of examination under anesthesia.

MANAGEMENT.   Only symptomatic hemorrhoids require treatment. Sixty-five percent of patients improve over weeks without any treatment, though two-thirds later experience recurrent disease. Controlled trials document that bulk laxatives such as psyllium decrease bleeding and discomfort over weeks; other sources of dietary fiber (fruits, vegetables, bran, whole grains) may be equally effective. Nonprescription creams/suppositories and sitz baths have not been scientifically tested, although they are safe and effective, according to many patients. If symptoms fail to resolve with conservative treatment (bulk laxatives, sitz baths), patients should be referred to a surgeon for any of a number of outpatient procedures designed to fix the anal cushions and prevent prolapse. Rubber band ligation, injection sclerotherapy, infrared coagulation, bipolar diathermy and D.C. electrotherapy are all safe (producing minimal temporary pain and bleeding) and effective (80% response). Fewer than 7% of all patients referred for fixation procedures fail to respond and ultimately require hemorrhoidectomy.

Most patients with thrombosed external hemorrhoids or pain from fissures improve after 2 to 3 days of conservative management (rest, bulk laxatives, sitz baths), although the fissure itself may require weeks to heal. Patients with persistent pain or chronic fissures may require surgery (excision for thrombosed hemorrhoids, lateral sphincterotomy for fissures).

FOLLOW-UP.   Hemorrhoids and fissures rarely result in hospitalization. Long-term studies demonstrate that fixation procedures reduce hemorrhoidal recurrence rates in the few patients who have unresponsive symptoms. Complications of chronic fissures, which affect less than 10%, are anal fistula and perirectal abscess.

Cross-references: Colorectal Cancer Screening (Section 91), Inflammatory Bowel Disease (Section 98), Sigmoidoscopy and Colonoscopy (Section 105).

REFERENCES

1. Jensen SL, Harling H, Arseth-Hansen P, Tange G. The natural history of symptomatic haemorrhoids. Int J Colorect Dis 1989;4:41–44.
    Randomized trial of rubber band ligation vs. no treatment in 189 patients with their first episode of second-degree hemorrhoids; at 4-year follow-up, 25% of untreated and 60% of treated patients remained asymptomatic.

2. Lieberman DA. Common anorectal disorders. Ann Intern Med 1984;101:837–846.
    Scientific overview of hemorrhoids, fissures, pruritus ani, and fecal incontinence.

3. Moesgaard F, Nielsen ML, Hansen JB, Knudsen JT. High-fiber diet reduces bleeding and pain in patients with hemorrhoids. Dis Colon Rectum 1982;25:454–456.
    Double-blind, randomized, placebo-controlled trial in 52 patients; 6 weeks of psyllium reduced hemorrhoidal symptoms. The drug was effective whether or not the patient was constipated.

4. Shub HA, Salvati EP, Rubin R. Conservative treatment of anal fissure. Dis Colon Rectum 1978;21:582–3.
    Of 317 patients with fissures (mean duration of 24 weeks), over one-half responded to conservative nonsurgical treatment.

5. Thomson WHF. The nature of haemorrhoids. Br J Surg 1975;62:542–552.
    Classic anatomic and clinical study suggesting that hemorrhoids are not simple venous varicosities but instead are the normal vascular anal cushions that have lost their fibromuscular support.

105 SIGMOIDOSCOPY AND COLONOSCOPY

Procedure

TIMOTHY E. LITTLE

SIGMOIDOSCOPY

INDICATIONS AND CONTRAINDICATIONS.   Endoscopic evaluation of the rectosigmoid colon or distal colon is indicated in the following settings: (1) bright red hematochezia (along with careful inspection of the anal canal for fissures and internal hemorrhoids), (2) microscopic intestinal blood loss in asymptomatic patients (sigmoidoscopy combined with barium enema examination is appropriate when full colonoscopy is not available), (3) suspected antibiotic-associated colitis, (4) suspected inflammatory bowel disease, (5) chronic bloody or inflammatory diarrhea, (6) tenesmus, rectal or perineal pain, (7) fistuli in ano, perirectal abscess, and atypical rectal fissures, and (8) chronic small-volume diarrhea. Mass screening for colorectal neoplasia by sigmoidoscopy is discussed in Section 91.

The only absolute contraindication to sigmoidoscopy is suspected or impending bowel perforation (e.g., toxic megacolon, acute diverticulitis). Relative contraindications include hemodynamic instability, an uncooperative patient, and colonic distention.

RATIONALE.   Most pathology responsible for hemodynamically insignificant, recurrent bright red hematochezia is located within reach of a sigmoidoscope. Direct visualization of the pseudomembranes of antibiotic-associated colitis or the characteristic ulcerations of inflammatory bowel disease, along with histologic confirmation, is often diagnostic of these diseases. Both rigid and, more recently, flexible instruments have been developed to examine the most distal aspect of the rectosigmoid colon. The rigid instrument is cheap and partly disposable, easy to clean, easier to use than flexible instruments, and of proven efficacy in finding colonic neoplasia. In addition, the rigid sigmoidoscope may be used in the unprepared rectosigmoid of patients with normal bowel habits, often with good visualization of mucosa. The flexible sigmoidoscope examines more of the colon area and is thus more sensitive in diagnosing colonic neoplasms, but is relatively expensive ($14,000), difficult to clean, and requires more training to learn to use.

METHODS.   *Rigid Sigmoidoscopy.*   Patient acceptance of rigid sigmoidoscopy is increased if the patient is placed in a modified left lateral decubitus position with the pelvis and buttocks extending well out over the operator's side of the table and the shoulders brought forward over the opposite side of the table for balance and security. Although the traditional jackknife-prone position is useful when liquid stool or blood is encountered, it requires a special table and places the patient in an unusual and psychologically vulnerable position. After a careful digital rectal examination, the lubricated plastic disposable instrument is inserted very slowly through the anal sphincters with the obturator in place. After the sphincter mechanism has been traversed, usually only after the first 2 to 3 cm, the instrument must be pointed immediately toward the patient's back to follow the rectum along the sacral curve. Failure to follow this normal anatomy can result in perforation of the anterior rectal wall. The obturator is then removed, the lens cap closed, and the path of the colon is followed, with the instrument advanced only after direct visualization of the judiciously inflated colonic lumen ahead. Particular care must be taken to inspect the capacious distal rectal vault just proximal to the anal canal, where low-lying lesions may be missed. Liquid obscuring the view can be removed with long cotton pledgets or a plastic suction catheter. A clean suction catheter can be used to stiffen a flexible cup biopsy forceps, as is used in flexible endoscopy, to obtain superficial mucosal biopsy specimens. The procedure should take about 5 minutes.

Flexible Sigmoidoscopy.   After two cleansing enemas, the flexible sigmoidoscope is introduced under direct vision as far as is comfortably possible (usually 30–60 cm), as described above, with inspection of the mucosa usually occurring during withdrawal. Procedure time should be 10 to 15 minutes.[2]

Cost/Complications.   The usual charge for flexible sigmoidoscopy is $400 to $600 (physician and hospital charges). One major complication of these procedures is perforation (<0.015%). Mortality is extraordinarily rare. The use of cautery to remove neoplasms by flexible sigmoidoscopy is not recommended because of the risk of colonic explosion in the enema-prepared bowel and the high incidence of synchronous neoplasia proximal to the area examined, obligating fully prepared colonoscopy. A potentially serious but unquantified complication is failure to diagnose significant and treatable neoplasia in the area screened.

COLONOSCOPY

Indications and Contraindications.   Indications include (1) asymptomatic microscopic gastrointestinal blood loss or unexplained iron deficiency anemia, (2) suspected neoplasia found on barium enema examination or sigmoidoscopy (performed to remove polyps or to screen the entire colon for neoplasia), (3) ulcerative pancolitis present for longer than 10 years (to screen for dysplasia), (4) a history of adenomatous polyps (screening usually recommended every 3 to 5 years after the last colonoscopy that either demonstrated no polyps or removed all lesions), (5) a strong family history of colon cancer, and (6) preoperative evaluation for synchronous neoplasia in patients being considered for curative colon cancer surgery.

The contraindications to colonoscopy are similar to those for sigmoidoscopy. Additional contraindications include the concurrent use of anticoagulants or aspirin, or a history suggestive of bleeding disorders.

RATIONALE.   Colonoscopy is the most specific and sensitive method for screening the colon for mucosal abnormalities and provides the opportunity for definitive therapy in some patients with localized neoplasia.

METHODS.   The bowel must be formally prepared for colonoscopy by having the patient adhere to a liquid diet for several days and ingest a purgative, usually 4 to 6 liters of an osmotically balanced sodium sulfate solution containing polyethylene glycol (GoLytely or Colyte). Many patients find this preparation mildly unpleasant. Patients should discontinue oral iron intake at least 1 week before the procedure. Because parenteral sedation is usually provided during colonoscopy to prevent and treat abdominal cramps, the patient should be instructed to bring a driver. The procedure typically requires 30 to 60 minutes, and is an outpatient procedure in most cases. Patients are usually able to resume a regular diet immediately after the procedure.

COST/COMPLICATIONS.   Colonoscopy is expensive, currently $1000 to $1500 in total charges. The incidence of bacteremia in colonoscopy, even with polypectomy, is very low, and recommendations for endocarditis prophylaxis are the same as those for upper endoscopy[3] (see Section 106, Upper Gastrointestinal Endoscopy).

The most significant complications of bowel preparation with polyethylene glycol–containing solutions are nausea (6%) and vomiting (2%). Perforation occurs in 0.17% of diagnostic studies and 0.30% of cases with polypectomy. Bleeding occurs in 0.03% of diagnostic studies and 1.5% of cases with polypectomy and rarely leads to surgical intervention.[1] Overall, mortality has been estimated to be 0.03%. Cardiopulmonary complications related to oxygen desaturation, vagally mediated bradycardia, and sedation do occur but are rarely life-threatening.

Cross-references: Periodic Health Assessment (Section 7), Colorectal Cancer Screening (Section 91), Diarrhea (Section 92), Inflammatory Bowel Disease (Section 98), Hemorrhoids and Fissures (Section 104), Upper Gastrointestinal Endoscopy (Section 106).

REFERENCES

1. Habr-Gama A, Waye JD. Complications and hazards of gastrointestinal endoscopy. World J Surg 1989;13:193–201.
    Morbidity and mortality data on colonoscopy in more than 30,000 patients (compiled studies).

2. Katon RM, Keefe EB, Melnyk CS. Flexible Sigmoidoscopy. Grune & Stratton, Orlando, Fla., 1985, p. 192.

Additional comparative data for rigid sigmoidoscopy, flexible sigmoidoscopy, and colonoscopy as well as specific techniques for performing flexible sigmoidoscopy.

3. Neu HC, Fleischer D. Recommendations for antibiotic prophylaxis before endoscopy. Am J Gastroenterol 1989;84:1488–1491.
    Broader discussion of endocarditis prophylaxis than that given by the American Heart Association (JAMA 1990;264:2919–2922).

106 UPPER GASTROINTESTINAL ENDOSCOPY

Procedure

TIMOTHY E. LITTLE

INDICATIONS/CONTRAINDICATIONS.   During upper GI endoscopy, a flexible fiberoptic or video endoscope is passed orally for direct visualization of the hypopharynx, esophagus, stomach, and proximal duodenum.

The most important indications for upper GI endoscopy in the ambulatory care setting are the following:

1. *Dyspepsia unresponsive to acid suppression therapy.* Most patients with acute or subacute dyspepsia do not require immediate diagnostic tests unless they have sustained weight loss, diarrhea, anemia, or symptoms that suggest a systemic or prolonged process (see Section 96, Dyspepsia). Most symptoms of acid peptic disease respond to treatment over several weeks, even before complete healing occurs. Patients with dyspepsia who do not respond require diagnostic tests (endoscopy or upper gastrointestinal radiography) to exclude complicated benign ulcer disease requiring surgical therapy, gastric neoplasia, nonpeptic inflammatory disease, or esophagitis requiring additional maneuvers for healing. Endoscopy is not routinely indicated solely to detect *Helicobacter pylori* colonization of gastric mucosa, since the value of eradicating this organism in chronic dyspepsia is not established.

2. *Reflux symptoms not responding to treatment.* These patients often require more expensive or hazardous treatment, such as chronic omeprazole or, rarely, surgical intervention. Endoscopy will define the degree of mucosal inflammation and exclude other diagnoses such as cancer.

3. *Dysphagia preferentially for solid food.* The clinician should simultaneously obtain an esophagogram and plan for endoscopic consultation. Solid food

dysphagia almost always indicates significant esophageal pathology that is best identified with early endoscopy. Esophagography provides complementary information because it evaluates the cervical esophagus better than endoscopy (e.g., diverticuli), and it studies the region of esophagus distal to tight strictures that prevent passage of an endoscope.

4. *Gastric ulceration.* Large solitary gastric ulcerations, irrespective of a benign radiographic appearance, should be biopsied to exclude cancer. Waiting to see if the ulcer heals with acid suppression therapy may be inappropriate, since 15% of neoplastic ulcers heal temporarily with standard ulcer therapy.[2] Duodenal ulceration without mass effect is rarely neoplastic and does not routinely justify endoscopy.

5. *Masses in the upper GI tract.*

6. *Occult blood loss.* Evaluation of the colon is the usual first test in asymptomatic patients with GI blood loss. Upper endoscopy should follow if that evaluation is unrevealing.

7. *Small bowel biopsy.* If small bowel pathology is suspected (e.g., nonpancreatic steatorrhea), a large-channel endoscope may rapidly obtain small bowel biopsy specimens from the third portion of the duodenum.

Contraindications to endoscopy include (1) severe dysphagia or suspected tracheoesophageal fistula, until after contrast radiography is performed, (2) suspected gastric or esophageal perforation, (3) severe dyspnea, (4) atlantoaxial instability, (5) profound anemia, and (6) suspected myocardial ischemia. Inadequate circulating clotting factors or platelet counts below 60,000/mm³ are contraindications to mucosal biopsy. Most authorities recommend stopping aspirin 7 days before elective endoscopy.

RATIONALE.   Endoscopy is more sensitive and specific than contrast radiography in the diagnosis of most if not all upper GI mucosal diseases. Diagnostic endoscopy is safe, with a morbidity of 0.1% to 0.2% and a mortality of less than 0.0006%.[3] Patients tolerate endoscopy well, and many prefer it to contrast radiography. A major advantage of endoscopy is the ability to perform mucosal biopsies.

Endoscopy is relatively expensive ($500–$900) compared with upper GI radiography ($300), and some subgroups of patients, particularly young adults, tolerate endoscopy poorly without heavy sedation. Moreover, its diagnostic sensitivity is operator dependent, and even experienced endoscopists may miss serious lesions.

METHODOLOGY.   Before endoscopy, the history and physical examination should focus on bleeding disorders, cardiac valvular pathology, use of anticoagulants, swallowing disorders, drug intolerance, and signs of unstable dentition. Patients are generally instructed to avoid oral intake for 6 to 8 hours before the procedure, except to take their medication with a small amount of water up to 2 hours before the procedure. To allay anxiety, the procedure should be discussed well beforehand. The patient should be instructed to bring a driver to the procedure as some patients, depending on their culture, age, and expectations, will require parenteral sedation.

The routine diagnostic procedure should require no more than 15 minutes and usually can be done in the outpatient setting.

COMPLICATIONS.   Some transient oxygen desaturation usually occurs during intubation with the endoscope, even in normal subjects; oximetry monitoring is advisable in patients with severe cardiopulmonary disease or who require substantial parenteral sedation. Significant retropharyngeal trauma occurs during intubation in a small but unknown number of patients. Other complications are aspiration (0.08%), perforation (0.033%–0.1%), and bleeding (0.03%). The risk of endocarditis is exceedingly small and endocarditis prophylaxis is not required for patients with valvular heart disease undergoing routine upper endoscopy with biopsy unless the risk of bacteremia is abnormally high, as in esophageal dilation or sclerotherapy.[1] Since very few data exist, however, many clinicians choose to give antibiotic prophylaxis to high-risk patients (prosthetic valve, prior endocarditis) even during the low risk of routine endoscopy. Prophylaxis is not recommended for patients with nonvalvular prostheses such as prosthetic joints, pacemakers, shunts, and mature vascular grafts. Transmission of HIV or hepatitis B virus via endoscopes has not been reported, but outbreaks of *Pseudomonas* infection have occurred related to poor endoscope cleaning. Cardiopulmonary complications, including respiratory arrest due to the parenteral sedation, are very rare.

Cross-references: Dyspepsia (Section 96), Dysphagia and Heartburn (Section 97), Peptic Ulcer Disease (Section 103).

REFERENCES

1. Dajani AS, et al. Prevention of bacterial endocarditis: Recommendations by the American Heart Association. JAMA 1990;264:2919–2922.
    Recent recommendations.

2. Erickson RA. Impact of endoscopy on mortality from occult cancer in radiographically benign gastric ulcers: A probability analysis model. Gastroenterology 1987;93:835–845.
    Cost-effective approaches to the radiographically diagnosed gastric ulcer.

3. Shahmir M, Schuman BM. Complications of fiberoptic endoscopy. Gastrointest Endosc 1980;26:86–91.

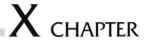

X CHAPTER

MUSCULOSKELETAL DISORDERS

---

107 GENERAL APPROACH TO ARTHRITIC SYMPTOMS

Symptom

RICHARD H. WHITE

EPIDEMIOLOGY. Nontraumatic joint pain is a common problem in all age groups. There are more than 200 different causes of arthritis, many with their own unique epidemiology. The prevalence of osteoarthritis varies markedly with age. The radiographic changes of osteoarthritis are noted in less than 5% of individuals under age 35 and in over 70% of those age 65 and older. The annual incidence of rheumatoid arthritis is approximately 2 to 4 per 100,000 adults; the prevalence of definite rheumatoid arthritis is approximately 1%. The prevalence of gout increases with age and with the serum uric acid concentration; in men aged 45 to 64 years the prevalence is approximately 34 per 1000, and in women is approximately 14.5 per 1000. The incidence of systemic lupus erythematosis (SLE) is approximately 4 to 6 per 100,000 persons per year, with a prevalence of approximately 50 per 100,000; the disease occurs much more frequently in women and more commonly in blacks.

Synovitis (tender, thickened, palpable synovium, with or without heat and redness) is to be distinguished from traumatic injury, tendinitis (e.g., lateral epicondylitis, or heel spur), the myofascial pain syndromes, and fibromyalgia. Synovitis can be classified as **monarticular** or **polyarticular.**

MONARTICULAR ARTHRITIS

EPIDEMIOLOGY. The incidence of acute monarticular synovitis increases with advancing age, as crystal-induced arthritides (gout, pseudogout) become

327

more common. Patients with three or fewer affected joints should usually be approached as though they have a monarticular problem.

ETIOLOGY.   In individuals less than 40 years old, the most common causes of monarticular synovitis are septic arthritis (particularly gonococcal arthritis), reactive arthritis (Reiter's syndrome), gout, a peripheral manifestation of spondylitis, and as the initial manifestation of a polyarticular disorder (e.g., rheumatoid arthritis) (Table 107–1). After age 40 the most common causes are gout, pseudogout, septic arthritis, and reactive arthritis.

Chronic monarticular arthritis should prompt an evaluation for infection, particularly tuberculous or fungal. Chronic crystal-induced arthritis, primary osteoarthritis, posttraumatic degenerative arthritis, and a persisting reactive arthritis can also lead to chronic monarticular synovitis.

CLINICAL APPROACH.   The patient should be carefully questioned about sexual activity, history of ocular inflammation (reactive arthritis), pulmonary symptoms (pneumonia, sarcoidosis), bowel symptoms (inflammatory bowel disease, reactive arthritis), genitourinary symptoms (gonococcal disease, reactive arthritis), and previous skin rash (erythema nodosum with sarcoid and

TABLE 107–1.   CAUSES OF MONARTICULAR SYNOVITIS

Acute
1. Septic arthritis
    a. *N. gonorrhoeae*
    b. *S. aureus*
    c. Streptococci
    d. *H. influenzae*
    e. Other gram-negative rods
2. Gout
3. Pseudogout (calcium phosphate deposition disease)
4. Reactive arthritis
    a. Reiter's syndrome
    b. Inflammatory bowel disease
    c. Acute sarcoidosis
    d. Acute rheumatic fever
5. Spondylitis (HLA B-27 related)
6. Psoriatic arthritis
7. Aseptic necrosis
8. Other: Hemarthrosis, mechanical problem, initial manifestation of a connective tissue disease, metastatic cancer, lymphoma.

Chronic
1. Septic arthritis
    a. Tuberculosis
    b. Fungal arthritis
    c. Lyme disease
2. Chronic gout
3. Chronic pseudogout
4. Posttraumatic degenerative arthritis
5. Reactive arthritis
6. Loose body, mechanical derangement
7. Neuropathic arthropathy
8. Pigmented villonodular synovitis
9. Sarcoid arthritis

inflammatory bowel disease, erythema chronicum migrans with Lyme disease, psoriasis with psoriatic arthritis). Fever commonly accompanies acute monarticular synovitis associated with septic arthritis, gout, pseudogout, and reactive arthritis. Several days of migratory polyarthralgias may precede the characteristic hemorrhagic skin pustules and synovitis of gonococcal arthritis, which occurs more commonly in women. Acute gout characteristically develops abruptly with striking erythema over the affected joint(s).

Physical examination of the affected joint(s) may reveal, in addition to an effusion, exquisite pain on motion in any plane (septic arthritis), marked overlying redness (gout), or an adjacent subcutaneous tophus (gout). Other important findings include metastatic lesions (septic arthritis), oral ulcerations (reactive arthritis), ocular inflammation (reactive arthritis, sarcoid), tophi (gout), or signs of skin breakdown (portal of entry for septic arthritis). Although septic arthritis can affect any joint, involvement of certain joints is characteristic of certain diagnoses: the first metatarsophalangeal joint (gout, rarely pseudogout), the isolated small joints of the foot (psoriatic arthritis, reactive arthritis), the midtarsal joints (gout), the ankle (reactive arthritis, gout), the knee (gout, pseudogout, reactive arthritis), and the wrists (pseudogout).

Aspiration of the joint is mandatory to diagnose septic and crystal-induced arthritis. If only a few drops of fluid are available, one drop should be submitted for crystal examination (followed by Gram stain), while the remainder is sent for bacterial and fungal culture. A joint fluid white blood cell (WBC) count less than 15,000 cells/mm³ is uncommon in septic arthritis; a count of greater than 100,000 cells/mm³ is characteristic of infection, but is also seen in crystal-induced and reactive arthritis. Polarizing microscopy may reveal intracellular negatively birefringent needle-shaped crystals characteristic of gout, or smaller, rhomboidal positive birefringent crystals characteristic of pseudogout. Plain radiographs are usually unremarkable but may show findings consistent with gout (erosion with an overhanging lip, tophus), pseudogout (chondrocalcinosis), a neuropathic process (advanced joint destruction), or a loose body. In puzzling cases, a radiograph of the pelvis may reveal bilateral or unilateral sacroilitis, suggesting that the peripheral arthritis is a manifestation of one of the spondylitides (ankylosing spondylitis, reactive arthritis).

Pending the results of synovial fluid culture and analysis, any patient with fever, severe joint pain, and an elevated synovial fluid WBC count should be admitted to the hospital and treated for septic arthritis.

If crystal-induced arthritis is diagnosed, treatment with a nonsteroidal antiinflammatory agent (NSAID) is usually effective (see Section 120, Gout/Hyperuricemia). When NSAID therapy is contraindicated, a tapering dose of prednisone is the treatment of choice. Intra-articular injection of a long-acting corticosteroid preparation is not recommended until a firm diagnosis is established and the arthritis is unresponsive to rest and NSAID therapy.

FOLLOW-UP.   Any patient not admitted to the hospital requires close follow-up because the possibility of infection is not excluded until synovial cultures have proved sterile and joint symptoms begin to resolve. The clinician should telephone the patient and schedule a follow-up visit for 2 to 3 days after the initial evaluation. Resolution of crystal-induced arthritis may require several weeks, and in cases of reactive arthritis, weeks to months.

POLYARTICULAR ARTHRITIS

EPIDEMIOLOGY/ETIOLOGY.   Acute polyarticular synovitis is relatively uncommon in all age groups. Polyarthralgias are common, especially in patients with generalized osteoarthritis.

The most common causes of polyarticular synovitis are (1) postinfectious arthritis (e.g., influenza, coxsackievirus, rubella), (2) rheumatoid arthritis, (3) SLE, (4) reactive arthritis, and (5) psoriatic arthritis (Table 107–2).

CLINICAL APPROACH.   In patients with physical signs of polyarticular synovitis, the initial diagnostic goal is to exclude life-threatening conditions such as subacute bacterial endocarditis, SLE, and systemic vasculitis. Other useful findings, in addition to the pattern of joint involvement, include (1) new onset of severe hypertension (vasculitis), (2) fever (SLE, endocarditis, Still's disease, vasculitis, disseminated gonorrhea, gout), (3) rash (SLE, Still's disease, vasculitis, dermatomyositis, endocarditis, gonococcal arthritis, Behçet's disease), (4) oral ulceration (SLE, viral, Behçet's disease, reactive arthritis), (5) dry eyes and dry mouth (primary Sjögren's syndrome, rheumatoid arthritis, SLE), (6) Raynaud's phenomena (scleroderma, mixed connective tissue disease, SLE), (7) ocular inflammation (SLE, reactive arthritis, Behçet's, sarcoid), and (8) serositis (SLE, vasculitis, familial Mediterranean fever). Certain combinations of findings may be diagnostic (e.g., malar rash, serositis, and arthritis for SLE; diarrhea, arthritis, and uveitis for reactive arthritis).

Initial laboratory testing should include a complete blood count (CBC), platelet count, urinalysis, and serum creatine phosphokinase (CPK), creatinine, and liver function tests. Hemolytic anemia or thrombocytopenia suggests SLE; leukopenia is compatible with SLE or HIV infection. An elevated CPK level suggests myositis or vasculitis. Proteinuria or urinary casts suggest a systemic immune complex process (subacute bacterial endocarditis, SLE, vasculitis). Radiographs of the involved joints are not usually helpful unless symptoms persist for weeks to months, after which findings typical of rheumatoid arthritis, psoriatic arthritis, or erosive osteoarthritis may appear.

Other tests include the following: (1) blood cultures if there is *any* suspicion of endocarditis, (2) arthrocentesis and synovial fluid analysis, including WBC count, crystal examination, and culture, (3) antinuclear antibody (ANA) assay (see Section 124, Interpretation of Serologic Tests), (4) rheumatoid factor assay, (5) chest radiography to look for infiltrates, fibrosis, hilar adenopathy, or pleural effusion, and (6) serum complement levels (C3 and CH_{50}). Low levels of serum complement are consistent with immune complex formation (SLE, serum sickness, endocarditis, hepatitis); high levels indicate an acute phase reactant (reactive arthritis, rheumatoid arthritis, polymyalgia rheumatica).

TABLE 107–2.   CAUSES OF ACUTE POLYARTICULAR SYNOVITIS

Causes	Common Features
Common Causes	
1. Acute viral syndrome	Polyarthralgias, resolution in days to weeks
2. Rheumatoid arthritis	Metacarpophalangeal joints, wrists, knees, ankles, forefoot, positive RF assay
3. Systemic lupus erythematosus	Hands and large joints, positive ANA assay, other features of SLE
4. Reactive arthritis	Oligoarticular, especially joints in the lower extremities
5. Psoriatic arthritis	Psoriatic rash, oligo- or polyarticular disease
Less Common Causes	
1. Gout	Usually asymmetric, oligoarticular; tophi often present
2. Pseudogout	Usually oligoarticular, in knees, wrists, elbows
3. Gonococcal	True synovitis present in only a few joints
4. Acute rheumatic fever	Lower extremity joints, migratory, elevated ASO titer
5. Sarcoidosis	Erythema nodosum, hilar adenopathy
6. Systemic rheumatic diseases	
a. Sjögren's syndrome	Dry eyes, dry mouth, positive ANA assay
b. Polymyositis/dermatomyositis	Proximal weakness, characteristic rash, elevated CPK levels
c. Scleroderma/CREST syndrome	Sclerodactyly, Raynaud's, telangectasias
d. Mixed connective tissue disease	Raynaud's, myositis, positive ANA assay, positive anti-(U_1)RNP
e. Still's (adult) disease	Sore throat, fever, evanescent macular rash
f. Vasculitis	Signs and symptoms of a multisystem disorder
g. Polymyalgia rheumatica	Age > 50, high ESR, shoulder/hip girdle pain
7. Serum sickness	After exposure to foreign protein
8. Subacute bacterial endocarditis	Murmur, low-grade fever, positive blood cultures
9. Erosive osteoarthritis	Swelling, heat in interphalangeal joints, radiographic changes

Other more specific serologic tests should be ordered only when clinical findings indicate an appreciable probability (e.g., pretest probability > 20%) that a particular disease is present (e.g., antineutrophil cytoplasmic antibody in patients with suspected Wegener's granulomatosis).

MANAGEMENT.   If the symptoms of the polyarthritis are mild, and if endocarditis or sepsis is unlikely, outpatient management is appropriate. If sepsis or endocarditis is suspected, or if an acute multisystem disorder (SLE or vasculitis) is likely, the patient should be admitted to the hospital. Pending the results of initial studies, outpatients can be managed with NSAIDs and bed rest; physical therapy with daily range of motion exercises should be ordered as soon as possible to preserve the function of the involved joints. If joint inflammation is profound and does not respond to the above measures, referral for rheumatologic evaluation is recommended. Low-dose prednisone (7.5 mg/day) can be given to patients with suspected rheumatoid arthritis who do not respond to nonsteroidal therapy.

FOLLOW-UP. Outpatients started on anti-inflammatory drugs should be followed in 2 to 3 days to monitor the patient's response to therapy.

Cross-references: Psoriasis (Section 32), Redness of the Eye (Section 37), Dry Eyes and Excessive Tearing (Section 38), Pleural Effusion (Section 65), Inflammatory Bowel Disease (Section 98), Low Back Pain (Section 108), Shoulder Pain (Section 109), Hip Pain (Section 110), Wrist and Hand Pain (Section 111), Knee Pain (Section 112), Ankle and Foot Pain (Section 113), Polymyalgia Rheumatica and Temporal Arteritis (Section 118), Osteoarthritis (Section 119), Gout/Hyperuricemia (Section 120), Interpretation of Serologic Tests (Section 124), Sexually Transmitted Diseases (Section 178).

REFERENCES

1. Arnett FC. Revised criteria for the classification of rheumatoid arthritis. Bull Rheum Dis 1989;38(5):1–6.

    Reports diagnostic performance of the 1987 revised criteria for rheumatoid arthritis using both the traditional format and a classification tree. The sensitivity is approximately 92% and specificity approximately 89%.

2. Goldenberg DL, Cohen AS. Acute infectious arthritis. Am J Med 1976;60:369–377.

    Classic article on the bacteriology of acute infectious arthritis and the response to antibiotic treatment plus needle aspiration.

3. Hochberg MC, Ed. Epidemiology of Rheumatic Diseases. Rheum Clin North Am 1990; 16:499–781.

    Entire volume devoted to the epidemiology of common rheumatic diseases.

4. McCune WJ. Monarticular arthritis. Sargent JS. Polyarticular arthritis. In Kelly WN, Harris ED, Ruddy S, Sledge CB, Eds. Textbook of Rheumatology. W.B. Saunders, Philadelphia, 1989, pp. 442–461.

    Exhaustive discussion.

5. Resnick D, Williams G, Weisman MH, Slaughter L. Rheumatoid arthritis and pseudorheumatoid arthritis in calcium pyrophosphate dihydrate crystal deposition disease. Radiology 1981;140:615–621.

    Emphasizes that CPPD deposition can mimic rheumatoid arthritis.

108 LOW BACK PAIN

Symptom

RICHARD A. DEYO

EPIDEMIOLOGY. Nearly 80% of adults have low back pain at some time during their lives. About 14% have an episode of back pain that persists longer than 2 weeks, but only 2% have back pain associated with sciatica, the symptom associated with most cases of herniated disks or spinal stenosis. Lumbar disk herniation occurs most often in 30- to 50-year-old adults, while spinal stenosis is most common after age 50.

ETIOLOGY. Pain may result from "mechanical" back problems, systemic diseases that affect the spine, and visceral diseases that cause back pain. At least 95% of all back pain is due to mechanical causes, most commonly muscle sprains and strains, degenerative disk disease, and, in older adults, osteoporosis with compression fractures. Herniated disks and spinal stenosis account for only a small proportion of these cases. Less common causes include anatomic abnormalities such as spondylolisthesis, severe scoliosis, and some transitional vertebrae. Because an exact diagnosis is often impossible to establish, as many as 85% of patients with back pain will never receive a definitive diagnosis.

"Systemic" causes, which account for less than 2% of cases, include neoplastic, infectious, and inflammatory diseases. Metastatic breast, lung, and prostate cancer are the most common malignancies. Osteomyelitis and epidural abscesses are occasionally found in patients with risk factors such as urinary tract infection, skin infection, or intravenous (IV) drug abuse. The prototypic inflammatory disorder is ankylosing spondylitis. Visceral diseases that cause low back pain include prostatitis, endometriosis, pyelonephritis, nephrolithiasis, and aortic aneurysms.

CLINICAL APPROACH. Because definitive diagnosis is often impossible, the initial evaluation should focus on three basic questions: (1) Is there a systemic or visceral cause of pain? (2) Is there neurologic compromise that may require surgical referral? (3) Are other findings present that influence the choice of therapy, regardless of the precise etiology?

Features that raise the suspicion of systemic causes include age over 50 years, a previous history of cancer, unexplained weight loss, fever, drug or alcohol abuse, corticosteroid use (predisposing to infection), and pain unresponsive to conservative therapy within a few weeks. Ankylosing spondylitis is rare; it occurs most often in men under age 40 and is characterized by morning stiffness, improvement with exercise, and a gradual onset.

333

The only true surgical emergency is the cauda equina syndrome, characterized by urinary retention, saddle anesthesia, and bilateral leg weakness and numbness.

Sciatica is usually the first clue to nerve root irritation and possible neurologic compromise. Sciatica is a sharp or burning pain, usually associated with numbness, that radiates down the posterior or lateral leg and is often aggravated by coughing or sneezing. Radiation below the knee is a more specific indicator of sciatica than is isolated thigh pain.

The most common cause of sciatica is herniated disks, 95% of which occur at the L4–5 or L5–S1 levels. L5 nerve root involvement results in weakness of the great toe extensors and other dorsiflexors of the foot, and in sensory loss along the medial aspect of the foot and in the web space between the first and second toes. Compromise of the S1 nerve root leads to a diminished ankle reflex, weak plantar flexors of the foot, and sensory deficits of the posterior calf and lateral foot. Almost 90% of patients with a herniated disk will have either weak foot dorsiflexion or diminished ankle reflexes. Abnormal straight leg raising (less than 60 degrees) is found in approximately 80% of patients with a herniated disk, but is nonspecific (i.e., it is found in other conditions as well).

Other factors may also influence the choice of therapy, regardless of specific pathoanatomic derangements. For example, narcotic analgesics, highly appropriate in patients with acute severe sciatica, should be avoided in patients with chronic pain syndromes (see Section 13, Chronic Pain Syndrome). A neurologic deficit probably mandates longer and stricter bed rest. Chronic pain may be an indication for antidepressant drug therapy even in the absence of overt depression. Frank depression or inconsistent physical findings suggest a need for psychological evaluation. Disability compensation proceedings may strongly influence patient perceptions, expectations, behavior, and prognosis.

Plain radiographs of the spine, often unhelpful or even misleading, are recommended only after trauma or when systemic disease is likely (Fig. 108–1). An erythrocyte sedimentation rate (ESR) greater than 20 mm/hr is relatively sensitive for metastatic cancer (about 80%) or infection (90%), but nonspecific. It may be a useful "screening" test for systemic diseases. Computed tomography (CT) or magnetic resonance imaging (MRI) may be misleading, demonstrating herniated disks in about 20% of normal persons without back pain. These studies are indicated only when surgery is a serious consideration (Table 108–1).

MANAGEMENT.   The most common error in management is failure to provide patients with strong reassurance and an explanation of their symptoms. The prognosis of acute low back pain is excellent. Discussions with the patient should avoid frightening labels such as "ruptured" disk, "degenerative" spine disease, or even "injury," since these terms imply serious tissue damage that often cannot be documented. Nonthreatening terms such as "muscle strain" or "changes due to wear and tear" are preferable.

For most patients without neurologic deficits, brief bed rest (2–3 days) helps alleviate pain but probably does not alter the natural history. Some patients

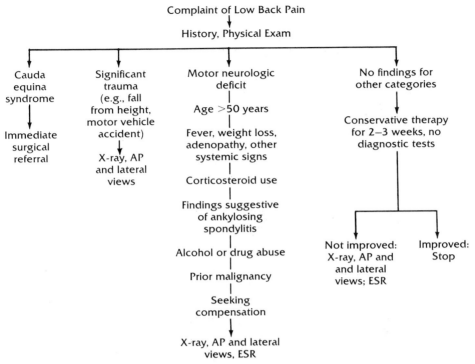

FIGURE 108—1. Algorithm for the initial approach to a patient with low back pain. Subsequent diagnostic testing is highly individualized, depending on results of the tests shown here, clinical findings, and response to initial therapy. ESR = erythrocyte sedimentation rate. (From Deyo RA. Early diagnostic evaluation of low back pain. J Gen Intern Med 1986;1:328–338. Reproduced by permission.)

may reasonably prefer to remain active. Patients with neurologic deficits should probably be prescribed longer and stricter bed rest (e.g., 1 week), with brief periods of ambulation beginning on day 3. Nonsteroidal anti-inflammatory drugs, including aspirin, relieve pain. Muscle relaxants such as carisoprodol are occasionally beneficial. Use of muscle relaxants and narcotic analgesics should be strictly time-limited (e.g., 1 week).

After the acute phase (usually within 2 weeks), patients should be encouraged to begin an exercise program. Stretching exercises for the back and lower extremities as well as general aerobic fitness exercises improve mobility, reduce fatigue, and decrease the likelihood of recurrences. Weight loss and smoking cessation should be encouraged, since obesity and cigarette smoking have been implicated in epidemiologic studies as causal factors for back pain (nicotine may impair diskal nutrition, raise intradiskal pressure due to coughing, or simply be a marker for anxiety and depression, which prolong pain symptoms).

Complete cure of chronic back pain (greater than 3 months) is an unrealistic expectation. Prolonged pain does not warrant surgery in the absence of neu-

**TABLE 108–1.   INDICATIONS FOR SURGICAL REFERRAL IN
THE PATIENT WITH SCIATICA**

1. Cauda equina syndrome (a surgical emergency): characterized by bowel and bladder dysfunction (usually urine retention), saddle anesthesia, bilateral leg weakness and numbness.
2. Progressive or severe neurologic deficit.
3. Persistent neuromotor deficit after 4–6 weeks of conservative therapy.
4. Persistent sciatica, sensory deficit, or reflex loss after 4–6 weeks in a patient with positive straight leg raising sign, consistent clinical findings, and favorable psychosocial circumstances (e.g., realistic expectations; no evidence of depression, substance abuse, or excessive somatization).

Source: Deyo RA, Loeser JD, Bigos SJ. Herniated lumbar intervertebral disk. Ann Intern Med 1990;112:598–603. Reproduced by permission.

rologic and imaging findings that indicate surgically reversible disease. Antidepressant drugs (even in the absence of overt depression), physical therapy, and specific pain treatment programs are all modalities that may help to restore function.

Hospitalization is rarely necessary for patients with low back pain unless surgery is scheduled. Indications for surgical referral appear in Table 108–1.

FOLLOW-UP.   Patients should be advised to schedule a return visit if they are not improved within 3 weeks. The prognosis of acute low back pain is excellent, with about 80% experiencing substantial improvement within 2 to 3 weeks. Even patients with herniated disks and neurologic deficits usually improve, and most do not require surgery. Approximately one-fourth of patients will experience recurrence of back pain within 3 to 4 years. Chronic pain carries a less favorable prognosis but may still respond to appropriate management. Other poor prognostic factors include a low educational status, self-perception as a sick person, disability compensation proceedings, and inflexible or unpleasant job circumstances.

Cross-references: Determining Disability: The Primary Physician's Role (Section 5), Smoking Cessation (Section 11), Chronic Pain Syndrome (Section 13), Obesity (Section 15), Osteoporosis (Section 117), Back Pain in the Cancer Patient (Section 208).

REFERENCES

1. Deyo RA. Early diagnostic evaluation of low back pain. J Gen Intern Med 1986;1:328–338.
   Focuses on details of the history and physical examination and the value of plain radiography. The algorithm in Figure 107–1 was suggested by this review.

2. Deyo RA, Diehl AK. Cancer as a cause of back pain: Frequency, clinical presentation, and diagnostic strategies. J Gen Intern Med 1988;3:230–238.
   Documents the prevalence of cancer among primary care patients, the most helpful history and physical examination findings, and a economical diagnostic strategy.

3. Deyo RA, Loeser JD, Bigos SJ. Herniated lumbar intervertebral disc. Ann Intern Med 1990;112:598–603.

Reviews the primary care approach to patients with sciatica and suspected disk herniations, including indications for surgery.

4. Scavone JG, Latshaw RF, Weidner WA. Anteroposterior and lateral radiographs: An adequate lumbar spine examination. AJR 1981;136:715–717.
    Documents the low yield of plain radiography and the limited value of oblique and coned lateral views.

5. Spitzer WO, LeBlanc FE, Dupuis M. Scientific Approach to the Assessment and Management of Activity-Related Spinal Disorders: A Monograph for Clinicians. Report of the Quebec Task Force on Spinal Disorders. Spine 1987;12(suppl 7):S16–S21.
    An exhaustive synthesis of the diagnostic and therapeutic literature for low back pain. Provides summary ratings of the efficacy of various treatments based on careful methodologic review of existing literature, and concludes with a management algorithm.

109 SHOULDER PAIN

Symptom

STEPHAN D. FIHN

EPIDEMIOLOGY/ETIOLOGY.   Shoulder pain is common, particularly among the elderly. Probably the most common cause is inflammation of the subacromial bursa, which is between the deltoid muscle and the rotator cuff tendon (a conjoint tendon of the supraspinatus, infraspinatus, teres minor and the subscapularis muscles). **Subacromial bursitis**, also known as rotator cuff tendinitis, supraspinatus tendinitis, and painful arc syndrome, usually affects patients over age 60, often as a result of occupational overuse of the shoulder or, in younger patients, sports such as swimming.

Another relatively common problem is **partial or complete rotator cuff tears,** which predominantly occur in patients over age 50. The supraspinatus is the tendon most often involved. Overuse is often a predisposing factor, although abrupt tears may occur in patients with weakened rotator cuffs who then sustain a strain or fall.

Frozen shoulder (adhesive capsulitis) is most common during middle age and is more prevalent in women than in men. It generally follows a period of immobilization that results from trauma to the shoulder, rotator cuff or bicipital tendinitis, rheumatoid arthritis, stroke, myocardial infarction, cervical radiculopathy, herpes zoster, distal injuries to the arm, mastectomy, or chest wall surgery. It is also associated with diabetes. Originally thought to be an adhesive bursitis, frozen shoulder is now considered to be a neuromuscular problem within the spectrum of reflex sympathetic dystrophy (see below).

As described in Section 123, **myofascial pain** is a controversial entity of unknown etiology that may involve the shoulder musculature. It typically develops after carrying heavy objects or using the shoulder in an unaccustomed fashion.

It is often erroneously assumed that many cases of shoulder pain are due to **osteoarthritis of the glenohumeral joint**. In fact, in the absence of prior direct trauma, isolated degenerative arthritis of the joint is rare and almost always occurs in association with disease of the rotator cuff.

Bicipital tendinitis usually occurs in conjunction with rotator cuff tendinitis and is relatively uncommon as an isolated condition. When it does occur, it is typically the result of a repetitive stress such as overhead painting or ball throwing.

Reflex sympathetic dystrophy (shoulder-hand syndrome, Sudek's atrophy) is an uncommon disorder that manifests with shoulder pain accompanied by signs and symptoms involving the arm, forearm, and hand. These include pain and swelling in the upper extremity, trophic skin changes (atrophy, hyperpigmentation, hypertrichosis, hyperhidrosis, nail changes), and evidence of vasomotor instability. The condition is almost always bilateral to some degree and, as with frozen shoulder, there is usually a precipitating event. The etiology is unknown but is postulated to be related to autonomic dysfunction that causes rapidly progressive osteopenia and erosions plus a proliferative synovitis.

Exceedingly rare causes of shoulder pain include amyloidosis, acromegaly, hemophilia, thoracic outlet syndrome, and brachial neuritis. Pain may be referred to the shoulder in a variety of diseases, including diaphragmatic irritation from gallbladder disease, subphrenic processes, pulmonary infarction, or ruptured viscus, as well as cervical radiculopathy, Pancoast tumor, and myocardial infarction.

CLINICAL APPROACH. Most causes of shoulder pain can be identified from the history and physical examination; radiographs are not always necessary. Key elements of the history are acuteness of onset, types of recent activity, a history of distant or recent trauma, stiffness, pain at night, and weakness. Both shoulders should be examined, with the unaffected side used for comparison. The presence of atrophy, swelling, deformity, or tenderness, should be noted, with particular attention paid to the area of the supraspinatus tendon (immediately caudal and anterior to the acromion) and to the bicipital groove (points anteriorly with the arm in 10 degrees of internal rotation). Active range of motion should be observed with the patient sitting and moving the arm through forward flexion. External rotation is measured with the arm fully adducted and the elbow flexed to 90 degrees. Internal rotation is checked by having the patient move the thumb up the spine as far as possible, with assistance from other hand if necessary. Passive range of motion should be performed with patient supine to eliminate rotation of the thorax and relax guarding.

There is usually no history of trauma in patients with subacromial bursitis. The pain begins gradually over several days and is more severe at night, particularly when the patient lies on the affected side. Pain may be limited to the subacromial region or may extend around the shoulder girdle or down the arm. Subacromial tenderness is present and occasionally extends into the bicipital groove. A classic finding is a "painful arc" of abduction between 40 to 120 degrees. The patient will limit true abduction by elevating the shoulder. Internal rotation is painful, external rotation is normal. The "impingement sign" may be positive, producing subacromial pain when the arm is forwardly elevated to the maximum while the shoulder girdle is depressed. The diagnosis is confirmed by subacromial injection of 5 to 10 ml of 1% lidocaine, which greatly improves pain and function. In straightforward cases, radiographs are unnecessary, but they may demonstrate calcium in the supraspinatus tendon if obtained.

The pain of rotator cuff tears is indistinguishable from that of rotator cuff tendinitis. Following acute tears there may be accumulation of fluid in the subacromial bursa, causing swelling. In more long-standing cases, atrophy of the supra- and/or infraspinatus may be detectable. Passive range of motion is usually normal, but pain and limitation of active range of motion are present. Subacromial instillation of lidocaine relieves the pain but weakness persists, demonstrated by the patient's inability to maintain the arm at 90 degrees of abduction. Plain radiographs of the shoulder may show the humeral head to be osteopenic and to ride high against the acromion. Arthrography shows extravasation of contrast material from the glenohumeral joint into the subacromial bursa.

Symptoms of frozen shoulder overlap with those of rotator cuff tendinitis and tears. Patients present with mild to moderate shoulder pain or stiffness of subacute onset. Atrophy of the shoulder girdle may be present. There is restricted range of active and passive range of motion in *all* planes. Typically abduction is limited to less than 40 degrees and external rotation to no more than 30 degrees. Instillation of lidocaine in the subacromial space does not substantially improve function. Radiographs may show calcification of the rotator cuff tendon or may be normal. Osteoporosis of the humeral head is common. Arthrography is not required for diagnosis but demonstrates a small, tight joint capsule.

Patients with myofascial shoulder pain usually give no history of prior shoulder problems. The pain may be localized around the shoulder or may extend down the arm. Trigger points may be identified in one or more locations, including the supraspinatus, infraspinatus, and teres minor. Radiographs are normal.

In bicipital tendinitis, pain is the predominant symptom and may involve the entire shoulder girdle. Active and passive range of motion are usually normal, although the patient may be tentative in these actions. Resisted flexion and supination of the forearm is painful (Yergason's sign). There is tenderness in the bicipital groove, but unless it is extreme, this finding is nonspecific. Calcifications of the biceps tendon are uncommon.

In reflex sympathetic dystropy there is often burning pain of the shoulder and hand, occasionally with swelling. Radiographs demonstrate osteopenia and radionuclide bone scans often demonstrate marked uptake on the affected side.

MANAGEMENT. Treatment of shoulder pain is largely empiric, since there are almost no well-designed trials with adequate statistical power. Initial treatment for subacromial bursitis consists of nonsteroidal anti-inflammatory drugs, avoidance of stressful use of the shoulder, and exercises. The latter include Codman's pendulum exercises and "walk-ups" (walking fingers up a wall as high as possible while standing perpendicularly). Instillation of an aqueous steroid preparation may help some patients who do not respond to these measures (see Section 128, Injection of the Shoulder). Chronic pain lasting more than 3 to 6 months suggests chronic impingement of the acromion on the rotator cuff or a rotator cuff tear and should prompt orthopedic referral. Arthrography, ultrasonography, or computed tomography (CT) may be warranted. Small tears may heal with conservative treatment similar to that for tendinitis or bursitis. Larger tears require surgical repair.

Physical therapy is the mainstay of treatment for frozen shoulder and consists of daily firm but gentle range of motion exercises. The patient may begin by "loosening up" the shoulder with a warm shower. In the supine position, the contralateral arm is then used to range the affected shoulder, with a stick used if necessary to gain external rotation. Steroid injections appear to be of no benefit.

Therapy for myofascial pain involves cessation of the aggravating activity, nonsteroidal anti-inflammatory drugs, and heat. If symptoms fail to abate with these measures, stretch and spray with vapocoolant may be applied or the trigger point may be injected with 1% lidocaine.

Treatment of bicipital tendinitis is similar to that for rotator cuff tendinitis. Injection of steroids may be helpful in stubborn cases.

Early treatment of reflex sympathetic dystrophy with high-dose corticosteroids (i.e., 60 mg of prednisone per day, tapered over 4–6 weeks) appears beneficial. When this approach fails, sympathetic blocks and, in refractory cases, sympathectomy may be considered.

Cross-references: Myofascial Pain Syndromes (Section 123), Principles of Physical Therapy (Section 126), Trigger Point Injection (Section 127), Injection of the Shoulder (Section 128).

REFERENCES

1. Bland JH, Merrit JA, Boushey DR. The painful shoulder. Semin Arthritis Rheum 1977;7:21–47.

   An older but still useful review of anatomy and clinical approach.

2. Kozin F, McCarty DJ, Sims J, Genant H. The reflex sympathetic dystrophy syndrome: 1. Clinical and histologic studies. Evidence for bilaterality, response to corticosteroids and articular involvement. Am J Med 1976;60:321–338.

   A classic study of 11 patients, delineating clinical and radiologic features and demonstrating improvement with prednisolone, 60–80 mg/day for 2 weeks and tapered over 12 weeks. Unfortunately, the evaluation of treatment was uncontrolled.

3. Matsen FA 3d, Kirby RM. Office evaluation and management of shoulder pain. Orthop Clin North Am 1982;13:453–475.

   An orthopedist's view. Describes examination of the shoulder and illustrates shoulder exercises.

4. Rogers LF, Hendrix RW. The painful shoulder. Radiol Clin North Am 1988;26:1359–1371.
    Describes the radiographic appearance of common and uncommon problems of the shoulder with plain radiographs, arthrograms, and computed tomographs.

5. Simkin PA. Tendinitis and bursitis of the shoulder: Anatomy and therapy. Postgrad Med 1983;73:177–190.
    Excellent description of the anatomy, pathophysiology, diagnosis, and management of these problems.

110 HIP PAIN

Symptom

GREGORY L. GARDNER

ETIOLOGY.   Hip pain may originate from disease within the joint or from conditions outside the joint (Table 110–1). Most patients seen by the primary care physician will have bursitis, myofascial conditions, or osteoarthritis.

CLINICAL APPROACH.   Examination should focus on range of motion of the patient's hip, palpation of surrounding structures, stance, and gait. It is especially important to recognize soft tissue causes of pain.

Arthritis.   Arthritis of the hip joint itself usually manifests with groin pain, sometimes radiating to the knee. Although **osteoarthritis** generally causes pain aggravated by weight bearing, advanced disease may cause rest pain that is especially severe at night. Physical examination in early osteoarthritis reveals loss of hip extension and internal rotation. Radiographs may show characteristic changes. The pain of **inflammatory arthritis** is sometimes continuous and is accompanied by morning stiffness that lasts hours but improves with use. To

TABLE 110–1.   DIFFERENTIAL DIAGNOSIS OF PAIN IN THE HIP REGION

Arthritis	**Neuropathy**
Osteoarthritis	Lateral femoral cutaneous nerve
Rheumatoid arthritis	
Ankylosing spondylitis	**Miscellaneous**
Infectious arthritis	Femoral/inguinal hernias
	Referred pain
Bursitis	Fractures
Trochanteric	Osteonecrosis
Iliopsoas	Tumors
Ischial	
Myofascial Syndromes	
Tensor fascia lata fasciitis	
Fibromyalgia	
Muscle/tendon strains	

distinguish rheumatoid arthritis from ankylosing spondylitis, the two most common causes of inflammatory arthritis of the hip, the pattern of other joints affected and radiographs are helpful. Patients with **infectious arthritis** of the hip usually experience fever and intense groin pain. During examination they hold the hip in slight flexion and resist any attempt to move it. The most common responsible organism is *Staphylococcus aureus*.

Bursitis.   Of eighteen bursae found around the hip, only three typically cause hip pain. Patients with **trochanteric bursitis** usually complain of pain during ambulation or when lying on the affected side. On examination the trochanteric bursa, located just posterior and superior to the greater trochanter, is tender. The **iliopsoas bursa** lies behind the iliopsoas muscle, lateral to the femoral vessels and just anterior to the hip joint. When inflamed, pain may be felt in the thigh, pelvis, or groin. On examination the bursa is tender, and patients hold the hip in flexion to avoid painful extension. Computed tomography (CT) is rarely indicated but may help distinguish iliopsoas bursitis from intra-articular pathology in refractory cases. **Ischial bursitis,** or "weaver's bottom," is most often caused by prolonged sitting. Tenderness is found over the ischial tuberosity.

Myofascial Conditions.   The tensor fascia lata is a wide band of fascia that begins at the lateral ilium and ends at the lateral knee. The taut fascia may slip over the greater tuberosity and cause painless snapping of the hip. In others, the fascia becomes inflamed, causing a dull ache at the lateral hip and thigh. Stretching the fascia reproduces the pain and confirms the diagnosis: the patient lies with the affected side up while the straightened leg is adducted and drawn over the edge of the examining table. **Iliac apophysitis** describes a condition in which maximal tenderness is found over the iliac crest at the insertion of the tensor fascia lata.

Fibromyalgia occurs most often in women and leads to generalized body pain, sleep disturbances, fatigue, headache, and irritable bowel symptoms (see Section 122). Of the many tender points present, two near the hip are located at the trochanteric bursa and high gluteal areas.

A variety of muscle strains may produce hip pain, including strains of the hip adductors, abductors, and hamstrings. The patient interview usually uncovers injury or overuse. Maximal tenderness is located in the specific muscles or their insertions, and isometric contraction of the specific muscles reproduces the pain.

Entrapment Neuropathy.   Entrapment of the lateral femoral cutaneous nerve at the anterior superior iliac spine (**meralgia paresthetica**) causes painful paresthesia in the groin and lateral thigh (see Section 146, Entrapment Neuropathies).

Miscellaneous.   Femoral or inguinal hernias may cause groin pain and are easily found during examination. Pain from sacroiliac joint arthritis, lumbar radiculopathies (especially L3–4 disk herniations), and renal colic may be referred to the hip region.

Although most hip fractures cause acute pain, stress fractures may be more insidious and may be apparent on bone scans long before radiographs are abnormal.

Risk factors for **osteonecrosis of the femoral head** include corticosteroid use, alcohol abuse, hemoglobinopathies, scuba diving, and systemic lupus erythematosus (SLE). Patients note pain with weight bearing and at night. Radiographs, normal in early disease, eventually show progressive collapse of the femoral head. Magnetic resonance imaging (MRI) is the most sensitive test for early diagnosis.

A variety of **tumors** may metastasize to the acetabulum and femoral head, including prostate, breast, thyroid, renal, and lung cancer. Osteoid osteoma, a benign tumor, may involve the femoral head or neck and cause severe pain that sometimes dramatically responds to aspirin. Bone scans are the most sensitive diagnostic tests for osteoid osteoma and metastatic tumors.

MANAGEMENT. *Arthritis.* Treatment of arthritis of the hip depends on the specific cause (see Section 119, Osteoarthritis). Because septic arthritis of the hip can cause rapid destruction of the hip, hospitalization, parenteral antibiotic administration, and urgent consultation with an orthopedic surgeon is mandatory.

Bursitis. Treatment of bursitis includes local heat and ultrasound, massage, gentle stretching exercises, and anti-inflammatory medication. Local corticosteroid injections are often helpful (see Section 129, Injection of the Trochanteric Bursa).

Myofascial Conditions. The treatment for tensor fascia lata tendinitis includes physical therapy with stretching, massage, local application of heat and ultrasound, and anti-inflammatory medication. Injection of a local anesthetic into particularly tender areas is also helpful (see Section 123). Most muscle strains are self-limited. Analgesic medication and local application of ice relieve acute pain. If symptoms persist, physical therapy and anti-inflammatory medications are beneficial.

Miscellaneous. When osteonecrosis is recognized early, before radiographic changes appear, femoral core decompression biopsy frequently reduces pain, slows progression of disease, and prevents collapse of the femoral head. Patients with advanced disease may require joint replacement for pain relief.

The treatment of osteoid osteoma is surgical excision.

Cross-references: Low Back Pain (Section 108), Osteoporosis (Section 117), Osteoarthritis (Section 119), Fibromyalgia (Section 122), Myofascial Pain Syndromes (Section 123), Trigger Point Injection (Section 127), Injection of the Trochanteric Bursa (Section 129), Entrapment Neuropathies (Section 146).

REFERENCES

1. Cushner FD, Friedman RJ. Osteonecrosis of the femoral head. Orthop Rev 1988;17:29–34.
   Discusses the pathophysiology, classification, and treatment options for osteonecrosis of the femoral head.

2. Polisson RP. Sports medicine for the internist. Med Clin North Am 1986;70:469–489.
   Discusses various musculoskeletal problems commonly encountered in athletes (including hip pain) and provides otherwise hard to find information on iliac apophysitis.

111 WRIST AND HAND PAIN

Symptom

GREGORY L. GARDNER

ETIOLOGY. Table 111–1 lists the most common conditions causing wrist and hand pain, organized by anatomic abnormality. Traumatic conditions are not covered in this section.

CLINICAL APPROACH. Evaluation of the hand and wrist focuses on careful inspection for swelling and deformity, palpation, and range of motion testing.

Arthritis. Although it may be difficult to distinguish arthritis from tenosynovitis, passive movement of the affected joint causes pain in arthritis but not in tenosynovitis. Active movement causes pain in both conditions.

The pattern of joint involvement differentiates the various forms of arthritis. Helpful laboratory tests include assays for antinuclear antibodies (ANA) and rheumatoid factor (RF), ESR, and synovial fluid crystal analysis and culture. **Osteoarthritis** involves the distal interphalangeal joints and proximal interphalangeal joints, sparing the metacarpophalangeal joints. Heberden's and Bouchard's nodes are often found. **Rheumatoid arthritis** involves the metacarpophalangeal and proximal interphalangeal joints and wrists in a symmetric pattern. Patients with **gout** may have tophaceous deposits about the digits. **Psoriatic arthritis** may involve any joint of the hand or wrist, usually asymmetrically, and often associated with a characteristic skin rash.

The clinician must have a high degree of suspicion for **infectious arthritis,** especially when monarthritis affects the wrist. Bacterial arthritis rarely affects the small joints of the hand except following puncture wounds (e.g., human bites). Disseminated gonococcal infection may cause an acute arthritis associated with tenosynovitis and vesiculopustular skin lesions.

TABLE 111–1. CONDITIONS CAUSING WRIST AND HAND PAIN

Arthritis	Neuropathy
Osteoarthritis	Carpal tunnel syndrome
Rheumatoid arthritis	Ulnar nerve entrapment
Psoriatic arthritis	
Systemic lupus erythematosus	**Cutaneous Inflammation**
Crystal arthropathies	Paronychia
Infectious arthritis	Felon
	Cellulitis/lymphangitis
Tenosynovitis	
Flexor tenosynovitis	**Miscellaneous**
de Quervain's tenosynovitis	Raynaud's phenomenon
Ganglions	Reflex sympathetic dystrophy

Tenosynovitis.   **Flexor tenosynovitis** may produce a trigger finger, which occurs when the inflamed tendon, often with a palpable nodular thickening, impinges on the flexor pulley located at the base of the finger. Tenosynovitis of the abductor pollicis longus and the extensor pollicis brevis tendons (*de Quervain's*), results in a tender distal radius and positive Finkelstein's test (with the thumb gripped beneath the fingers, ulnar deviation of the wrist reproduces the pain). **Ganglions** are synovial cysts that are typically located on the dorsum of the wrist but may also occur over metacarpophalangeal joints. They are occasionally painful and may interfere with joint motion.

Neuropathy.   **Carpal tunnel syndrome** (median nerve entrapment) and **ulnar nerve entrapment** cause numbness, tingling, and sometimes weakness in the distribution of the affected nerve (see Section 146, Entrapment Neuropathies).

Skin Conditions.   **Paronychia,** a common infection located at the nail fold, is usually due to staphylococci. Examination reveals swelling, erythema, and tenderness at the margins of the nail bed. A **felon** is an infection of the distal finger pulp, usually marked by severe pain and tenderness. **Cellulitis** of the hand, common in IV drug abusers or after trauma, may cause fever, lymphangitis, or axillary adenopathy.

Miscellaneous.   **Raynaud's phenomenon** is relatively common and affects women more often than men. After exposure to cold, patients classically develop pain and blanching of the fingers, followed by cyanosis and redness. **Reflex sympathetic dystrophy** is a condition characterized by burning pain, swelling, and exquisite tenderness of the hand, often with similar involvement of the shoulder (hand-shoulder syndrome). The skin of the affected hand is sweaty and thin, and its temperature may alternate between warm and cold. Patients frequently have a history of diabetes, previous trauma, hand or wrist surgery, or myocardial infarction. Radiographs demonstrate mottled osteopenia; bone scans may show markedly increased uptake in the affected extremity.

MANAGEMENT.   Specific therapy for arthritis depends on an accurate diagnosis (see Section 107, General Approach to Arthritic Symptoms; Section 119, Osteoarthritis; and Section 120, Gout/Hyperuricemia).

Both flexor tenosynovitis and de Quervain's tenosynovitis may respond to wrist splinting and nonsteroidal anti-inflammatory medication. Refractory cases may require local injections of corticosteroids (5–10 mg of triamcinolone preparation). If ganglions become problematic, needle aspiration followed by steroid injection may help temporarily, but recurrence is common. Surgery is usually curative.

The treatment of paronychia or felons includes warm soaks and antibiotics. Incision and drainage may be necessary, especially with felons. Hospital admission and parenteral antibiotic administration are indicated for most patients with cellulitis, especially if lymphangitis, adenopathy, and fever are present. Abscesses require surgical drainage.

The treatment of reflex sympathetic dystrophy is prednisone, 60 mg/day in divided doses, slowly tapered over a month. Patients who relapse may require a second course. If steroids are ineffective, patients may experience prolonged relief with a series of sympathetic blocks. If the blocks produce only transient relief, surgical sympathectomy should be considered. To be effective, treatment should begin early and include physical therapy.

Cross-references: Psoriasis (Section 32), General Approach to Arthritic Symptoms (Section 107), Shoulder Pain (Section 109), Osteoarthritis (Section 119), Gout/Hyperuricemia (Section 120), Interpretation of Serologic Tests (Section 124), Raynaud's Syndrome (Section 132), Sexually Transmitted Diseases (Section 178).

REFERENCES

1. Cardelli MB, Kleinsmith DM. Raynaud's phenomenon and disease. Med Clin North Am 1989;73:1127–1141.

    Discusses the significance of a positive ANA assay associated with Raynaud's phenomenon; excellent discussion on differential diagnosis and treatment.

2. Dorwart BB. Carpal tunnel syndrome: A review. Semin Arthritis Rheum 1984;14:134–140.

    A concise article containing good sections on differential diagnosis and treatment.

3. Kozin F. Reflex sympathetic dystrophy. Bull Rheum Dis 1986;36:1–8.

    A good review of reflex sympathetic dystrophy and its treatment. The author has been responsible for a considerable amount of original work delineating this syndrome.

112 KNEE PAIN

Symptom

GREGORY L. GARDNER

ETIOLOGY.   The knee is one of the most frequently injured joints in athletes who participate in weight-bearing sports. It is also a common site for nontraumatic arthritis (Table 112–1).

CLINICAL APPROACH.   With the patient recumbent, the clinician observes the patient's knees for alignment. The examination, which should include the popliteal fossa, focuses on palpation for warmth, effusions, and joint line tenderness.

Arthritis.   **Chondromalacia patellae** is a common condition that affects women more than men. The patella of affected patients is not aligned in its track

TABLE 112–1.   COMMON CONDITIONS CAUSING KNEE PAIN

Arthritis	**Tendinitis**
Chondromalacia patellae	Patellar tendinitis
Meniscal tear	Popliteal region tendinitis
Osteoarthritis	
Rheumatoid arthritis	**Miscellaneous**
Psoriatic arthritis	Osgood-Schlatter disease
Gout	Osteonecrosis
Pseudogout	
Septic arthritis	
Bursitis	
Prepatellar bursitis	
Pes anserine bursitis	
Baker's cyst	

and moves abnormally (i.e., overpull of the vastus lateralis muscle leads to abnormal lateral pull on the patella), causing excessive compression, softening, and fibrillation of the cartilage. Patients report anterior knee pain especially when using stairs or getting up from a chair. Examination may reveal patellofemoral compartment crepitation, a knee effusion, or abnormal patellar tracking. Pressure placed on the patella while the patient contracts the quadriceps muscles may reproduce the pain. Sunrise and lateral radiographs of the knee show the patellofemoral compartment and may demonstrate joint space narrowing or alignment abnormalities.

Meniscal tears usually occur after trauma, especially a twisting injury. Patients usually complain of acute pain, swelling, locking, or episodic "giving way" of the knee. Depending on the site of the tear, the medial or lateral joint lines may be tender. The McMurray test may be positive (i.e., starting with the knee flexed, slow extension with simultaneous internal or external rotation on the tibia produces pain and clicking). Arthrography, magnetic resonance imaging (MRI), or arthroscopy will confirm the diagnosis.

Osteoarthritis usually involves the medial compartment, but lateral or patellofemoral disease also occurs (see Section 119, Osteoarthritis).

The pattern of joint involvement and the presence of psoriatic skin lesions or a positive rheumatoid factor assay distinguish **rheumatoid** (symmetric polyarthritis) from **psoriatic** arthritis (usually asymmetric). **Gout,** a common cause of knee pain, is discussed in Section 120. Calcium pyrophosphate dihydrate crystal–induced synovitis, or **pseudogout,** mimics acute gout of the knee and often afflicts patients bedridden because of acute medical disease or surgery. A thin line of calcified cartilage (chondrocalcinosis) often appears on anteroposterior knee radiographs in patients with pseudogout, and arthrocentesis reveals characteristic crystals (rhomboid and positively birefringent).

Because the knee is the most common joint that becomes infected, any acute inflammatory knee monarthritis should be regarded as septic arthritis until examination and culture of the joint fluid prove otherwise. *Staphylococcus aureus* is the usual organism, followed by streptococci, gonococci, and other gram-negative organisms. Patients experience fever and severe pain, and often guard against any movement of the knee joint. To diagnose gonococcal arthritis, cultures of both joint fluid and other potentially infected sites (urethra, cervix, rectum) are helpful.

Bursitis.   **Prepatellar bursitis** is covered in Section 121.

Inflammation of the pes anserine bursa, which is located at the medial knee, usually affects patients with osteoarthritis. Knee pain with walking and nocturnal pain are common; examination reveals local tenderness. Although **medial collateral ligament strain** resembles anserine bursitis, nocturnal pain is less common.

A **Baker's cyst** occurs when knee effusions from any cause accumulate and distend the gastrocnemius and semimembranosa bursae located in the popliteal fossa. Patients typically complain of fullness and pain in the popliteal fossa, especially with walking. A palpable cyst in the medial popliteal fossa may be the only finding, although some cysts may grow quite large and obstruct venous return or even rupture, causing lower extremity swelling (pseudothrombophlebitis, see Section 131, Painful and Swollen Calf). Ultrasound of the popliteal fossa or arthrography confirms suspected cysts.

Tendinitis.   **Suprapatellar** and **infrapatellar tendinitis** result from overuse, abnormal patellar tracking, or malrotation of the tibia or femur. Infrapatellar tendinitis may also occur in athletes after repetitive jumping ("jumper's knee"). Pain worsens when the patient climbs stairs, and the involved tendon is tender on examination.

Popliteal pain may reflect strain of the hamstring tendons. In these patients posterior knee pain worsens with the straight leg maneuver (i.e., with the hip and knee flexed, the knee is slowly extended).

Miscellaneous.   **Osgood-Schlatter disease** affects teenage males who are active in sports. Anterior knee pain is typical and is aggravated by activities such as climbing stairs, kicking, or kneeling. Tenderness and swelling over the tibial tubercle may be present. Radiographs may show avulsion of the tubercle.

Of the two types of **osteonecrosis** of the knee, **osteochondritis dissecans** involves the lateral portion of the medial knee compartment and typically affects young men following an episode of trauma. The inflammation may heal spontaneously or may lead to formation of a loose body and symptoms of locking. Radiographs are diagnostic. The second type of osteonecrosis affects the elderly and those taking corticosteroids, and involves the medial and lateral femoral condyles. Both knees are affected in over 50% of patients. Patients experience sudden severe knee pain, especially with weight bearing, and have a small to moderate effusion. Radiographs become abnormal only after several months and are not as useful for early diagnosis as are bone scans or MRI.

MANAGEMENT.   *Arthritis.*   **Chondromalacia patellae** is managed with anti-inflammatory medications and quadriceps strengthening exercises (the patient extends the knee while sitting or lying, gradually adding ankle weights to improve conditioning). Rarely, surgery may be necessary.

Meniscal tears initially require rest and anti-inflammatory medications. Arthroscopic surgery is indicated when patients experience locking of the knee or persistent symptoms.

Therapy for **inflammatory arthritis** (e.g., rheumatoid, psoriatic, and crystal-induced arthritis) includes combinations of anti-inflammatory medications, local corticosteroid injections, and disease-modifying agents. Consultation is advised in difficult cases.

Cases of **infectious arthritis** require hospitalization, high doses of parenteral antibiotics, and frequent joint drainage. Consultation with an orthopedic surgeon is advised.

Therapy for osteoarthritis is covered in Section 119.

Bursitis.   Therapy for **prepatellar bursitis** is covered in Section 121.

Pes anserine bursitis responds to physical therapy (gentle stretching, ultrasound, massage) and, in unresponsive cases, corticosteroid injection.

Corticosteroid injections into the knee joint may benefit patients with **Baker's cysts,** irrespective of whether the underlying arthritis is inflammatory or noninflammatory. In some patients with noninflammatory conditions (e.g., osteoarthritis), the cyst itself may require aspiration and instillation of a corticosteroid preparation (a large-bore needle, e.g., 19-gauge needle, is needed to aspirate the thick fluid). Surgical excision is sometimes necessary but is difficult, and recurrence is common. Most cysts, even if recurrent, respond to intermittent aspirations and injections. Some patients with Baker's cysts have internal derangements of the knee (i.e., chronic meniscal tear) that require specific therapy.

Tendinitis.   Most forms of tendinitis respond to rest, physical therapy, and anti-inflammatory medications. Corticosteroid injections into the areas of the large tendons about the knee are not recommended because of the risk of rupture.

Miscellaneous.   **Osgood-Schlatter disease** is treated with rest, discontinuation of athletic activity, and anti-inflammatory medications. Casting is useful in resistant cases.

Treatment of **osteochondritis dissecans** (usually arthroscopic removal of the loose body) is necessary only in those with persistent symptoms.

Osteonecrosis in the elderly or in those taking corticosteroids is initially treated with rest (to reduce stresses on the joint) and analgesics. Surgical treatment in advanced cases includes bone grafts or total joint replacement.

Cross-references: Psoriasis (Section 32), General Approach to Arthritic Symptoms (Section 107), Osteoarthritis (Section 119), Gout/Hyperuricemia (Section 120), Prepatellar and Olecrannon Bursitis (Section 121), Interpretation of Serologic Tests (Section 124), Principles of Physical Therapy (Section 126), Aspiration/Injection of the Knee (Section 130), Painful and Swollen Calf (Section 131).

REFERENCES

1. Raskas D, Lehman RC. Meniscal injuries in athletes: Pinpointing the diagnosis. Musculoskel Med 1988;00:20–28.

   Discusses normal knee anatomy, mechanism of meniscal injury, physical examination for detection of a tear, and management.

2. Rozing PM, Insall J, Nohne WH. Spontaneous osteonecrosis of the knee. J Bone Joint Surg 1980;62A:2–7.

   Details the diagnosis and treatment of spontaneous osteonecrosis in ninety affected knees, and the diagnostic utility of bone scans.

113 ANKLE AND FOOT PAIN

Symptom

GREGORY L. GARDNER

ETIOLOGY.   The most common causes of ankle and foot pain are listed in Table 113–1. Although not discussed here, the physician should always consider trauma in the differential diagnosis.

CLINICAL APPROACH.   With the patient standing as well as sitting, the examination should focus on the presence of swelling, deformity or tenderness, and the patient's footwear.

Arthritis.   In the foot, osteoarthritis affects either the first metatarsophalangeal joint (**hallux valgus**) or previously injured joints. Hallux valgus, which causes pain with walking, is especially common in women who wear narrow-

TABLE 113–1.   COMMON CONDITIONS CAUSING ANKLE AND FOOT PAIN

Arthritis	**Neuropathy**
Osteoarthritis	Tarsal tunnel syndrome
Rheumatoid arthritis	Peroneal neuropathy
Psoriatic arthritis	Morton's neuroma
Reiter's disease	Diabetic neuropathy
Gout	
Septic arthritis	**Miscellaneous**
	Pes planus
Tendinitis/Fasciitis	Stress fracture
Achilles tendinitis	Metatarsalgia
Posterior tibial tendinitis	
Plantar fasciitis	

toed shoes. During examination the first metatarsophalangeal joint is tender and protrudes medially, frequently with an adventitious bursa (bunion). Radiographs show typical osteoarthritic changes. **Hallux rigidus** describes a form of osteoarthritis that markedly limits extension of the great toe. **Rheumatoid arthritis** may produce pain and swelling in the ankle, subtalar, or metatarsophalangeal joints. **Psoriatic arthritis** may cause ankle arthritis, metatarsophalangeal joint arthritis, or "sausage digits" (diffuse phalangeal swelling from interphalangeal joint involvement). Characteristic psoriatic skin and nail changes are often present. **Reiter's disease** mimics psoriatic arthritis, but urethral discharge, conjunctivitis, oral ulcerations, characteristic skin changes, plantar fasciitis, or Achilles tendinitis are also found. **Gout** usually affects the first metatarsophalangeal joint and less often the ankle (see Section 120). Because **septic arthritis** may also involve the ankle, any acute arthritis at the ankle joint warrants arthrocentesis and culture of the joint fluid.

Tendinitis/Fasciitis. Conditions causing **Achilles tendinitis** include athletic overuse, the spondyloarthropathies (e.g., ankylosing spondylitis, Reiter's disease), rheumatoid arthritis, and, if the tendinitis is recurrent, familial hypercholesterolemia. Pain worsens with ankle dorsiflexion, and the tendon is tender and sometimes thickened. Inflammation that is maximal 2 to 6 cm distant from the tendon's insertion into the calcaneum is typical of overuse, while inflammation maximal at the insertion, a finding called *enthesopathy,* is characteristic of the spondyloarthropathies. Chronic tendinitis may lead to tendon rupture. Laboratory testing for lipid abnormalities is indicated in unexplained cases or if the family history suggests hyperlipidemia.

The **posterior tibialis** tendon lies posterior to the medial malleolus and may become inflamed after athletic overuse or with Reiter's disease or rheumatoid arthritis. Resisted inversion or passive eversion of the ankle provokes the pain, and localized swelling and tenderness may be present. Tendon rupture may occur, leading to progressive flat foot deformity.

Plantar fasciitis afflicts obese patients, those with flat feet, and, less often, patients with rheumatoid arthritis, Reiter's disease, or ankylosing spondylitis. Patients complain of painful soles, usually beginning immediately with walking. Dorsiflexion of the toes tenses the plantar fascia and may reveal localized tender points anywhere between the calcaneum and metatarsal heads. Radiographs may reveal heel spurs, but their significance is unknown because they are also commonly found in asymptomatic people.

Neuropathy. **Posterior tibial nerve entrapment** occurs at the tarsal tunnel, which is a space confined by the flexor retinaculum just posterior and inferior to the medial malleolus. Risk factors include valgus heel deformity and ankle fracture; women are more often affected than men. The patient typically complains of burning and numbness that extends from the toes and sole to the medial malleolus. Findings include a positive Tinel's sign (pressure over the nerve reproduces the pain) and diminished two-point discrimination and pinprick sensation. Electrodiagnostic studies are diagnostic.

Peroneal neuropathy, which causes a foot drop, may result from local compression or a systemic vasculitis (see Section 146, Entrapment Neuropathies).

Morton's neuroma is common in middle-aged women and results from entrapment of the interdigital nerve, usually between the third and fourth toes. Toe numbness and burning worsen with walking on hard surfaces or wearing tight shoes. Tenderness is maximal between, rather than upon, the metatarsal heads.

Peripheral neuropathy is discussed in Section 149.

Miscellaneous.   **Pes planus,** or flat feet, is usually inherited but may result from trauma, generalized hypermobility, or rupture of the posterior tibial tendon. Although usually asymptomatic, pes planus may cause pain in the soles during prolonged standing or walking. Examination reveals an absent longitudinal arch, valgus heel deviation, and a prominent navicular bone.

Stress fractures usually involve the shafts of the metatarsal bones, especially the second metatarsal neck, but may also occur at the calcaneum. Predisposing conditions include trauma or exercise (e.g., long marches of new military recruits), obesity, and osteoporosis. Localized pain and swelling may be present. Although initial radiographs are normal, films several weeks later may reveal callous formation. Bone scan is the most sensitive test for early diagnosis.

Metatarsalgia ("pain at the metatarsals") results from wearing high-heeled shoes, obesity, high-arched feet, rheumatoid arthritis, and trauma. Pain is aggravated by standing, and findings of metatarsal tenderness and calluses are common. Simple metatarsalgia must be distinguished from inflammatory arthritis of the metatarsophalangeal joint. Examination will uncover swelling or synovial hypertrophy in cases of inflammatory arthritis.

MANAGEMENT. *Arthritis.*   The treatment of hallux valgus includes using proper shoes (wide toe box, rigid soles, no high heels—some recommend good running shoes), pads to cushion the bunion, and placement of a rocker bar under the metatarsal portion of the shoe. The best candidates for surgical repair are patients with refractory pain despite conservative treatment, not those with isolated cosmetic deformity.

The treatment of inflammatory arthritis includes combinations of anti-inflammatory medication, steroid injections, and specific disease-modifying agents (see Section 107, General Approach to Arthritic Symptoms). Patients with septic arthritis require hospitalization, appropriate antibiotics, and consideration of surgical drainage.

The treatment of gout is described in Section 120.

Tendinitis/Fasciitis.   Achilles tendinitis is managed by rest, gentle stretching, and, especially with spondyloarthropathies, anti-inflammatory medication. Steroid injections are not recommended. Overuse Achilles tendinitis may require casting or splinting to rest the tendon. Refractory overuse tendinitis may improve after surgical stripping of the tendon.

Posterior tibialis tendinitis responds to rest, anti-inflammatory medications, and, in certain cases, splinting or local corticosteroid injection.

Plantar fasciitis usually responds to arch supports, soft-soled shoes, anti-inflammatory medications, and, in some patients, heel cup orthoses and local steroid injection. Less than 2% of patients require surgery.

Neuropathy.   Tarsal tunnel syndrome may resolve with corticosteroid injections and, if there is a valgus ankle deformity, shoe modifications or orthoses. Most patients, however, require surgical release. Management of peroneal neuropathy appears in Section 146.

Morton's neuroma may respond to shoes with a wide toe box, metatarsal bars, and local corticosteroid injections, or, if pain persists, surgical excision.

Miscellaneous.   Symptoms of pes planus may improve with the Thomas heel (a device that aligns the heel), firm shoes, and toe-grasping exercises that strengthen the intrinsic muscles. Some patients require rigid-molded inserts, which can be quite expensive.

Stress fractures are treated with rest, decreased weight bearing, weight loss if appropriate, and analgesic medication. Most fractures resolve within 6 to 8 weeks.

Metatarsalgia responds to metatarsal pads or bars placed behind the metatarsal heads, well-fitting shoes with a wide toe box, weight reduction, softening of the calluses, and toe-grasping exercises.

Cross-references: Corns and Calluses (Section 24), Psoriasis (Section 32), General Approach to Arthritic Symptoms (Section 107), Osteoarthritis (Section 119), Gout/Hyperuricemia (Section 120), Entrapment Neuropathies (Section 146), Peripheral Neuropathy (Section 149), Hyperlipidemia (Section 155).

REFERENCES

1.   Gerber L. Foot and ankle problems in the arthritides. J Musculoskel Med 1989.
     An excellent review article detailing the anatomy of the ankle and foot region, arthritides that affect this area, and treatment.

2.   Mann R. Acquired flatfoot in adults. Clin Orthop 1983;181:46–51.
     Reviews the major causes of flatfoot, including posterior tibial rupture.

3.   Nelen G, Martens M, Burssens A. Surgical treatment of chronic Achilles tendonitis. Am J Sports Med 1989;17:754–759.
     Review of a large series of patients with chronic idiopathic or overuse Achilles tendinitis. If conservative treatment failed, 90% had an excellent or good response to surgery.

4.   Sheon RP, Moskowitz RW, Goldberg VM. Ankle and foot. In: Soft Tissue Rheumatic Pain. Philadelphia, Lea & Febiger, 1982.
     A useful discussion of common soft tissue foot and ankle problems, with an emphasis on treatment.

114 RESTLESS LEGS SYNDROME

Symptom

STEVEN R. McGEE

EPIDEMIOLOGY. Patients with restless legs syndrome experience creeping, aching, or writhing sensations in their lower extremities; the sensations appear only during rest (usually at night) and subside immediately after movement of the legs. Estimates of prevalence are 2% to 5%.

ETIOLOGY. The cause of restless legs syndrome is unknown, although many investigators attribute it to an underactive dopaminergic system. Strong associations occur with iron deficiency anemia, pregnancy, rheumatoid arthritis, and uremia.

CLINICAL APPROACH. The clinician should exclude anemia, confirm that the neurologic examination is normal, and consider withdrawing any medication that has been associated with the development of restless legs syndrome (neuroleptics, phenytoin, methsuximide, and antidepressants).

MANAGEMENT. Carbamazepine, levodopa plus benserazide (a peripheral decarboxylase inhibitor), bromocriptine, and clonazepam all are superior to placebo in randomized double-blind trials of patients with restless legs syndrome. Forty percent of patients treated with carbamazepine, however, had unwanted side effects, despite less than 5 weeks of treatment.

The clinician should reassure patients with restless legs syndrome that the condition spontaneously waxes and wanes over years, and may remit for long periods. In the very few patients with severe and refractory symptoms, clonazepam or levodopa preparations may be the treatments with the fewest side effects.

Cross-references: Chronic Renal Failure (Section 181), Anemia (Section 201), Diagnosis of Pregnancy (Section 209).

REFERENCES

1. Gibb WRG, Lees AJ. The restless legs syndrome. Postgrad Med J 1986;62:329–333.
   Reviews clinical features, differential diagnosis, and treatment.
2. McGee SR. Restless legs syndrome. JAMA 1991;265:3014.
   Concise, up-to-date review.
3. Von Scheele C. Levodopa in restless legs. Lancet 1986;2:426–427.
   Of twenty patients, seventeen preferred levodopa plus benserazide to placebo.

115 MUSCLE CRAMPS

Symptom

STEVEN R. McGEE

ETIOLOGY. Painful skeletal muscle contractions, or cramps, result from several distinct clinical entities: true cramp, contracture, tetany, and dystonia (Table 115–1).

Isolated bursts of motor neuron action potentials characterize true cramps. The most common example, ordinary cramp or "charley horse," usually develops while the subject is resting at night, may be accompanied by fasciculations, affects calf and ventral foot muscles unilaterally, and is relieved by muscle stretching. Lower motor neuron diseases may cause weakness, atrophy, fasciculations as well as true cramps in affected muscles. Dehydration also produces true cramps, usually associated with hyponatremia; examples include overdiuresis, hemodialysis (excessive ultrafiltration), or heavy muscular activity in high environmental temperatures (heat cramps).

Contractures, in contrast to true cramps, are uncommon, develop not at rest but during exercise, and are characterized by electromyographic silence during the muscle spasm. In metabolic myopathies such as McArdle's disease, exer-

---

TABLE 115–1. MUSCLE CRAMPS: ETIOLOGY

True Cramp—Motor Unit Hyperactivity
Ordinary cramps
Lower motor neuron disease
Hemodialysis
Saline depletion (e.g., heat cramps)
Drug-induced
    Nifedipine
    Beta-agonists (terbutaline, salbutamol)

Contracture—Electrically Silent
Metabolic myopathy (e.g., McArdle's disease)
Thyroid disease

Tetany—Motor Unit and Sensory Hyperactivity
Hypocalcemia
Hypomagnesemia
Respiratory alkalosis
Hypokalemia, hyperkalemia

Dystonia
Occupational cramp
Phenothiazines, butyrophenones, metoclopramide

Source: McGee SR. Muscle cramps. Arch Intern Med 1990;150:511–518. Adapted with permission.

cise depletes available energy stores more rapidly than normal. Because muscle requires energy to relax, contracture occurs. Hypothyroid and hyperthyroid patients may experience either contractures or true cramps.

Tetany consists of characteristic distal extremity muscle cramps (carpopedal spasm) associated with paresthesias and positive Trousseau's and Chovstek's signs. Causes appear in Table 115–1.

Dystonia produces sustained postures, not always painful, which result from simultaneous contraction of agonistic and antagonistic muscles. After years of practice, musicians, writers, and typists, among others, may develop muscle spasms and incoordination, all focal dystonias, during attempts to perform their occupation-specific fine-motor tasks. These occupational cramps may ruin careers. Focal dystonias also occur during treatment with antipsychotic and antidopaminergic medications.

CLINICAL APPROACH.   Symptoms confused with cramps are myotonia, which is a painless disorder marked by percussion myotonia on examination, and claudication, which, although described by patients as cramps, does not produce palpable hardening of the muscle. The diagnosis of cramps depends largely on the patient interview: the nocturnal calf cramp relieved by stretching of the muscle (ordinary cramp), the steelworker's arm cramp (heat cramps), the asthmatic's cramps provoked by inhalant treatments (beta-agonist cramps), or the exercise-induced cramp associated with dark urine (metabolic myopathy). Physical examination emphasizes the search for dehydration, thyroid disease, tetany (Trousseau's and Chovstek's signs), and neurologic disease. If the condition is still undiagnosed, appropriate laboratory tests include electrolyte calcium, and magnesium determinations and, if suggested by signs and symptoms, thyroid function tests.

MANAGEMENT.   The physician should withdraw responsible medications, if possible, and treat underlying fluid, electrolyte, or endocrine abnormalities. Patients with newly suspected lower motor neuron disease (weakness and atrophy), dystonia unrelated to medication, or suspected contracture should be referred to a neurologist.

Muscle stretching exercises performed periodically during the day may reduce ordinary nocturnal cramps. In double-blind placebo-controlled trials, quinine effectively relieved ordinary cramps, sometimes with prolonged effects after a single dose (200–300 mg PO). Adverse reactions to quinine, uncommon with the recommended dose, include cinchonism (nausea, vomiting, tinnitus), hypoglycemia, immune thrombocytopenia, and retinal toxicity.

Simple writing aids may benefit patients with writer's cramps.

Cross-references: Muscular Weakness (Section 139), Common Thyroid Disorders (Section 156), Chronic Renal Failure (Section 181), Electrolyte Abnormalities (Section 184).

REFERENCES

1. Daniell HW. Simple cure for nocturnal leg cramps. N Engl J Med 1979;301:216.
    Forty-four patients with nocturnal calf cramps were cured after 1 week of calf-stretching exercises performed three times per day.

2. Fung M, Holbrook JH. Placebo-controlled trial of quinine therapy for nocturnal leg cramps. West J Med 1989;151:42–44.
    In a double-blind crossover trial in eight patients, quinine reduced cramp severity and frequency.

3. Layzer RB. Motor unit hyperactivity states. In Vinken PF, Bruyn GW, Eds. Handbook of Clinical Neurology. North-Holland, Amsterdam, 1980, vol. 41, pp. 295–316.
    Encyclopedic review that includes descriptions of exotic cause of cramps such as tetanus, strychnine poisoning, stiff-man syndrome, and black widow spider bite.

4. McGee SR. Muscle cramps. Arch Intern Med 1990;150:511–518.
    Thorough overview of cramping conditions and treatments.

116 PAGET'S DISEASE

Problem

DENNIS ANDRESS

EPIDEMIOLOGY/ETIOLOGY.   Paget's disease is characterized by localized areas of enhanced bone turnover, which lead to enlargement and vascularization of compact bone and increased susceptibility to deformity and fracture. Although the etiology is unknown, a viral infection of the bone-resorbing cells (osteoclasts) is suspected. It is more commonly observed in Europe, North America, and Australia, with clinical manifestations usually beginning by the fifth decade. In the United States, Paget's disease is present in 4% of those over 45 years and in 8% of those over 80 years of age. There is a slight male predominance.

SYMPTOMS AND SIGNS.   Most patients are asymptomatic, especially with early disease. The most common symptom is localized pain over affected bone. Bowing deformities of the femur or tibia cause pain from either secondary arthritis or abnormal gait and consequent mechanical stresses. Back pain may be due to vertebral compression fractures, lumbar spinal stenosis, or degenerative changes of the spine. Motor and sensory changes may occur with spinal involvement, while cranial nerve palsies or headache occur in 33% with skull involvement. Long bone involvement produces localized tenderness and warmth. Vertebral disease may cause kyphosis. Extreme skull involvement may produce bone softening and basal flattening that rarely leads to brain stem compression.

CLINICAL APPROACH.   In asymptomatic patients the only clue to Paget's disease may be the incidental finding of an elevated serum alkaline phosphatase level. When suspected, pagetic bone is most easily identified with scintigraphy. Because bone scans are nonspecific, it is necessary to obtain a radiograph of areas positive on bone scan to identify the characteristic changes. Occasionally, metastatic bone disease becomes a consideration and can only be ruled out by biopsy.

MANAGEMENT.   Indications for treatment in asymptomatic patients include a serum alkaline phosphatase level more than three times the upper normal limit. Treatment at this stage prevents severe and prolonged bone resorption and symptoms. In the United States, approved agents for treatment include etidronate and calcitonin. Both are effective, but etidronate is usually preferred because of oral administration and few side effects; the recommended dose is 5 mg/kg/day for 6 months, followed by no treatment for 6 months to prevent osteomalacia. Aminohydroxypropylidene will likely be the diphosphonate of choice once it has been approved in the United States. Calcitonin requires self-injection subcutaneously and causes nausea in 15% but is the preferred choice in severe disease of weight-bearing bones. In 20% of patients, resistance to calcitonin develops. A combination of calcitonin and etidronate may be required in resistant cases.

FOLLOW-UP.   An acceptable biochemical response is a 50% reduction in the serum alkaline phosphatase level. Declines in urinary hydroxyproline excretion precede the change in the alkaline phosphatase level. Etidronate has a more long-lasting effect; calcitonin's effect is usually lost within 1 year. Both forms of therapy will ameliorate bone pain in the majority of patients but will not correct bone deformities or improve pain from secondary arthritis. Potential long-term problems include fractures, which usually heal normally, and neoplastic degeneration of pagetic bone (<1% incidence).

Cross-references: Low Back Pain (Section 108), Hip Pain (Section 110).

REFERENCES

1. Harinck HIJ, Bijvoet OLM, Vellenga CR, et al. Relation between signs and symptoms in Paget's disease of bone. Q J Med 1986;58:133–151.
    Good review.

2. Harinck HIJ, Papapoulos SE, Blanksma HJ, et al. Paget's disease of bone: Early and late responses to three different modes of treatment with aminohydroxypropylidene bisphosphonate (APD). Br Med J 1987;295:1301–1305.
    Short-term (10-day) intravenous APD appears to be as effective as long-term oral treatment.

117 OSTEOPOROSIS

Problem

DENNIS ANDRESS

EPIDEMIOLOGY/ETIOLOGY. Osteoporosis is defined clinically as a reduced bone mass that results in bone fragility and fractures. Approximately 30% of women have one or more fractures following menopause; 25% of these fractures involve the distal radius (Colles fracture), 50% the vertebrae, and 25% the hip. One-third of all women and 17% of all men suffer a hip fracture before age 90, and 20% of those who sustain a fracture die within 3 months of the event. The major cause of osteoporosis in women is estrogen deficiency (postmenopausal, oophorectomy, prolonged amenorrhea). In women and men, osteoporosis also results from age-related declines in bone cell function. Risk factors for osteoporosis include caucasian or Asian race, family history of osteoporosis, small body frame, chronic low calcium intake, excessive alcohol intake, and cigarette smoking. Clearly defined secondary causes of osteoporosis include hyperparathyroidism, hyperthyroidism, Cushing's syndrome, multiple myeloma, thyroid replacement therapy, and corticosteroid therapy.

SYMPTOMS AND SIGNS. Prior to the occurrence of a fracture, osteoporosis is asymptomatic. Although most fractures are painful, 35% of vertebral fractures are asymptomatic and are manifested only by loss of height or kyphosis (dowager's hump).

CLINICAL APPROACH. General screening of all asymptomatic women with measurements of bone density is not appropriate. Such measurements are advocated, however, for the following groups of patients: (1) estrogen-deficient women, (2) patients with vertebral abnormalities or roentgenographic osteopenia, (3) patients receiving glucocorticoids, and (4) patients with asymptomatic primary hyperparathyroidism. Spinal bone density measurements are also appropriate for patients with a vertebral fracture. Dual-photon absorptiometry, CT, and dual-energy radiography all measure the bone density of the spine or hip and can be used to diagnose osteoporosis (i.e., bone density > 1 standard deviation (SD) below normal mean bone density). Dual-energy x-ray absorptiometry (cost: $75–$150) appears to be superior because of its precision, accuracy, and low radiation exposure.

In patients with documented osteoporosis, routine laboratory tests include determinations of serum calcium (for hyperparathyroidism), serum thyroid hormone, serum protein electrophoresis (for multiple myeloma), testosterone (to document male hypogonadism), and alkaline phosphatase (to rule out osteomalacia). A normal serum 25-hydroxyvitamin D level excludes the most common form of osteomalacia. Bone biopsy (following tetracycline labeling) is necessary whenever osteomalacia is suspected (e.g., in subjects with skeletal pain and elevated alkaline phosphatase levels, with or without hypocalcemia).

MANAGEMENT. The initial management of vertebral fractures consists of analgesic therapy and bed rest. Prolonged bed rest increases bone resorption and is discouraged. A back brace may help reduce pain in some patients.

The recommended daily calcium intake for all patients is 1000 to 1200 mg. If calcium supplements are required, calcium citrate provides optimal gastrointestinal absorption. Other preventive measures include regular moderate exercise (30 minutes of walking three times per week) and avoidance of medications that may precipitate falling.

In mild to moderate osteoporosis (bone mass 1–2 SD below the normal mean), antiresorptive agents such as estrogens and calcitonin prevent further declines in bone mass. Oral estrogen, 0.625 mg/day, is recommended soon after menopause and for an 8- to 10-year minimum duration, with annual cervical Papanicolaou smears to monitor for the development of neoplasia (see Section 164, Menopausal Symptoms). The addition of cyclical progesterone produces menstrual cycles and appears to decrease the risk of estrogen-induced endometrial cancer, but may negate the cardiovascular benefit of estrogen therapy. Calcitonin, though effective, has not been widely accepted because of the need for frequent subcutaneous injections. The future availability of nasally administered calcitonin may make it the preferred choice when estrogen therapy is contraindicated (e.g., in subjects with a history of estrogen-dependent tumor or endometrial cancer, venous embolic disease, fibrocystic breast disease, or abnormal liver function).

For patients with severe bone demineralization (bone mass > 2 SD below the normal mean), effective restoration of bone mass is possible only through long-term treatment with agents not yet approved by the FDA. These agents, which include sodium fluoride and the diphosphonate, etidronate, should be given intermittently over years only by clinicians experienced in their use. The apparent effectiveness and virtual lack of adverse effects may make etidronate the future treatment of choice for severe osteoporosis.

FOLLOW-UP. Although bone density measurements at yearly intervals may be helpful in assessing treatment efficacy, and especially in identifying rapid bone loss, follow-up guidelines are lacking. Ongoing treatment studies utilizing dual energy x-ray should soon provide specific follow-up protocols. In patients receiving calcium supplements, twice yearly documentation of urinary calcium excretion below 250 mg/day should prevent nephrocalcinosis and renal stones.

Cross-references: Periodic Health Assessment (Section 7), Low Back Pain (Section 108), Hip Pain (Section 110), Common Thyroid Disorders (Section 156), Menopausal Symptoms (Section 164).

REFERENCES

1. Kiel DP, Felson DT, Anderson JJ, et al. Hip fracture and the use of estrogens in postmenopausal women: The Framingham Study. N Engl J Med 1987; 317:1169–1174.

   Women who began taking estrogens within 4 years of menopause were protected against subsequent hip fracture.

2. Melton LJ, Eddy DM, Johnston CC Jr. Screening for osteoporosis. Ann Intern Med 1990;112:516–528.

   Extensive review of the clinical utility of bone mass measurements as a screening method. Mass screening is not recommended because treatment guidelines have not been generally accepted.

3. Munk-Jensen N, Pors Nielsen S, Obel EB, et al. Reversal of postmenopausal vertebral bone loss by oestrogen and progestogen: A double blind placebo controlled study. Br Med J 1988;296:1150–1152.

   Sequential or continuous administration of estrogen and progestogen for 1 year reversed vertebral bone loss.

4. Riggs BL, Hodgson SF, O'Fallon WM, et al. Effect of fluoride treatment on the fracture rate in postmenopausal women with osteoporosis. N Engl J Med 1990;322:802–809.

   Sodium fluoride, 75 mg/day for 3 years continuously, did not decrease the vertebral fracture rate despite significant increases in spine density. Controversy exists regarding the high dose and continuous mode of treatment.

5. Watts NB, Harris ST, Genant HK, et al. Intermittent cyclical etidronate treatment of postmenopausal osteoporosis. N Engl J Med 1990;323:73–79.

   Etidronate taken orally for 2 weeks every 13 weeks caused increased spinal bone density and decreased vertebral fractures in 1 to 2 years without significant side effects.

118 POLYMYALGIA RHEUMATICA AND TEMPORAL ARTERITIS

Problem

GREGORY L. GARDNER

POLYMYALGIA RHEUMATICA

EPIDEMIOLOGY.   Both polymyalgia rheumatica and temporal arteritis primarily affect elderly patients, with a mean age at onset of 70 years. These conditions are rare before the age of 50, affect women more than men, and, although data are incomplete, are rare in blacks. The reported annual incidence of polymyalgia rheumatica is 30 to 50 cases per 100,000 per year; the prevalence in predominantly white populations is 500 per 100,000.

SYMPTOMS AND SIGNS.   Patients with polymyalgia rheumatica complain of pain and stiffness (often profound and worse in the morning) of the neck, shoulders, thighs, and hips. Fatigue, weight loss, and lassitude may accompany the pain and stiffness, rendering simple tasks such as getting out of bed extremely difficult. Patients often recall the exact day that symptoms began.

Physical examination is usually unremarkable; muscle weakness is *not* found. As many as 20% of patients have synovitis (usually transient) of the shoulders, wrists, or knees.

CLINICAL APPROACH.   Because other causes of proximal muscle symptoms include hypothyroidism, polymyositis, early rheumatoid arthritis in the elderly, and fibromyalgia, important initial laboratory tests are the erythrocyte sedimentation rate (ESR), rheumatoid factor and creatine phosphokinase (CPK) determinations, and thyroid function tests. In polymyalgia rheumatica, the ESR is very high, often exceeding 100 mm/hr, though rare cases with a normal ESR exist. Other laboratory abnormalities seen in polymyalgia rheumatica are anemia, thrombocytosis, and elevated liver alkaline phosphatase levels. Clinicians should question all patients with suspected polymyalgia rheumatica about symptoms suggestive of temporal arteritis (see below).

MANAGEMENT.   Most patients with polymyalgia rheumatica respond dramatically in 1 to 2 days to 10 to 20 mg/day of prednisone, although some require up to 1 week of treatment before improvement becomes noticeable. The diagnosis should be questioned if there is no response after 1 week. After 1 month of treatment, the prednisone dose is gradually reduced to a maintenance dose of 5 to 7.5 mg/day. Most patients need 2 years of treatment, although some relapse even after as long as 10 years of prednisone.

Any patient who takes more 7.5 mg/day of prednisone for 6 months or more is at increased risk for steroid-induced osteoporosis. Such patients should take calcium supplements (800–1500 mg/day). Many authorities also prescribe vitamin D supplements if the 24-hour urinary excretion of calcium remains low despite calcium supplementation. Patients who receive vitamin D supplementation should be carefully monitored for hypercalcemia and hypercalciuria.

FOLLOW-UP.   Patients who fail to initially respond to corticosteroids or who become steroid dependent should be referred to a rheumatologist. Steroid-dependent patients may be candidates for methotrexate.

TEMPORAL ARTERITIS

EPIDEMIOLOGY.   Temporal arteritis, a giant cell arteritis of the medium to large arteries, is less common than polymyalgia rheumatica, with an incidence of 2 to 18 cases per 100,000 and a prevalence of 234 per 100,000. Although the specific relationship is unclear, most authorities regard temporal arteritis and polymyalgia rheumatica as different manifestations of the same disease process.

SYMPTOMS AND SIGNS.   Inflammation of the extracranial arteries causes headache, scalp tenderness, jaw claudication, and visual symptoms (diplopia, ptosis, and transient or permanent visual loss). Inflammation of the vessels of the aortic arch, although infrequent, leads to upper extremity claudication, transient ischemic attacks, or strokes. Polymyalgia rheumatica accompanies temporal arteritis in 40% to 60% of cases.

Physical findings may include prominent temporal arteries, absent temporal artery pulsations, or bruits over large vessels, especially of the upper extremities. Brushing the temporal scalp may elicit tenderness. Eye examination is usually normal unless ischemia has occurred.

CLINICAL APPROACH. The ESR in temporal arteritis is frequently very high (often 100 mm/hr), although cases with less impressive elevations exist. The clinician should suspect temporal arteritis in any person over 50 years of age with an unexplained elevation of the ESR and a new headache or transient visual changes. When temporal arteritis is suspected, the best diagnostic test is temporal artery biopsy, an outpatient procedure in which a specimen 2 to 4 cm long is removed from the symptomatic side. Multiple pathologic sections are necessary because the inflammation may involve only small isolated portions of the vessel. If the biopsy results are normal but temporal arteritis is still likely, the other side should be biopsied.

MANAGEMENT. When temporal arteritis is strongly suspected, immediate treatment with prednisone while awaiting biopsy is appropriate. Treatment for as long as 1 week does not alter the biopsy results. High doses of prednisone (60 mg/day in divided doses) are initially used to prevent blindness, a complication that may affect patients suddenly and without warning. Some authorities believe that 1 month of high-dose prednisone precludes future relapses.

After 1 month of treatment, the prednisone dosage is slowly reduced over 6 months to 5 to 7.5 mg/day and is continued at this level as recommended above for patients with polymyalgia rheumatica. Once the daily dose has been reduced to 30 mg, it can be consolidated to a single daily dose. With both polymyalgia rheumatica and temporal arteritis, the best clinical guide to steroid dosing is the patient's symptoms and signs, not the ESR. Although patients without visual symptoms may respond to lower doses of prednisone, this is under investigation and not yet generally recommended.

Recommendations for calcium and vitamin D supplementation are the same as for patients with polymyalgia rheumatica. Other potential complications of large doses of corticosteroids include cataracts, infection, and hyperglycemia.

Cross-references: General Approach to Arthritic Symptoms (Section 107), Interpretation of Serologic Tests (Section 124), Muscular Weakness (Section 139), Headache (Section 140).

REFERENCES

1. Delecoeuillerie G, Joly P, Cohen De Lara A, Paolaggi JB. Polymyalgia rheumatica and temporal arteritis: A retrospective analysis of prognostic features and different corticosteroid regimens. Ann Rheum Dis 1988;47:733–739.

In a large retrospective study, patients with symptoms of polymyalgia rheumatica but without symptoms of temporal arteritis responded to low-dose prednisone even when the temporal biopsy results were positive. The authors suggest that biopsy is unnecessary in this setting and that temporal arteritis without visual symptoms may respond to lower doses of steroids (see text).

2. Healey LA. Rheumatoid arthritis in the elderly. Clin Rheum Dis 1986;12:173–179.

The clinical presentation of elderly patients with seronegative rheumatoid arthritis was similar to that of patients with polymyalgia rheumatica. They responded well to low doses of steroids.

3. Lauter SA, Reece D, Avioli LV. Polymyalgia rheumatica. Arch Intern Med 1985;145:1273–1275.

A concise and well-written summary of polymyalgia rheumatica and temporal arteritis.

4. Sonnenblick M, Nesher G, Rosin A. Nonclassical organ involvement in temporal arteritis. Semin Arthritis Rheum 1989;19:183–190.

Article reviewing involvement of unusual organ systems. The hepatic alkaline phosphatase level was elevated in up to 60% of patients with temporal arteritis/polymyalgia rheumatica.

119 OSTEOARTHRITIS

Problem

GREGORY L. GARDNER

EPIDEMIOLOGY.   In the United States, approximately 60 million people have osteoarthritis. The prevalence rises sharply after the age of 50; by age 60, 50% of people have clinical osteoarthritis and 80% have some radiologic evidence of osteoarthritis. Not all radiographic changes are symptomatic, however; some studies suggest that only 9% of men and 25% of women with moderate to severe radiographic osteoarthritis of the distal interphalangeal joints report symptoms, while 56% and 80%, respectively, with radiographically demonstrated knee involvement have symptoms.

Risk factors depend on the joint affected and include a family history of hand osteoarthritis (especially in women), prior congenital or acquired hip abnormalities (hip arthritis), and obesity and previous trauma (knee arthritis).

A simple classification of osteoarthritis appears in Table 119–1.

SYMPTOMS AND SIGNS.   Primary osteoarthritis most commonly affects the hands (distal interphalangeal joints, proximal interphalangeal joints, first carpometacarpal joints), followed by the cervical spine, lumbar spine, hips, knees, and first metatarsophalangeal joints. Pain occurs with use of the joint and is associated with mild morning stiffness (less than 15 minutes) that is most pronounced after rest ("gelling"). Severe disease may lead to rest pain or nocturnal

TABLE 119–1. CLASSIFICATION OF OSTEOARTHRITIS

Primary
Localized
Generalized (three or more joint areas affected)
Erosive (inflammatory osteoarthritis of the hands)

Secondary
Trauma
Congenital anomaly
  Perthes disease
  Congenital hip dysplasia
Metabolic
  Calcium pyrophosphate dihydrate deposition disease
  Ochronosis
  Hemachromatosis
  Acromegaly
  Gout
Post-inflammatory arthritis
  Rheumatoid arthritis
  Infection
Other
  Avascular necrosis
  Charcot joint

pain. Loose bodies or degenerative meniscal tears in the knee may cause symptoms of locking or catching.

Some patients may initially notice asymptomatic deformity of the hand, especially at the distal interphalangeal joints (Heberden's nodes), less commonly at the proximal interphalangeal joints (Bouchard's nodes). Knee effusions are common, while erosive osteoarthritis may cause tender swelling of hand joints. Osteoarthritis of the spine may cause compression of the spinal cord (spinal stenosis) or nerve roots.

CLINICAL APPROACH.   The diagnosis of primary osteoarthritis depends on (1) involvement of characteristic joints, (2) morning stiffness that is brief (prolonged stiffness suggests other active inflammatory forms of joint disease), (3) laboratory data that are normal [normal ESR, negative rheumatoid factor (RF) assay], and (4) radiographs that are characteristic for osteoarthritis (nonuniform joint space narrowing, osteophytes, bone sclerosis, and subchondral cysts).

Rheumatoid arthritis, psoriatic arthritis, and tophaceous gout may all affect the proximal and distal interphalangeal joints. Calcium pyrophosphate deposition (CPPD) disease, a secondary form of osteoarthritis, should be considered when osteoarthritis affects joints not typically involved by primary osteoarthritis. Radiographs of joints with CPPD often reveal chondrocalcinosis (linear calcification of the cartilage parallel to the underlying bone); aspirated joint fluid shows positively birefringent crystals when viewed with compensated polarized microscopy.

MANAGEMENT.   The most effective medications for osteoarthritis are the nonsteroidal anti-inflammatory agents (NSAIDs) (Table 119–2). All NSAIDs

TABLE 119–2. NONSTEROIDAL ANTI-INFLAMMATORY DRUGS

Drug	Dose Range (mg/day)	Divided Doses (No./day)	Comments	Cost[1]
Salicylates				
Aspirin	2400–6000	2–4	Tinnitus	0.06
Salicylsalicylic acid (Disalcid)	2000–5000	2–4	Tinnitus	0.38
Diflusinal	500–1000	2	Use reduced dose in elderly; longer half-life with higher doses	1.60
Propionic acids				
Ibuprofen	600–3200	3–4		0.10
Naproxen	500–1500	2–3		1.26
Fenoprofen	1200–3200	3–4	Interstitial nephritis	1.30
Ketoprofen	100–400	3–4		1.74
Flurbiprofen	200–300	2–3		1.92
Indoleacetic acids				
Indomethacin	50–200	3–4	Headache	0.06
Sulindac	300–400	2	Relative renal sparing?	1.06
Tolmetin	800–1600	3–4	Rare anaphylaxis	1.50
Pyrazoles				
Phenylbutazone	200–400	1–3	Blood dyscrasias	0.11
Fenamates				
Meclofenamate	200–400	4	Diarrhea in up to 15%	1.45
Diclofenac	100–200	2–4		1.50
Oxicams				
Piroxicam	10–20	1	Rash	1.95

[1]Daily cost for lower dose range listed, generic if available; average wholesale price, 1991 *Drug Topics Red Book.*

except for the nonacetylated salicylates have potential gastrointestinal toxicity (dyspepsia, gastric ulceration or perforation) and renal toxicity (fluid retention, renal insufficiency, renal failure). Low-dose tricyclic antidepressants such as amitriptyline may benefit patients with nocturnal pain.

Intra-articular steroids, especially when injected in the first carpometacarpal joint, knee, or ankle joints, may result in prolonged benefit. Injections more frequent than every 3 to 4 months, however, should be avoided because they may hasten joint destruction. The usual dose of triamcinolone or equivalent is 30 to 40 mg in the knee, 20 to 30 mg in an ankle, and 10 mg in the small joints of the hand. There is presently no role for oral steroids in the treatment of osteoarthritis.

Physical therapy maintains range of motion and muscle strength around affected joints. In addition, physical therapy manages the painful surrounding bursae and tendons, especially the pes anserine bursae at the medial knee, that are affected by the altered joint mechanics of osteoarthritis. Use of a cane in the hand opposite the affected hip or knee can improve walking.

Joint replacement surgery should be considered in those with refractory pain or markedly altered joint mechanics. In the knee, arthroscopy can remove loose bodies or trim degenerative menisci that may be limiting motion.

Cross-references: General Approach to Arthritic Symptoms (Section 107), Low Back Pain (Section 108), Hip Pain (Section 110), Wrist and Hand Pain (Section 111), Knee Pain (Section 112), Ankle and Foot Pain (Section 113), Gout/Hyperuricemia (Section 120), Principles of Physical Therapy (Section 126), Aspiration/Injection of the Knee (Section 130).

REFERENCES

1. Brandt KD. Osteoarthritis. Clin Geriatr Med 1988;4:279–293.
   The most important theories concerning the pathogenesis of osteoarthritis.

2. Davis MA. Epidemiology of osteoarthritis. Clin Geriatr Med 1988;4:241–255.
   Risk factors for and the natural history of osteoarthritis.

3. Hammerman D. The biology of osteoarthritis. N Engl J Med 1989;320:1322–1330.
   Biology of normal articular cartilage and the changes that occur with osteoarthritis.

4. Paulus HE, Furst DE. Aspirin and other nonsteroidal antiinflammatory drugs. In McCarty D, Ed. Arthritis and Allied Conditions. Lea & Febiger, Philadelphia,1989, pp. 507–543.
   Outlines the mechanism of action of NSAIDs and discusses each NSAID individually, detailing their reported adverse reactions.

120 GOUT/HYPERURICEMIA

Problem

DOUGLAS S. PAAUW

EPIDEMIOLOGY.   Approximately 1.5% of the population experiences an attack of gout. Gout is far more common in men (90% of cases). The average age at onset for men is 48. Women usually do not develop gout until after menopause (average age, 54). Most patients (94%) who develop gout have elevated uric acid levels (hyperuricemia). Patients who are not taking drugs that raise serum uric acid and have a level between 7 and 8 mg/dl have a 20% risk of developing gout, while those with levels over 9 mg/dl have a 90% risk.

Of the many drugs that elevate uric acid, diuretics and alcohol are the most common (Table 120–1). Uncommonly, lead exposure due to drinking "moonshine" produces arthritis (saturnine gout).

SYMPTOMS AND SIGNS.   In 90% of cases, the initial attack of gout is acute, extremely painful, and affects a single joint. Polyarticular involvement is more

TABLE 120–1.   DRUGS THAT INCREASE SERUM URIC ACID

Ethanol	Cyclosporin
Nicotinic acid	Ethambutol
Diuretics	Pyrazinamide
Thiazides	Salicylates (low dose, e.g., <600 mg/day)
Furosemide	
Chlorthalidone	
Amiloride	
Triamterene	

common in women. An attack frequently follows minor trauma, with symptoms often beginning at night as bedsheets pull against the toe and produce the first awareness of pain. More than 50% of initial attacks affect the first metatarsophalangeal joint (podagra). Other sites commonly involved are the knees, metatarsophalangeal joints, tarsal joints, arch of the foot, and ankles. In patients with osteoarthritis, gout can occur in Heberden's nodes.

Periarticular erythema and edema are common. Dramatic erythema and warmth as well as low-grade fever and chills may accompany the attack and lead to a mistaken diagnosis of cellulitis or septic arthritis. Desquamation of periarticular skin frequently occurs as the attack resolves.

CLINICAL APPROACH.   Before instituting therapy, especially long-term preventive therapy, the clinician should establish the diagnosis of gout by finding monosodium urate crystals in tophi or synovial fluid leukocytes. Urate crystals are found in 85% of patients with acute gout. The crystals appear yellow under a polarized light microscope with a red compensator when oriented parallel to the axis of the compensator (negatively birefringent).

Because it may be technically difficult to tap a small joint such as the metatarsophalangeal or tarsal joint, a presumptive diagnosis of gout may be made if these joints are affected and the patient is hyperuricemic.

MANAGEMENT.   NSAIDs are effective for acute gouty arthritis (Table 120–2). Indomethacin is the most widely used. These medications should be avoided in patients with congestive heart failure, cirrhosis, or renal disease. Colchicine is effective but produces adverse gastrointestinal effects in 70% to 80% of patients taking the drug for acute gout. Colchicine should be avoided in patients with renal or hepatic insufficiency. Prednisone is an effective alternative for patients with monarticular gout and contraindications to NSAIDS and colchicine, as are intra-articular steroid injections (e.g., aqueous or repository methylprednisone, 20–40 mg). Drugs that lower uric acid levels should not be started until 4 to 6 weeks after an initial attack, as they may prolong or worsen the attack or precipitate a relapse.

Treatment of elevated uric acid levels should not be considered unless the patient has tophi, nephrolithiasis, or recurrent gouty arthritis. The cause of hyperuricemia should be sought and any drugs that elevate the uric acid level should be eliminated if possible (see Table 120–1). A 24-hour urine collection

TABLE 120–2.   TREATMENT OF GOUT: ACUTE ATTACKS AND PROPHYLAXIS

Clinical Setting	Drug	Dose and Administration	Cost $ (per Pill)[1]
Acute Gout	Indomethacin	25–50 mg t.i.d. PO	0.05 (25 mg)
	Ibuprofen	800 mg t.i.d. PO	0.20 (800 mg)
	Naproxen	750 mg followed by 250 mg t.i.d. PO	0.63 (250 mg)
	Sulindac	200 mg b.i.d.	0.80 (200 mg)
	Colchicine	0.6 mg PO q.h. up to 12 doses until relief or diarrhea/nausea	0.04 (0.6 mg)
	Prednisone	30–50 mg q.d. with rapid taper (over 10 days)	0.05 (10 mg)
	Triamcinolone hexacetamide	5–20 mg injected into joint	7.77 (20 mg)
Prophylaxis	Probenecid	Begin 250 mg b.i.d. increase to 1–3 g/day	2.40[3]
	Sulfinpyrazone	100 mg b.i.d.	7.80[3]
	Allopurinol	300 mg q.d.[2]	3.00[3]
	Colchicine	0.6 mg b.i.d.	2.40[3]

[1]Average wholesale price, 1991 *Drug Topics Red Book.*
[2]Dosage should be reduced in renal insufficiency.
[3]Cost per month.

measures uric acid production (normal 24-hour urate excretion is 600 mg). The vast majority of hyperuricemic patients are underexcretors of uric acid who respond well to the uricuouric agents probenecid and sulfinpyrazone. These drugs, however, should not be used in overproducers (indicated by the presence of tophi or a 24-hour urate excretion > 600 mg), in the presence of impaired renal function (creatinine > 1.5), or in patients with nephrolithiasis. Allopurinol effectively treats both overproducers and underexcretors of uric acid by decreasing uric acid production but can cause an exfoliative dermatitis that is occasionally life-threatening. Uric acid–lowering drugs should be started while the patient is still taking colchicine or an NSAID, and the anti-inflammatory agent should be continued for an additional 2 to 4 weeks to prevent a gouty flare. Treatment of asymptomatic hyperuricemia is rarely indicated.

Occasionally the clinician will encounter a patient who has been started on a uric acid–lowering drug without having had uric acid crystals demonstrated in joint aspirates. It is reasonable to continue the drug if the patient has a history of hyperuricemia and recurrent monarticular arthritis affecting typical joints and if the arthritis has responded to colchicine or NSAIDs. Otherwise, the patient should be given a trial off therapy to determine whether gouty arthritis recurs.

FOLLOW-UP.   A single gout attack requires no follow-up as long as the patient remains asymptomatic. Patients with recurrent attacks should consider treatment of hyperuricemia, with the goal of reducing the serum uric acid below 6 mg/dl. Patients with hyperuricemia and hypertension should avoid diuretics if at all possible.

Cross-references: General Approach to Arthritic Symptoms (Section 107), Wrist and Hand Pain (Section 111), Knee Pain (Section 112), Ankle and Foot Pain (Section 113), Aspiration/Injection of the Knee (Section 130), Nephrolithiasis (Section 176).

REFERENCES

1. Groff GD, Frank WA, Raddatz DA. Systemic steroid therapy for acute gout: A clinical trial and review of the literature. Semin Arthritis Rheum 1990;19(6):329–336.
    Addresses issue of steroid use for acute gout. A 10-day taper of prednisone resulted in clinical resolution without rebound arthropathy.

2. Lin HY, Rocher LL, et al. Cyclosporine-induced hyperuricemia and gout. N Engl J Med 1989;321:287–292.
    Hyperuricemia is a common complication of cyclosporin therapy. Gouty arthritis occurred in 7% of the patients in this study.

3. Roberts WN, Liang MH, Stern SH. Colchicine in acute gout: Reassessment of risks and benefits. JAMA 1987;257:1920–1922.
    Discusses the dangers of IV colchicine, including reports of two deaths related to neutropenia.

4. Wallace SL, Singer JZ. Therapy in gout. Rheum Dis Clin North Am 1988;14(2):441–457.
    Reviews standard therapies for gout.

121 PREPATELLAR AND OLECRANON BURSITIS

Problem

DAVID L. SMITH

EPIDEMIOLOGY/ETIOLOGY.   The olecranon bursa is situated over the extensor tissue of the elbow; the prepatellar bursa (including the infrapatellar bursa) is located anterior to the knee. These bursae facilitate motion of adjacent tendons but are subject to injury from trauma or infection. Repetitive trauma of the elbow or knee, incurred by laborers such as carpenters, mechanics, or carpet layers, predisposes to both septic and nonseptic bursitis. Alcoholic patients with neurologic disorders (e.g., seizures, ataxia) or impaired host defense mechanisms and those with bursal involvement by rheumatoid nodules or gouty tophi are also at risk for bursitis. Dermatitis overlying the bursa increases the risk of infection. The incidence of olecranon or prepatellar bursitis is between 0.03% and 0.1% of hospital admissions, outpatient or urgent clinic visits. The ratio of nonseptic to septic cases is 3:1; the ratio of olecranon to prepatellar bursitis is 8:1.

Pathogens that typically cause septic bursitis are *Staphylococcus aureus* or *S. epidermidis* and several streptococcal species. The etiology of nonseptic cases is idiopathic in 60% of patients, traumatic in 35%, and crystal-induced in 5%. Crystal-induced cases, secondary to monosodium urate or calcium pyrophosphate deposition, may be precipitated by trauma.

SYMPTOMS, SIGNS, AND LABORATORY FINDINGS. *Septic Bursitis.* Except for immunocompromised patients, bursal warmth and a surface temperature difference of 2.2°C or greater compared to the contralateral side is observed in virtually all patients (Table 121–1). Peribursal edema or cellulitis is noted in about 60% of cases. Spontaneous purulent or serosanguinous drainage occurs in 36%. The fluid aspirated from the bursa ranges from purulent to serous. The mean WBC count of the aspirated fluid varies between 2,000 and 60,000 WBC/

TABLE 121–1.   UTILITY OF SELECTED CHARACTERISTICS IN DISTINGUISHING SEPTIC FROM NONSEPTIC BURSITIS[1]

Characteristic	Sensitivity (%)	Specificity (%)	Positive Predictive Value (%)	Negative Predictive Value (%)	Positive Likelihood Ratio
History of trauma	54	60	30	80	1.4
Warmth on palpation	100	50	38	100	2.0
Surface temperature difference between involved and control sides (≥2.2°C)	100	94	85	100	16.7
Tenderness	80	63	60	93	1.7
Skin lesion	64	80	54	90	3.2
WBC count > 2000/mm³	78	75	53	90	3.1
≥50% of WBCs are PMNs	82	77	53	93	3.6
Positive Gram stain	54	100	100	88	∞

Source: Smith DL, McAfee JH, Lucas LM, Kumar KL, Romney DM. Septic and nonseptic bursitis: Utility of the surface temperature probe in the early differentiation of septic and nonseptic cases. Arch Intern Med 1989; 149:1581–1585.

[1]These features appear to have similar utility in prepatellar bursitis (unpublished observation, DL Smith).

mm^3, with polymorphonuclear leukocytes predominating. The Gram stain is positive in only 60% of cases.

Nonseptic Bursitis.   Bursal warmth is found in 50%, tenderness in 20%, and an overlying skin lesion (e.g., dry or cracked skin) in 17% of cases. Aspirated bursal fluid ranges from clear to bloody. The leukocyte count in the aspirated fluid is approximately 2,500 WBC/mm^3 but ranges from 200 to 27,000 cells/mm^3, with mononuclear cells predominating. An olecranon bone spur is radiographically present in 30% of olecranon cases.

CLINICAL APPROACH.   In all cases of newly diagnosed olecranon and prepatellar bursitis, the bursa should be aspirated. A 20-gauge 1-inch needle attached to a 10-ml syringe is adequate to aspirate the bursal contents after skin cleansing. A lateral approach helps to avoid bacterial inoculation through the skin when these areas are exposed to pressure after aspiration.

In some cases the history, examination, and bursal fluid aspirate do not distinguish between septic and nonseptic bursitis. The individual clinical features listed in Table 121–1 assist in determining whether infection is present before culture results are available. When there is uncertainty, antibiotic treatment is usually prudent.

MANAGEMENT.   *Septic Bursitis.*   In cases of localized infection, an antistaphylococcal penicillin (e.g., dicloxacillin, 500 mg every 6 hours) or cephalosporin should be given for 14 days. Sterilization of the bursa may be delayed in patients with impaired host defenses. Warm soaks, arm elevation, daily dressing changes, and repeated bursal aspiration are also of value. The patient should be admitted for IV antibiotics (e.g., nafacillin, 1 g every 4 hours) when extensive arm or leg cellulitis, lymphadenitis, or chills and fever are present. IV antibiotic therapy is administered for 1 to 2 weeks, followed by 10 to 14 days of oral antibiotic therapy.

Nonseptic Bursitis.   Idiopathic or traumatic bursitis usually responds to complete evacuation of the sterile bursal sac contents, use of a compression dressing, injection of an intrabursal steroid preparation (e.g., 20 mg of methylprednisolone acetate), and use of extensor area protective pads. Bursal sterility must be assured by culture. In olecranon bursitis, the steroid injection shortens the course and minimizes recurrences. A 10-day course of an oral NSAID is effective for crystal-induced cases. Treatment of underlying gout is essential. When rheumatoid nodules involve the bursa, appropriate systemic treatment is required.

FOLLOW-UP.   Patients with septic bursitis should be reevaluated within several days. Repeat aspiration may be required to evacuate a recurrent or persistent effusion. Normally, complete resolution occurs within 4 weeks. In protracted septic cases, referral to an orthopedic surgeon for incision and drainage is indicated if parenteral antibiotic use is unsuccessful. Patients with nonseptic bursitis should be reevaluated in 7 to 10 days. Recurrent or chronic cases due to repetitive trauma may respond to temporary splinting of the affected joint. Resection of the bursa or underlying bone spur is reserved for particularly chronic cases.

Cross-references: General Approach to Arthritic Symptoms (Section 107), Knee Pain (Section 112), Gout/Hyperuricemia (Section 120).

REFERENCES

1. Ho G, Tice AD. Comparison of nonseptic and septic bursitis: Further observations on the treatment of septic bursitis. Arch Intern Med 1979;139:1269–1273.
    Helpful analysis of bursal fluid findings.

2. Ho KG, Tice AD, Kaplan SR. Septic bursitis in the prepatellar and olecranon bursae: An analysis of 25 cases. Ann Intern Med 1978;89:21–27.
    Useful features of septic cases and their treatment.

3. McAfee JH, Smith DL. Olecranon and prepatellar bursitis: Diagnosis and treatment. West J Med 1988;149:607–610.
    Review of anatomy, clinical features, and management of olecranon and prepatellar bursitis.

4. Smith DL, McAfee JH, Lucas LM, Kumar KL, Romney DM. Septic and nonseptic bursitis: Utility of the surface temperature probe in the early differentiation of septic and nonseptic cases. Arch Intern Med 1989;149:1581–1585.
    A surface temperature probe reading helps distinguish septic from nonseptic cases.

5. Smith DL, McAfee JH, Lucas LM, Kumar KL, Romney DM. Treatment of nonseptic olecranon bursitis. Arch Intern Med 1989;149:2527–2530.
    Controlled prospective clinical trial demonstrated efficacy of intrabursal methylprednisolone acetate compared to an oral anti-inflammatory agent.

122 FIBROMYALGIA

Problem

JOHN B. STIMSON

EPIDEMIOLOGY.   Fibromyalgia is a clinical syndrome of generalized aching and stiffness, associated with the finding of numerous tender points in characteristic locations (Table 122–1). The terms "fibrositis" and "primary" or "secondary" fibromyalgia have been abandoned. In contrast to myofascial pain syndrome, patients with fibromyalgia experience generalized instead of focal discomfort, have no trigger points on examination, and respond less well to treatment (see Section 123). Although no cause or characteristic laboratory abnormality has been identified, the clinical syndrome of fibromyalgia is characteristic enough that most physicians accept it as a real entity. The number of

TABLE 122–1.   AMERICAN COLLEGE OF RHEUMATOLOGY 1990 CRITERIA FOR THE CLASSIFICATION OF FIBROMYALGIA

1. Widespread pain for more than 3 months.

   "Widespread" requires both right- and left-sided pain, pain above and below the waist, and axial skeletal pain. Low back pain is regarded as being below the waist.

2. Pain on palpation in at least 11 of 18 of the following tender point sites:

   Occiput: bilateral, at the suboccipital muscle insertions.
   Low cervical: bilateral, at the anterior aspects of the intertransverse spaces at C5–C7.
   Trapezius: bilateral, at the midpoint of the upper border.
   Supraspinatus: bilateral, at origins, above the scapula spine near the medial border.
   Second rib: bilateral, at the second costochondral junctions, just lateral to the junctions on upper surfaces.
   Lateral epicondyle: bilateral, 2 cm distal to the epicondyles.
   Gluteal: bilateral, in upper outer quadrants of buttocks in anterior fold of muscle.
   Greater trochanter: bilateral, posterior to the trochanteric prominence.
   Knee: bilateral, at the medial fat pad proximal to the joint line.

Source: Wolfe F, Smythe HA, Yunus MB, et al. The American College of Rheumatology 1990 criteria for the classification of fibromyalgia: Report of the Multicenter Criteria Committee. Arthritis Rheum 1990;33:160–172.

---

individuals with fibromyalgia in the United States was estimated at 3 million in 1983, making it third among rheumatic disorders, behind osteoarthritis and rheumatoid arthritis. Five percent of unselected patients in a general medical clinic satisfy criteria for fibromyalgia. Approximately 70% to 90% of affected patients are women.

SYMPTOMS AND SIGNS.   The most common symptom is prolonged (i.e., > 3 months) multifocal pain, accompanied by fatigue, morning stiffness, and non-restorative sleep. Patients may report prolonged morning stiffness similar to that seen in rheumatoid arthritis. The pain typically worsens with acute stress, exposure to cold, inactivity or overactivity, and changes in barometric pressure. Less common complaints are headaches, irritable bowel symptoms, sensations of numbness or swelling, reactive hyperemia of the skin, and Raynaud's phenomenon.

Tender points, the hallmark of fibromyalgia, are discrete areas over muscle, ligaments, or fat pads that produce local pain when moderately firm pressure is applied with a single finger or thumb. The appropriate technique uses pressure insufficient to produce pain in normal individuals or uninvolved sites in affected individuals. In contrast to the trigger points seen in myofascial pain syndromes, palpation of tender points generally does not cause referred pain, and tender points are not confined to muscle.

Depression is no more common than among patients with rheumatoid arthritis, although patients with fibromyalgia do report higher stress levels.

CLINICAL APPROACH.   The patient interview does not reliably differentiate fibromyalgia, rheumatoid arthritis, and osteoarthritis. Chronic generalized pain refractory to anti-inflammatory medications suggests fibromyalgia. Low back pain is common and hand involvement is rare in fibromyalgia, in contrast to rheumatoid arthritis. Physical examination in fibromyalgia patients, however, is remarkable for the absence of joint abnormalities (unless a coincidental arthritic disorder is present) and the presence of characteristic tender points. Control areas not expected to be tender in fibromyalgia (e.g., middle of the forehead, fingertips) should be examined to exclude psychogenic pain or malingering.

Diagnostic criteria for fibromyalgia are listed in Table 122–1. Laboratory evaluation is unnecessary unless a coexisting condition is suspected. A normal ESR helps exclude most inflammatory conditions, such as rheumatoid arthritis, polymyalgia rheumatica, ankylosing spondylitis, myositis, lupus erythematosus, and vasculitis. Although hypothyroidism can cause generalized aching, tender points are unusual on examination.[1]

MANAGEMENT.   Therapy for fibromyalgia is generally disappointing. Far greater benefit is achieved by reassurance than by any pharmacologic therapy currently available. Patients benefit from learning they have a recognizable condition that does not progress or cripple and that does not warrant further diagnostic testing. Various medications produce minor benefit in some patients. Low-dose amitriptyline (10–50 mg q.h.s.) or cyclobenzaprine (10–40 mg/day) may improve sleep and slightly lessen daytime fatigue and aching. Nonsteroidal anti-inflammatory medications can help some patients, but the small benefit may not justify the risks. A controlled trial of prednisone, 20 mg/day, showed no benefit. Low-impact cardiovascular conditioning (e.g., stationary cycling) helps some patients, although initial worsening for 2 weeks is the rule.[2] Use of narcotics for pain management is to be avoided.

Cross-references: Chronic Pain Syndrome (Section 13), General Approach to Arthritic Symptoms (Section 107), Myofascial Pain Syndromes (Section 123), Common Thyroid Disorders (Section 156).

REFERENCES

1. Carett S, Lefrancois L. Fibrositis and primary hypothyroidism. J Rheumatol 1988;15:1418–1421.
    Hypothyroid patients frequently have diffuse aching, but multiple tender points were no more frequent than in the general medical clinic population.

2. McCain GA, Bell DA, Mai FM, Halliday PD. A controlled study of the effects of a supervised cardiovascular fitness training program on the manifestations of primary fibromyalgia. Arthritis Rheum 1988;31:1135–1141.
    Some 50% of patients with fibromyalgia who underwent a 5-month cardiovascular fitness training program significantly improved, compared with 10% of patients who underwent a simple stretching program.

3. Wolfe F, Smythe HA, Yunus MB, et al. The American College of Rheumatology 1990 criteria for the classification of fibromyalgia: Report of the Multicenter Criteria Committee. Arthritis Rheum 1990;33:160–172.
    293 patients considered to have fibromyalgia and 265 controls with rheumatic conditions most likely to be confused with fibromyalgia were examined in a standardized and blinded fashion. The information was used to develop the 1990 criteria for the diagnosis of fibromyalgia.

123 MYOFASCIAL PAIN SYNDROMES

Problem

JOHN B. STIMSON

EPIDEMIOLOGY.   Myofascial pain syndromes usually affect overused or injured muscles, may persist long after the actual muscle injury, and are associated with discrete, tender areas within muscle called trigger points. The pathophysiology is unknown. A given trigger point, which may be further stimulated by moderate pressure or needle insertion, causes referred pain in characteristic patterns, just as ischemic foci in cardiac muscle cause referred neck, jaw, or arm pain. The overall prevalence of myofascial pain syndrome is unknown but is reportedly as high as 55% to 85% in patients attending pain clinics.

SYMPTOMS AND SIGNS.   Myofascial pain is poorly localized and can include sensations of tingling, numbness or skin hyperalgesia. In the involved muscle, trigger points are often found within palpable firm bands, which may visibly twitch during palpation or needle puncture. Because stretching of affected muscles causes pain, patients often keep muscles in a shortened position and restrict motion of nearby joints.

Common clinical syndromes and associated trigger points include (1) temporomandibular joint syndrome from masseter muscle trigger points, (2) arm or shoulder pain from scapular muscle trigger points, (3) occipital headache and neck pain from trapezius or posterior neck muscle trigger points, (4) anterior chest pain from sternalis, pectoralis, sternocleidomastoid, or serratus anterior muscle trigger points (at times misdiagnosed as ischemic cardiac pain),[2] (5) low back pain from lumbar spinal muscle trigger points, and (6) sciatica from gluteal muscle trigger points.

CLINICAL APPROACH.   Familiarity with common trigger points and their referred pain patterns is essential to the diagnosis.[1] The examiner strokes his fingers perpendicular to the affected muscle fibers and searches for palpable bands. Moderately firm pressure over these bands may identify the actual trigger point. If the examination fails to elicit discrete tenderness and produce referred pain, a true trigger point and a myofascial cause for pain are unlikely.

Other causes of soft tissue pain appear in Table 123–1. Joint or tendon crepitation, tenderness over bony structures, reflex loss, or muscle wasting are not features of myofascial pain syndromes and will generally point to the correct diagnosis.

MANAGEMENT.   Established myofascial pain responds poorly to conventional therapy for musculoskeletal pain, such as heat and anti-inflammatory agents. Instead, measures directed at the responsible trigger point are most

TABLE 123–1. CAUSES OF SOFT TISSUE PAIN

Trigger points in muscle
Bursitis, tendinitis, tenosynovitis, arthritis
Phlebitis or deep venous thrombosis
Hematoma in muscle
Nerve entrapment syndromes
Reflex dystrophies
Referred pain syndromes from viscera
Mononeuritis multiplex
Central nervous system pain syndromes

effective: vapocoolant spray (chlorofluoromethane) or trigger point injection with a local anesthetic, followed by stretch of the involved muscle (see Section 127, Trigger Point Injection). A single treatment may be effective, but often treatments repeated every 2 to 4 days are necessary until sustained improvement is achieved. Correction of postural abnormalities or occupational overuse may prevent relapses.

Cross-references: Chest Pain (Section 74), General Approach to Arthritic Symptoms (Section 107), Low Back Pain (Section 108), Shoulder Pain (Section 109), Hip Pain (Section 110), Fibromyalgia (Section 122), Trigger Point Injection (Section 127), Headache (Section 140).

REFERENCES

1. Simons DG, Travell JG. Myofascial pain syndromes. In Wall PD, Melzack R, Eds. Textbook of Pain. Churchill Livingstone, New York, 1984, pp. 263–276.
    Excellent maps of referred pain patterns for common trigger points.

2. Travell J, Rinzler SH. Pain syndromes of the anterior chest muscles: Resemblance to effort angina and myocardial infarction, and relief by local block. Can Med Assoc J 1948;59: 333–338.
    Case reports illustrating that myofascial pain can mimic pain from ischemic cardiac muscle, resulting in hospital admission.

3. Travell JG, Simons DG. Myofascial Pain and Dysfunction: The Trigger Point Manual. Williams & Wilkins, Baltimore, 1983.
    Comprehensive review of location and treatment techniques for trigger points in the most important muscles in the upper body. Includes otherwise difficult to find techniques for stretching each muscle.

124 INTERPRETATION OF SEROLOGIC TESTS

Procedure

RICHARD H. WHITE

INDICATIONS/CONTRAINDICATIONS. Numerous serologic tests are available that may aid in the diagnosis of specific rheumatic diseases. Those serologic tests with high *specificity* should be ordered to verify suspected diagnoses. For example, a high level of antibody to double-stranded DNA or to the Smith (Sm) antigen is specific for systemic lupus erythmatosis (SLE), and an elevated level of antibody to neutrophil cytoplasmic antigens (ANCA) is specific for Wegener's granulomatosis and related disorders (polyarteritis nodosa and crescentic glomerular nephritis). Tests with high *sensitivity* should be ordered to help exclude a diagnosis when clinical findings are equivocal. For example, a negative antinuclear antibody (ANA) assay essentially excludes the diagnosis of SLE.

METHODS. The serologic tests most frequently ordered are listed in Table 124–1, together with the sensitivity, specificity, and clinical utility of each test. It should be emphasized that each laboratory has a different range for normal and abnormal values.

TEST INTERPRETATION. Results of a fluorescent ANA test are usually reported as a titer, together with a pattern. A **rim** pattern is rare and is specific for SLE. A **speckled** pattern is common, nonspecific, and frequently present in high titer in patients who have no manifestations of a rheumatic disease. A **nucleolar** pattern is less common and is nonspecific. A **centromere** pattern is rare and is not the same as a positive test for anticentromere antibody. A **homogeneous** pattern is common, nonspecific, usually present in low titer (less than 1:640), and characteristic for drug-induced ANA.

In the absence of signs and symptoms of the rheumatic disease under consideration, a positive serologic test is not diagnostic. For example, in patients with isolated chronic fatigue, a positive Lyme titer (ELISA for IgG) is not diagnostic for Lyme disease. A positive ANA assay without findings of lupus is meaningless, and sometimes occurs with subclinical autoimmune disease or with certain medications.

Cross-references: Principles of Screening (Section 12), General Approach to Arthritic Symptoms (Section 107).

TABLE 124–1.   INTERPRETATION OF SEROLOGIC TESTS

Serologic Tests	Sensitivity	Specificity	Clinical Utility
ANA	SLE (95%), mixed connective tissue disease (MCTD) (99%), drug-induced SLE (99%)	Low; associated with many disorders	A negative test helps to exclude SLE, MCTD, and drug-induced SLE
RF	RA (85%–90%)	Low; associated with many disorders	A positive test helps classify patients with polyarthritis for greater than 3 mo
Anti-dsDNA	SLE (50%–60%) (with active disease)	High, >95% for SLE	A positive test helps to diagnose SLE
Anti-Sm (Smith)	SLE (30%–40%)	High, >98% for SLE	A positive test helps to diagnose SLE
Anti-(U1) RNP	MCTD (100%)	Low, seen in SLE, PSS, RA, discoid lupus	A negative test excludes MCTD
Antihistone	Drug-induced SLE (100%)	Low, seen in SLE, RA	Not helpful
Anti-Ro (SSA)	Sjögren's (60%–70%)	Low, seen in SLE, RA	Associated with aggressive Sjögren's, neonatal SLE, neonatal heart block
Anti-La (SSB)	Sjögren's (50%–60%)	Low, seen in SLE	Not useful
Anticentromere	CREST syndrome (50%–90%)	High for CREST, PSS, or Raynaud's	Minimal value over clinical findings alone
Anti-SCL$_{70}$ (Anti-Topo 1)	Scleroderma (20%)	High, >95% for scleroderma	Positive test is helpful in the diagnosis of scleroderma
Anti-JO$_1$	Polymyositis (30%)	?	Associated with myositis and interstitial fibrosis
ANCA	Wegener's granulomatosis: Generalized (95%) Limited (67%)	High, >99% for Wegener's granulomatosis	A positive test helps diagnose Wegener's granulomatosis and related disorders (e.g., polyarteritis)
Lyme titer	High for subacute and chronic Lyme disease	Low, <90%	Helpful when there is a high titer *and* clinical manifestations of Lyme disease

REFERENCES

1. Barbour AG. The diagnosis of Lyme disease: Rewards and perils. Ann Intern Med 1989;110:501–502.

   Summary of the current status regarding the role of serologic testing in the diagnosis of Lyme disease. The test should be ordered solely to confirm a diagnosis based on epidemiologic and clinical evidence.

2. Falk RJ, Hogan S, Carey TS, Jennette C, Glomerular Disease Collaborative Network. Clinical course of anti-neutrophil cytoplasmic autoantibody–associated glomerulonephritis and systemic vasculitis. Ann Intern Med 1990;113:656–663.

   Prospective study of 70 patients with ANCA documenting its specificity for Wegener's granulomatosis and the related disorders, crescentic glomerulonephritis and polyarteritis nodosa.

3. Tsokos GC, Pillemer SR, Klippel JH. Rheumatic disease syndromes associated with antibodies to the Ro (SS-A) ribonuclear protein. Semin Arthritis Rheum 1987;16:237–244.

   Reviews associations between anti-Ro antibody and (1) ANA-negative SLE, (2) subacute cutaneous SLE, (3) neonatal SLE, and (4) extraglandular Sjögren's syndrome.

4. Wade JP, Sack B, Schur PH. Anticentromere antibodies: Clinical correlates. J Rheumatol 1988;15:1759–1763.

   The presence of anticentromere antibody is less specific than previously thought in the screening of unselected patients with rheumatic disease.

5. White RH, Robbins DL. Clinical significance and interpretation of antinuclear antibodies. West J Med 1987;147:210–213.

   Reviews the diagnostic utility of the antinuclear antibody test.

125 DIABETIC FOOT CARE EDUCATION

Procedure

JESSIE H. AHRONI

INDICATIONS/CONTRAINDICATIONS. All diabetic patients should be taught the basic principles of foot care, although there is no evidence that young persons with healthy feet require detailed advice.

RATIONALE. For the patient with a neuropathy, orthopedic deformity, history of foot infection, or ulceration, a simple education program can reduce the incidence of recurrent ulceration and limb amputation.[1]

METHODS. The clinician should review the principles of foot care with diabetic patients at every visit. One way to emphasize the importance of foot care is to say, "People with diabetes have a 15 times higher risk of a foot or leg amputation than nondiabetic individuals, but with a few simple steps most of these amputations can be prevented." The main points of self care for persons with diabetic feet are the following:

1.   Inspect the feet and interdigital areas daily, e.g., whenever putting on or taking off socks. A mirror may be helpful. If the patient is unable, a family member should perform the inspection.

2.   Wash and dry the feet thoroughly, especially between the toes. A thin layer of lamb's wool can be used to separate overlapping or contacting toes and help prevent maceration. The clinician should caution the patient about avoiding hot-water burns by checking the bath water temperature with the forearm or elbow. Routine soaking is not recommended.

3.   Moisturize dry skin (except between the toes) with an emollient such as lanolin or hand lotion.

4.   Cut or file toenails straight across the contour of the toe, being sure all sharp edges are filed smooth. If the patient does not see well or has difficulty reaching his feet, this may be done by a family member, nurse, or podiatrist.

5.   Avoid self-treatment of corns, calluses, athlete's foot, or ingrown toenails. Chemicals, sharp instruments, or razor blades should never be used on the feet by a patient. Flaky fungal debris can be loosened and removed with a soft nail brush during regular bathing.

6.   Wear well-fitting soft cotton or wool socks. The patient should not use hot water bottles or heating pads for cold feet.

7.   Avoid walking barefoot (to avoid puncture wounds and burns from hot sand or pavement).

8.   Examine the shoes daily for internal cracks, loose linings, pebbles, and other irregularities that may irritate the skin. Soft leather or canvas shoes that have cushioned insoles and fit well at the time of purchase are best. Changing shoes during the day can limit repetitive local pressure.

9.   Seek prompt medical attention for any problems (e.g., cuts, blisters, calluses, and any wounds that do not heal, or signs of infection such as redness, swelling, pus, drainage, or fever).

Cross-references: Leg Ulcers (Section 134), Local Care of Diabetic Foot Lesions (Section 135), Peripheral Neuropathy (Section 149), Diabetes Mellitus (Section 157).

REFERENCES

1.   Malone JM, Snyder M, Anderson G, Bernhard VM, Holloway GA Jr, Bunt TJ. Prevention of amputation by diabetic education. Am J Surg 1989;158:520–524.
     A prospective randomized study found the incidence of lower extremity amputation to be three times higher in the "no foot care education" group.

2.   Most R, Sinnock P. The epidemiology of lower extremity amputations in diabetic individuals. Diabetes Care 1983;6:87–91.
     Diabetes Control Activity programs in six states provide profiles of diabetic lower extremity amputations.

3. National Diabetes Advisory Board. The national long-range plan to combat diabetes. U.S. Government Printing Office, Washington, D.C., 1987, p. ix.

126 PRINCIPLES OF PHYSICAL THERAPY

Procedure

CAROLYNN PATTEN
SUSAN STEINDORF

INDICATIONS/CONTRAINDICATIONS.   Physical therapy may benefit patients with a wide variety of acute and chronic medical conditions. Some of these patients, many with acute self-limited injuries, never see a physical therapist and are primarily managed by the primary physician. Table 126–1 lists groups of patients who should see a physical therapist, preferably early in the course of their illness or injury.

TABLE 126–1.   INDICATIONS FOR REFERRAL TO A PHYSICAL THERAPIST

1. Patients with musculoskeletal pain that persists longer than 1 week and is unresponsive to medical treatment
2. Patients with musculoskeletal pain that requires immediate and specific treatment:
    Reflex sympathetic dystrophy
    Shoulder and hip problems that may cause capsular limitation (bursitis, impingement syndromes)
    Competitive athletes
    Overuse syndromes (patellofemoral joint dysfunction)
3. Patients at risk for falling or who have difficulty walking, difficulty transferring, or other disability that may benefit from a cane, walker, crutches, or a wheelchair
4. Patients who may benefit from specific procedures:
    Electrotherapy
       Transcutaneous nerve stimulation
       Neuromuscular electric stimulation
       Laser
    Phonophoresis or ultrasound
    Supervised exercise
    Manual therapy
    Biofeedback
    Traction
5. Patients with any other disability that interferes with daily activities

TABLE 126–2. COMMON PHYSICAL THERAPY PROCEDURES

Treatment	Indications	Contraindications	Method	Comments
Heat	Muscle spasm/contracture	First 24–48 hr after acute injury Sensory neuropathy Hemophilia Malignancy Hemorrhage	Duration 15–30 min Wet heat penetrates better than dry heat	Decreases spasm, increases blood flow, inhibits nerve conduction, counterirritant to pain May increase swelling
Cold	Acute injury (first 24–48 hr)	Peripheral vascular disease Raynaud's syndrome Cold urticaria Open wounds	Duration 10–30 min	Causes vasoconstriction, inhibits pain fiber conduction, counterirritant to pain Prevents swelling, decreases pain May increase stiffness
Hydrotherapy	Wound debridement Exercise against resistance	Acute injury Fever or active infection Severe cardiac or pulmonary disease Malignancy	Duration 20 min	Usually an inpatient treatment; may be prescribed for outpatient use
Contrast	Subacute injuries (>48 hr old) Edema	See Heat/Cold above	Start with heat, end with cold Heat duration longer than cold (ratio usually 4:1–2:1)	
Massage	Limited range of motion Myofascial pain Muscle spasm	Acute injury Hemorrhage Open wound Active infectious, cardiac, venous, renal disease	Usually provided by a massage therapist	Gentle stretching breaks up adhesions, promotes venous and lymphatic flow, decreases spasm Helpful after immobilization or traumatic injuries

Table continued on following page

TABLE 126–2. COMMON PHYSICAL THERAPY PROCEDURES *Continued*

Treatment	Indications	Contraindications	Method	Comments
Deep friction massage	Acute muscle tear Sprains Trigger points in tendon, muscle, ligaments	Active local inflammation or infection Tissue calcification Rheumatoid arthritis	Duration 5 min Massage applied perpendicular to muscle fibers Massage often followed by cold treatment	See Massage Treatment is uncomfortable
Splint	Joint injury requiring rest		Must be combined with range of motion exercises	Excessive use causes contracture
Stretching and active assisted range of motion	Hypomobility	Unhealed fracture Joint fusion Active joint disease	Sustain stretch 30–60 sec Use at least 2–3 times/day	20–30 min of continuous stretching required to lengthen tissues
Passive range of motion	Acute injury, severe pain	None	Exercise works within pain-free range Includes pendulum exercises, cane exercises	
Active exercise	Muscle weakness Joint swelling Hypermobility	Recent surgery Severe cardiac disease	Exercise works within pain-free range More aggressive exercises after recovery of normal range of motion	Improves joint stability, endurance, and coordination Soreness lasting 24–48 hr after treatment may occur and is acceptable
Isometric exercise	Movement of joint not desirable or possible (e.g., cast, active arthritis, overuse injury)	None	Patient should use 60%–80% of maximal strength, maintain for at least 6 sec	Convenient, good for home use, requires no equipment Some authorities question benefit because exercises compress joints with considerable force and may not improve active function

RATIONALE.   Physical therapy, when properly applied to the injured patient, facilitates recovery, prevents complications, and, through patient education, averts similar injuries in the future. Patients in the groups listed in Table 126–1 should be referred to a physical therapist not only because early physical therapy prevents complications (e.g., appropriately treated deltoid bursitis will prevent a frozen shoulder), but because physical therapists often discover important diagnostic information and assist in the integrated treatment of the patient.

The rationale behind several commonly employed physical therapy treatments (e.g., heat, cold, hydrotherapy) and their applications are given in Table 126–2.

METHODS.   When referring patients to physical therapists, the clinician should keep three important principles in mind:

1.   Physical therapists legally are autonomous professionals in most states, but are legally required to carry out the clinician's specific treatment recommendation. To allow physical therapists to be most effective, therefore, it is often preferable for the clinician to avoid prescribing specific treatments on the referral form and instead make general recommendations. When the diagnosis is unclear, the referral may simply state "evaluate and treat."

2.   The clinician should include on the referral information about the patient's relevant medical history, especially cardiac problems or infectious diseases, and precautions against exercise or bearing weight on a specific extremity.

3.   While clinicians often focus on specific diagnoses (e.g., gout, disk herniation, vascular insufficiency), physical therapists focus more on specific symptoms or signs (pain, swelling, hypo- or hypermobility, altered sensation, function, weakness, muscle imbalance, balance and coordination). Figure 126–1 shows an example of a completed referral form.

COSTS AND COMPLICATIONS.   Most private insurers cover a portion of physical therapy costs. Customary charges for outpatient treatment are in the range

---

Problem: Low back pain radiating in R. L5 dermatome; onset = 3 weeks ago s/p motor vehicle accident.

Precautions and/or other pertinent medical information: Patient has pacemaker; long-standing history of cardiac problems. Lumbar spine x-rays are normal.

Recommended treatment: _____Ice   _____Massage

X Treat appropriately   X Discuss patient with me

__ Treat only as requested   __ No precautions

Doctor Signature: _____ MD Phone: _____

FIGURE 126–1.   Sample of a physical therapy referral form.

of $50 to $60 per hour. Preferred provider plans and health maintenance organizations typically limit coverage, e.g., 10 visits per complaint or 20 visits per year.

Cross-references: Chronic Pain Syndrome (Section 13), General Approach to Arthritic Symptoms (Section 107), Low Back Pain (Section 108), Shoulder Pain (Section 109), Knee Pain (Section 112).

REFERENCES

1. Hertling D, Kessler RM. Management of common musculoskeletal disorders. In: Physical Therapy: Principles and Methods, 2nd ed. J.B. Lippincott, Philadelphia, 1990.
    Excellent overview of functional anatomy, concepts of management, and specific treatment techniques.

2. Hoppenfeld S. Physical Examination of the Spine and Extremities. Appleton-Century-Crofts, Norwalk, Conn., 1976.
    Clear, concise review of the physical examination of the spine and extremities.

3. Magee DJ. Orthopedic Physical Assessment. W.B. Saunders, Philadelphia, 1987.
    Thoughtful discussion of functional anatomy and specific diagnostic techniques.

4. Michlovitz SL. Thermal Agents in Rehabilitation. F.A. Davis, Philadelphia, 1986.
    The present definitive text discussing efficacy of treatment with modalities.

5. Scully RM, Barnes MR. Physical Therapy. J.B. Lippincott, Philadelphia, 1989.
    In-depth review of physical therapy.

127 TRIGGER POINT INJECTION

Procedure

JOHN B. STIMSON

INDICATIONS/CONTRAINDICATIONS.   Prolonged myofascial pain syndromes with reproducible trigger points (see Section 123, Myofascial Pain Syndromes) justify trigger point injection. Soft tissue pain or tender muscles without trigger points are unlikely to respond to injection and should not be treated in this manner. Tender points seen in fibromyalgia also respond poorly to injection. True allergy or a previous idiosyncratic reaction to local anesthetics are the only contraindications to trigger point injection. Coagulopathy and anticoagulant therapy render patients more likely to develop small hematomas at injection sites and are relative contraindications.

RATIONALE.   Whether abnormalities of muscle, nerves, or both cause trigger points is unknown. Nonspecific therapy with analgesics, rest, and heat is generally ineffective. Empirical treatment of trigger points with local anesthetic injections or chlorofluoromethane spray, however, reduces pain and restores normal muscle length and function. Interestingly, needle insertion without injection or saline injection alone is also sometimes effective, though local anesthetic injections are probably superior.

METHODS.   A reproducible discrete trigger point is a prerequisite to trigger point injection. Following palpation, a 22- to 25-gauge needle is inserted into the muscle to locate the exact spot that reproduces the patient's pain. Once the trigger point is located, 1 to 2 ml of anesthetic is injected. If the trigger point cannot be located with the needle, a larger amount of anesthetic should be infiltrated in the general area. When the site is anesthetic, the muscle is passively stretched to restore full range of motion. Short-acting anesthetics without epinephrine, such as 1% procaine or lidocaine, are preferred because they produce less muscle necrosis at the injection site than long-acting anesthetics (e.g., bupivacaine) or those containing epinephrine. A 1½-inch needle is sufficient to reach essentially all trigger points in the upper body. Lumbar and gluteal trigger points may require longer needles and more expertise to locate. Repeated treatments every few days are sometimes necessary to achieve sustained improvement, though no specific guidelines exist.

COMPLICATIONS.   Trigger point injection is quite safe if simple precautions are observed. If not properly performed, intravascular or intraneural injections can occur. Pneumothorax is an uncommon complication of injections in the thorax. Up to 50 ml of 1% procaine or lidocaine can be safely infiltrated into soft tissues before concerns about neurologic or cardiac toxicity arise. These volumes far exceed those required for multiple trigger point injections.

Cross-references: Low Back Pain (Section 108), Shoulder Pain (Section 109), Myofascial Pain Syndromes (Section 123).

128 INJECTION OF THE SHOULDER

Procedure

STEPHAN D. FIHN

INDICATIONS/CONTRAINDICATIONS. For the primary care provider, injection of the shoulder usually refers to injection of the subacromial bursa. Injection of the glenohumeral joint itself is usually only performed during arthrography. The response to injection of the subacromial bursa with 1% lidocaine is useful in differentiating subacromial bursitis from other causes of shoulder pain, particularly rotator cuff tears and frozen shoulder. Patients with subacromial bursitis who fail to respond to treatment with nonsteroidal agents, heat, and exercise may respond favorably to injection of a long-acting steroid preparation into the bursa.

Contraindications to injection include suspected infection of the shoulder joint, surrounding structures, or overlying skin and the presence of a prosthetic shoulder joint. Contraindications to steroid injection are a suspected rotator cuff tear or a history of repeated steroid injections.

RATIONALE. Injection of lidocaine into the subacromial bursa can be helpful in deciding which patients with significant shoulder pain should have an early referral to an orthopedic surgeon or for arthrography. Injection of a corticosteroid into an inflamed bursa can provide substantial relief of pain and improvement in range of motion to patients with otherwise stubborn symptoms.

METHODS. The patient should be seated comfortably with his hands folded in his lap. After thorough hand washing, the clinician should locate the acromion. The area immediately anterior and inferior to the acromion should be palpated with the index finger of the same hand as the side of the patient being examined (e.g., right index finger on right shoulder). The area of maximal tenderness should be pressed firmly with the examining finger while the clinician holds the patient's elbow with his other hand and passively abducts and adducts the arm. At the point of maximal tenderness or in the immediate vicinity, the clinician should feel his finger enter the space between the lower border of the acromion and the humeral head. This spot should be marked using gentle pressure with a retracted ball-point pen or the open end of a pen cap. The location marked is usually 1 to 2 cm below the acromion and 1 to 2 cm anterior to it. If there is marked disparity between the point of maximal tenderness and the spot marked, the shoulder should be reexamined to confirm the diagnosis. Otherwise, the shoulder should be scrubbed with an iodine-povidine solution and allowed to dry.

Meanwhile, the examiner should place 6 to 8 ml of 1% lidocaine (without epinephrine) into a 10-ml syringe. If a corticosteroid is to be injected in addition, it should be mixed with the lidocaine in the syringe. Suitable steroid preparations include aqueous methylprednisonolone acetate, 20 to 40 mg, aqueous dexamethasone phosphate, 2 to 6 mg, or triamcinolone acetonide, 20 to 40 mg.

Wearing sterile gloves, the physician may then raise a skin wheal with 1 to 2 ml of 1% lidocaine at the previously marked location, although in most cases this is unnecessary. If a steroid is being injected, the physician should then briskly shake the syringe to disperse the steroid suspension in the lidocaine. A 23- to 27-gauge, 1½-inch needle should be placed on the syringe and then, taking lateral approach to the previously marked spot, the needle is angled 45 degrees downward and 10 to 15 degrees posteriorly (aiming for the inferior tip of the ipsilateral scapula). The needle is slowly advanced through the deltoid muscle until it reaches a hard surface, which may be the humerus or, more likely, the rotator cuff tendon. The needle is then withdrawn slightly to avoid injecting directly into the tendon. After gentle aspiration, the contents of the syringe are slowly instilled. Only minimal resistance should be felt. When 3 or 4 ml has been inserted, the needle should be withdrawn 2 to 3 cm and redirected slightly more posteriorly, maintaining the 45-degree downward angle. Again, when firm resistance is encountered, the needle is withdrawn slightly. The remaining contents of the syringe should then be injected, the needle removed and placed in an appropriate disposal container, and a Band-aid placed over the injection site.

Following injection, the patient should be asked to actively move the shoulder to distribute the injected materials and to determine whether the pain is diminished. If the purpose of the injection was solely diagnostic (i.e., no steroids were given), the examiner should passively abduct the shoulder. If pain is still present, the injection may have been performed improperly or the differential diagnosis was inaccurate. If there is full range of motion without pain, a frozen shoulder is excluded. In this case, strength of the shoulder girdle should be tested. If strength is normal, the diagnosis is most likely subacromial bursitis. If there is weakness in abduction and external rotation, a rotator cuff injury is probable.

If steroids have been instilled, the same maneuvers should be performed. Patients should be forewarned that when the effect of the lidocaine wears off, in several hours, the pain may recur for a day or so before the full effect of the steroid is felt. If no relief is obtained, the patient should be reexamined and the diagnosis reconsidered. If pain disappears but recurs in several weeks or months, the injection may be repeated. Steroid injections should not be given more than once every 6 months (and less often if possible).

COST/COMPLICATIONS.   Injection of the subacromial bursa is generally a very safe procedure with few adverse effects. Occasional patients may find their pain made worse by injection. Injection directly into the rotator cuff tendon, especially the supraspinatus tendon, may cause rupture. Repeated injections may contribute to thinning of the rotator cuff. Infection or hematomas following injection are exceedingly rare. The cost of injection varies widely, depending on physician fees although an average charge is $70 to $100.

Cross-reference: Shoulder Pain (Section 109).

REFERENCES

1. Bulgen DY, Binder AI, Hazleman BL, Dutton J, Roberts S. Frozen shoulder: Prospective clinical study with an evaluation of three treatment regimens. Ann Rheum Dis 1984;43:353–360.

    A small randomized trial that compared intrarticular steroids, physiotherapy, ice therapy, and no therapy in forty-two patients. Shortly after entry, the steroid-treated group showed more improvement in pain and function, although at 6 months the groups were all equally improved.

2. White RH. Diagnosis and management of shoulder pain. In Stults BM, Dere WH, Eds. Practical Care of the Ambulatory Patient. W.B. Saunders, Philadelphia, 1989, pp. 490–500.

    An illustrated description of procedures for injecting the shoulder, along with a comprehensive review of shoulder pain.

3. White RH, Paull DM, Fleming KW. Rotator cuff tendinitis: Comparison of subacromial injection of a long acting corticosteroid versus oral indomethacin therapy. J Rheumatol 1986;13:608–613.

    A small controlled trial involving forty patients failed to demonstrate a benefit beyond that provided by indomethacin.

129 INJECTION OF THE TROCHANTERIC BURSA

Procedure

RICHARD H. WHITE

INDICATIONS/CONTRAINDICATIONS.   The only indication for injection of the trochanteric bursa is to diagnose and treat suspected trochanteric bursitis.

RATIONALE.   When hip pain is associated with exquisite tenderness over the lateral/posterior aspect of the greater trochanter, inflammation of one or more of the bursae that lie between the gluteus maximus, gluteus medius, and the greater trochanter is likely. The best way to confirm the diagnosis of trochanteric bursitis is to inject 8 to 10 ml of lidocaine 1% into the region of the bursa, which should ameliorate most of the pain in 5 to 10 minutes.

The cause of bursal inflammation is unknown but is thought to be mechanical in nature. It is not due to infection or a crystal-induced process but instead is associated with low back pain and osteoarthritis of the hip. Injection is necessary for diagnosis, because tenderness over the greater trochanter is nonspecific and is sometimes seen in degenerative or inflammatory arthritis of the hip and with aseptic necrosis of the femoral head.

METHODS.   Choosing the exact location for the injection is critical. With the patient lying on the opposite hip and the underwear removed, the femur should be palpated, working from the midthigh upward. The upper extent of the femur (trochanter) should be identified and a small mark made on the skin. The iliac crest should also be identified 4 or 5 inches cephalad. The area of maximal tenderness should be over the *posterior* aspect of the trochanter, and may extend caudad 10 to 14 cm.

In obese patients, the trochanter may be difficult to palpate. In addition, the bursa is usually located over 1 1/2 inches from the surface of the skin, making use of a spinal needle (usually 21 gauge) necessary. In many instances, even the tip of the spinal needle may not reach the trochanter until the hub of the spinal needle touches the skin.

After locating and marking the area of greatest tenderness, the clinician cleans the overlying skin with alcohol and anesthetizes the epidermis and dermis with 1 ml of lidocaine 1%. The patient should be approached from the back, so that he does not see the long spinal needle. Sterile gloves are required since insertion of the spinal needle requires two hands. After the skin is prepared with an iodine solution, the needle is inserted directly perpendicular to the trochanter. Numerous points of resistance and sudden "pops" or giving sensations are felt as the needle passes through fascial planes. Once the bone has been touched, the clinician may be confident that the basic direction of the injection is correct. Failure of the spinal needle to touch the bone by the time the needle hub reaches the skin suggests that the angle of the search was incorrect. The needle should be redrawn and reinserted until the needle tip touches the femur.

Injections of lidocaine should be "fanned out," with 3 ml placed right over the trochanter, 3 ml placed several centimeters superiorly, and the final 3 ml placed several centimeters caudally.

Only patients who respond to the initial lidocaine injection will benefit from additional injection of 40 mg of a long-acting form of methylprednisolone or its equivalent. Corticosteroids should be injected at the time of the initial visit. Most patients with trochanteric bursitis experience marked relief of pain for many months; return of the pain in several days suggests either that the injection was not made in the correct location or that there is another etiology for the pain.

COSTS/COMPLICATIONS.   The complications associated with injection of the trochanteric bursa are local pain and bacterial infection. If proper technique is employed, the risk of introducing infection is very low.

Cross-reference: Hip Pain (Section 110).

REFERENCES

1. Gordon ET. Trochanteric bursitis and tendinitis. Clin Orthop 1961;20:193–202.
    Review of the clinical manifestation of trochanteric bursitis.

2. Larsson L-G, Baum J. The syndromes of bursitis. Bull Rheum Dis 1986;36:1–8.
    Review of common bursitis syndromes and their treatment.

3. Ramon D, Haslock I. Trochanteric bursitis: A frequent cause of "hip" pain in rheumatoid arthritis. Ann Rheum Dis 1982;41:602–603.
    Trochanteric bursitis was present in 15% of an unselected group of 100 patients with rheumatoid arthritis.

4. Schapira D, Nahir M, Scharf Y. Trochanteric bursitis: A common clinical problem. Arch Phys Med Rehab 1986;67:815–817.
    Most patients also had lumbar spine arthrosis or ipsilateral hip damage.

130 ASPIRATION/INJECTION OF THE KNEE

Procedure

RICHARD H. WHITE

INDICATIONS/CONTRAINDICATIONS.   The principal indications for arthrocentesis are (1) to obtain joint fluid for analysis in the setting of monarticular or polyarticular arthritis of unknown etiology, (2) to remove joint fluid as a therapeutic maneuver, or (3) to inject a therapeutic agent, usually a corticosteroid preparation, to treat an inflammatory arthritis. The only contraindication is suspected hemarthrosis due to an uncorrectable coagulopathy, such as acquired antibody to von Willebrand factor, because bleeding may be impossible to control. Overlying cellulitis is not a contraindication to aspiration of the knee, which should be performed if there is any suspicion of septic arthritis; IV antibiotics should be administered to treat the cellulitis as soon as arthrocentesis is completed.

RATIONALE.   Analysis and culture of synovial fluid can aid in the diagnosis of a number of causes of arthritis, including (1) septic arthritis, based on Gram stain and culture results, (2) gout, based on the finding of negatively birefringent crystals, (3) pseudogout, based on the presence of small, positively bire-fringent crystals, (4) inflammatory arthritis, based on a joint fluid WBC count greater than 2000 cells/mm^3, with no crystals and a negative culture, (5) non-inflammatory arthritis, based on a synovial WBC count less than 2000 cells/mm^3, and (6) hemarthrosis. Synovial fluid should be aspirated whenever there is an unexplained arthropathy leading to an effusion, particularly if infection is suspected.

Although a large number of joint fluid tests are available (protein level, glucose, quality of the mucin clot, etc.), only a microbiologic culture, examination for crystals, and determination of the synovial white and red blood cell counts provide useful information. Even these tests, however, are imperfect: culture results may be falsely positive (contamination) or false negative; crystals may be seen in cases of septic arthritis; crystals, especially calcium pyrophosphate, may be difficult to see; the synovial fluid WBC count may lead to inaccurate classification. The entire clinical picture, only one part of which is synovial fluid analysis, forms the basis for diagnosis.

METHODS. Prior to aspirating a knee joint, the clinician cleans the point of entry with alcohol and anesthesizes the skin with 0.5 to 1 ml of lidocaine 1%. An injection of lidocaine into deep subcutaneous tissues is unnecessary. The skin is then cleaned with an iodine-containing solution. Because joint fluid can be very viscous, a No. 18 or No. 19 needle is needed for aspiration. Appropriate collection tubes should be available, including a tube for cell count and differential, a tube to save fluid for synovial crystal analysis, and an appropriate container for microbiologic culture. A 5-ml syringe is adequate for small effusions; larger collections should be removed with a 50-ml syringe.

To obtain joint fluid from the knee, the easiest and safest site to insert a needle is the medial or lateral suprapatellar recess. The joint fluid is forced into the suprapatellar recess by the clinician applying pressure with the nondominant hand, positioning the palm just below the patella, with the thumb running along one edge of the patella and the fingers along the opposite edge. With the syringe in the dominant hand, the clinician inserts the needle above the superior edge of the patella, aimed to pass just beneath the cartilaginous surface of the patella. Often there is a popping sensation when the joint space has been entered. The dominant hand withdraws the plunger to remove the joint fluid. If an assistant is available to compress the joint fluid, the physician is freed to operate the syringe with both hands.

Joint fluid may be difficult to aspirate, particularly in patients with rheumatoid arthritis. Hypertrophied synovium, which may be mistaken for joint fluid, consists of thousands of microvilli that can occlude the lumen of a needle when too much negative pressure is applied. If no joint fluid is retrieved, reducing the negative pressure being applied to the syringe and rotating the needle often results in a successful tap.

Occasionally one may want to inject a therapeutic agent into the joint after removing the joint fluid. This requires either the use of a three-way stopcock or removing the syringe from the needle hub while the needle tip remains in the joint space. Any exchange of syringes must be performed using sterile technique; the first syringe should be only gently tightened on the needle, allowing easy removal during the procedure.

After aspiration, the iodine solution should be wiped off the skin with alcohol to prevent skin sensitization.

COSTS/COMPLICATIONS.   The complications associated with aspiration of the knee are pain and bacterial contamination. Avoiding needle contact with the patella minimizes pain. If aseptic technique is followed, the likelihood of introducing bacteria in the joint space is less than one in 2000 aspirations.

Cross-references: General Approach to Arthritic Symptoms (Section 107), Knee Pain (Section 112), Osteoarthritis (Section 119), Gout/Hyperuricemia (Section 120).

REFERENCES

1. Bomalaski JS, Lluberas G, Schumacher HR Jr. Monosodium urate crystals in the knees of patients with asymptomatic nontophaceous gout. Arthritis Rheum 1986;29:1480–1484.
    In fifty patients with a prior diagnosis of gout, aspiration of nonflammatory joint fluid revealed monosodium urate crystals in twenty-nine (58%).

2. Moll JMH. Management of Rheumatic Diseases. Chapman and Hale, London, 1983, pp. 213–238.
    A chapter describing local injection/aspiration techniques.

3. Schmerling RH, Delbanco TL, Tosteson ANA, Trentham DE. Synovial fluid tests: What should be ordered? JAMA 1990;264:1009–1014.
    Chemistry studies, including glucose, protein, and lactic dehydrogenase levels, provided misleading or redundant information in classifying inflammatory versus nonflammatory joint fluid.

4. Schumacher HR Jr. Synovial fluid analysis and synovial biopsy. In Kelly WN, Harris ED Jr, Ruddy S, Sledge CB, Eds. Textbook of Rheumatology. W.B. Saunders, Philadelphia, 1989, pp. 637–664.
    A thorough overview of synovial fluid analysis.

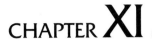
VASCULAR DISORDERS

131 PAINFUL AND SWOLLEN CALF

Symptom

STEVEN R. McGEE

EPIDEMIOLOGY. Acute deep venous thrombosis (DVT) occurs with an annual incidence of 1 per 1000 in the general population. The mean age of affected patients is 60 years. Men are affected as often as women, the left leg is involved more often than the right. Risk factors include prolonged immobility, surgery or trauma (especially of the lower limb or pelvis), malignancy, congestive heart failure, pregnancy, estrogen therapy, and deficiencies of antithrombin III, protein C, or protein S.

ETIOLOGY. The most important causes of the acutely painful and swollen calf are cellulitis, DVT, Baker's cysts, and muscle hematoma. When outpatients with acute calf swelling are studied with both venography and arthrography (cellulitis is clinically excluded), Baker's cysts are found in about 30%, acute DVT in 25%, both Baker's cyst and DVT in 10%, and neither diagnosis in 35%.

Acute DVT usually originates in the venous sinuses of the soleus muscle. When confined to the calf (i.e., "distal" DVT), clinically significant pulmonary emboli are unlikely. DVTs that propagate from the calf to involve at least the popliteal vein ("proximal" DVT) cause symptomatic pulmonary emboli in as many as 50% of untreated patients, sometimes with a fatal outcome. **Baker's cysts** are distended gastrocnemius-semimembranosus bursae that usually communicate with the knee joint and may enlarge from any cause of knee arthritis (e.g., rheumatoid arthritis, osteoarthritis, loose body). Baker's cysts may cause acute swelling that is indistinguishable from DVT ("pseudothrombophlebitis"), either because of dissection or rupture of the cyst into the calf or because of pressure from the enlarging cyst on the popliteal vein. **Muscle hematomas** may result from tears in the calf muscles, often following trauma or

395

excessive exercise. **Cellulitis** is a spreading infection of the skin and subcutaneous tissues, usually caused by group A streptococcus or *Staphylococcus aureus*.

CLINICAL APPROACH.   The most important diagnosis to address is acute DVT, not only because untreated patients may die, but because empirical anticoagulation without a firm diagnosis may promote bleeding in patients with unsuspected Baker's cysts or muscle hematomas.

Most muscle hematomas are beneath the deep muscle fascia and cause no leg discoloration, although some patients have a hemorrhagic crescent near either malleolus as the only clue. Cellulitis may cause shaking chills and high fever, with the findings of a hot extremity, bright well-demarcated redness, lymphangitis, and tender local lymph nodes. Other history, symptoms and signs, such as prolonged immobility, prior DVT, recent swelling behind the knee, palpable cord on examination, or a positive Homan's sign, do not reliably distinguish DVT from other diagnoses. Therefore, other diagnostic tests are necessary.

Although contrast venography is the reference standard test for DVT, it has several disadvantages, including expense, radiation exposure, invasiveness, and the tendency to induce DVT (1%–2% of cases). Further, as many as 10% of studies are inadequate for interpretation, and in another 10%, radiologists differ on the test's interpretation.

Noninvasive tests are now commonly used for the outpatient diagnosis of DVT (Table 131–1). Two large studies of outpatients with acute calf swelling have demonstrated that it is safe to withhold anticoagulant therapy if serial **impedance plethysmography** (three studies over 7 days) remains negative. Because noninvasive tests only detect proximal DVTs with any reliability, these studies support the view that DVTs confined to the calf rarely cause significant pulmonary emboli even without anticoagulation. A single impedance plethysmogram is inadequate, however: 25% of proximal DVTs are first identified on the second or third test, which suggests that some distal DVTs, missed on the first test, propagate over time to above the popliteal vein and would only be detected with serial testing. **Duplex ultrasonography** (US) combines Doppler US, which measures the flow in the vein, with real-time US, which directly visualizes the vein and its compressibility (clots make veins noncompressible). Because results with duplex US are so promising, many authorities acknowledge that duplex US may be substituted for impedance plethysmography. One advantage of duplex US is that in 5% to 10% of patients, other diagnoses such as Baker's cysts or muscle hematomas are identified. **Doppler US** is popular

TABLE 131–1.   NONINVASIVE DIAGNOSTIC TESTS FOR PROXIMAL DVT

Test	Sensitivity[1]	Specificity[1]
Doppler ultrasound	0.76–0.95	0.84–0.95
Impedance plethysmography	0.95	0.83–0.95
Duplex ultrasound	0.95	0.98–1.0

[1]Contrast venography is the reference standard.

because the device is hand-held and portable, but published results vary and probably depend heavily on the operator's experience.

Several points regarding noninvasive tests are important: (1) Clinicians should determine their own hospital's experience, compared to contrast venography, and not rely entirely on published data. (2) Until studies demonstrate otherwise, patients with persistent symptoms should be tested serially over 1 week before the clinician concludes that no DVT is present. (3) False-positive results occur, usually with Doppler US and impedance plethysmography, in patients with extrinsic compression of the vein by a mass or with prior history of DVT. In patients with suspected recurrent DVT or with abdominal or pelvic masses on examination, therefore, contrast venography may be the preferred test. Alternatively, many clinicians repeat noninvasive testing when patients with documented DVT complete their anticoagulation regimen, to have a baseline examination on hand in case recurrent disease is later suspected.

To diagnose a Baker's cyst, real-time US is equivalent to arthrography in most studies. US of the popliteal fossa is indicated if symptoms persist despite therapy (whether or not a DVT is documented). Patients with obvious knee effusions on examination require arthrocentesis (see Section 130, Aspiration/Injection of the Knee).

MANAGEMENT.   Patients with proximal DVTs require hospital admission and heparin anticoagulation. Those with cellulitis, especially when fever or lymphangitis is present, are best managed in the hospital with parenteral antibiotics. The remaining patients with an acutely swollen leg usually respond to leg elevation and nonsteroidal anti-inflammatory agents over 1 to 2 weeks.

FOLLOW-UP.   A common reason for recurrent cellulitis is untreated tinea pedis.

Section 203 reviews chronic anticoagulation therapy, which is usually recommended for 3 to 6 months following the first DVT, and for longer periods if DVT is recurrent. In patients with DVT the prevalence of deficiencies of protein C, protein S, antithrombin III, or plasminogen is too low (8.5%) to justify mass screening.

Cross-references: Pleuritic Chest Pain (Section 61), Knee Pain (Section 112), Aspiration/Injection of the Knee (Section 130), Chronic Anticoagulation (Section 203).

REFERENCES

1. Heijboer H, Brandjes DPM, Buller HR, Sturk A, Cate JW. Deficiencies of coagulation-inhibiting and fibrinolytic proteins in outpatients with deep-vein thrombosis. N Engl J Med 1990;323:1512–1516.
    See text. In patients with DVT that was recurrent, familial, or occurred before the age of 41 years, abnormalities were present in 9%, 16%, and 12%, respectively.

2. Hirsh J, Hull RD, Raskob GE. Clinical features and diagnosis of venous thrombosis. J Am Coll Cardiol 1986;8:114B–127B.
    Excellent review that includes a differential diagnosis.

3. Huisman MV, Buller HR, Cate JW, Vreeken J. Serial impedance plethysmography for sus-
    pected deep venous thrombosis in outpatients: The Amsterdam general practitioner study.
    N Engl J Med 1986;314:823–828.
    A study of 426 outpatients with suspected DVT that demonstrated the accuracy of impedance plethys-
    mography and the safety of withholding anticoagulation therapy when serial tests performed over sev-
    eral days were negative (see companion study, Arch Intern Med 1989;149:511–513).

4. White RH, McGahan JP, Daschbach MM, Hartling RP. Diagnosis of deep-vein thrombosis
    using duplex ultrasound. Ann Intern Med 1989;111:297–304.
    Reviews the accuracy of duplex ultrasonography and compares it with other diagnostic tests.

5. Wigley RD. Popliteal cysts: Variations on a theme of Baker. Semin Arthritis Rheum
    1982;12:1–10.
    Excellent review of Baker's cysts.

132 RAYNAUD'S SYNDROME

Symptom

STEVEN R. McGEE

EPIDEMIOLOGY.   Raynaud's syndrome (intermittent vasospasm of the fingertips) affects up to 5% of the population. The mean age at onset is 30 years.
The disease is more common in women (70%–90% of cases), in northern climates, during colder months, and in users of hand-held vibratory tools (e.g.,
jackhammers, grinders, chainsaws).

ETIOLOGY.   Raynaud's syndrome is either **primary** ("vasospastic," formerly
termed "Raynaud's disease") or **secondary** to systemic disease that affects the
small arteries of the hand ("obstructive," formerly termed "Raynaud's phenomenon"). Large surveys from vascular surgery clinics suggest that 40% of
cases are primary and 60% are secondary, with two-thirds of the secondary
cases resulting from connective tissue disease, most commonly systemic sclerosis, the CREST syndrome (calcinosis, Raynaud's, esophageal hypomotility,
sclerodactyly, telangiectasia), or systemic lupus erythematosus (SLE). Other
secondary causes, among many, include arterial diseases (atherosclerosis,
Buerger's disease), cryoglobulinemia, multiple myeloma, myxedema, and
frostbite. However, because of the high prevalence of Raynaud's syndrome
(5%) and the low incidence of systemic sclerosis (5–10 new cases per 1 million
population per year), these data probably reflect referral bias and overestimate
the prevalence of secondary cases seen in general practice settings.

Medications associated with an increased incidence of Raynaud's syndrome
include beta blockers, sympathomimetics, ergotamine, vinblastine, and bleomycin.

CLINICAL APPROACH.   The diagnosis depends entirely on a characteristic history: following emotional upset or exposure to cold, patients experience attacks of discrete pallor that extend at least to the distal interphalangeal joint. Cyanosis and rubor may sequentially follow the pallor, although only 20% have the full triphasic color response. The syndrome usually affects both hands and sometimes involves the toes, ears, and cheeks, but typically spares the thumbs. Numbness, tingling, or burning frequently accompany the attack, which usually lasts 30 to 60 minutes; severe pain is rare. The differential diagnosis includes cyanotic diseases of the central (hypoxemia, hemoglobin abnormalities) or peripheral (low cardiac output, peripheral vascular disease) type. These diseases differ because they lack discrete attacks of pallor; furthermore, central cyanosis may worsen with warming of the extremity, and involves the tongue and buccal mucosa.

The patient interview focuses on the patient's medications (including non-proprietary cold remedies), occupation, and symptoms suggestive of connective tissue disease (arthralgia, rash, dysphagia, tight skin, sicca symptoms of dry eyes and mouth). The clinician should closely examine the patient's pulses and skin (ulcers, sclerodactyly, telangiectasia). Routine laboratory tests include a complete blood cell count, erythrocyte sedimentation rate (ESR), chemistry profile, urinalysis, and antinuclear antibody assay. Because vasospasm alone never causes digital ulcers or gangrene, patients with these findings, as well as those with absent pulses on examination, should be referred to a vascular surgeon for consideration of arteriography.

MANAGEMENT.   About 90% of patients respond to (1) discontinuing offending medications and cigarette smoking, (2) limiting occupational exposure to vibratory tools, and (3) using mittens and insulated fabrics to minimize exposure to cold.

Pharmacologic therapy for Raynaud's syndrome, given during the colder months, is appropriate for the few patients who have frequent disabling symptoms despite the measures listed above. Double-blind placebo-controlled trials document the efficacy of nifedipine (10 mg PO t.i.d.), diltiazem (30–120 mg t.i.d.), and prazosin (slowly advanced to 1 mg PO t.i.d.). In one study, nifedipine was superior to prazosin.

Surgery is indicated only for documented proximal arterial stenosis. Upper extremity sympathectomy has been abandoned because relapses were common.

FOLLOW-UP.   The frequency of attacks waxes and wanes over years. The course of primary Raynaud's syndrome, present at least 2 years, is benign: 9 years later, fewer than 5% of patients have signs of connective tissue disease.[2]

Cross-references: Smoking Cessation (Section 11), General Approach to Arthritic Symptoms (Section 107), Wrist and Hand Pain (Section 111), Interpretation of Serologic Tests (Section 124).

REFERENCES

1. Cardelli MB, Kleinsmith DM. Raynaud's phenomenon and disease. Med Clin North Am 1989;73:1127–1141.

    Overview of etiology, pathophysiology, and management.

2. Gerbracht DD, Steen VD, Ziegler GL, Medsger TA, Rodnan GP. Evolution of primary Raynaud's phenomenon (Raynaud's disease) to connective tissue disease. Arthritis Rheum 1985;28:87–92.

    Only four of eighty-seven patients with primary Raynaud's syndrome had developed signs of connective tissue disease a decade later. ANA and anticentromere antibody assays did not help predict who would develop connective tissue disease.

3. Houtman PM, Kallenberg CGM, Fidler V, Wouda AA. Diagnostic significance of nailfold capillary patterns in patients with Raynaud's phenomenon. J Rheumatol 1986;13:556–563.

    Although a decrease in nail fold capillary loops helped distinguish primary from secondary Raynaud's syndrome (sensitivity = 46%, specificity = 92%), the diagnosis of connective tissue disease was obvious from other clinical findings.

4. Jobe JB, Sampson JB, Roberts DE, Beetham WP. Induced vasodilation as treatment for Raynaud's disease. Ann Intern Med 1982;97:706–709.

    A controlled study demonstrating the efficacy of pavlovian conditioning: simultaneous exposure of the body to cold and the hands to warm, repeated over 3 weeks, resulted in lasting benefit.

5. Rodeheffer RJ, Rommer JA, Wigley F, Smith CR. Controlled double-blind trial of nifedipine in the treatment of Raynaud's phenomenon. N Engl J Med 1983;308:880–883.

    Moderate or marked improvement occurred in 60%.

133 PERIPHERAL ARTERIAL DISEASE

Problem

KAJ JOHANSEN

EPIDEMIOLOGY/ETIOLOGY.   Most patients with symptoms and signs of peripheral arterial disease have atherosclerosis. The age-adjusted prevalence of claudication is 0.3% in men and 0.1% in women. Claudication is five times more common in diabetics. Patients with peripheral arterial disease are generally over 50 years of age, and almost all have an extensive smoking history. Many are hypertensive, and various forms of hyperlipidemia are more common in this patient population. Although only a minority are diabetic, such patients are at high risk for complications related to arterial occlusive disease. For example, over half of the lower extremity amputations in the United States are performed in diabetics.

Abdominal aortic aneurysm (AAA) is found in 20% of unselected autopsy series and in at least 10% of patients attending a vascular surgery clinic. AAA rarely occurs before the age of 60; it is predominantly a disease of elderly men with a past or current history of smoking. Hypertension is common in AAA patients, and first-degree relatives of AAA patients have at least an eightfold higher likelihood of developing AAA themselves, in comparison with an age-matched control population.

SYMPTOMS AND SIGNS.   Claudication is exercise-related muscle discomfort. Classically, patients are asymptomatic at rest and begin walking without difficulty, but at distances of from four to six blocks down to as little as a few feet, they note the onset of calf muscle distress characterized as "aching," "tiredness," or "burning." Symptoms appear sooner with uphill walking or walking up stairs, because such activity uses the gastrocnemius and soleus muscles.

Claudication is usually diagnostic of a high-grade atherosclerotic stenosis or occlusion of the superficial femoral artery in the thigh. Less common distributions of atherosclerotic arterial occlusive disease may cause claudication in the gluteal or thigh muscles, which when associated with absent femoral pulses, impotence in men, and thigh muscle atrophy (the Leriche syndrome) suggests aortoiliac occlusive disease.

Very rarely, instep claudication is noted in patients with diffuse tibial artery occlusive disease. This almost always occurs in young male patients addicted to cigarette smoking and is virtually pathognomonic for thromboangiitis obliterans (Buerger's disease). Much less commonly, patients with peripheral arterial disease present with nocturnal rest pain or tissue loss (heel or toe gangrene or a nonhealing arterial ulcer of the foot). Virtually all such patients have a prior history of claudication, and examination of their lower extremities typically shows retarded capillary refill, loss of hair growth, and thickened nails. Advanced cases manifest dependent rubor, pallor with elevation, and coolness.

The absence of diabetes or a smoking history should suggest another diagnosis (e.g., lumbar spinal stenosis, trauma, myositis, or another nonvascular cause). Neurogenic or pseudoclaudication may occur in individuals with lumbar spinal stenosis or osteophytic impingment on lumbosacral nerve roots. Such patients may have few or no symptoms at rest, but may develop calf pain after walking or even standing for a period of time. These individuals' pain is characteristically sharper and more burning. Such individuals usually have normal pulses on physical examination, normal Doppler pressure indices (see below), and history, physical examination findings, and spinal imaging studies consistent with chronic back disease (e.g. degenerative disk disease, past fractures, or operations).

AAA is rarely symptomatic prior to rupture. About 50% of patients with AAA ultimately die of aneurysmal rupture. Hospital mortality rates from AAA rupture vary from 30% to 70%; overall, the mortality (including those who die at home or en route to the hospital) exceeds 90%.[3] On the other hand, the operative mortality associated with elective repair of AAAs discovered prior to rupture is less than 5%, even in octogenarians.

CLINICAL APPROACH.   The diagnosis of peripheral arterial disease in the patient with claudication is implied by absent popliteal and pedal pulses on physical examination and by diminished Doppler pressures at the ankle. Ankle/brachial indices (ABIs) (see Section 136) are diminished in direct proportion to the walking distance. A normal ABI is about 1.0; one to two-block claudication is generally associated with an ABI of 0.6 to 0.8, while patients with severe (less than one-block) claudication have an ABI of 0.4 to 0.6. Patients with rest pain, arterial ulcers or gangrene have an ABI below 0.4.

Although claudication is diagnostic of significant arterial occlusive disease, patients with claudication are at greater risk of subsequent cardiovascular mortality than of limb loss. In one study, limb loss following onset of claudication occurred in only 7% of claudicants during the next 5 years, and in only 12% by 10 years, whereas cardiovascular mortality was 27% during the first 5 years and 63% at 10 years. Accordingly, close attention to the cardiac and cerebrovascular status of patients with claudication is warranted.

A single abdominal ultrasound (US) examination performed at age 60 in men or women with a history of smoking, peripheral vascular disease, or a relative with a known AAA should detect more than 90% of all AAAs. Individuals with a normal abdominal aortic US study at the age of 60 need be evaluated no further. Those with a small AAA, less than 4 cm in diameter, should undergo repeat abdominal US every 6 months and should be referred to a vascular surgeon when the size of the AAA exceeds 4 cm. Patients with an AAA of any size should be instructed to seek medical attention immediately should new abdominal, flank, or back pain occur.

MANAGEMENT.   Claudication in most patients stabilizes or improves with simple measures such as weight loss, daily aerobic exercise, and, most important, cessation of cigarette smoking. In compliant patients, pentoxifylline (Trental) may be useful: a prospective multicenter trial showed a small but significant improvement in walking distance.[4] Gastrointestinal upset accompanies the administration of pentoxifylline in 5% to 10% of patients. A 3-month supply (400 mg PO t.i.d.) costs approximately $114.

A very small number of patients with severe claudication may be considered for arterial reconstruction. Because such operative or endovascular procedures are only moderately successful, they should be proposed only if all nonoperative means, including smoking cessation, have failed and the patient's employability or quality of life is significantly affected. Arteriography is warranted only when a therapeutic intervention—balloon dilation or surgical reconstruction—is contemplated.

By contrast, *all* individuals with rest pain, arterial ulcers, or gangrene require an intervention, either arterial reconstruction or amputation. Lower extremity arteriography always shows atherosclerotic occlusions at two or more sites. Because their coronary or cerebrovascular occlusive disease is proportionately more advanced as well, the 5-year survival rate after the onset of rest pain or lower extremity gangrene in the nondiabetic patient is substantially less than 50%.

No nonoperative therapy exists for AAA. All AAAs larger than 5 cm should be repaired, and AAAs with diameters of 4 cm or greater should be repaired in younger or healthy patients, or those living in remote locales. Few contraindications to surgery exist, other than rapidly terminal conditions such as metastatic cancer or severe chronic pulmonary disease. Occasional long-term survivors develop graft complications, such as anastomotic pseudoaneurysm.

FOLLOW-UP. The clinician should monitor the patients' symptoms, and ankle pressures or ABIs every 3 to 6 months. Any improvement in ankle pressures and symptoms can be appropriately ascribed to exercise or smoking cessation programs; such positive feedback is often very encouraging to the patient. After an arterial reconstructive procedure, regular follow-up (usually by the vascular surgeon) is important to detect vessel or graft reocclusion (from arterial neointimal hyperplasia).

Because aneurysmal arterial degeneration is a systemic disorder, follow-up of patients with AAAs should include surveillance of femoral and popliteal arteries for asymptomatic dilation.

Cross-references: Smoking Cessation (Section 11), Ankle and Foot Pain (Section 113), Diabetic Foot Care Education (Section 125), Leg Ulcers (Section 134), Doppler Measurement of Ankle Pressures (Section 136), Hyperlipidemia (Section 155), Diabetes Mellitus (Section 157), Preoperative Cardiovascular Problems (Section 217).

REFERENCES

1. Boyd AM. Natural course of arteriosclerosis of lower extremities. Proc R Soc Med 1962; 55:591–599.
    A classic study from the pre-vascular surgery era documenting that lower extremity claudication is a relatively insensitive predictor of limb loss but a very good indicator of an early coronary demise. For a modern study corroborating Boyd's findings, see Surgery 1975;78:795–799.

2. Collin J. Screening for abdominal aortic aneurysms. Br J Surg 1985;72:851–852.
    Because AAAs are usually asymptomatic and are diagnosed on physical examination in less than half of cases, screening of populations at risk seems warranted. Such an approach, however, requires consideration of the resource expenditures necessary to manage the large number of asymptomatic lesions thus discovered.

3. Johansen K, Kohler TR, Nicholls S, Zierler RE, Clowes AW, Kazmers A. Ruptured abdominal aortic aneurysm: The Harborview experience. J Vasc Surg 1991;13:240–247.
    Despite (or perhaps because of) skilled prehospital paramedic care, rapid diagnosis, timely operation, and expert postoperative care, 70% of patients with ruptured AAAs died. This toll, and the extraordinary utilization of health care resources used to try to salvage patients with ruptured AAA, underscores the importance of AAA screening programs.

4. Porter JM, Cutler BS, Lee BY, et al. Pentoxifylline efficacy in the treatment of intermittent claudication: Multicenter controlled double-blind trial with objective assessment of chronic arterial occlusive disease patients. Am Heart J 1982;104:66–72.
    A multicenter trial found a small but significant benefit of this agent in altering whole blood viscosity and red cell deformability when administered to patients with claudication.

134 LEG ULCERS

Problem

STEVEN R. McGEE

EPIDEMIOLOGY.   Venous ulcers, which account for up to 90% of all leg ulcers, affect 0.2% to 0.4% of the population.

ETIOLOGY.   Table 134–1 lists the most important causes of leg ulceration. Some 50% to 75% of patients with sickle cell disease have leg ulcers.

Venous ulcers result from chronic venous hypertension. Although the exact cause is debatable, many authorities attribute venous ulcers to capillary leakage of fibrin, with subsequent impairment of oxygen diffusion and tissue ischemia.

CLINICAL APPROACH.   The clinician should ask the patient how rapidly the ulcer developed, and whether there is associated trauma, claudication, edema, or symptoms of systemic disease (e.g., fever, weight loss). Pain is common to all etiologies except neuropathic ulcers. The examination focuses on the ulcer's location and appearance (base and edge), and on associated skin, vascular, and neurologic findings.

Venous ulcers, which may appear abruptly, are classically located over the medial malleolus but may occur over the lateral malleolus, distal leg, or dorsal surface of the foot. Affected patients have findings of underlying venous insufficiency, such as edema or venous (stasis) dermatitis (pruritic erythematous rash on distal third of calf, skin hyperpigmentation from hemosiderin and melanin). The ulcer base consists of granulation tissue (red pebbly tissue, reflecting

TABLE 134–1.   ETIOLOGY OF LEG ULCERS[1]

Venous*
Arterial*
Neuropathic*
Vasculitis
Hemoglobinopathy
  Sickle cell disease
Infectious
  Sporothrix schenckii
  Mycobacterium marinum
Pyoderma gangrenosum
Tumors
  Squamous cell carcinoma
  Mycosis fungoides

[1]A more complete differential diagnosis appears in reference 4.
*Most common causes.

new capillary tufts of wound healing) and frequently contains abundant yellow-green exudate. **Arterial ulcers** develop gradually, affect the foot distal to the ankle (tips of toes, "kissing ulcers" between toes, heel, plantar metatarsal heads), and have a necrotic base without granulation tissue. Affected patients have claudication; some also experience rest pain that improves with dangling of the leg. Associated findings include absent pulses, delayed capillary refill, thin hairless skin, and dependent rubor. When arterial ulcers occur in male smokers less than 40 years old, especially if associated with superficial thrombophlebitis, the diagnosis of thromboangiitis obliterans (Buerger's disease) should be considered. **Neuropathic ulcers** occur from pressure against bony prominences (metatarsal heads, heel, toes) and affect patients with peripheral sensory neuropathy.

Vasculitic ulcers, which resemble arterial ulcers, may be associated with a blue, nonpalpable, lacelike discoloration of the extremity (livedo reticularis), and sometimes with the associated findings of subcutaneous nodules and systemic disease (fever, weight loss, abnormalities of kidneys, joints, nerves, or gastrointestinal system). Ulcers of **sickle cell disease** resemble venous ulcers. The ulcer of **pyoderma gangrenosum** (may be associated with inflammatory bowel disease) appears abruptly (over days), is very painful, and is diagnosed clinically (not by biopsy) from its characteristic violet, undermined edge, ragged heaped-up border, and surrounding red halo.

MANAGEMENT.　The treatment of venous ulcers should reduce the venous hypertension and leg edema with measures such as leg elevation, elastic bandages, elastic support stockings, or the Unna's boot. For most patients, over-the-counter support hose is probably as effective as the more expensive custom-made stockings. Patients should put on the stockings before arising in the morning and wear them the entire day. When patients have arthritis or other debilities that make dressing with these stockings difficult, elastic bandage wraps are an alternative. Unna's boot is a generic term for bandages impregnated with glycerin, sorbitol, gelatin, zinc oxide, and calamine that are wrapped around the leg (Dome-Paste, GeluCast). One advantage of the Unna's boot is that it is left in place and removed 1 week later in the doctor's office, allowing the physician to follow the progress of the ulcer closely and preventing the patient from manipulating or scratching the ulcer during the week.

One relatively recent advance in the treatment of venous ulcers is the application of synthetic occlusive dressings (e.g., DuoDerm) directly to the ulcer. These dressings help debride the ulcer, significantly reduce pain, promote healing, and, because patients often learn to change them themselves, facilitate outpatient management. They should cover the ulcer and at least a 3-cm margin of surrounding skin, and should be changed only after they start to leak exudate at the edges (an average of every 5 days, range, 1–10 days). The patient should learn that this accumulation of exudate (which is sometimes foul-smelling) is normal, that infection is rare, and that premature removal of the dressing may pull off the new epithelium and retard healing. Because some form of compression therapy must accompany occlusive dressings in patients with significant edema, many clinicians combine the Unna's boot with occlusive dressings. The only major contraindication to occlusive dressings is an established infection.

No study clearly demonstrates the superiority of any of these treatments. Most ulcers heal in 6 to 12 weeks. Despite the typical yellow-green exudate that often is colonized with bacteria, randomized controlled trials demonstrate that *routine* administration of antibiotics does not promote healing of venous ulcers. When the patient has signs of infection (fever, lymphangitis, rapidly spreading erythema, tenderness), antibiotics are clearly indicated.

Patients with arterial ulcers should be referred to a vascular surgeon for consideration for a revascularization procedure. The care of diabetic foot ulcers is described in Section 135. Patients with suspected pyoderma gangrenosum should be seen by a dermatologist; if the diagnosis is confirmed, corticosteroids are the preferred treatment.

FOLLOW-UP. The patient should be seen every 1 to 2 weeks until the ulcer is clearly healing and the patient understands the treatment regimen, when the follow-up intervals may be increased. At each visit the clinician should measure the size of the ulcer (maximum length by width). Any ulcer that fails to improve or develops a nodular or heaped-up edge should be biopsied to exclude cancer, vasculitis, or infection. Large ulcers may require skin grafting.

Cross-references: Principles of Dermatologic Diagnosis and Therapy (Section 22), Eczema (Section 28), Edema (Section 77), Inflammatory Bowel Disease (Section 98), Diabetic Foot Care Education (Section 125), Peripheral Arterial Disease (Section 133), Local Care of Diabetic Foot Lesions (Section 135), Doppler Measurement of Ankle Pressures (Section 136), Diabetes Mellitus (Section 157), Sickle Cell Disease (Section 202).

REFERENCES

1. Falanga V. Occlusive wound dressings: Why, when, which? Arch Dermatol 1988;124:872–877.
    Practical review of the various occlusive dressing materials available.

2. Fitzpatrick JE. Stasis ulcers: update on a common geriatric problem. Geriatrics 1989; 44:19–31.
    Excellent overview. [Because stagnation of blood flow probably does not occur, many authorities are replacing the term "stasis ulcers" with "venous ulcers."]

3. Rijswijk L, Brown D, Friedman S, Degreef H, Roed-Petersen J, et al. Multicenter clinical evaluation of a hydrocolloid dressing for leg ulcers. Cutis 1985;35:173–176.
    Uncontrolled study of DuoDerm in 152 leg ulcers refractory to other treatment measures, including the Unna's boot; 62% healed over a mean of 51 days and 80% of patients achieved significant pain relief. No patient developed infection.

4. Young JR. Differential diagnosis of leg ulcers. Cardiovasc Clin 1983;13:171–193.
    Encyclopedic review with many clinical points.

135 LOCAL CARE OF DIABETIC FOOT LESIONS

Procedure

JESSIE H. AHRONI

INDICATIONS AND CONTRAINDICATIONS. Foot lesions are common in patients with diabetes, particularly the elderly and those with sensory neuropathy. In one study 86% of amputations followed potentially preventable minor trauma and cutaneous injury. To prevent progression to chronic nonhealing wounds, gangrene, or refractory infections, all diabetic foot lesions—discrete ulcers, blisters, calluses, abscesses, or fissures—require prompt and aggressive care.

RATIONALE. Healing requires a bed of clean granulation tissue, treatment and drainage of infections, dressings for protection, and control of edema.

METHODS. Thorough debridement with a sharp instrument should remove superficial debris, fibrin, and remnants of necrotic or nonviable tissue, including eschar. Topical debriding and cleansing applications cannot replace proper surgical debridement. If a sinus tract, abscess, or deep infection is discovered, it must be incised to provide drainage. Clinicians are sometimes hesitant to incise lesions on diabetic feet for fear of nonhealing. However, undrained pus and devitalized, infected tissue represent a greater hazard; early complete drainage of deep infections affords the best chance of saving the foot. Callus around an ulcer, especially in the plantar area, should be carefully pared with a scalpel to create a flat, saucerized area. Despite differences of opinion and the lack of good data on the details of local care, wound dressings should be applied according to accepted principles for such care. Dressings are used to protect the area from trauma, to protect the wound from contamination, and to contain wound drainage. They should not contain materials that harm growing cells or predispose to sensitization, and they should be easy to apply, comfortable, and nonadherent. At the present time, occlusive dressings (e.g., Duoderm) are not recommended for diabetic foot lesions.

For most lesions, a sterile applicator dipped in a 50:50 mixture of 3% hydrogen peroxide and normal saline can be gently rolled over the wound once daily as a form of mild chemical debridement. This peroxide solution is allowed to foam, and the wound is blotted dry with a sterile gauze. Release of oxygen radicals by tissue catalase is weakly germicidal; the effervescence mechanically cleans and debrides the wound. Hydrogen peroxide does not appear to retard wound healing.

A single layer of nonadherent dry sterile fine mesh gauze dressing (Owens Non-Adherent Dressing or equivalent) is cut to the size of the ulcer with sterile

407

scissors and placed evenly over the wound with forceps. The gauze should touch the entire wound surface but should not overlap onto healthy skin. This fine mesh gauze is then covered with a plain gauze pad and gauze wrap (Kerlix or equivalent) and taped in place.

When necessary, damp to dry dressings can be used to provide additional gentle debridement of lesions and remove wound debris that remains after instrument debridement. A saline-moistened gauze pad opened to two-ply thickness can be laid over the wound and air dried for 1 to 2 hours twice a day, for 2 or 3 days. Removing the dried dressing debrides necrotic tissue, but because it can also damage newly forming epithelium, damp to dry dressings should be discontinued as soon as exudation is minimal. Soaking should be avoided because it macerates the skin, damages granulation tissue, opens small fissures that are portals to infection, and may result in hot-water burns.

In noncytotoxic concentrations, Dakin's solution (sodium hypochlorite) is a chlorine-releasing agent that is bactericidal and loosens necrotic tissue to aid in local debridement. Damp to dry dressings with quarter-strength Dakin's solution used as the wetting agent have been safely used on diabetic ulcers. To avoid maceration caused by prolonged application of wet dressings, damp to dry quarter-strength Dakin's dressing during the night can be alternated with the half-strength hydrogen peroxide cleansing and dry sterile dressing (described above) during the day.

Leg edema, whether from local infection or systemic causes, can adversely effect local cutaneous circulation and wound healing. Elevating the affected extremity may be sufficient to control local edema, but in some cases diuretics are required. When arterial flow is severely compromised, the leg should be elevated only to the level of the heart. Elastic wraps or compression hose, fitted so as not to restrict arterial flow, may also be useful.

Pressure from walking can increase edema, prevent a wound from healing, or cause further foot problems. Patients should be instructed to avoid walking, even around the house, except as absolutely necessary until skin closure occurs. When ambulation is essential, appropriate footwear is crucial. Optimal footwear should provide the following: (1) correct width sizing, (2) even weight distribution over the plantar surface of the foot, (3) a rounded, fairly high toe box, (4) a removable padded insole with energy-absorbing properties under which accommodative pads may be placed, (5) soft upper materials, (6) relatively low cost, (7) aesthetic acceptability, and (8) comfort. Protective temporary shoes, such as Dermaplast or Darco with moldable insoles, should be used when the patient's usual footwear is inappropriate for necessary ambulation. After healing, patients without major foot deformities may use good-quality running shoes. In some cases specially constructed shoes, molded insoles, metatarsal bars, or rocker bottoms may be needed.

The basic principles of diabetic foot care which all patients must be taught are described in Section 125, Diabetic Foot Care Education.

COMPLICATIONS.   Patients who cannot perform or obtain good outpatient local care, who have signs of systemic toxicity (e.g., high fever, hypotension, severe hyperglycemia, acidosis), or who have an infection that is immediately threatening to life or limb (i.e., accompanied by extensive cellulitis, lymphangitis, deep space infection, gangrene, crepitus, gas in the tissues, or osteomyelitis) should be admitted to the hospital for treatment.

Cross-references: Edema (Section 77), Diabetic Foot Care Education (Section 125), Peripheral Arterial Disease (Section 133), Doppler Measurement of Ankle Pressures (Section 136), Diabetes Mellitus (Section 157).

REFERENCES

1. Katz S, McGinley K, Leyden JJ. Semipermeable occlusive dressings: Effects on growth of pathogenic bacteria and reepithelialization of superficial wounds. Arch Dermatol 1986; 122:58–62.
    Six commercially available semiocclusive dressings used on experimentally induced wounds in humans all provided microenvironments conducive to the growth of resident and pathogenic bacteria; there were no differences in the rates of reepithelialization.

2. Kozak G, Hoar CJ, Rowbotham J, Wheelock F, Gibbons G, Campbell D, Eds. Management of Diabetic Foot Problems. W.B. Saunders, Philadelphia, 1984.
    Overview of the management of diabetic foot problems.

3. Lineaweaver W, Howard R, Soucy D, et al. Topical antimicrobial toxicity. Arch Surg 1985;120:267–270.
    Three topical antibiotics and four antiseptics applied to cultured human fibroblasts and an animal model of wound healing varied in toxicity and bactericidal potency.

4. Lipsky BA, Pecoraro RE, Larson SA, Hanley ME, Ahroni JH. Outpatient management of uncomplicated lower-extremity infections in diabetic patients. Arch Intern Med 1990; 150:790–797.
    Previously untreated infections are usually caused by aerobic gram-positive cocci and generally respond well to outpatient management with oral antibiotics.

5. Pecoraro RE, Reiber GE, Burgess E. Pathways to diabetic limb amputation: A basis for prevention. Diabetes Care 1990;13:513–521.
    Defines the causal pathways to diabetic limb amputation in 80 patients.

136 DOPPLER MEASUREMENT OF ANKLE PRESSURES

Procedure

KAJ JOHANSEN

INDICATIONS/CONTRAINDICATIONS.   The hand-held Doppler ultrasonic probe allows rapid, accurate, and noninvasive measurement of lower extremity arterial pressure, which is a reasonable indicator of tissue perfusion. Use of this technique is indicated to confirm suspected peripheral arterial disease, to exclude the diagnosis in others, and to evaluate patients serially during exercise programs or following arterial reconstructive surgery.

Contraindications include a recent limb operation or other conditions that make use of a pneumatic pressure cuff painful. Doppler pressures cannot, of course, be measured when the limb has been amputated, and are unreliable in diabetics, whose arterial medial sclerosis renders their calf arteries noncompressible.

RATIONALE.   In the normal adult, systolic arterial pressure at the ankle equals brachial artery pressure, and pedal pulses should be palpable. Because it is difficult to palpate a pedal pulse with a pressure of less than 70 or 80 mm Hg, a simple noninvasive means of measuring pressure in arteries with atherosclerotic stenoses or occlusions is necessary. Individuals with symptoms (e.g., claudication) suggesting arterial occlusive disease but whose ankle pressures are normal may have another cause for the pain, such as lumbar spinal stenosis.

Ankle pressure measurement and calculation of the ankle/brachial index (ABI) reliably indicate perfusion to the level of the muscular arteries of the ankle in patients with atherosclerosis (excluding diabetics).

METHODS.   The technique is simple and rapid. A standard arm blood pressure cuff is placed on the calf just above the ankle. A dollop of ultrasound gel is placed over the posterior tibial artery (just behind the medial malleolus) and over the dorsalis pedis artery (one to three fingerbreadths lateral to the meridian of the foot on its dorsal surface), and the arterial signal is located with the hand-held Doppler device. The cuff is then inflated to suprasystolic levels, and the higher of the two systolic pressures (either the dorsalis pedis or the posterior tibial artery) is recorded just as for measuring arm blood pressure (i.e., by the first sounds of arterial flow as the blood pressure cuff is "bled" down toward normal). The higher of the two brachial artery pressures is then measured in the same fashion. The ABI equals the highest pedal systolic pressure divided by the higher of the two brachial systolic pressures.

The normal ABI should be approximately 1.0 (range, 0.90–1.2). Patients with one-block claudication generally have an ABI of approximately 0.6 to 0.8, those with severe (less than one-block) claudication have an ABI of 0.4 to 0.6, and those with limb-threatening ischemia (rest pain, gangrene, nonhealing ulcers) have an ABI of less than 0.4.

COST/COMPLICATIONS. No significant complications have been reported with this technique. This method is highly reliable in standard lower extremity arterial occlusive disease, but may be unreliable in diabetics (in whom measurement of toe blood pressure by strain-gauge plethysmography in the vascular laboratory appears to be much more dependable). A hand-held ultrasonic flow detector can be purchased for $300 to $600 and should last at least 5 years. Because costs of measuring the ABI in a vascular laboratory setting may range from $60 to $200, measurement of Doppler pressures and ABI calculation in the office setting can be both clinically useful and cost-effective.

Cross-references: Peripheral Arterial Disease (Section 133), Leg Ulcers (Section 134).

CHAPTER XII

NEUROLOGIC DISORDERS

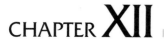

137 SCREENING FOR DEMENTIA

Screening

DANIEL L. KENT

EPIDEMIOLOGY. Dementia is a generalized loss of mental functions in a patient who is not delirious, psychotic, or obtunded. The prevalence of dementia rises from under 1% in 50-year-old adults to 30% in the very elderly, those aged 80 to 90 years. The two most prevalent types of dementia are vascular dementia and Alzheimer's disease. These are irreversible, progressive conditions. Only 10% of all dementias are considered treatable. Patients with human immunodeficiency virus (HIV) infection do not develop dementia until late in the course of infection, at the onset of AIDS.

After age 60, natural aging includes subtle deterioration in the ability to manage simultaneous tasks or to complete complex spatial reasoning problems. Basic cognitive functions of orientation, registration, and recall of long-term memories do not deteriorate.

RATIONALE. Dementia affects four components of cognition: recall, orientation, ability to follow multistep commands, and language abilities. Apparent cognitive impairment may be caused by delerium, deafness, visual impairment, or depression. These conditions cause false-positive results on formal cognitive screening tests. False-negative results occur because testing instruments do not use sensitive probes for all areas of cognition. The Folstein Mini-Mental Status Examination (Table 137–1) and other short cognitive status testing instruments have sensitivities of 50% to 80% and specificities of 80% to 95%. These tests use probes of complex language, task completion, and spatial reasoning that are not very challenging.

STRATEGY. Primary screening for dementia in the population cannot be recommended. No test offers high sensitivity, and all have high false-positive rates. No efficacious treatment can be offered to most asymptomatic patients

TABLE 137–1. THE MINI-MENTAL STATE EXAMINATION

	Score[1]
Orientation	
What is the year, season, month, day of month, and day of week?	5
Where are we (i.e., state, county, town, building, floor)?	5
Registration	
Examiner names three objects, then asks patient to repeat them.	3
Attention and Calculation	
Serial sevens (five successive subtractions from 100), or spell "world" backwards.	5
Recall	
What were the three objects learned earlier? (One point for each correct answer)	3
Language and Praxis	
Examiner points to a pencil and a watch and asks patient to name them.	2
Patient is asked to:	
Repeat "no ifs, ands, or buts."	1
Follow the three-stage verbal command, "take this piece of paper in your right hand, fold it in half, and put it on the floor."	3
Follow the written command, "close your eyes."	1
Make up and write a sentence.	1
Copy a simple figure (e.g. intersecting pentagons).	1
Maximum Total Score:	30

Source: Folstein M, et al. J Psychiatr Res 1975;12:189–198. Adapted with permission.
[1]Scores less than 24 generally signify dementia or delerium.

found to have dementia by screening. Some instruments designed primarily to measure general health status in the elderly include items related to cognitive functioning. The clinical utility of these measures in routine practice remains uncertain.

Early detection of dementia in a patient with symptoms of forgetfulness may be valuable, but no studies document net positive benefits of early detection programs. Early diagnosis may help patients manage family affairs and plan for sheltered living situations with a minimum of social crises.

A diagnosis of dementia raises certain legal concerns. If the patient is custodian of a minor or an estate, these roles may be challenged. Powers of attorney may be null and void if a patient becomes incompetent; the dementia diagnosis may be taken as evidence of incompetency. Patients and families should review legal concerns before obtaining a firm diagnosis of dementia.

ACTION.   Clinicians can form strong diagnostic hypotheses from the history and the patient's ability to converse and follow examination procedures. Positive results on a screening instrument (see Mini-Mental Status Examination in Table 137–1) confirm a cognitive impairment. Comprehensive neuropsychiatric testing may resolve cases in which screening tests are negative but the clinical suspicion of dementia is high.

Once a diagnosis of dementia is accepted, the clinician, patient, and family must accept a high degree of uncertainty about prognosis. About half of dementia patients will become incontinent and dependent in basic activities of daily living within 2 to 3 years of the diagnosis. Section 142 reviews the diagnosis and treatment of dementia.

Cross-references: AIDS (Section 14), Dementia (Section 142), Common Thyroid Disorders (Section 156).

REFERENCES

1. Albert MS. Cognition and aging. In Hazzard WR, Andres R, Bierman EL, Blass JP, Eds. Principles of Geriatric Medicine and Gerontology, 2nd ed. McGraw-Hill, New York, 1990, pp. 913–919.
    The natural process of aging and cognition.

2. Nelson A, Fogel BS, Faust D. Bedside cognitive screening instruments: A critical assessment. J Nerv Ment Dis 1986;174:73–83.
    Reviews five short interview instruments, indicates adequate reliability and correspondence with disease states, and concludes there is no evidence that instruments enhance the accuracy of clinical diagnoses. False-negative and false-positive errors are common with all instruments.

3. Selnes, et al. HIV-1 infection: No evidence of cognitive decline during the asymptomatic stages. Neurology 1990;40:204–208.
    A longitudinal study found no dementia; first of two articles from a multicenter study.

4. Siu AL. Screening for dementia and investigating its causes. Ann Intern Med 1991;115:122–132.
    Reviews the value of mental status findings and ancillary tests in diagnosing dementia or its causes.

5. Strub RL, Black FN. The Mental Status Examination in Neurology, 2nd ed. F.A. Davis, Philadelphia, 1985.
    Details of the classic mental status examination.

138 TREMOR

Symptom

THOMAS D. BIRD

EPIDEMIOLOGY.   The prevalence of tremor in the general population or in the outpatient clinical setting has never been precisely determined. However, it is a relatively common symptom or sign. Approximately 500,000 Americans suffer from Parkinson's disease, and this represents only one of several relatively common causes of tremor.

ETIOLOGY.   The most common cause of a **resting tremor** is Parkinson's disease. Phenothiazines and other dopaminergic blocking agents may also produce a resting tremor. The most common causes of a **postural tremor** are anxiety, benign essential tremor, toxins or medication (e.g., alcohol, caffeine, lithium, β-adrenergic agonists, phenytoin, and mercury), and metabolic disorders (e.g., hyperthyroidism). An **intention** or **action tremor** is usually associated with benign essential tremor or diseases of the cerebellar system such as multiple sclerosis, alcoholic cerebellar degeneration, primary or metastatic tumors of the cerebellum, postanoxic syndrome, and paraneoplastic cerebellar degeneration (usually seen with carcinoma of the lung or ovary).

CLINICAL APPROACH.   **Postural tremor** is a fine regular movement of the fingers or hands when the arms are outstretched. It is usually not present at complete rest. Anxiety, the side effects of medication, or an underlying metabolic disturbance are the most common explanations. The major problem in the differential diagnosis of tremor is distinguishing Parkinson's disease from essential tremor or disorders of the cerebellum. The tremor of Parkinson's disease is rapid, rhythmic, most evident in the fingers ("pill rolling"), *present at rest, and often improved with intention or action.* Most important, the tremor of Parkinson's disease rarely occurs in isolation, but rather is associated with other characteristics of the parkinsonian syndrome. These include bradykinesia, cogwheel rigidity, masked facies, stooped posture, a festinating gait, a tendency toward retropulsion when standing, micrographia, and decreased voice volume (see Section 147). Parkinsonian tremor may be asymmetric and may involve the head and lower extremities. Note that a parkinsonian syndrome may be caused by neuroleptic dopaminergic blocking agents used to treat psychosis.

Benign **essential tremor** is rarely if ever present at rest, is present with the arms outstretched, and is much *worse with action or intention.* Essential tremor may also produce a horizontal or vertical head tremor and a "quivering voice," and is often familial. It is usually bilateral, but may be worse on one side. It does not usually involve the lower extremities or produce gait ataxia. The handwriting of patients with essential tremor is large and irregular compared to the micrographia of Parkinson's disease. Patients with essential tremor may have considerable difficulty with handwriting, drinking from a cup or glass, or any activity involving hand movement. In fact, a useful clinical test is to observe the patient with tremor drinking from a full cup of water. The patient with essential tremor will often have great difficulty and spill the liquid, whereas the patient with Parkinson's disease will be slow but successful in the maneuver, except in the late stages of the disease. Furthermore, the patient with essential tremor will not have the other associated clinical signs of Parkinson's disease.

Both Parkinson's disease and essential tremor are slowly progressive over many years. Parkinson's disease generally becomes much more handicapping because of rigidity, bradykinesia, and an approximately 20% incidence of dementia.

As an isolated finding, the hand tremor of essential tremor is indistinguishable from the hand tremor of other cerebellar disorders. However, other disorders of the cerebellum are much more likely to also be associated with nystagmus, dysarthria, and gait ataxia, none of which is expected with benign essential tremor.

The assessment of tremor may also involve the question of the presence of asterixis, myoclonus, or chorea. **Asterixis** refers to brief recurring lapses in muscle contraction, best demonstrated with the arms outstretched and the hands dorsiflexed at the wrist. This is commonly seen in metabolic disorders such as azotemia and early hepatic encephalopathy. **Myoclonus** usually refers to brief, lightning-like contractions or jerks of an isolated limb or the entire trunk. **Chorea** refers to sudden, irregular, sometimes "semi-purposeful" jerking of the limbs that may also involve the face or trunk. Chorea may be a side effect of levodopa medications used to treat Parkinson's disease.

MANAGEMENT.   The tremor of Parkinson's disease may improve with levodopa preparations or anticholinergic agents (such as trihexyphenidyl or benztropine) or a combination of the two (see Section 147). Selegiline (a monoamine oxidase-B inhibitor) may also be of value early in the course of Parkinson's disease; detailed clinical trials are in progress. Mild (truly benign) essential tremor often requires no treatment. However, essential tremor may not be "benign" and may interfere with daily activities. The observation that essential tremor often improves with a small amount of alcohol is a useful point in the history, but usually not appropriate therapy. No medication completely eliminates the tremor, and side effects often prevent increases in dosage. However, several drugs ameliorate essential tremor, including low doses of phenobarbital (30–90 mg/day), benzodiazepines (chlordiazepoxide, 20–50 mg/day), and beta-blocking agents (propranolol, 40–160 mg/day). Patients with tremor should avoid caffeine.

Cross-references: Parkinsonism (Section 147), Generalized Anxiety (Section 188).

REFERENCES

1. Cleeves L, Findley LJ, Koller W. Lack of association between essential tremor and parkinson's disease. Ann Neurol 1988:24:23–26.
    A useful comparison of the features of Parkinson's disease and essential tremor.

2. Elble RJ, Koller WC. Tremor. Johns Hopkins University Press, Baltimore, 1990.

3. Findley LJ, Koller WC. Essential tremor: A review. Neurology 1987;37:1194–1197.
    Discusses the clinical characteristics and various suggested treatments of essential tremor.

4. Sumi SM, Ruff RL, Swanson PD. Motor disturbances. In Swanson PD, Ed. Signs and Symptoms in Neurology. J.B. Lippincott, Philadelphia, 1984, pp. 132–205.
    A review of the differential diagnosis of tremor in a practical text of clinical neurology for the general physician.

139 MUSCULAR WEAKNESS

Symptom

JOHN RAVITS

ETIOLOGY/SYMPTOMS AND SIGNS.   **Weakness,** an objective loss of muscle strength, is a frequent problem seen by primary care clinicians and by neurologists. It is often confused with **lassitude,** a feeling of weariness without actual weakness, or with other kinds of neurologic dysfunction such as pain, incoordination, rigidity, and apraxia. **Paresis** refers to incomplete loss of strength, and **plegia** or **paralysis** refers to complete loss of strength. **Upper motor neuron weakness** is caused by lesions in the central nervous system (CNS) and is characterized by weakness affecting groups of muscles (usually extensor muscles in the arms and flexor muscles in the legs), loss of fine-skilled movements, increased muscle tone (spasticity), increased reflexes, and extensor plantar responses. **Lower motor neuron weakness** is caused by lesions in the peripheral nervous system and is characterized by weakness in specific distributions (such as a ventral root or a peripheral nerve), fasciculations, muscle atrophy, decreased muscle tone (flaccidity), and decreased reflexes.

Lassitude and fatigue (distinct from true muscular weakness) may result from a variety of metabolic diseases (e.g., thyroid disease, Addison's disease, diabetes), systemic inflammatory conditions (e.g., polymyalgia rheumatica), anemia, hepatic disease, renal disease, infections (e.g., subacute bacterial endocarditis, urosepsis, flulike illnesses, mononucleosis, tuberculosis, HIV), malignancy, chronic fatigue syndrome, and psychiatric problems (previously called neurasthenia) (see Section 21, Fatigue).

The distribution of true muscle weakness provides clues to its cause. **Monoparesis** refers to a weakness in a single limb and usually is of the lower motor neuron type. It is caused by radiculopathy, plexopathy, or mononeuropathy. Monoparesis of an upper motor neuron type indicates a discrete lesion in the CNS, usually from strokes, neoplasms, or multiple sclerosis. **Hemiparesis** refers to weakness on one side of the body and usually indicates a CNS lesion contralateral to the weak side. The more typical etiologies are stroke, neoplasms, infections, trauma, or perinatal injury. **Quadriparesis** refers to weakness in the arms and legs. If it is of the lower motor neuron type, it indicates peripheral nervous system dysfunction. **Distal weakness** with relative sparing of proximal muscles is the hallmark of polyneuropathy. It is usually caused by toxic-metabolic neuropathies such as diabetes, vitamin B_{12} deficiencies, demyelinating neuropathies such as Guillain-Barré syndrome, paraproteinemic neuropathies, and hereditary neuropathies. **Proximal muscle weakness** with relative sparing of distal muscles is the hallmark of myopathy. The usual causes of myopathy are polymyositis, toxic-metabolic myopathy (e.g., thyroid disease, Cushing's syndrome), and muscular dystrophy. Also, defective neuromuscular transmission such as myasthenia gravis or myasthenic syndrome may simulate myopathy. If quadriparesis has the features of upper motor neuron weakness, it indicates spinal cord disease (myelopathy) at or above the cervical level. The most common causes of myelopathy include compression from spondylosis or disk disease, trauma, tumors (either primary tumors or metastatic disease), myelitis, and multiple sclerosis.

Paraparesis refers to weakness of the legs. If it is of the lower motor neuron type, it indicates polyneuropathy, Guillain-Barré syndrome, myopathy, multiple mononeuropathies, or abnormalities of the cauda equina (usually from neoplasms, lumbar stenosis, or lumbar disk disease). If paraparesis is of the upper motor neuron type, it indicates myelopathy at the thoracic or upper lumbar levels; the usual etiologies are compression from spondylosis or disk disease, trauma, tumors (either primary or metastatic), myelitis, and multiple sclerosis.

Diffuse weakness may indicate, in addition to any of the above conditions, multiple sclerosis, multiple strokes, posterior circulation strokes, and degenerative conditions such as motor neuron disease. **Episodic weakness** may indicate transient ischemic attacks, multiple sclerosis, myasthenia gravis, and periodic paralysis.

CLINICAL APPROACH.   In addition to the character and pattern of weakness, the patient interview should identify associated symptoms and signs. In particular, the presence or absence of ocular bulbar symptoms, sensory disturbance, pain, sphincter dysfunction, and autonomic dysfunction must be noted. One must know the clinical context, such as the patient's general medical health, age, other systemic diseases such as diabetes, malignancy, arthritis, vascular disease, alcoholism, and medications. The family history may shed light on some patients' weakness. The physician should identify associated orthopedic problems (e.g., kyphoscoliosis) and cutaneous markings (e.g., café au lait spots), and examine the axial, shoulder, hip girdle and appendicular muscles for atrophy, fasciculations, muscle tone, and weakness. "Give-way weakness" is ratchety rather than smooth and is often seen in the patient who is co-contracting other muscles other than those being examined. While this usually represents functional overlay or malingering, it may accompany a frightened patient with an underlying organic problem. Patients in pain often will not make a full effort, especially if the muscle contraction puts the body part into a position of greater pain; these patients are best examined isometrically, as contraction of the muscle does not produce movement about a joint. Reflexes must be carefully tested and compared for symmetry; the Jendrassik's maneuver (i.e., the patient contracts a muscle group other than that being tested) may help elicit an otherwise absent reflex.

Laboratory testing includes a complete blood cell (CBC) count, erythrocyte sedimentation rate (ESR), chemistry panel, muscle enzymes, and acetylcholine receptor antibodies (when myasthenia gravis is suspected). Radiographs of the chest and spine may be particularly important. Magnetic resonance imaging (MRI) of the head or relevant regions of the spinal axis may ultimately be necessary to define the etiology of weakness, but because of its expense there should be a clear definition of the weakness, its differential diagnosis, and the need for MRI. Electromyography, nerve conduction studies, muscle biopsies, and nerve biopsies may identify neuromuscular abnormalities in selected cases. Examination of the cerebrospinal fluid (CSF) may demonstrate a cytoalbuminologic dissociation in Guillain-Barré syndrome, abnormal immunoglobins in multiple sclerosis or myelitis, or abnormal cytologies in carcinomatous infiltration of the meninges.

One of the most dreaded and treatable complications of weakness is respiratory weakness. In rapidly evolving weakness or weakness in which respiratory compromise is apparent or possible, hospitalization and mechanical ventilation may be appropriate.

Cross-references: Fatigue (Section 21), Low Back Pain (Section 108), Multiple Sclerosis (Section 143), Entrapment Neuropathy (Section 146), Peripheral Neuropathy (Section 149), Electromyography and Nerve Conduction Studies (Section 151).

REFERENCES

1. Adams RD, Victor M, Eds. Principles of Neurology, ed 4. McGraw-Hill Information Services Co., Health Professions Division, New York, 1989.
   A standard textbook of neurology. The first half discusses cardinal manifestations of disease and differential diagnosis, the second half discusses the various disease processes.

2. Rowland LP, Ed. Merritt's Textbook of Neurology, ed 8. Lea & Febiger, Philadelphia, 1989.
   Another very good standard neurology textbook.

140 HEADACHE

Symptom

JOYCE E. WIPF

EPIDEMIOLOGY. Headaches affect 90% of the population, accounting for about 2% of all visits to emergency rooms or primary care physicians. About 50% of adults will experience a severe or disabling headache at some time; 1% have daily headaches. Headaches in patients older than 65 years are less common, affecting only 40%, and are more likely to be due to serious pathology.

ETIOLOGY. Over 80% of headaches are idiopathic and benign, including (1) tension-type headaches (e.g., psychogenic, muscle contraction headaches), (2) vascular-type headaches (e.g., migraine with or without aura, cluster headache, carotidynia), or (3) mixed headaches with features of both tension and vascular types. **Tension-type headaches** are usually bilateral (90%) and located at the vertex, temporal, or frontal areas; less than 20% are occipital. They may be episodic or chronic, often feature prominent fatigue, and usually respond within hours to analgesics. A typical **migraine** consists of unilateral throbbing discomfort that lasts 1 to 3 days. Associated mood changes and gastrointestinal symptoms may precede the headache by minutes to hours. Reversible neurologic auras (most commonly visual scotomata or flashing lights; less commonly focal weakness, numbness, tingling, mild aphasia, or confusion) may precede, accompany, or even follow the pain phase of the headache. Migraines rarely occur more often than once or twice a week. **Cluster headaches,** usually seen in middle-aged men, are characterized by paroxysms of severe unilateral pain, usually of the orbit, and associated ipsilateral autonomic changes, such as lacrimation, erythema of the eye, nasal congestion, and Horner's syndrome. Cluster headaches often recur in groups over consecutive days or weeks. **Carotidynia** is characterized by unilateral anterior neck pain with tenderness of the ipsilateral carotid artery and floor of the mouth.

Factors that may precipitate idiopathic headaches include dietary items (strong or aged cheeses containing tyramine, alcohol, chocolate, canned figs, cured meats containing nitrate, monosodium glutamate, caffeine), sleep deprivation or excess, stress, menstruation, and various medications (oral contraceptives, vasodilators such as hydralazine, minoxidil, prazosin, and nifedipine, and beta blockers with sympathomimetic or partial agonist activity such as acebutolol and pindolol).

Organic causes of headache include **mass lesions** (e.g., brain tumor, abscess, subdural hematoma, subarachnoid or intracerebral hemorrhage), **meningitis, sinusitis, vascular etiologies** (carotid or basilar artery stenosis, aneurysm, temporal arteritis), **intracranial hypertension** (hydrocephalus, pseudotumor cere-

420

bri), **medical conditions** (malignant hypertension, pheochromocytoma, carbon monoxide poisoning, hypoxia, hypercapnia, anemia, glaucoma), **neuralgia,** and miscellaneous diseases of the bones, joints, and teeth.

CLINICAL APPROACH.   The clinician's goal is to distinguish the common idiopathic headaches from the uncommon organic causes. A careful patient interview identifies the pattern and location of headache with open-ended questions, and determines previous treatments for headaches, associated symptoms, and precipitating factors. Symptoms traditionally associated with migraine, such as throbbing, photophobia, and gastrointestinal distress, may be seen in a severe headache of any type.

Features that are worrisome for organic causes include the patient's complaint of "worst headache ever"; a headache that is "different" from before; a headache precipitated by position change, cough, or exertion; a history of trauma or fever; and abnormal mentation or other neurologic findings. Features that suggest benign headaches include young age (<35), a history of a previous identical headache, normal vital signs, normal neurologic findings, and pain relieved by oral analgesics.

Routine laboratory tests include a CBC, chemistry screen, and, in patients over 40, an ESR (to exclude temporal arteritis) and screening for glaucoma. Computed tomography (CT) of the head is indicated in patients with trauma, worrisome historical features, or focal neurologic findings. MRI may better evaluate those with suspected posterior fossa lesions. Lumbar puncture is indicated in patients with acute fever and headache. If bacterial meningitis is strongly suspected, antibiotics should be administered without delay, even before completion of the diagnostic workup.

MANAGEMENT.   The clinician should initially clarify the patient's specific concerns. Although physicians often assume that relief of headache is the patient's primary concern, studies suggest that patients more often seek medical attention for reassurance that no serious pathology exists. Therapy for headache encompasses (1) avoidance of precipitating factors, (2) treatment of acute attacks, and (3) prophylaxis for migraine headaches (Table 140–1).

Patients with headaches that persist beyond 72 hours (status migrainosus) are frequently volume depleted and should receive intravenous (IV) fluids prior to drug treatment. Ergotamines, which are available in oral, sublingual, aerosolized, rectal, and parenteral forms, are most effective when given early during a migraine headache, are contraindicated in patients with atherosclerotic cardiovascular disease, and may actually promote headaches if used more than 2 days per week. Narcotic medications are best avoided in both acute and chronic headaches. Other effective medications include nonsteroidal anti-inflammatory agents, which are underutilized, and prochlorperazine, which also relieves the nausea and vomiting of severe headaches. Preliminary data suggest that parenteral dexamethasone (8–20 mg) may also benefit patients with acute headaches. Finally, subcutaneous injection of sumatriptan, a new drug, has proven effective for both migraine and cluster headaches.

TABLE 140–1. THERAPY FOR HEADACHES—ACUTE ATTACK

Drug	Dose	Side Effects	Cost ($)[1]
Oral			
Nonsteroidal anti-inflammatory		Gastrointestinal distress, ulceration and bleeding, rash, renal effects, tinnitus, edema	
Aspirin	650 mg q.4h.		0.01 (325 mg)
Naproxen	250–375 mg t.i.d.		0.64 (250 mg)
Indomethacin	75–150 mg q.d.		0.03 (25 mg)
Acetaminophen	650 mg q.4h.	Overdose: nausea, vomiting, hepatotoxicity	0.03 (325 mg)
Barbiturates			
Fiorinal (50 mg Butalbital, caffeine, and aspirin)	1–2 tabs q.4h. (max. 6 tabs/day)	Nausea and vomiting, constipation, sedation, dizziness, drug dependency	0.32 (tab)
Ergotamines (vascular headaches)			
Cafergot (1 mg ergotamine and caffeine)	2 tablets PO at start of attack, 1 additional tablet every 1/2 hour (max. 6/day or 10/wk)	Vasoconstriction[2], nausea, vomiting, transient bradycardia or tachycardia	0.76 (tab)
Ergostat (2 mg ergotamine)	1 sublingual tablet at first symptoms, then repeat q.1/2h. × 2, PRN (max. 3/24 hr or 5/wk)		0.52 (tab)
Parenteral			
Dihydroergotamine (vascular)	1 mg IM or IV (preceded by 10 minutes with 10 mg IM or IV metoclopramide)	Coronary vasospasm[2], nausea and vomiting, flushing, drowsiness, anxiety	
Prochlorperazine	10 mg slow IV × 1 (max. 5mg/min), used alone or with other therapies	Drowsiness, orthostatic hypotension (extrapyramidal symptoms are rare)	
Chlorpromazine	7.5 mg IV over 3 min, may repeat × 3 at 7-min intervals	Hypotension	
Meperidine	25–75 mg IM with 25–50 mg hydroxyzine	Hypotension, drug dependency	

[1]Average wholesale price, 1991 *Drug Topics Red Book.*
[2]Ergotamines are contraindicated in patients with coronary artery disease, peripheral vascular disease, hypertension, and impaired renal/hepatic function.

A 3- to 6-month trial of prophylactic medications (Table 140–2) is reasonable when migraines are frequent, complicated (associated reversible neurologic deficitis), or refractory to abortive treatments. Beta-blocker medications are useful prophylactic agents but do not alleviate prodromes and may even aggravate them. Pindolol and acebutolol should not be used because of their sympathomimetic effects. Patients with refractory migraines should be referred to a neurologist. Treatment with the lysergic acid derivative, methysergide, is rarely necessary and should be limited to 4 months, followed by a 1-month period without the medication because of its potentially severe side effects.

Treatment of cluster headaches includes ergotamines, lithium, tricyclic antidepressants, and methysergide. Nondrug therapies, including behavioral modification and stress-coping relaxation training, may benefit patients with either vascular or tension headaches.

FOLLOW-UP. Within a few weeks of starting a new drug, a follow-up appointment should be scheduled to monitor the patient's response and side effects. Those with frequent severe migraines should be given prophylaxis for a limited period of 3 to 6 months. Headaches refractory to therapy deserve further evaluation for an intracranial lesion despite a normal neurologic examination, since occasional mass lesions present without localizing findings and respond temporarily to drug therapies. Although controversial, current evidence does not conclusively demonstrate that migraine is a risk factor for stroke.

TABLE 140–2. PROPHYLAXIS OF MIGRAINES

Drug	Dose	Side Effects	Cost ($)[1]
Beta blockers Propranolol	80–320 mg/day	Bronchospasm, hypotension, fatigue, impotence	0.03 (40 mg)
Tricyclic antidepressants Amitriptyline	50–175 mg/day	Anticholinergic sx, orthostatic hypotension	0.03 (50 mg)
Calcium channel blockers Verapamil Nifedipine Diltiazem	80–120 mg t.i.d. 10–20 mg t.i.d. 60–120 mg t.i.d.	Postural hypotension, edema, constipation, facial flushing	0.16 (80 mg) 0.40 (10 mg) 0.53 (60 mg)
Cyproheptidine (Periactin)	6–12 mg b.i.d.	Sedation, weight gain, appetite stimulation	0.03 (4 mg, generic) 0.33 (4 mg, Periactin)
Methysergide (Sansert)	2 mg b.i.d.	Vivid dreams, hallucinations; pericardial, cardiac, pulmonary, and retroperitoneal fibrosis with long-term use	1.14 (2 mg)

[1]Average wholesale price, 1991 *Drug Topics Red Book.*

Cross-references: Screening for Glaucoma (Section 35), Polymyalgia Rheumatica and Temporal Arteritis (Section 118), Myofascial Pain Syndromes (Section 123).

REFERENCES

1. Edmeads J. The worst headache ever: Ominous causes. Postgrad Med 1989;86:(1)93–104.

    Good discussion of organic causes of headache, with descriptions of the typical presenting features of an intracranial mass, subarachnoid hemorrhage, and meningitis.

2. International Headache Society. The classification and diagnosis criteria for headache disorders, cranial neuralgia and facial pain. Cephalalgia 1988;8(suppl 7):1–96.

    1988 changes in classification of headaches. The muscle contraction type is now included under tension headache, and migraines are no longer categorized as "classic" or "common" types, but as migraine with or without aura.

3. Jones J, Sklar D, Daugherty J, White W. Randomized double-blind trial of intravenous prochlorperazine for the treatment of acute headache. JAMA 1989;261:1174–1176.

    Eighty-two adults under age 65 with severe headache (tension or migraine) were given a single dose of 10 mg IV prochlorperazine; 74% had a complete response and 14% a partial response.

4. Larson EB, Omenn GS, Lewis H. Diagnostic evaluation of headache. JAMA 1980;243:359–362.

    In an analysis of 161 patients (average age 41) CT, skull films, and angiography were unnecessary if the neurologic examination was normal.

5. Smith MJ, Jensen NM. The severity model of chronic headache. J Gen Intern Med 1988;3:396–409.

    A convincing argument for classification of idiopathic headache based on severity rather than type; points out similarities between various causes of headache.

141 SEIZURES

Symptom

JAMES J. COATSWORTH

EPIDEMIOLOGY/ETIOLOGY.   Between 0.5% and 1% of the population suffer from epilepsy, and up to 5% have a single seizure. The incidence is about 20 to 50 per 100,000 population per year, increasing after age 60. Seizures result from a wide variety of primary CNS diseases (e.g., brain tumors, infection, and degenerative diseases), or systemic disturbances (e.g., drug withdrawal, electrolyte imbalance, renal or hepatic failure, or hypoxia). In patients with a known seizure disorder, certain factors increase susceptibility to seizures (e.g., sleep deprivation, stress, menstruation, drugs). The term *epilepsy* refers to chronic recurrent seizures, whether or not the cause is known.

SYMPTOMS AND SIGNS.   Seizures are classified as either focal (partial) or generalized; focal seizures may or may not impair consciousness (Table 141–1). A detailed history relying on witnesses is important to characterize events immediately preceding and following a suspected seizure. For example, focal motor or sensory manifestations before or after the seizure suggest a seizure caused by a localized cerebral structural lesion. Additional historical points of importance include evidence of head trauma, use of drugs or alcohol, and compliance with seizure medications.

A careful neurologic examination may yield clues that the episode was a seizure (tongue biting, incontinence) or that a structural problem is present (mild hemiparesis, reflex asymmetry, extensor plantar response). Careful physical examination may help identify skin lesions of tuberous sclerosis (adenoma sebaceum) or neurofibromas suggesting associated von Recklinghausen's disease.

CLINICAL APPROACH.   The practitioner should classify the type of seizure and define any underlying pathology that may require specific treatment. An electroencephalogram (EEG) may assist in confirming the clinical diagnosis and help differentiate partial from generalized seizures. Videotape monitoring in combination with EEG may help differentiate true seizures from pseudoseizures.

Patients with seizures related to alcohol or drug withdrawal who have normal neurologic findings and no head trauma need not undergo EEG, computed tomography (CT), or magnetic resonance imaging (MRI), because these studies are almost always normal. Patients with partial seizures, focal abnormalities on the EEG, or other unexplained neurologic signs should undergo head CT or MRI to evaluate potential pathologic causes.

Laboratory testing is rarely useful but should exclude hypoglycemia, hypocalcemia, and hyponatremia. Hospitalization is indicated in patients with electrolyte abnormalities or who have multiple seizures that recur within a short period of time.

TABLE 141–1.   CLASSIFICATION OF SEIZURES

Generalized seizures (no focal onset)
    Absence (petit mal)
    Tonic-clonic (grand mal)
    Myoclonic
Partial seizures (focal onset)
    Simple (consciousness not impaired)
        Motor
        Sensory
        Autonomic
        Psychic
    Complex (consciousness impaired)

MANAGEMENT.   A single seizure does not constitute a diagnosis of epilepsy and does not necessarily require treatment. Because 40% of adults will experience recurrent seizures within 2 to 3 years of their first seizure, those with a progressive cerebral disorder or clearly abnormal EEGs should usually receive medication after the initial event. Patients with postconcussion, alcohol withdrawal or drug-related seizures do not require anti-epileptic treatment.

Therapy should begin with the least toxic drug at a relatively low dose that is increased gradually if seizures recur. Primary generalized seizures respond best to phenytoin, carbamazepine, or valproic acid. Partial seizures should be treated with the same drugs, starting with carbamazepine and moving to phenytoin or valproic acid as required.

Primidone and phenobarbital are less frequently used because of their sedating side effects. Patients who experience recurrent seizures despite an adequate serum level of an initial anti-epileptic medication sometimes require the addition of a second anti-epileptic medication. Phenobarbital is a commonly used second drug, especially in patients with partial seizures. Patients requiring two or more drugs require careful monitoring of symptoms and drug levels to prevent toxicity (Table 141–2).

Pregnant epileptic women appear to have more obstetric complications, and their children, more fetal abnormalities. Seizure medications themselves are likely responsible for some of these complications. Although withdrawal of anti-epileptics prior to pregnancy is advisable in women with prolonged remissions from epilepsy, most patients require medication despite the risks. Treatment with phenytoin, valproic acid, and combinations of agents should be avoided if possible. Serum drug levels should be monitored monthly during the last trimester and again after delivery.

FOLLOW-UP.   During the first few weeks of therapy, toxic effects and compliance should be carefully monitored. Once stabilized, the patient should return to the clinic every 6 to 12 months. It must be remembered that symptoms may be satisfactorily controlled with lower than therapeutic serum levels, and conversely, many patients tolerate high serum levels without complications. Therapeutic drug levels are therefore an adjunct to drug evaluation rather than an absolute guide.

Discontinuing medications is best done in consultation with an experienced neurologist. Most authorities recommend repeat EEG prior to discontinuing medications. Up to 40% of patients who are seizure-free on medication for 2 or more years will relapse with discontinuation. The chance of relapse decreases with the passage of time after withdrawal. Other factors favoring successful withdrawal include a normal EEG at the time of withdrawal, generalized epilepsy, and an epileptic history of short duration. Drugs should be discontinued gradually over 4 to 6 weeks to avoid precipitating seizures. Patients with structural brain diseases as a cause of seizures are best continued on treatment.

Well-controlled patients do not need repeated imaging studies or EEGs. Those who fail treatment or show progressive neurologic abnormalities require reevaluation.

TABLE 141–2. COMMONLY USED ANTI-EPILEPTIC MEDICATIONS IN ADULTS

Drug	Usual Daily Dose (mg)	Plasma t$_{1/2}$ (hr)	Therapeutic Range (µg/ml)	Adverse Effects	Cost ($)[1]
Phenytoin	300–400	24	10–20	Ataxia, diplopia, gingival hyperplasia, hirsutism, low folate level	0.51
Carbamazepine	600–1200	12–17	4–12	Dizziness, leukopenia	1.05
Primidone	750–1250	12	5–15	Drowsiness	0.45
Valproic acid	1000–1500	5–20	50–100	Nausea, vomiting, sedation	1.00
Phenobarbital	90–120	48–144	20–40	Sedation	0.15

[1]Cost per day, average wholesale price, 1991 *Drug Topics Red Book*, for lower range of common daily dose.

Cross-references: Alcohol Withdrawal (Section 144), Electroencephalography (Section 150).

REFERENCES

1. Engel J Jr. Seizures and Epilepsy. Contemporary Neurology Series, No. 31. F.A. Davis Co., Philadelphia, 1989.
    The best textbook on seizures in English.

2. Penry JK, Ed. Epilepsy: Diagnosis, Management and Quality of Life. Rover Press, New York, 1986.
    An excellent review on epilepsy for the primary care physician.

3. Porter RJ. Epilepsy—100 elementary principles. Major Problems in Neurology, 2nd ed. W.B. Saunders, Philadelphia, 1989.
    A thoughtful compendium on the treatment of seizures, suitable for both students and experienced clinicians.

4. Scheuer ML, Pedley TA. The evaluation and treatment of seizures. N Engl J Med 1990;323:1468–1474.
    Excellent review.

142 DEMENTIA

Symptom

DAVID G. FRYER

EPIDEMIOLOGY.   Dementia refers to the gradual loss of cognitive function that occurs over many months or years, eventually resulting in total dependency. It is most common in older patients. About 15% of patients over 75 years of age suffer from some degree of dementia; in 5% of cases, the dementia is severe.

ETIOLOGY.   Alzheimer's disease is the most common cause of dementia, followed by multi-infarct dementia. Less common causes include AIDS, head injury, alcohol-related cerebral degeneration, and Parkinson's disease. Communicating hydrocephalus, hypothyroidism, hyperparathyroidism, CNS vasculitis, brain tumor, vitamin B_{12} deficiency and Jakob-Creutzfeldt disease are rare.

CLINICAL APPROACH.   Only the demonstration at autopsy of excessive numbers of neurofibrillary tangles and senile plaques containing amyloid beta protein confirms the diagnosis of Alzheimer's disease. Because brain biopsy is almost never justified or helpful, and because no laboratory test for Alzheimer's disease exists, the diagnosis during life depends on demonstration in the patient of (1) impaired short- and long-term memory, (2) altered abstract thinking, judgment, or personality, sufficient to interfere with social activities or work, and (3) exclusion of factors that cause delirium.

Although older patients have more difficulty with memory and tasks requiring spatial organization, this normal deterioration differs from dementia because it preserves vocabulary and spelling and improves with offered cues. The abnormal memory of Alzheimer's disease, in contrast, is always associated with some degree of dysphasia and does not improve by use of association. For example, unlike normal elderly people, patients with Alzheimer's disease can recall a list of related words no better than random words.

A simple questionnaire will measure the degree of dementia (Table 142–1). This test is similar to the Folstein Mini-Mental State Examination (see Section 137, Screening for Dementia) but has some advantages in that it partially adjusts for age, race, sex, education, and motor or visual impairment.[5]

The neurologic examination is otherwise normal in Alzheimer patients until late in the disease. Headache, seizures, or focal neurologic deficits (e.g., hemiparesis) suggest different etiologies such as tumor and subdural hematoma, while gait disturbance and urinary incontinence suggest communicating hydrocephalus.[4]

The clinician should inquire about cardiovascular disease, head trauma, alcohol consumption, HIV exposure, and current medications. Routine laboratory tests include a complete blood count (CBC), ESR, chemistry profile, and determination of thyrotropin and vitamin B_{12} levels. Although lumbar puncture, EEG, and computed tomography (CT) or magnetic resonance imaging (MRI) are not helpful as routine tests, they are appropriate in cases with unusual findings, such as (1) abrupt onset of dementia, (2) onset before age 60 years, (3) associated focal neurologic signs, or (4) recent seizures or new-onset headache. Indium cysternography may be helpful to confirm normal pressure hydroceph-

---

TABLE 142–1.   MENTAL STATUS QUESTIONNAIRE

1. What is the name of this place?
2. What is today's date?
3. What day of the week is it?
4. What is your telephone number?
5. How old are you?
6. What year were you born?
7. Who is the president of the United States?
8. Who was the previous president?
9. What was your mother's maiden name?
10. Subtract 3 from 20 and keep subtracting all the way down.

Nine to ten correct answers indicate no dementia; six to eight, slight dementia; three to five, moderate dementia; and none to two, severe dementia.

alus. Single-photon emission computed tomography (SPECT) often shows decreased blood flow in the parietal cortex in Alzheimer's disease, but its place in the evaluation of dementia is not yet established.

Clues to the diagnosis of multi-infarct dementia are (1) a stepwise progression of dementia, (2) associated hypertension or diabetes, (3) findings of peripheral vascular disease or previous cerebrovascular accidents, and (4) emotional incontinence (exaggerated crying or laughing).[2]

The differential diagnosis of dementia includes delirium and depression ("pseudodementia"). **Delirium** also involves defective memory and cognitive function, but unlike dementia is characterized by clouding of consciousness, disordered sleep pattern, and more abrupt development over hours or days.[3] Types of delirium include the agitated type, where patients are excited and distractible, often with hallucinations that provoke unpredictable or violent behavior (followed by amnesia for such episodes), and the retarded type, where patients are lethargic and apathetic, with depressed mood and motor activity. The evaluation of patients with delirium emphasizes the search for medication intoxication (especially anticholinergic, antiparkinsonian, antidepressant, nonsteroidal anti-inflammatory, antihistamine, and narcotic medications) and acute physical illnesses (such as urinary tract infection, pneumonia, uremia, volume depletion, hypokalemia, hypoxia, hypoglycemia, and hepatic failure).

Pseudodementia refers to a memory disturbance that results from depression and responds to antidepressive drug therapy. In pseudodementia, the depression usually precedes the abnormal memory, the onset may be abrupt, the severity may plateau rather than progress, and the mental status examination is often characterized by profound apathy. Depression may also occur in true dementia.

MANAGEMENT.   Although most causes of dementia are untreatable, many patients improve following treatment of associated conditions, such as adverse drug reactions, depression, and malnutrition.[1]

Treatable causes of dementia are hydrocephalus, subdural hematoma, hyperparathyroidism, vitamin B_{12} deficiency, hypothyroidism, and chronic CNS infections. Sedatives, neuroleptic drugs (e.g., haloperidol), and antidepressants (e.g., amitriptyline) may provide some relief of symptoms for agitated, paranoid, or depressed patients but require careful dosage adjustment in order to avoid accentuating confusion and disorientation.

Demented patients benefit from repeated explanations that reinforce orientation, for example, reminders of what has been done, what is going to happen, what building they are in, and other points of reference. In those with dysphasia, the clinician and family should emphasize nonverbal aspects of communication (e.g., gestures). Patients with dementia are often inclined to wander and should wear an identification bracelet or necklace. Other helpful measures include attaching neck chains to eyeglasses, illuminating the bedroom at all times, labeling drawers and appliances at home, and establishing a toileting program in which the patient is reminded to go to the bathroom at regular intervals. Family members often benefit from community support groups and, if burdened by the responsibilities of caring for the patient, short respites during which the patient is temporarily admitted to a nursing home.

Cross-reference: AIDS (Section 14), Screening for Dementia (Section 137), Parkinsonism (Section 147), Cerebrovascular Disease (Section 148), Screening for Thyroid Disease (Section 153), Screening for Depression (Section 187), Management of Depression (Section 192).

REFERENCES

1. Barry PP, Moskowitz MA. The diagnosis of reversible dementia in the elderly: A critical review. Arch Intern Med 1988;148:1914–1918.
    Although many studies have methodologic flaws, the authors conclude that demented patients often benefit from a search for treatable conditions that judiciously uses selected tests.

2. Hachinski VC, Lassen NA, Marshall J. Multi-infarct dementia: A cause of mental deterioration in the elderly. Lancet 1974;2:207–209.
    Describes multi-infarct dementia and how it differs from Alzheimer's disease.

3. Lipowski ZJ. Delirium in the elderly patient. N Engl J Med 1989;320:578–582.
    Excellent review of clinical findings, differential diagnosis, and treatment.

4. Martin RA, Guthrie R. Office evaluation of dementia: How to arrive at a clear diagnosis and choose appropriate therapy. Postgrad Med 1988;84:176–187.
    Includes a table of physical examination clues.

5. McCormick WC, Larson EB. Pragmatism and probabilities in dementia. Hosp Pract 1990;25:93–114.
    Outstanding practical review.

143 MULTIPLE SCLEROSIS

Problem

JAMES B. MACLEAN

EPIDEMIOLOGY.   The precise etiology of multiple sclerosis is unknown but current scientific evidence suggests that it may result from immunologic alterations triggered by a viral infection in genetically susceptible individuals. Multiple geographic studies have shown an increased incidence in more northern latitudes, particularly with exposure in the early years of life. Familial studies have shown a significantly increased incidence in family members of patients with multiple sclerosis, perhaps five times higher than in the general population at large.

SYMPTOMS AND SIGNS.   Multiple sclerosis is classically defined by the appearance of CNS lesions that are separated in both time and place. There is an enormous variety in the presenting symptoms and signs of multiple sclerosis since the pathologic lesions, plaques in the white matter, may appear anywhere in the CNS or even in the peripheral nervous system. The more common symptoms include monocular visual loss, focal numbness with clumsiness, imbalance, bilateral leg weakness with sensory distortion, double vision, and autonomic symptoms (particularly bowel and bladder dysfunction). Less frequent symptoms include trigeminal neuralgia, vertigo, hearing loss, peripheral neuropathic patterns, and hypothermia. Helpful diagnostic signs are internuclear ophthalmoplegia, monocular optic atrophy, incomplete myelopathy (particularly Brown-Sequard patterns), bilateral horizontal and vertical nystagmus, an evolving spastic hemiparesis, focal ataxia, and midline ataxia with various gait abnormalities. Seventy-two percent of patients present with a single symptom, with attacks recurring about once per year. Some 20% to 40% of patients have a benign course without progression, while the remainder develop progressive disease, usually within 6 or 7 years after onset. About 10% to 15% of patients have a malignant course. Symptoms lasting more than 1 year are usually permanent.

CLINICAL APPROACH.   Because there is no definite diagnostic test, the diagnosis of multiple sclerosis is based on clinical findings. Although its role in diagnosis is not truly defined, magnetic resonance imaging (MRI) is used to display patchy lesions of demyelination in the paraventricular white matter. MRI with gadolinium may differentiate active disease from more chronic disease. MRI is less useful for identification of plaques in the optic nerve or spinal cord. About 95% of patients with definite clinical multiple sclerosis have abnormal MR scans. MRI changes, however, are not specific and may be caused by tumor nodules or vasculitis. This lack of specificity, combined with wide use of MRI in patients who lack definite symptoms of multiple sclerosis, has led to overdiagnosis, particularly in the elderly.

In 90% of patients with definite multiple sclerosis, CSF studies demonstrate an increase in immunoglobulin G. Evoked potentials, including visual, somatosensory, and auditory, may identify definite sites of abnormalities and help meet the criteria of lesions separated in space. At present, MRI is the most useful, with CSF changes the second most useful in confirming a clinical suspicion of multiple sclerosis.

MANAGEMENT.   There is no cure for multiple sclerosis, and management involves symptomatic therapy only. Diazepam or baclofen (Lioresal) help control spasticity, and amantidine (Symmetrel) (100 mg two to three times a day) or clonazepam (0.5 mg at night) may help reverse the fatigue that commonly occurs with multiple sclerosis. Some experimental therapies, including IM adrenocorticotropin or IV methylprednisolone (500 mg for 5 days), appear to hasten resolution of active symptoms but do not improve the overall prognosis. Cyclophosphamide with or without adrenocorticotropin has not proved successful and may actually be quite toxic. Interferon-α, cyclosporin, colchicine, azathioprine, and plasmapheresis are ineffective and may be harmful. Copolymer-1, a synthetic polypeptide with some antigens similar to myelin-basic protein, has recently been dismissed as being helpful in chronic multiple sclerosis. The efficacy of total lymphoid irradiation and monoclonal antibodies is under study.

FOLLOW-UP. Regular follow-up is essential to confirm the diagnosis and to assist families and patients with the numerous psychosocial problems that arise. Indicators of a favorable prognosis include an intermittent course with asymptomatic intervals, early onset (before the age of 40), isolated optic neuritis or sensory symptoms, a long first remission time, and lack of malignant progression within 5 years. Poor prognostic indicators include a rapidly progressive course, late onset of multiple sclerosis, and an initial presentation with motor, cerebellar, or sphincter impairment. Prognosis is unrelated to sex, number of attacks, psychological symptoms, or any laboratory or imaging findings.

Cross-reference: Muscular Weakness (Section 139).

REFERENCES

1. Papadopoulos FM, McFarlin DE, Pationas NJ, et al. A comparison between chemical analysis and MRI with the clinical diagnosis of multiple sclerosis. Am J Clin Pathol 1987;88:365–368.
    MRI revealed findings suggestive of multiple sclerosis in forty-eight of fifty-one patients with definite multiple sclerosis (as determined by clinical examination), four of four with possible multiple sclerosis, and one of six without multiple sclerosis.

2. Rolak L. Multiple sclerosis. In Appel SH, Ed. Current Neurology, vol. 9, chap. 4. Year Book Medical Publishers, Chicago, 1989.
    Excellent current information on multiple sclerosis.

3. Scheinberg L, Smith CR. Rehabilitation of patients with multiple sclerosis. Neurol Clin 1987;5:585–600.
    Important suggestions, often forgotten, that help in the management of chronic multiple sclerosis.

4. Shapiro RT. Symptom Management in Multiple Sclerosis. Demos Publications, New York, 1987.
    Helpful clinical suggestions in the care of multiple sclerosis patients.

5. Thompson AJ, Hutchinson M, Brazil J, et al. A clinical and laboratory study of benign multiple sclerosis. Q J Med 1986; 58:69–80.
    In a study of 400 patients, 42% of those with disease for more than 10 years had a benign course. Early onset of disease and long first remission correlated with a favorable prognosis.

144 ALCOHOL WITHDRAWAL

Problem

STEVEN R. McGEE

EPIDEMIOLOGY. The abrupt interruption of any sustained exposure to alcohol may produce the alcohol withdrawal syndrome. Risk factors for major withdrawal (or delirium tremens) include a prior history of major withdrawal, infection, and prolonged exposure to alcohol.

SYMPTOMS AND SIGNS. Alcohol withdrawal consists of minor and major syndromes (Table 144–1). As little as 3 weeks of drinking may precede major withdrawal.

Most patients experience minor symptoms such as irritability, tremor (6–8 cps, an exaggeration of the physiologic tremor), anorexia, and insomnia. These symptoms usually last days and are easy to treat. In a few patients, minor symptoms blend over days into major withdrawal.

Hallucinations (more often visual than auditory) occur early after the last drink (<48 hours) and appear in 25% of those with minor withdrawal. Withdrawal seizures are generalized seizures that also appear early (< 48 hours). Although 50% of seizures are single, multiple bursts of two to six seizures over several hours may occur. In minor withdrawal, fever is unusual (<25% of cases) and indicates infection (usually pneumonia). In major withdrawal, fever is common (>80%), though infections are found in 50%; in the remainder, the fever presumably occurs because of autonomic and motor hyperactivity.

CLINICAL APPROACH. Outpatient management is most appropriate for patients who voluntarily decide to stop drinking. Table 144–2 lists the indications for patient hospitalization. Detoxification centers in some communities provide alternatives to inpatient care when, for example, a patient has only minor symptoms without associated illness (favoring outpatient treatment), but is unknown to the physician and has no stable residence (favoring inpatient treatment).

TABLE 144–1. MINOR VS. MAJOR WITHDRAWAL

	Minor	Major
Onset (hours from last drink)	Early (6–48 hr)	Late (>48 hr)
Frequency	Common	Uncommon
Disorientation?	No	Yes
Autonomic hyperactivity? (tachycardia, hypertension, fever, mydriasis, diaphoresis)	Mild	Marked

434

TABLE 144–2.   OUTPATIENT VS. INPATIENT CARE

Inpatient care indicated
Associated illness (infection, fever, liver disease, pancreatitis, gastrointestinal bleeding, dehydration, ataxia, head trauma)
Major withdrawal present
Hallucinations
Previous history of major withdrawal
Social factors (isolation)
Abuse of other drugs (barbiturates, cocaine)
First seizure

Outpatient care appropriate
Minor symptoms only
Absence of significant associated illness
Availability of physician daily during withdrawal
Commitment to abstinence
Adequate social support (friends/family)

The history and physical examination should focus on the search for associated illnesses that require treatment and increase risk of major withdrawal (see Table 144–2). Wernicke's encephalopathy—ophthalmoplegia (usually lateral rectus palsies), ataxia, and/or encephalopathy (somnolence, confusion)—responds to thiamine, though 80% of patients ultimately develop Korsakoff's psychosis. Computed tomography (CT) of the head adds little to the evaluation of withdrawal seizures, unless (1) the seizure is atypical for withdrawal (multiple seizures over days, focal seizure), (2) the neurologic examination reveals asymmetric findings, or (3) there is evidence of head trauma.

MANAGEMENT.   Patients should receive thiamine (100 mg PO × 3) and a loading dose of a sedating medication that is subsequently slowly withdrawn. In several placebo-controlled trials, benzodiazepines were superior to other sedating medications in calming the patient and reducing the progression to seizures and delirium. The doses of benzodiazepines listed in Table 144–3 apply only to minor withdrawal; treatment of major withdrawal requires hospital admission and parenteral benzodiazepines.

TABLE 144–3.   DRUG TREATMENT OF MINOR WITHDRAWAL[1]

Drug	Dose (mg)[2]	Cost ($)[3]
Lorazepam	2 mg PO t.i.d. (+2 mg)[4]	0.05
Oxazepam	30 mg PO t.i.d. (+30 mg)	0.15
Chlordiazepoxide	50 mg PO t.i.d. (+50 mg)	0.04
Diazepam	10 mg PO t.i.d. (+10 mg)	0.02

[1]Only the first day's dose is listed. Doses are tapered over 4 days.
[2]Average doses listed. Physicians should monitor the patient's course daily to determine whether more or less sedation is necessary.
[3]Per dose listed, generic if available; average wholesale price, 1991 *Drug Topics Red Book*.
[4]For example, patient receives 18 1-mg lorazepam tablets: day 1 dose is 2 mg q.8h. plus an additional 2 mg as needed (e.g., at bedtime), day 2 dose is 2 mg in A.M. 1 mg in afternoon, 2 mg in evening; day 3 dose is 1 mg q.8h.; day 4 dose is 1 mg in A.M. 1 mg in evening.

Long-acting benzodiazepines (chlordiazepoxide, diazepam) and their active metabolites have elimination half-lives as great as 50 hours. Innovative recipes exist that allow patients to receive loading doses alone of long-acting benzodiazepines; further doses are unnecessary because the drug self-tapers over days.[4] The use of long-acting agents is not recommended in patients with liver disease because significant drug accumulation and oversedation occur. Short-acting benzodiazepines (lorazepam, oxazepam) have no active metabolites and are safe in those with liver disease.

Atenolol (50–100 mg/day, based on pulse and blood pressure), when given *with* benzodiazepines, results in more rapid normalization of vital signs and may reduce alcohol craving.[3] Clonidine also restores normal vital signs more quickly, but, like atenolol, does not prevent seizures or delirium and should not be used alone. Drugs to avoid during withdrawal include propranolol (which increases hallucinations) and phenothiazines (which increase seizures). Seizure prophylaxis with phenytoin is unnecessary.

FOLLOW-UP.   All patients should enter alcohol rehabilitation treatment. Frequent visits with the primary physician during subsequent months provide important emotional support to the patient.

Cross-references: Diagnosis and Management of Alcoholism (Section 8), Tremor (Section 138), Seizures (Section 141).

REFERENCES

1. Feussner JR, Linfors EW, Blessing CL, Starmer CF. Computed tomography brain scanning in alcohol withdrawal seizures. Ann Intern Med 1981;94:519–522.
    CT adds little unless there are focal neurologic findings or head trauma.

2. Guthrie SK. The treatment of alcohol withdrawal. Pharmacotherapy 1989;9:131–143.
    Extensive review of all drug trials (excellent table).

3. Horwitz RI, Gottlieb LD, Kraus ML. The efficacy of atenolol in the outpatient management of the alcohol withdrawal syndrome. Arch Intern Med 1989;149:1089–1093.
    Although all received benzodiazepines, atenolol resulted in more rapid normalization of vital signs, less craving for alcohol, and fewer treatment failures. Atenolol did not affect seizures, delirium, or tremor.

4. Sellers EM, Naranjo CA, Harrison M, et al. Diazepam loading: Simplified treatment of alcohol withdrawal. Clin Pharmacol Ther 1983;34:822–826.
    In a trial of placebo vs. diazepam (loading method, 20 mg q.2h. until calm, no taper; mean number of doses = 3), diazepam was superior in calming and in the prevention of seizures and hallucinations.

5. Turner R, Lichstein P, Peden J, Busher J, Waivers L. Alcohol withdrawal syndromes: A review of pathophysiology, clinical presentation, and treatment. J Gen Intern Med 1989;4:432–444.
    Outstanding up-to-date overview.

145 IDIOPATHIC FACIAL PALSY (BELL'S PALSY)

Problem

STEVEN R. McGEE

EPIDEMIOLOGY.   Bell's palsy, the acute onset of facial weakness, occurs with an annual incidence of 25 per 100,000. The age-associated incidence increases until age 30, after which it levels off. The palsy occurs equally in both men and women, on both sides of the face, and during all seasons of the year. *Bell's palsy* refers only to those facial palsies of unknown cause.

SYMPTOMS AND SIGNS.   Unilateral facial weakness usually appears abruptly, though symptoms in some may progress over 1 or 2 days. Associated symptoms include facial pain (33%–62%), increased (34%–68%) or decreased (2%–17%) tearing, facial numbness (26%–32%), hyperacusis (21%–29%), and alterations of taste (19%–57%). The pain centers around the ear and usually lasts 3 days, rarely longer than 1 week. Increased tearing occurs because the weak orbicularis oculi muscle cannot contain and direct tears down the nasolacrimal duct. Decreased tearing reflects damage to the greater superficial petrosal nerve, which accompanies the facial nerve through the skull. Hyperacusis, the perception of sounds as louder and brasher in the ipsilateral ear, results from involvement of the stapedius branch of the facial nerve. Abnormal taste is variably found and probably reflects the examiner's diligence; in other settings, after surgical section of the chorda tympani, most patients do not notice alterations of taste.

Physical examination reveals that on the affected side there is a less prominent nasolabial fold, a widened palpebral fissure, and weakness of the eyebrow, eyelid, and mouth muscles. One-third of patients experience only incomplete paralysis, a harbinger of quick and complete recovery. Upward rotation of the eyeball during attempted bilateral eye closure ("Bell's phenomenon") has dual significance: it convinces the examiner that the patient is indeed trying to close the eye, and it helps protect the cornea during sleep even when the eyelid muscles are weak. Hypesthesia of the trigeminal (facial sensation) and glossopharyngeal (degree of gag reflex) may occur on either side of the face.

CLINICAL APPROACH.   Topographic testing of lacrimation, hearing, and taste to pinpoint the site of discrete facial nerve lesions has limited value in Bell's palsy, probably because the lesion is patchy and incomplete. All patients with eye pain should undergo slit-lamp examination to search for corneal abrasions and ulcers.

The differential diagnosis of facial paralysis includes trauma, infections or tumors of the ear or parotid gland, Lyme disease, Ramsey-Hunt syndrome, sarcoid, and central facial palsy. The gradual development of weakness over several days or weeks suggests infection or tumor. Ramsey-Hunt syndrome, a herpes zoster infection of the geniculate ganglion, produces facial paralysis with vesicles in the auricle. In Lyme disease, 10% of patients develop facial palsies, usually weeks to months after the tick bite. These palsies may be bilateral, may be associated with other cranial nerve abnormalities, and may recover without treatment. Serology provides the diagnosis.

Any disease of the CNS that interrupts the supranuclear fibers to the facial nucleus produces central facial palsy. In contrast to Bell's palsy, central facial palsy preserves voluntary movements of the upper face. Further, emotional movements of the mouth, such as during laughter or crying, are paradoxically unaffected by central palsies.

MANAGEMENT. The physician should reassure the patient that facial paralysis does not represent a stroke. Eye protection includes the use of artificial tears during the day (one to two drops four times a day) and ophthalmic ointments at night. Massage and facial nerve electrical stimulation do not hasten recovery. Although steroids may decrease facial pain and produce few complications in Bell's palsy, two double-blind placebo-controlled studies have failed to document a beneficial effect on recovery of muscle strength. Surgical decompression of the facial nerve is not helpful and may be harmful.

FOLLOW-UP. Fifty percent of patients begin to recover within 2 weeks and return to normal within 2 months. The remaining half improve slowly over months. Predictors of incomplete recovery include complete facial paralysis, age greater than 40, pain other than ear pain, and the Ramsey-Hunt syndrome. Although minor degrees of weakness may persist, 90% are satisfied their face has returned to normal. Careful examination after recovery may reveal two complications: contracture (increased muscle tone) and associated movements (e.g., the ipsilateral eye may wink when the patient smiles, or the corner of the mouth may curl when the patient closes the eye). Abnormal reinnervation of the lacrimal gland with regenerating salivary gland nerves occurs in 5% and causes crocodile tears (tearing during eating).

Cross-references: Herpes Zoster (Section 30), Redness of the Eye (Section 37), Foreign Bodies and Corneal Abrasions (Section 42).

REFERENCES

1. Adour KK. Diagnosis and management of facial paralysis. N Engl J Med 1982;307:348–351.
   In one of the largest series of facial palsy cases, 80% had associated dysesthesia or hypesthesia of the trigeminal or glossopharyngeal nerve, or both.

2. Caruso VG. Facial paralysis from Lyme disease. Otolaryngol Head Neck Surg 1985;93:550–553.
   Suspect Lyme disease when there is bilateral paralysis.

3. Gates GA. Facial paralysis. Otolaryngol Clin North Am 1987;20:113–131.
    Outstanding review of anatomy, pathophysiology, clinical evaluation, and treatment of facial paralysis.
4. Taverner D. Bell's palsy: A clinical and electromyographic study. Brain 1955;78:209–228.
    Excellent photographs of the complications of synkinesis and contracture.
5. Wolf SM, Wagner JH, Davidson S, Forsythe A. Treatment of Bell palsy with prednisone: A prospective randomized study. Neurology 1978;28:158–161.
    Most recent steroid trial: 88% of treated patients and 80% of control patients completely recovered, an insignificant difference.

146 ENTRAPMENT NEUROPATHIES

Problem

LAIRD G. PATTERSON

MEDIAN NERVE ENTRAPMENT NEUROPATHY

EPIDEMIOLOGY/ETIOLOGY.   The carpal tunnel syndrome is the most common nerve entrapment syndrome, affecting 0.1% of the general population. It is found in 15% of workers in high-risk industries and is most frequent in middle-aged women. Associated conditions include congenitally small carpal tunnels, wrist trauma, tenosynovitis, collagen vascular disease, diabetes, hypothyroidism, pregnancy, paraproteinemias, and Raynaud's syndrome. Other median nerve entrapment syndromes are rare.

SYMPTOMS AND SIGNS.   The median nerve arises from the C6-T1 nerve roots and innervates the flexor muscles of the wrist and fingers. Sensory symptoms are classically confined to the thumb, index, and middle fingers, although paresthesias may affect the entire hand, forearm, or even upper arm. Nocturnal dysesthesias may awaken the patient, and activities such as sewing, kneading dough, washing dishes, writing, or driving may precipitate or aggravate symptoms. Actual weakness is often minimal because the abductor pollicis brevis is the only primary muscle involved; however, complaints of diminished grip strength and poor dexterity are often voiced. Symptoms are commonly unilateral and affect the dominant hand, but may be bilateral.

In more severe carpal tunnel syndrome, the abductor pollicis brevis muscle is weak and the thenar eminence appears atrophic. Altered sensation may be detected in all median nerve–innervated fingers, especially the index and middle fingers. Phalen's maneuver (hyperflexion of the wrist) for 1 minute may reproduce symptoms. Tinel's sign (tingling or pain produced by gentle percussion of the median nerve at the wrist) may be elicited. Both tests have a sensitivity of approximately 50% and a specificity of approximately 80%. These tests by themselves do not make the diagnosis of carpal tunnel syndrome, but provide additional confirmatory clinical information.

Conditions that resemble carpal tunnel syndrome include cervical radiculopathy (C6 or C7), middle brachial plexus lesions, and median nerve lesions at or above the elbow. Rarely, cervical cord abnormalities such as demyelinating disease, syringomyelia, or mass lesions may mimic carpal tunnel syndrome. Findings that suggest other sources of hand numbness include sensory or motor abnormalities proximal to the wrist, asymmetric deep tendon reflexes, or neck pain.

CLINICAL APPROACH.   The patient interview and physical examination will identify most patients with carpal tunnel syndrome. Electrodiagnostic studies are positive in 90% of cases if both sensory and motor conduction are tested. Electromyography (EMG) rarely contributes to the diagnosis. In selected cases, laboratory tests should include ESR, antinuclear antibody and rheumatoid factor assays, fasting glucose level determinations, thyroid function studies, and serum protein electrophoresis.

MANAGEMENT.   Symptoms respond to rest, application of a wrist splint, and use of anti-inflammatory medications. Some patients, particularly those who continue to have pain as a major symptom, may benefit from steroids injected under the flexor retinaculum.

About one-third of patients fail conservative management and should be considered for surgery. Ninety percent of these patients, if they have persistent pain or weakness, as well as classic neurologic findings and abnormal electrophysiologic tests, will benefit from surgery performed by experienced surgeons. Patients with thenar atrophy are less likely to recover. If both hands are affected, the most symptomatic hand should be treated first.

FOLLOW-UP.   A neurologic consultation is recommended if surgery is contemplated, to confirm the diagnosis and perform necessary electrophysiologic tests. The physician should assess the patient's symptoms, weakness, and atrophy at monthly intervals so that a timely decision regarding surgical therapy can be made if conservative treatment fails.

ULNAR NERVE ENTRAPMENT NEUROPATHY

EPIDEMIOLOGY/ETIOLOGY.   Ulnar entrapment, the second most common entrapment syndrome, may result from elbow trauma, chronic subluxation of the nerve at the ulnar groove, arthritis, or osteophyte formation at the elbow. Other risk factors are diabetes and chronic confinement to bed. Approximately 30% to 50% of cases are idiopathic.

SYMPTOMS AND SIGNS. The ulnar nerve arises from the C8–T1 roots, passes behind the elbow through the ulnar groove into the cubital tunnel (formed by the two heads of the flexor carpi ulnaris), and then enters the hand via Guyon's canal at the wrist. The nerve supplies all intrinsic motor function of the hand except for the abductor pollicis brevis, part of the opponens pollicis, and the first and second lumbricals, and supplies sensation to the fifth finger and the ulnar aspect of the fourth finger and hand.

The nerve is most susceptible to trauma at the ulnar groove, cubital tunnel, wrist, and palm. The usual initial symptoms are nocturnal paresthesias in the ulnar distribution or numbness accompanying repetitive elbow flexion. Grip strength may be gradually and subtly affected. Sensory symptoms usually reflect entrapment at the elbow, whereas pure motor involvement usually represents injury to the deep palmar branch, but may occur with injury at the elbow or wrist as well.

Elbow entrapment causes weakness of the intrinsic muscles of the hand (abduction of the index finger and of the little finger against resistance are simple tests) and classic sensory loss in the ulnar distribution. Palm or wrist entrapment does not affect sensation because the sensory branches bifurcate before the ulnar nerve passes into the hand. Percussion at the ulnar groove or wrist as well as elbow or wrist flexion may provoke symptoms and help localize the ulnar entrapment.

CLINICAL APPROACH. Other conditions mimic ulnar entrapment, such as infiltration or compression of the inferior brachial plexus by tumor, motor neuron disease, syringomyelia, lesions of the cervical roots or cords, or, rarely, thoracic outlet syndrome. The presence of Horner's syndrome (unilateral ptosis, myosis and anhydrosis of the face); sensory abnormalities proximal to the wrist, weakness outside of the ulnar nerve distribution, or asymmetric reflexes suggests causes other than ulnar nerve entrapment.

Electrophysiologic studies (nerve conduction studies and EMG) help to distinguish the various causes of weakness and numbness in the hand. Chest radiography or imaging studies of the cervical cord and brachial plexus may be necessary when more proximal lesions are suspected. The clinician should also consider generalized polyneuropathy due to diabetes or alcohol abuse, which may be superimposed on ulnar neuropathy.

MANAGEMENT. Conservative measures, such as elbow splinting or padding, and avoidance of aggravating positions or activity will often reverse symptoms. If the condition progresses despite conservative treatment, it may be necessary to refer the patient to an experienced orthopedic or neurologic surgeon for nerve decompression or transposition.

FOLLOW-UP. Monthly follow-up during the early phases of the condition is advisable. Weakness may progress without symptoms, and any decision regarding surgery should be made within 6 months of the onset of symptoms to assure a good outcome. Ulnar neuropathy due to a single traumatic event will usually recover without surgery, though it may take 6 to 12 months. Neurologic consultation to confirm the diagnosis of ulnar neuropathy is recommended. Neurologic follow-up is also recommended, since progressive ulnar nerve dysfunction can be relatively silent and may result in a useless hand if surgical intervention is delayed.

RADIAL NERVE ENTRAPMENT NEUROPATHY

EPIDEMIOLOGY/ETIOLOGY.   Radial entrapment is uncommon, representing only 1% of upper extremity entrapment neuropathies. Most lesions are proximal to the elbow and usually result from trauma to the axilla or humerus. Approximately 10% to 15% of fractures of the humerus result in radial neuropathy. The use of crutches, hyperextension of the arm during surgery, or pressure in the axilla or upper arm during sleep or coma account for most cases.

SYMPTOMS AND SIGNS.   The radial nerve arises from the C5-T1 nerve roots and innervates the triceps, brachioradialis, and the extensor muscles of the wrist and fingers. Patients note weakness but rarely have sensory complaints. Pain is uncommon, though trauma to the nerve as it passes through the supinator muscle may be accompanied by severe pain and tenderness, resembling "tennis elbow."

Weakness is generally limited to wrist and finger extensor muscles, although proximal entrapment weakens the triceps and brachioradialis. Sensory loss is usually confined to the dorsal web space between the thumb and forefinger.

CLINICAL APPROACH.   Because of technical difficulties, electrophysiologic studies are less helpful in radial entrapment than in other entrapment neuropathies. Lesions of the brachial plexus, nerve roots, cervical cord, or cerebral cortex may mimic the distal extensor weakness of a radial neuropathy.

MANAGEMENT.   Most radial entrapment neuropathies, whether proximal or distal, will recover with time and avoidance of aggravating positions or activity. In cases of severe wrist drop and finger extensor weakness, a cock-up wrist splint provides comfort and improves function. Although rarely necessary, some patients with persistent pain require exploration and decompression of the radial nerve as it passes through the supinator muscle.

FOLLOW-UP.   Recovery from ulnar lesions takes 6 to 24 weeks. Follow-up appointments every 1 or 2 months are adequate. The use of nerve conduction studies or EMG for prognostic purposes is rarely necessary.

LATERAL FEMORAL CUTANEOUS NERVE ENTRAPMENT NEUROPATHY (MERALGIA PARESTHETICA)

EPIDEMIOLOGY/ETIOLOGY.   Entrapment of the lateral femoral cutaneous nerve (LFCN) occurs as the nerve passes through the lateral portion of the inguinal ligament at the anterosuperior iliac spine. Entrapment may be idiopathic or the result of chronic injury from tight clothing, obesity, pregnancy, or frequent leaning against a bench or cupboard at waist height.

SYMPTOMS AND SIGNS. The LFCN is a purely sensory nerve and is composed of fibers from the L1–L3 nerve roots. Entrapment causes burning, stinging, itching, tingling, or numbness in an ovoid area of the anterolateral thigh. The pain is often aggravated by standing, hyperextending the leg, or lying flat. Hyperpathia may occur, causing discomfort when clothing or bedclothes lightly touch the affected area. Dysesthesias gradually subside, often to be replaced by painless anesthesia.

Examination demonstrates sensory loss confined to the anterolateral thigh. Testing temperature or light touch sensation often identifies the sensory loss more easily than testing with a pin.

CLINICAL APPROACH. The typical history and examination are usually sufficient to make the diagnosis of LFCN entrapment. Electrophysiologic studies can confirm the diagnosis but are difficult to perform and usually unnecessary.

Other uncommon conditions may mimic LFCN entrapment, such as intrapelvic or retroperitoneal processes that infiltrate the LFCN or a high lumbar root lesion that manifests with purely sensory symptoms. CT or MRI is useful in selected cases.

TREATMENT. Initial treatment includes weight loss, if appropriate, and avoidance of tight clothing and positions that exacerbate symptoms. If pain is severe, it may be relieved by a nerve block at the inguinal ligament with Depo-Medrol, 60 to 80 mg, and a local anesthetic. Although rarely necessary, patients with persistent pain may require surgical decompression.

PERONEAL NERVE ENTRAPMENT NEUROPATHY

EPIDEMIOLOGY/ETIOLOGY. Injury to the peroneal nerve usually occurs at the fibular head, either from direct trauma, fracture of the fibula, compression with casts or tight stockings, or prolonged pressure on the nerve that occurs in bedridden patients or those who repeatedly cross their legs, squat, or kneel. Occasionally a fibrous band or mass in the fibular tunnel entraps the nerve. It is the most common mononeuropathy in the leg.

SYMPTOMS AND SIGNS. The most common presentation is painless weakness of foot dorsiflexion and eversion, although pain may occur early in the course of entrapment or compression. Although the common peroneal nerve is affected in most, isolated deep branch involvement produces weakness and only minimal sensory loss in the dorsal web space between the first and second toes; isolated peripheral branch involvement results in weak foot eversion and extensive sensory loss of the lower calf, dorsal foot, and medial toes. Reflexes are not affected in peroneal entrapment.

CLINICAL APPROACH. The typical sensory loss and weakness of peroneal entrapment may be mimicked by sciatic nerve pathology, L5 root or even upper motor neuron lesions. The findings of absent ankle or patellar reflexes or of weak foot inversion, plantar flexion, or knee or hip movements all suggest conditions other than peroneal entrapment. EMG and nerve conduction testing help identify the lesion.

MANAGEMENT.   Removal of the identified risk factor usually allows recovery. An ankle-foot orthosis prevents ankle injury if the foot drop is severe. Conservative care will almost invariably lead to recovery, although rare patients have persistent weakness and may require exploration of the nerve at the fibular head. Electrophysiologic studies are useful to follow and predict recovery.

FOLLOW-UP.   The clinician should examine patients monthly until clear-cut recovery is documented, since a decision regarding surgery should be made within 3 to 6 months of the onset of symptoms.

Cross-references: Diagnosis and Management of Alcoholism (Section 9), Low Back Pain (Section 108), Hip Pain (Section 110), Wrist and Hand Pain (Section 111), Ankle and Foot Pain (Section 113), Myofascial Pain Syndromes (Section 123), Raynaud's Syndrome (Section 132), Peripheral Neuropathy (Section 149), Electromyography and Nerve Conduction Studies (Section 151), Screening for Thyroid Disease (Section 153), Common Thyroid Disorders (Section 156), Diabetes Mellitus (Section 157).

REFERENCES

1. Dawson DM, Hallett M, Millender LH. Entrapment Neuropathies. Little, Brown, Boston, 1983.
    Excellent comprehensive discussion of entrapment neuropathies.

2. Nakano KK. The entrapment neuropathies. Muscles Nerve 1978;1:264–279.
    Compact review of the important entrapment syndromes.

3. Spinner RJ, Bachman JW, Amadio PC. The many faces of carpal tunnel syndrome. Mayo Clin Proc 1989;64:829–836.
    Detailed clinical review of the most common entrapment neuropathy.

147 PARKINSONISM

Problem

LAIRD G. PATTERSON

EPIDEMIOLOGY/ETIOLOGY. Parkinson's disease affects approximately 1% of the population over the age of 50. The peak incidence is between the fifth and sixth decades, with men more likely to be affected than women in a ratio of 3:2. The disease is distributed worldwide, affects all ethnic groups, and has a prevalence that has been stable for at least 100 years. A single genetic cause is unlikely, and definite environmental causes have not been identified. Mortality was two to three times higher in the era before levodopa was available but is now similar to that in age-related cohort groups.

Extrapyramidal signs appear when dopamine levels in the putamen and caudate are reduced by 80% or more.

SYMPTOMS AND SIGNS. The onset is insidious and often unrecognized by the patient or family for several years. Many symptoms are nonspecific and include arthralgias, depression, vague sensory or balance complaints, stiffness, fatigue, and generalized slowing, all of which may be attributed to arthritis or aging.

Tremor is the first symptom in about 50% of patients but often appears late or not at all. Unilateral stiffness or clumsiness, diminished arm swing, dragging a leg, difficulty getting out of low seats or out of a car, poor postural reflexes, slowed gait, sialorrhea (excessive saliva), decreased facial expression, restless legs, or a dystonic foot may be presenting symptoms. Patients often report symptoms of seborrhea, micrographia, or flexed posture.

The signs of early Parkinson's disease may be subtle. A 4- to 6-Hz **tremor** is usually present at rest but can occur with activity. **Rigidity** is often minimal but can be elicited by reinforcement techniques such as making a fist with the hand contralateral to the limb being tested. Decreased blink rate (normal, 12–15 blinks per minute), infrequent postural adjustment, slowness in dressing or adjusting glasses, and difficulty getting out of a chair are all manifestations of **bradykinesia.** Gait is often shuffling or difficult to initiate. Festination, a tendency to chase the center of gravity when walking, and **loss of postural reflexes** appear as the disease progresses. Rapid alternating movements that progressively diminish in amplitude, micrographia, mumbling, and stammering may all be present. Deep tendon reflexes are generally normal but may become hyperactive in affected extremities. The plantar reflex is usually flexor. Eye movement abnormalities include restricted upward gaze and diminished saccadic movements. Other findings such as orthostatic hypotension, dementia, and ataxic gait may be seen, but if encountered early may signify other conditions. Despite sensory symptoms, the sensory examination is usually normal.

CLINICAL APPROACH. A clinical diagnosis of Parkinson's disease is possible in at least 80% to 90% of cases, although patients with atypical features may need further studies. Conditions that mimic Parkinson's disease include frontal and midline tumors, chronic subdural hemorrhage, multiple infarcts, normal pressure hydrocephalus, and Wilson's disease. Other degenerative diseases such as Huntington's chorea, multisystem atrophy, Shy-Drager syndrome, progressive supranuclear palsy, olivopontocerebellar atrophy, Creutzfeldt-Jakob disease, and even Alzheimer's disease can all exhibit parkinsonian features. Neuroleptic medications, metoclopramide, and hypnotic-sedative drugs all may produce extrapyramidal side effects. Intoxication with methyl-phenyl-tetrahydropyridine (MPTP), a toxic byproduct produced during illicit manufacture of a meperidine analogue, causes a striking parkinsonian syndrome.

Although the diagnosis of Parkinson's disease is based on clinical criteria, patients who are under the age of 50 or who have atypical features may require further studies. Magnetic resonance imaging (MRI) or computed tomography (CT) can exclude most structural causes of extrapyramidal dysfunction. A normal ceruloplasmin level and eye examination make Wilson's disease unlikely. A careful family history may reveal relatives with Huntington's chorea or olivopontocerebellar atrophy. Creutzfeldt-Jakob disease is suggested if the EEG shows myoclonic activity.

MANAGEMENT. The initial management of Parkinson's disease is straightforward but becomes quite complex as the disease progresses. Neurologic consultation is usually necessary to confirm the diagnosis and to aid in management. Patients are usually not treated until their symptoms begin to affect their life-style, job, or relationships. Education of the patient and family is an important aspect of treatment. Stretching and aerobic exercises should be utilized by all patients, including those on pharmacologic therapy. Vitamin E (800 units/day) is generally started at the time of diagnosis because of its theoretical neuroprotective effect as a free radical scavenger, although evidence confirming its benefit is lacking.

Pharmacologic therapy begins with levodopa and a decarboxylase inhibitor (Sinemet) (Table 147–1). A 1:4 ratio of inhibitor to levodopa is preferred, to minimize systemic dopaminergic side effects. An initial dose of Sinemet, 25/100 mg b.i.d. or t.i.d., is usually well tolerated and may provide symptom relief for several years in early disease. As the total dose of levodopa is increased up to 500 or 600 mg, a dopamine agonist, bromocriptine (Parlodel), is started in small doses, such as 1.25 mg t.i.d., and the total daily dose is then gradually increased to 15 to 20 mg. The combination of low-dose levodopa and dopamine agonist seems to prolong the period of effective therapy. After 3 to 5 years, however, most patients begin to have treatment complications such as early diminishment of the medication effect, rapidly fluctuating motor symptoms ("on-off phenomenon"), freezing, dyskinesias, and hallucinations, which require changing the frequency or size of the dose. The addition of selegiline (Eldepryl), 5 mg b.i.d., a monoamine oxidase (type B) inhibitor, may be war-

TABLE 147–1. ANTIPARKINSON MEDICATIONS

Agent	Daily Dose (mg)	Major Side Effects	Cost ($) per Tablet[1]
Sinemet 10/100 mg 25/100 mg 25/250 mg	30/100–150/1500	Dyskinesias, nausea, anorexia, orthostatic hypotension, cardiac arrhythmias, confusion, hallucinations	0.51 0.57 0.73
Trihexyphenidyl (Artane) 2 mg	1–20	Drowsiness, urine retention, constipation, confusion, hallucinations, tachycardia	0.03
Ethopropazine (Parsidol) 50 mg	50–200	Drowsiness, urine retention, constipation, confusion, hallucinations, tachycardia	0.08
Benztropine (Cogentin) 2 mg	1–6	Drowsiness, urine retention, constipation, confusion, hallucinations, tachycardia	0.04
Bromocriptine (Parlodel) 2.5 mg 5.0 mg	5–20	Nausea, dyskinesias, confusion, hallucinations, dizziness, syncope	1.11 1.69
Pergolide (Permax) 0.05 mg 0.25 mg 1.00 mg	1–5	Nausea, dyskinesias, confusion, hallucinations, dizziness, syncope	0.04 0.51 1.84
Amantadine (Symmetrel) 100 mg	200	Confusion, hallucinations, psychosis, hypotension, livedo reticularis, edema	0.21
Selegiline (Eldepryl) 5 mg	5–10	Exacerbates L-dopa side effects, headache, insomnia, fainting	1.88

[1]Average wholesale price, 1991 *Drug Topics Red Book*.

ranted since it often improves the effectiveness of Sinemet. Studies are underway to determine whether it delays progression of the disease as well.

Other medications that are used in Parkinson's disease are generally less effective but may contribute to further improvement in selected cases. These include amantadine or various anticholinergic medications such as trihexyphenidyl (Artane) or ethopropazine (Parsidol), which may partially alleviate symptoms but may cause some memory difficulty. Antidepressant therapy not only treats depression but may enhance the effectiveness of levodopa by decreasing synaptic dopamine re-uptake. Newer dopamine agonists, such as pergolide, are also being introduced. If the levodopa effect diminishes, a restricted protein diet may restore some of its potency.

FOLLOW-UP. Patients with early disease should be seen every 4 to 6 months. As the disease progresses and complications occur, closer follow-up becomes necessary. Disease complications in addition to those related to therapy include autonomic dysfunction, depression, inanition, sleep disturbances, dementia, delirium, and the dangers of immobility such as pneumonia and thrombophlebitis. Intercurrent illness or surgery often exacerbates the symptoms and signs of Parkinson's disease. Most patients with moderate to advanced disease will need to be managed with the help of a neurologist.

Cross-references: Tremor (Section 138), Dementia (Section 142), Electroencephalography (Section 150).

References

1. Calne DB, Stoessl AJ. Early parkinsonism. Clin Neuropharmacol 1986;9(suppl 2):S3–S8.
   Clinical observations regarding early symptoms.

2. Cederbaum JM, Silvestri M, Clark M, Harts A, Kutt H. L-deprenyl, levodopa pharmacokinetics, and response fluctuations in Parkinson's disease. Clin Neuropharmacol 1990; 13:29–35.
   Rationale for L-deprenyl therapy.

3. Kurlan R. Practical therapy of Parkinson's disease. Semin Neurol 1987;7:160–166.
   Good review of therapeutic strategy.

4. Obeso JA, et al. Motor complications associated with chronic levodopa therapy in Parkinson's disease. Neurology 1989;39(suppl 2):11–19.
   Discusses the difficulties of chronic levodopa therapy.

148 CEREBROVASCULAR DISEASE

Problem

LYNNE P. TAYLOR

EPIDEMIOLOGY/ETIOLOGY. **Stroke** refers to the sudden appearance of a focal neurologic deficit, caused by thrombotic (65%–80%) or embolic (5%–15%) arterial occlusion or cerebral hemorrhage (15%–20%). Stroke ranks third as a cause for death in the United States, where there are over 2 million stroke survivors and 500,000 new strokes each year.

The treatment of risk factors for stroke has reduced this incidence in recent years. Hypertension, cardiac disease, diabetes, polycythemia, and a history of transient ischemic attacks (TIA, episodes of focal neurologic dysfunction lasting less than 24 hours) all increase the risk of stroke. The risk of stroke is directly related to the level of systolic blood pressure. Cigarette smoking, excessive alcohol use, recreational drug use (cocaine), sedentary life-style, obesity, and hyperlipidemia also increase the risk, although it is uncertain whether intervention for these factors reduces the risk of stroke. The Framingham Study also suggested that an asymptomatic carotid bruit was a risk factor leading to a doubling of the risk of stroke, although this is controversial.

Atherothrombotic disease includes both extracranial (carotid stenosis) and intracranial occlusive disease (lacunar strokes). Lacunar strokes are small (1–20 mm in diameter), usually affect the deep hemispheric white matter or brain stem, and are associated with hypertension and diabetes. The pathology is distinct and thought to be related to lipohyalinosis of tiny penetrating blood vessels.

Emboli originate from arterial or cardiac thrombi. It is important to identify cardiogenic embolic disease, because these patients have a high risk of recurrent stroke (six to twelve times higher than stroke patients without a cardiac source), and 10% to 20% of recurrent emboli recur within the subsequent 2 weeks. Sources of cardioembolism are atrial fibrillation (45%), myocardial infarction or ventricular aneurysms (25%), rheumatic heart disease (10%), prosthetic heart valves (10%), and other sources such as bacterial endocarditis (10%).

Intracerebral hemorrhage may result from hemorrhage into an infarct, severe hypertension, or amyloid angiopathy.

SYMPTOMS AND SIGNS. It is useful to divide strokes into small vessel (lacunar infarcts) and large vessel occlusive disease, which can be further subdivided into anterior (carotid, middle cerebral, anterior cerebral arteries) or posterior (posterior cerebral, vertebrobasilar) circulation.

449

Because **lacunar** infarcts involve a small, dense area of white matter tracts, deficits tend to be limited and either pure motor or pure sensory. The face, arm, and leg are often equally affected. Common patterns include dysarthria–clumsy hand, ataxic hemiparesis, and pure motor stroke.

Stroke involving the **middle cerebral** artery distribution generally produces a mixed motor and sensory disturbance that maximally involves the face and arm, with relative sparing of the leg. Expressive or receptive aphasia may occur in left (dominant) hemisphere strokes and cortical neglect in right hemispheric (nondominant) strokes. Amaurosis fugax, a brief stereotypic monocular visual loss described by patients as a curtain descending over an eye, is typical of **carotid artery** disease. Strokes in the region of the **anterior cerebral artery** produce hemiparesis that is more pronounced in the leg.

Posterior cerebral artery strokes classically cause a contralateral homonymous visual field deficit, generally without other neurologic findings. **Vertebrobasilar system** symptoms include vertigo, headache, nausea, vomiting, or hiccoughs in association with a hemiparesis that may be unilateral, bilateral, or alternating. Typical neurologic findings, in addition to hemiparesis, include nystagmus, ocular motor palsies, and other cranial nerve findings.

Embolic strokes classically produce maximal deficit at onset and are noticed by the patient upon arising in the morning. A seizure occurs at the time of the embolic event in 5% to 10% of cases. Thrombotic strokes tend to pursue a more stuttering course with symptoms that wax and wane before the deficit becomes maximal. Cerebral hemorrhage produces symptoms abruptly at any time of the day, usually accompanied by headache.

CLINICAL APPROACH.   A proper diagnostic and therapeutic approach to stroke and TIA depends heavily on the correct identification of (1) the neuroanatomic location of the lesion, (2) the likely etiology, and (3) risk factors for stroke. The general physical examination focuses on peripheral blood vessels (hypertensive retinal changes and Hollenhorst plaques on ophthalmoscopic examination, blood pressure in both arms, pulse contour and bruits of the carotid and other arteries) and the heart (irregular rhythm, murmur).

The neurologic examination should detail the degree and distribution of motor and sensory findings as well as such "cortical" findings as apraxia, aphasia, neglect, or hemianopsia. Following the examination, the clinician should attempt to localize the lesion within the neuraxis, define its vascular distribution, and then exclude other diseases that mimic stroke (Table 148–1). Slowly progressive symptoms that worsen over days or weeks should be considered due to a tumor (or subdural hematoma) until proven otherwise.

Routine laboratory tests include electrocardiography (ECG), chest radiograph, blood glucose, complete blood count, prothrombin time, activated partial thromboplastin time, platelet count, and cholesterol level. In most cases computed tomography (CT) of the head with contrast agent is needed to exclude other abnormalities (see Table 148–1), confirm the size and site of the infarct, and evaluate for areas of previous silent ischemia in other vascular

TABLE 148–1.   DIFFERENTIAL DIAGNOSIS OF STROKE

Tumor
Subdural hematoma
Seizures
Migraine
Inner ear disturbance
Multiple sclerosis
Hypoglycemia

distributions that may suggest cardiogenic embolic disease. Magnetic resonance imaging (MRI) is more expensive and less available than CT and should be reserved for identification of lacunar infarcts too small to be seen on CT, or when lesions in the posterior fossa are suspected. When cardiogenic embolic disease is suspected (suspicious history or abnormal heart examination, ECG, or chest radiograph), echocardiography is necessary to look for left atrial enlargement, valvular disease, left ventricular dysfunction, and intracardiac clot. In unexplained cases of embolic stroke, echocardiography with bubble contrast and transesophageal echocardiography may identify a right-to-left shunt, and blood cultures may identify the bacteremia of endocarditis.

Duplex ultrasound, which uses pulsed echo imaging to visualize the carotid artery and a Doppler signal to measure blood flow, is indicated for patients with symptoms in the anterior circulation. Depending on the laboratory, it has a sensitivity of 85% to 100% and a specificity close to 90%. Carotid Doppler ultrasound, in combination with periorbital Doppler, is also useful when duplex ultrasound is unavailable. Patients with a history of TIA or stroke, if they have stenosis greater than 70% on noninvasive testing and are surgical candidates, should be further evaluated with carotid angiography. Intra-arterial digital subtraction technique is preferred to conventional angiography because a smaller catheter and a lower dose of contrast material are used. The morbidity from angiography should be less than 2% (stroke, wound hematoma, infection).

In young patients (less than 50 years old) with unexplained ischemic strokes, the physician should consider hematologic causes such as antithrombin III deficiency, polycythemia vera, lupus anticoagulant, and anticardiolipin antibodies. The prevalence of stroke attributed to hematologic disorders is zero to 7%.

MANAGEMENT.   Proper medical treatment depends on whether patients are (1) asymptomatic with normal neurologic findings, (2) previously symptomatic but now with normal neurologic findings, or (3) currently symptomatic.

Asymptomatic patients should be helped to modify risk factors such as smoking, excessive alcohol use, hypertension, poorly controlled diabetes, and perhaps hypercholesterolemia.

Patients with lone atrial fibrillation who are older than 60 years of age should be treated with 325 mg of aspirin each morning as prophylaxis against future stroke. Patients with atrial fibrillation associated with congestive heart failure, valvular heart disease, or a prosthetic valve may require treatment with war-

TABLE 148–2. ORAL ANTIPLATELET/ANTICOAGULANT DRUGS

Clinical Setting	Drug	Dose	Cost ($) per Day[1]
Atherothrombotic disease	Aspirin (enteric coated)	300–1200 mg/day	0.01–0.05
Cardiogenic emboli	Warfarin	See Section 203 (Chronic Anticoagulation)	0.44[2]
TIAs resistant to aspirin	Warfarin[3]	See Section 203 (Chronic Anticoagulation)	0.44[2]

[1]Average wholesale price, 1991 *Drug Topics Red Book.*
[2]Individual doses vary; price listed is for 5 mg/day.
[3]Data are lacking; treatment is empirical.

farin (see Section 83, Atrial Fibrillation, and Section 203, Chronic Anticoagulation). Asymptomatic patients with carotid bruits should learn about the symptoms of TIAs and modify their risk factors. The role of carotid duplex testing in these patients will remain unclear until studies on the value of endarterectomy in this patient group are completed.

Previously symptomatic but currently neurologically normal patients may have been having TIAs. Patients with crescendo TIAs (TIAs that occurred within the previous week and are increasing in frequency) should be admitted to the hospital for evaluation and possible anticoagulation. A patient with a more remote single neurologic event can be evaluated as an outpatient and managed with risk factor modification and initiation of aspirin therapy, 325 mg PO every morning (Table 148-2). All of these patients should also be referred to a neurologist to ensure that vascular pathology is correlated carefully with symptoms.

Patients with crescendo TIAs thought to be of cardiogenic origin (e.g., atrial fibrillation, after myocardial infarction) should be immediately anticoagulated with heparin, as long as the CT scan excludes hemorrhagic stroke, the systolic blood pressure is less than 170 mm Hg, and there is no large cerebral infarct that could increase the risk of an intraparenchymal hemorrhage. Data on anticoagulation of patients with TIAs in other settings are lacking.

There is rarely a role for anticoagulation in completed stroke if the deficit is profound. Management in these patients emphasizes supportive care and measures to prevent aspiration, deep venous thrombosis, and contracture. To avoid enlarging the ischemic area, hypertension should not be treated in an acute stroke unless the systolic pressure consistently exceeds 180 to 190 mm Hg and the diastolic pressure exceeds 100 mm Hg.

Symptomatic patients with hemodynamically significant carotid stenosis (70% or greater) and possibly those with an ulcerated plaque require carotid endarterectomy if it is ipsilateral to the site of TIA, as demonstrated in the North American Symptomatic Carotid Endarterectomy Trial.[5] Carotid endarterectomy is also appropriate for patients who have had a small completed stroke with good remaining functional abilities, although in this situation surgery is generally delayed for 6 weeks. Studies comparing endarterectomy to aspirin are currently underway for the asymptomatic patient group.

Lacunar strokes are generally treated with control of arterial hypertension. There is no role for anticoagulation, although a single aspirin a day is often prescribed empirically.

FOLLOW-UP. In the course of evaluation, patients are often discovered to have high-grade asymptomatic stenoses in the nonsymptomatic carotid artery. These patients should be followed closely for evidence of neurologic symptoms and with repeat Doppler studies as clinically indicated. The role of endarterectomy in asymptomatic carotid stenosis remains uncertain, although some authorities consider surgery when there is contralateral carotid occlusion.

Patients should be followed at 6-month intervals to monitor symptoms and reinforce risk factor modification.

Cross-references: Smoking Cessation (Section 11), Dizziness (Section 20), Visual Impairment (Section 36), Ophthalmoscopy (Section 46), Syncope (Section 75), Atrial Fibrillation (Section 83), Essential Hypertension (Section 86), Echocardiography (Section 90), Peripheral Arterial Disease (Section 133), Muscular Weakness (Section 139), Polycythemia (Section 200), Chronic Anticoagulation (Section 203).

REFERENCES

1. American College of Physicians. Position paper. Indications for carotid endarterectomy. Ann Intern Med 1989;111:675–677.
    A review of published evidence for and against carotid surgery.

2. Canadian Cooperative Study Group. A randomized trial of aspirin and sulfinpyrazone in threatened stroke. N Engl J Med 1978;299:53–59.
    Aspirin, 325 mg q.i.d., reduced the risk of subsequent stroke, TIA, or death by 19% (in men only); sulfinpyrazone was ineffective.

3. Dyken ML, et al. Risk factors in stroke. Stroke 1984;15:1105–1111.
    A good general review.

4. Mohr JP. Lacunes. Stroke 1982;13:3–10.
    Excellent clinical description of lacunar infarcts.

5. North American Symptomatic Carotid Endarterectomy Trial. N Engl J Med 1991;325:445–453.
    Demonstrated benefit of endarterectomy over medical treatment for *symptomatic* patients with 70% to 99% carotid stenosis by angiography.

149 PERIPHERAL NEUROPATHY

Problem

JOYCE E. WIPF

EPIDEMIOLOGY. Peripheral neuropathy is a disease of neural structures outside of the brain and spinal cord, which may involve abnormalities of axons (axonopathy) or myelin sheaths (demyelination), and may affect any combination of motor, sensory, or autonomic nerves. Although peripheral neuropathy may be congenital (e.g., the peroneal muscle atrophy of Charcot-Marie-Tooth disease), acquired neuropathy is much more common, occurring in a wide variety of medical disorders, including half of patients with long-standing diabetes and up to 15% with newly diagnosed diabetes.

SYMPTOMS AND SIGNS/ETIOLOGY. Because the causes are so diverse, peripheral neuropathy may be acute, subacute, or chronic, and symptoms may fluctuate or remain constant.

Common motor symptoms are weakness, muscle twitching, and cramps. Sensory symptoms include numbness, dysesthesia (painful sensations), cold feet, stumbling, and unsteady gait. Involvement of autonomic nerves may result in impotence, retrograde ejaculation, diaphoresis or loss of sweating, incontinence, urine retention, constipation, diarrhea, orthostatic dizziness, or flushing. Diabetics with autonomic neuropathy may become unaware of episodes of hypoglycemia or may develop symptoms of gastroparesis (postprandial nausea, vomiting, bloating, and early satiety).

Neurologic examination may reveal weakness, fasciculation, atrophy, ataxia, wide-based gait, abnormal sweating, diminished or absent reflexes, and orthostatic hypotension. Sensory findings include areas of hypesthesia (sometimes surrounded by a zone of hyperesthesia) or complete loss of sensation, with vibratory and position sensation usually disappearing before loss of pinprick and temperature sensation. Patients with neuropathic arthropathy may have diminished pulses and various foot abnormalities, including flat longitudinal arches, a tendency to evert and externally rotate the ankle, a shorter and wider foot, swelling, and painless punched-out ulcers. Signs of autonomic neuropathy include small dark-adapted pupil size, delayed pupillary response to light, resting tachycardia, and loss of sinus arrhythmia. The ECG may reveal evidence of silent myocardial ischemia.

It is helpful to classify the patient's peripheral neuropathy as polyneuropathy (the most common type), radiculopathy (compression of nerve roots), mononeuropathy, entrapment neuropathy, or mononeuropathy multiplex.

Polyneuropathy usually affects both legs in a symmetric "stocking-glove" distribution with varying combinations of motor, sensory, or autonomic find-

454

ings. Progressive disease may involve the thighs, trunk, and shoulders. Although diabetes is the most common cause, polyneuropathy may occur in many different systemic disorders. Sixty-five percent of patients in renal failure who are starting dialysis have a mixed sensorimotor polyneuropathy, often associated with the restless legs syndrome. Alcoholism and nutritional deficiencies (thiamine, pyridoxine, vitamin B_{12}, and pantothenic acid) cause a subacute polyneuropathy that may progress to severe weakness and atrophy. In vitamin B_{12} deficiency, the neuropathy may precede anemia.

Some 2% to 5% of all patients with malignancy have polyneuropathy, usually a mixed sensorimotor type, although other specific paraneoplastic syndromes occur (e.g., Lambert-Eaton syndrome with myasthenia-type weakness). Common associated tumors are small cell carcinoma of the lung (accounting for more than 50% of paraneoplastic neuropathy in some series) and those producing a paraproteinemia (e.g., plasmacytoma, multiple myeloma).

Although the neuropathy of rheumatologic diseases (e.g., vasculitis) is usually a mononeuropathy, 5% of patients with long-standing rheumatoid arthritis and 10% with systemic lupus erythematosus have polyneuropathy. Other important causes of polyneuropathy are medications and environmental toxins (Table 149–1), metabolic conditions (amyloidosis, hypothyroidism, and chronic liver failure), and HIV infection. Rapidly progressive sensorimotor polyneuropathy occurs in the Guillain-Barré syndrome.

Common **mononeuropathies,** which affect single nerves, are cranial nerve palsies, especially those of nerves III, IV, VI, and VII, and entrapment neuropathies, especially of the median nerve at the carpal tunnel, the ulnar nerve at the elbow or wrist, the lateral femoral cutaneous nerve at the inguinal ligament, and the posterior tibial nerve at the tarsal tunnel (see Section 146, Entrapment Neuropathies).

Mononeuropathy multiplex (asymmetric proximal motor neuropathy) involves several noncontiguous nerve trunks and is characterized by severe unilateral pain, followed by weakness and muscle atrophy, in the low back or hips, sometimes extending to the thigh and knee. Sensory loss, if any, is mild. Symptoms usually progress over days, but most experience gradual recovery. This neuropathy results from multifocal ischemic infarcts of the lumbar plexus and other regional nerve trunks and is associated with diabetes, leprosy, sarcoidosis, polyarteritis nodosa, and cryoglobulinemia.

Diabetic amyotrophy (symmetric proximal motor neuropathy), which is frequently associated with other neuropathies, features profound weight loss, wasting, and progressive weakness of the hip and thigh muscles bilaterally, often with proximal shoulder girdle involvement. It is often very painful, although sensory loss is unusual. Symptoms may progress rapidly over several weeks, and then slowly improve over months. **Diabetic neuropathic cachexia** is usually seen in middle-aged men and mimics metastatic cancer, with profound weight loss, severe diffuse pain, and absence of focal neurologic abnormalities. Recovery occurs after months to a year.

TABLE 149–1.   DRUGS AND TOXINS CAUSING PERIPHERAL NEUROPATHY[1]

Drugs	Toxins
Antibiotics	*Metals*
Nitrofurantoin	Lead (adults)
Chloramphenicol	Arsenic
Metronidazole	Lithium
Sulfonamides	Mercury
	Gold
Antituberculous	Platinum
Isoniazid	?Copper, zinc, bismuth
Ethambutol	
Ethionamide	*Occupational*
	Methyl-*n*-butyl ketone (solvent)
Antineoplastic	*n*-Hexane (contact cements)
Vincristine	Dimethylaminopropionitrile (manufacture of polyurethane foam)
Vinblastine	Carbon disulfide
Cisplatin	Allyl chloride (manufacture of epoxy resin, pesticides)
Procarbazine	Organophosphates (pesticides)
Etoposide (VP-16)	Thallium (rat poison)
Teniposide (VM-26)	Methyl and ethyl alcohol
Aramycin	
Nitrogen mustard	
Other	
Zidovudine	
Hydralazine	
Glutethimide	
Phenytoin	
Amiodarone	
Amitriptyline	
Imipramine	
Disulfiram	
Dapsone	

[1]Most cause axonal degeneration.

CLINICAL APPROACH.   The patient interview should focus on systemic diseases, medications, and exposure to toxins or chemicals. Genetic neuropathies are diagnosed from a careful family history and examination of blood relatives. The clinician's major diagnostic goals are to identify treatable diseases and potential environmental causes. Even individuals with diabetes or alcohol abuse may have other reasons for neuropathy and deserve careful evaluation. Routine laboratory tests should include a complete blood count, glucose, creatinine, urinalysis, thyroid function tests, VDRL, and vitamin B_{12} levels, and a recent chest radiograph. In patients with bone pain or elevated serum total proteins, an ESR and serum and urine protein electrophoresis are indicated.

Electrodiagnostic studies (see Section 151, Electromyography and Nerve Conduction Studies) distinguish demyelinating from axonal degeneration (e.g., most metabolic and toxic etiologies cause axonal degeneration) and are most useful in patients with unilateral neuropathies to confirm radiculopathy, entrapment, or mononeuropathy multiplex. Nerve biopsies are indicated in patients with unexplained asymmetric or multifocal neuropathies, or when nerves are enlarged on examination.

MANAGEMENT.   The clinician should treat the underlying disease and eliminate any causative agents. Whether diabetic neuropathy will improve with better control of hyperglycemia remains debated and is currently under study; present data suggest that tight control of the blood sugar level improves nerve conduction velocity, but without a measurable improvement in symptoms. Aldose-reductase inhibitors (e.g., sorbinil) may transiently improve nerve function in diabetic neuropathy, but with the potential of significant toxicity. Diabetic gastroparesis may respond to metoclopramide (10 mg PO q.i.d.) or, though data are preliminary, erythromycin (250 mg PO t.i.d.). If the evaluation of the patient's chronic diarrhea or constipation does not reveal a treatable cause, a bowel program may be beneficial.

The major concern for most patients with polyneuropathy is discomfort from dysesthesia. Nonnarcotic analgesics are most useful, including nonsteroidal anti-inflammatory agents, acetaminophen, and tricyclic antidepressants (amitriptyline, 50–150 mg PO q.d.; nortriptyline, 25–100 mg PO q.d.). If severe pain persists, a 3-month trial of anticonvulsant medication (e.g., phenytoin or carbamazepine) may be beneficial, following the same therapeutic drug levels used for patients with seizures.

Symptomatic orthostatic hypotension resulting from autonomic neuropathy may respond to the use of support hose, withdrawal of exacerbating drugs (e.g., tricyclic antidepressants, diuretics), and counseling the patient to rise slowly from a seated or supine position. Mineralocorticoid therapy (fludrocortisone, 0.1–0.2 mg b.i.d.) is helpful in refractory cases.

Many patients benefit from a referral to a physical therapist, who may recommend splints, specific exercise programs, transcutaneous electrical nerve stimulation for pain relief, or aids for ambulation. Nerve blocks for intractable focal pain are rarely required. Management of the specific entrapment neuropathies is discussed in Section 146.

FOLLOW-UP.   During regular follow-up visits, the clinician should carefully examine the skin for signs of infection or ulceration and should monitor for any progression of the neuropathy. All patients with polyneuropathy should inspect their feet daily, always wear shoes, and avoid testing water temperature with their feet. Any patient with new or persistent focal foot pain should undergo radiographic evaluation to exclude osteomyelitis, fracture, or dislocation.

Cross-references: Diagnosis and Management of Alcoholism (Section 9), Diarrhea (Section 92), Constipation (Section 94), Abdominal Pain (Section 95), Ankle and Foot Pain (Section 113), Restless Legs Syndrome (Section 114), Diabetic Foot Care Education (Section 125), Principles of Physical Therapy (Section 126), Leg Ulcers (Section 134), Local Care of Diabetic Foot Lesions (Section 135), Muscular Weakness (Section 139), Entrapment Neuropathies (Section 146), Electromyography and Nerve Conduction Studies (Section 151), Impotence (Section 171), Urinary Incontinence (Section 174).

REFERENCES

1. Brown MJ, Asbury AK. Diabetic neuropathy. Ann Neurol 1984;15:2–12.

   Reviews the various diabetic peripheral nerve disorders, including detailed clinical descriptions, pathologic changes, and electrodiagnostic findings.

2. Cohen JA, Gross KF. Autonomic neuropathy: Clinical presentation and differential diagnosis. Geriatrics 1990;45(7):33–42.

   Excellent overview of autonomic nervous system structure and function, with useful charts and diagrams.

3. Forman A. Peripheral neuropathy in cancer patients: Clinical types, etiology and presentation. Part II. Oncology 1990;4(2):85–89.

   Vincristine and cisplatin are commonly associated with peripheral neuropathy, with hypomagnesemia increasing the risk of cisplatin toxicity. Neuropathy may also result from tumor infiltration or compression of nerves (e.g., brachial or lumbosacral plexus).

4. He F. Occupational toxic neuropathies: An update. Scand J Work Environ Health 1985;11:321–330.

   Extensive review of environmental and work-related chemicals and toxins associated with peripheral neuropathy.

5. Lehtinen JM, Uusitupa M, Siitonen O, Pyörälä K. Prevalence of neuropathy in newly diagnosed NIDDM and nondiabetic control subjects. Diabetes 1989;38:1307–1313.

   Of 132 newly diagnosed non-insulin-dependent diabetics, 1.5% had symptomatic polyneuropathy, 2.3% had signs of polyneuropathy, and 15.2% had electrodiagnostic findings of polyneuropathy; 9.2% of the diabetic men and 3.3% of the diabetic women had autonomic dysfunction (i.e., reduced variation in heart rate during deep breathing).

150 ELECTROENCEPHALOGRAPHY

Procedure

JAMES J. COATSWORTH

INDICATIONS/CONTRAINDICATIONS. Electroencephalography is useful in evaluating patients with seizures or suspected seizures, recurrent loss of consciousness, metabolic disorders (delirium), sleep disorders, and brain injury. Computed tomography (CT) and magnetic resonance imaging (MRI) are superior to EEG in evaluating suspected brain tumors, stroke, multiple sclerosis, or arteriovenous malformations.

There are no contraindications to EEG, although tracings from uncooperative patients may include artifacts and be uninterpretable.

RATIONALE. The EEG records the cortical electrical activity of the brain. Two important types of EEG abnormalities are slowing (slow waves) and epileptiform activity (spike waves), either focal or generalized.

Even between actual seizures, patients with generalized epilepsy may exhibit generalized spike and slow wave discharges; those with focal (partial) epilepsy may have focal spikes or slow waves. Anterior temporal spikes are characteristic of patients with complex partial seizures. An accompanying slow wave focus suggests structural lesions such as tumor or infarct. Metabolic encephalopathy may cause generalized slow waves, a helpful finding in the assessment of the comatose patient.

Although a positive EEG confirms the diagnosis of epilepsy, some patients with documented epilepsy have normal EEGs between seizures.

All results require clinical correlation since minor abnormalities, while nonspecific, may be subtle indications of serious disease.

METHODS. Using 16 separate amplifying units, the EEG is very sensitive to artifacts produced by eye blinking, movement, sweating, and swallowing. A routine EEG takes 60 to 90 minutes to complete and is painless.

Certain procedures are used to activate latent seizure foci: hyperventilation (to produce alkalosis-induced cerebral vasoconstriction), stroboscopic stimulation, or sleep (with or without sedatives).

EEG by telemetry or with video monitoring may be useful in evaluating patients who have frequent seizures unresponsive to medications and in patients with pseudoseizures. Such patients should be referred to epilepsy centers where such monitoring is carried out.

COST. The cost of EEG is about $340.

Cross-references: Sleep Apnea Syndromes (Section 64), Syncope (Section 75), Seizures (Section 141), Dementia (Section 142).

REFERENCES

1. Kiloh LG, et al. Clinical Electroencephalography, 4th ed. Butterworth, London, 1981.
    A comprehensive textbook on electroencephalography.

2. Kooi KA, et al. Fundamentals of Electroencephalography, 2nd ed. Harper & Row, Haggerstown, Md, 1978.
    Discusses the usefulness of EEG in various settings.

151 ELECTROMYOGRAPHY AND NERVE CONDUCTION STUDIES

Procedure

JOHN RAVITS

INDICATIONS/CONTRAINDICATIONS. Electromyography and nerve conduction studies are specialized tests of neuromuscular function. These tests are often used to evaluate muscular weakness, sensory change (either hyperfunctioning, such as paresthesia, or hypofunctioning, such as anesthesia), or pain (especially when focal). There are no absolute contraindications to the test, although anticoagulated patients are at increased risk for hematomas.

RATIONALE. EMG and nerve conduction studies are often invaluable in the diagnosis of anterior horn cell disorders (such as amyotrophic lateral sclerosis and polio), radiculopathies, plexopathies, mononeuropathies (including nerve injuries and entrapment syndromes), polyneuropathies, myopathies, and disorders of neuromuscular junction transmission. These studies will (1) help confirm and measure abnormalities of the peripheral nervous system, especially when symptoms exist without signs, (2) help localize lesions (e.g., differentiate radiculopathy from plexopathy or myopathy from neuromuscular junction disorders), (3) assess the extent of disease when there are widespread abnormalities, not all of which are clinically apparent (e.g., anterior horn cell disease), (4) provide useful prognostic information (e.g., nerve injury and Guillain-Barré syndrome), and (5) monitor the course of a disease (e.g., nerve injuries, entrapment syndromes, and polyneuropathies).

Nerve conduction studies are extremely sensitive in detecting carpal tunnel syndrome, polyneuropathy, and entrapment syndromes, but are less sensitive for radiculopathy or myopathy. False-negative results may occur because the abnormalities are not continuously present, the techniques used are insensitive, the referral occurred early in the course of a disease (before diagnostic abnormalities appeared), or the electromyographer is inexperienced.

METHODS. EMG and nerve conduction studies are often referred to as "EMG," but they are two separate procedures. **Nerve conduction studies** evaluate nerve function and use an electrical impulse to depolarize nerves; electrodes placed over the skin record sensory or motor potentials. **Electromyography** evaluates muscle function and uses needle electrodes that are inserted into muscle to record muscle action potentials. Spontaneous activity, which refers to muscle potentials appearing while the muscle is inactive, is normally absent; abnormalities include fibrillations, fasciculations, and myotonic discharges. Voluntary activity refers to muscle potentials appearing during voluntary muscle activation. Voluntary activity is evaluated for size of the potentials (amplitude and duration), morphology of the potentials, and recruitment (as muscle is activated from minimal to maximal effort). Newer computerized techniques include a single-fiber EMG and quantitative EMG.

The neurophysiologist usually performs a combination of nerve conduction studies and EMG, depending on the particular clinical problem. For example, a patient with upper extremity radiculopathy may undergo nerve conduction studies to exclude peripheral nerve entrapments, followed by EMG to search for muscle denervated in a myotomal pattern.

COST/COMPLICATIONS.   EMG and nerve conduction studies are expensive: an EMG of two extremities costs approximately $350, and nerve conduction studies of two nerves (motor and sensory) costs about $390. Because this expense far exceeds that of a neurologic consultation, these studies should be obtained judiciously, often in consultation with a neurologist. Although the test may be uncomfortable, complications of local infection and local hematoma are extremely rare.

Cross-references: Low Back Pain (Section 108), Ankle and Foot Pain (Section 113), Muscular Weakness (Section 139), Entrapment Neuropathies (Section 146), Peripheral Neuropathy (Section 149).

REFERENCES

1. Kimura J. Electrodiagnosis in Diseases of Nerve and Muscle: Principles and Practice, ed 2. F.A. Davis Co., Philadelphia, 1989.
    Standard textbook on technical and clinical aspects of EMG and nerve conduction studies.

2. Warmolts JR. Electrodiagnosis in neuromuscular disorders. Ann Intern Med 1981;95:599–608.
    Reviews neuromuscular physiology and electrodiagnosis.

CHAPTER **XIII**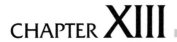

ENDOCRINE DISORDERS

152 CHOLESTEROL SCREENING

Screening

DOUGLAS EINSTADTER

EPIDEMIOLOGY. Coronary heart disease (CHD) is the major cause of mortality in the United States, responsible for more than 50% of the deaths in persons over age 65. CHD also causes significant morbidity and limitation among the more than 5 million survivors of myocardial infarction.

RATIONALE. Several studies, including the Seven Countries Study, the Multiple Risk Factor Intervention Trial (MRFIT), and the Framingham Heart Study, have demonstrated conclusively that cholesterol is a risk factor for CHD in middle-aged men. In the Lipid Research Clinics Coronary Primary Prevention Trial, treatment of middle-aged men with diet and cholestyramine reduced the cholesterol level and led to a 19% *relative* reduction in CHD events (fatal and nonfatal myocardial infarction), although no reduction in overall mortality was demonstrated. The *absolute* reduction in CHD events, however, was only 1.7% during the 7.4 years of study, from 9.8% among the controls to 8.1% among the treated patients. In men with a history of prior myocardial infarction, treatment with niacin reduced nonfatal myocardial infarctions by 27%; after 15 years (8 years after the close of the study) overall mortality decreased by 11% (Coronary Drug Project). Other studies have documented that aggressive cholesterol reduction can slow or sometimes reverse the progression of coronary artery lesions in men with established coronary artery disease.

STRATEGY. The United States Preventive Service Task Force and the National Cholesterol Education Program recommend screening of all adults older than 20 years of age for elevated cholesterol levels. A nonfasting serum cholesterol level should be determined on the first visit, to be repeated at least every 5 years if the prior determination was within the acceptable range. For individuals with a serum cholesterol level above 6.2 mmol/liter (240 mg/dl), or with a cholesterol between 5.2 and 6.2 mmol/liters (201–239 mg/dl) and at least two additional CHD risk factors (male sex, obesity, hypertension, cigarette smoking, or family history of CHD), the clinician should measure the patient's total cholesterol level, high-density lipoprotein (HDL) cholesterol, and triglycerides (TG). The low-density lipoprotein (LDL) cholesterol level is then calculated from the formula:

LDL C (mg/dl) = Total C (mg/dl) − HDL C (mg/dl) − (TG [mg/dl]/5).

This formula applies only when triglycerides are less than 400 mg/dl.

In asymptomatic persons older than 65 years, the value of treating elevated serum cholesterol is uncertain, and cholesterol screening in this group is controversial.

ACTION.   All individuals screened should receive counseling on CHD risk factor modification and advice about a prudent diet, such as the American Heart Association Step One diet. Whether cholesterol reduction, using diet or drugs, decreases the risk for CHD has not been demonstrated for groups other than middle-aged men at higher than average risk for CHD. Section 155 (Hyperlipidemia) reviews the management of hypercholesterolemia.

Cross-references: Periodic Health Assessment (Section 7), Principles of Screening (Section 12), Angina (Section 78), Hyperlipidemia (Section 155).

REFERENCES

1. Garber AM, Sox HC, Littenberg B. Screening asymptomatic adults for cardiac risk factors: The serum cholesterol level. Ann Intern Med 1989;110:622–639.
    Concise review of evidence supporting the use screening to identify adults at high risk for CHD.

2. Lipid Research Clinics Coronary Primary Prevention Trial Results. Part I. Reduction in incidence of coronary heart disease. JAMA 1984;251:351–364.
    One of the most influential and often cited articles in the cholesterol treatment literature.

3. Report of the National Cholesterol Education Program Expert Panel on Detection, Evaluation, and Treatment of High Blood Cholesterol in Adults. Arch Intern Med 1988;148: 36–69.
    Extensive report of the NCEP cholesterol screening program, with treatment recommendations.

4. Toronto Working Group. Asymptomatic hypercholesterolemia. J Clin Epidemiol 1990; 43:1029–1121.
    Entire issue devoted to the cholesterol screening debate.

153 SCREENING FOR THYROID DISEASE

Screening

ROBERT J. GRIEP

EPIDEMIOLOGY.   Depending on the diagnostic criteria, thyroid disease may be detected in more than 10% of the adult population over the age of 40. The prevalence of palpable thyroid nodules is 2% in individuals in their 20s and increases to 6% to 7% in persons over the age of 60. Approximately 7% to 10% of palpable nodules are malignant. Graves' disease, chronic thyroiditis, and thyroid nodules are five to eight times more common in females.

RATIONALE.   Screening tests for thyroid function include measurements of free thyroxine and a sensitive measurement of thyroid-stimulating hormone (TSH). The free thyroxine index, which measures the total thyroxine and thyroid binding ratio and corrects for protein binding abnormalities, detects thyroid function abnormalities with a sensitivity of 98%. Values in the high normal or low normal range require additional evaluation with a TSH measurement. Although TSH determination would be a more sensitive initial screening test, it costs two to three times more ($55 ± $8).

STRATEGY.   Thyroid function tests are rarely abnormal in asymptomatic patients under the age of 40 without palpable abnormalities of the thyroid. Individuals at greater risk include women over the age of 40, because of the high prevalence of autoimmune disease (4%–20%), and individuals with a personal or family history of autoimmune endocrine disease (e.g., type 1 diabetes, adrenal failure).

ACTION.   Minor abnormalities in TSH and thyroxine measurements may result from fever, other illnesses, or medications (e.g., corticosteroids). Repeat testing may be necessary to identify progressive with progressive thyroid disease. Section 156 reviews the management of thyroid nodules, goiter, hypothyroidism, and hyperthyroidism.

Cross-references: Sleep Apnea Syndromes (Section 64), Dementia (Section 142), Common Thyroid Disorders (Section 156), Thyroid Disorders in Pregnancy (Section 212), Preoperative Endocrine Problems (Section 219).

REFERENCES

See section on thyroid disease.

154 GYNECOMASTIA

Symptom

DOUGLAS S. PAAUW

EPIDEMIOLOGY.   Gynecomastia (enlargement of the male breast) is a common problem, affecting 30% to 40% of men. The prevalence of gynecomastia increases with advancing age, probably because of testicular failure.

ETIOLOGY.   Gynecomastia usually results from an increased ratio of estrogens to androgens, although in many cases the precise etiology is unknown. Transient gynecomastia is common during puberty (40%–70% of normal boys), probably because of a short-lived increase in plasma estrogens compared to androgens.

The broad range of recognized causes is given in Tables 154–1 and 154–2. Drug-induced gynecomastia is common and may occur because of the drug's intrinsic estrogen activity (digitalis, marijuana), inhibition of testosterone synthesis (spironolactone, ketoconazole), or direct damage to the testes (cytotoxic

---

TABLE 154–1.   CAUSES OF GYNECOMASTIA

Physiologic
Pubertal gynecomastia
Gynecomastia of aging

Decreased Androgen Production or Androgen Resistance
Congenital
   Congenital anorchia
   Klinefelter's syndrome
   Testicular feminization
Acquired
   Alcoholism
   Myotonic dystrophy
   Orchitis
   Renal failure

Increased Estrogen Production
Hermaphroditism
Testicular tumors
Bronchogenic carcinoma

Increased Peripheral Conversion to Estrogen
Congenital adrenal hyperplasia/adrenal tumors
Liver disease
Malnutrition
Thyrotoxicosis

Drugs (see Table 154–2)
Idiopathic Gynecomastia

TABLE 154–2.   MEDICATIONS ASSOCIATED WITH GYNECOMASTIA

Amiodarone	Estrogen*
Amphetamines	Isoniazid
Calcium channel blockers	Ketoconazole*
Human chorionic gonadotropin	Marijuana
Cimetidine	Methyldopa
Clomiphene	Phenothiazines
Cytotoxic agents	Reserpine
Digitalis	Spironolactone*
Diazepam	Tricyclic antidepressants

*More common.

agents) (see Table 154–2). Regular ingestion of milk or meat from estrogen-treated animals can cause gynecomastia.

CLINICAL APPROACH.   The history should emphasize the patient's present medications, use of alcohol, and reproductive history. The physical examination focuses on the breasts (size and consistency), the testes (size, nodules, and symmetry), and any evidence of hyperthyroidism or chronic liver disease. Gynecomastia may be asymmetric. A cushingoid appearance or the recent onset of hypertension suggests adrenal disease. Although breast cancer in males is rare (1% of all breast cancer cases), patients with signs suggestive of cancer (bleeding, fixation, regional adenopathy, eccentric breast mass) should have an immediate biopsy.

If the cause remains unknown despite a thorough history and physical examination, laboratory tests should include liver function tests, human chorionic gonadotropin determination (to exclude ectopic hCG from testicular and nontesticular tumors), thyroid function tests (30% of men with hyperthyroidism have gynecomastia), and measurement of testosterone levels (to exclude hypogonadism). If examination suggests Klinefelter's syndrome (small firm testes, euchanoid habitus, and long limbs), karyotyping is indicated.

MANAGEMENT.   If gynecomastia is drug induced, removal of the offending drug usually results in a decrease in breast size within several months. Reassurance and explanation are frequently all that is required in most cases of gynecomastia. Breast carcinoma is no more likely in patients with gynecomastia than in other males, except among patients with Klinefelter's syndrome, who are at increased risk.

Cross-references: Diagnosis and Management of Alcoholism (Section 9), Cirrhosis and Chronic Liver Failure (Section 100), Common Thyroid Disorders (Section 156), Male Infertility (Section 159), Impotence (Section 171), Scrotal Mass (Section 185).

REFERENCES

1.   Carlson HE. Gynecomastia. N Engl J Med 1980;303:795–799
     Excellent overall review of gynecomastia.

2. Dolsky RL. Gynecomastia: Treatment by liposuction subcutaneous mastectomy. Dermatol Clin 1990;8:469–478.
    Describes liposuction as a cosmetic treatment for gynecomastia. The operative complication rate is very low.

3. Tanner LA, Bosco LA. Gynecomastia associated with calcium channel blocker therapy. Arch Intern Med 1988;148:379–380.
    Thirty-one cases of gynecomastia with calcium channel blocker use were reported to the FDA. The underlying mechanism is unknown.

155 HYPERLIPIDEMIA

Problem

JAY W. HEINECKE
JOHN D. BRUNZELL

EPIDEMIOLOGY.   Hypercholesterolemia is strongly associated with premature atherosclerosis. In the Multiple Risk Factor Intervention Trial, 15% of middle-aged men had high total cholesterol levels (>240 mg/dl). To estimate the risk for coronary artery disease, elevated LDL levels and depressed HDL levels are better predictors than total cholesterol levels. Other abnormalities in lipid metabolism that increase the risk of atherosclerosis are increased apolipoprotein B100, the major protein carried by LDL; elevated levels of Lp(a), a lipoprotein that resembles LDL but carries an additional protein termed apolipoprotein (a); hypertriglyceridemia in patients with a family history of coronary artery disease; and low levels of apolipoprotein AI, the predominant HDL protein component. Tests for Lp(a) and apolipoprotein B100 abnormalities will become available to the clinician in the near future.

SYMPTOMS AND SIGNS.   Although generally asymptomatic, dyslipoproteinemia should be suspected in any patient with known coronary artery disease or with a family history of premature atherosclerosis (onset before age 60).

The physical examination may reveal tendon xanthomas, typically located in the extensor tendons of the hand or the Achilles tendon, which are pathognomonic for familial hypercholesterolemia (elevated LDL cholesterol levels and a strong family history of atherosclerosis). Palmar xanthomas are found in over half of patients with broad beta (type III) disease (both cholesterol and triglyceride levels are usually elevated). Xanthelasmas may be a marker for elevated apolipoprotein B100 levels but are also found in hypothyroidism, a common secondary cause of hypercholesterolemia.

In chylomicronemia syndrome, pancreatitis often occurs when triglyceride levels exceed 2000 mg/dl. Despite severe symptoms of nausea, vomiting, and epigastric pain radiating to the back, urine and blood amylase levels may be normal. Affected patients often have eruptive xanthomas over the extensor surface of the knees and elbows and on the buttocks. Their plasma is lipemic and resembles milk.

Clinical Approach.   Many physicians advocate the guidelines for the detection, evaluation, and treatment of hyperlipidemia proposed by the National Cholesterol Education Program (Fig. 155–1). Total cholesterol (which need not be fasting) is determined in children and adults of high-risk families in order to screen for individuals in whom fasting lipoproteins should be measured. Cholesterol levels above 240 mg/dl are considered high. Levels between 200 and 240 mg/dl are considered borderline, and levels below 200 mg/dl are "desirable."

The clinician should measure the patient's fasting cholesterol, triglyceride, and HDL cholesterol levels if the patient has (1) high total cholesterol levels, (2) borderline total cholesterol levels plus two or more risk factors for atherosclerosis or known atherosclerosis, or (3) a strong family history of atherosclerosis (onset before age 60 in a first-degree relative). Because of biologic variations in cholesterol levels (up to 20%) and analytic variations in HDL measurements, several determinations are necessary.

In units of mg/dl, the fasting LDL cholesterol level equals the total cholesterol level minus the HDL cholesterol level minus (triglyceride/5). This formula is not accurate if triglycerides are elevated above 400 mg/dl.

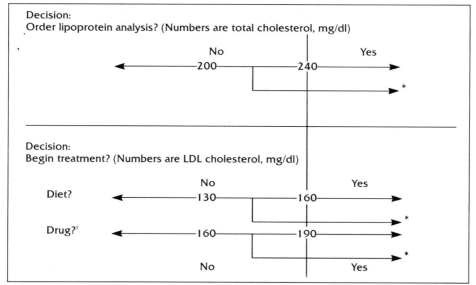

FIGURE 155–1.   Risk stratification based on cholesterol levels (see text). Borderline individuals with two or more risk factors are moved into the high-risk category (→ *). †LDL values are obtained after 3 to 6 months of a low-fat diet.

MANAGEMENT. Clinical studies indicate that lowering cholesterol levels reduces the incidence of coronary artery disease. Initially, patients with high LDL (>160 mg/dl) or those at high risk with borderline LDL levels (130–160 mg/dl) should begin the American Health Association Step 1 or Step 2 diet, which restrict the intake of saturated fat and cholesterol. The physician should counsel the patient and spouse regarding the diet, and may want to enlist help from a dietitian. Exclusion of secondary causes of hyperlipidemia (Table 155–1), such as hypothyroidism and selected medications, is essential.

Drug therapy is indicated when 3 to 6 months of a low-fat diet fails to lower the LDL cholesterol level to less than 190 mg/dl on several determinations in young and middle-aged adults, or to less than 160 mg/dl in those with known coronary artery disease or with more than one risk factor (see Fig. 155–1). The clinician should usually avoid drug therapy in those over the age of 65 and in patients with concurrent diseases that limit survival.

Drug treatment begins with a single agent (Table 155–2). For elevated LDL cholesterol levels, one to two scoops of a bile-binding resin once or twice a day with meals is often effective. Alternatively, crystalline nicotinic acid (500 mg) three times a day with meals or lovastatin (20 mg) each evening may prove effective. Nicotinic acid therapy is initially associated with bothersome symptoms, including flushing and pruritus. Initiation of treatment with 250 mg nicotinic acid once each day, with an increase by 250 mg each week, avoids most of these effects. Symptoms tend to lessen with time and may be prevented by taking one baby aspirin 30 minutes before each dose.

If such a regimen fails to lower LDL cholesterol levels adequately, higher doses of nicotinic acid (up to 1 g four times a day) or lovastatin (up to 40 mg twice a day) can be used, either alone or combined with resin therapy.

TABLE 155–1. ACQUIRED HYPERLIPIDEMIA

Etiology	Elevated Cholesterol (LDL)	Elevated Triglyceride (VLDL)	Elevated Cholesterol and Triglyceride
Disease State			
Diabetes		+	
Hypothyroidism	+		+
Nephrotic syndrome			+
Renal failure		+	
Monoclonal gammopathy	+	+	+
Medications			
Furosemide			+
Thiazides			+
Beta blockers		+	
Glucocorticoids			+
Estrogens		+	
Ethanol		+	
Isotretinoin		+	
Cyclosporin	+		

TABLE 155–2.   MEDICAL THERAPY OF HYPERLIPIDEMIA

Drug	Dose	Daily Cost ($)[1]
Bile-binding resin		
Colestipol	5 g q.d. to 10 g b.i.d.	0.83
Cholestyramine	5 g q.d. to 10 g b.i.d.	1.06
Nicotinic acid	0.5 g t.i.d. to 1.5 g q.i.d.	0.12
Lovastatin	20 mg q.h.s. to 40 mg b.i.d.	1.76
Fibric acids		
Clofibrate	1 g b.i.d.	0.84
Gemfibrozil	600 mg b.i.d.	1.66

[1]Average wholesale price, initial dose listed; 1991 *Drug Topics Red Book*.

Combinations of lovastatin with either nicotinic acid, cyclosporin, erythromycin, or fibric acids (clofibrate and gemfibrozil) are associated with a myositis syndrome and rhadomyolysis, and are best avoided. Therapy with nicotinic acid or lovastatin requires monitoring of the serum aspartate aminotransferase (AST) levels, initially each month and then semiannually on a stable treatment regimen. Creatine kinase levels should be monitored with lovastatin treatment. Liver disease, migraine headaches, and diabetes are contraindications to nicotinic acid therapy. Slow-release nicotinic acid should not be used because of associated hepatic dysfunction. Bile-binding resins alter the absorption of warfarin, digoxin, thyroxine, thiazides, and possibly other agents.

Patients with triglyceride levels above 2000 mg/dl are at risk for pancreatitis and the chylomicronemia syndrome. Acutely, instant breakfast mixes prepared with skim milk are useful. In addition to a low-fat diet, fibric acid derivatives (clofibrate or gemfibrozil) are often necessary to lower the triglyceride level. Bile-binding resins, ethanol, thiazide diuretics, beta blockers, glucocorticoids, and estrogens frequently exacerbate hypertriglyceridemia and are best avoided in moderate to severe hypertriglyceridemia.

FOLLOW-UP.   Drug treatment requires evaluation semiannually for adverse effects and efficacy. For young and middle-aged patients with desirable cholesterol levels, lipids may be reevaluated at 5-year intervals.

Cross-references: Periodic Health Assessment (Section 7), Diagnosis and Management of Alcoholism (Section 9), Obesity (Section 15), Angina (Section 78), Cholesterol Screening (Section 152), Screening for Thyroid Disease (Section 153), Common Thyroid Disorders (Section 156), Diabetes Mellitus (Section 157).

REFERENCES

1.   Brunzell JD. Disorders of lipoprotein metabolism. In Wyngaarden JB, Smith LH Jr, Eds. Cecil Textbook of Medicine, 18th ed. W.B. Saunders, Philadelphia, 1988, pp. 1137–1144. Overview of lipoprotein pathophysiology and treatment.

2. Lipoprotein and lipid metabolism disorders: In Scriver CR, Beaudet AL, Sly WS, Valle D, Eds. The Metabolic Basis of Inherited Disease. McGraw-Hill, New York, 1989, pp. 1129–1304.

   A comprehensive discussion of the hyperlipidemias, with an emphasis on the genetics and pathophysiology of these disorders.

3. Report of the National Cholesterol Education Program Expert Panel on Detection, Evaluation, and Treatment of High Blood Cholesterol in Adults. Arch Intern Med 1988;148: 36–69.

   Extensive review of the NCEP guidelines and treatment recommendations.

156 COMMON THYROID DISORDERS

Problem

ROBERT J. GRIEP

GOITER

EPIDEMIOLOGY/ETIOLOGY.   Goiter refers to enlargement of the thyroid, not necessarily associated with hypothyroidism or hyperthyroidism. Goiters may be diffusely enlarged or multinodular, although most become nodular with time. The incidence of endemic goiter has decreased in populations with additional iodine in their diets, but remains high in other areas of the world. Other causes include autoimmune disorders (chronic thyroiditis) and congenital enzymatic defects.

SYMPTOMS AND SIGNS.   Smaller goiters often are asymptomatic and are found on physical examination. Large goiters may cause a feeling of constriction or discomfort in certain body positions.

CLINICAL APPROACH.   Because hypo- and hyperthyroidism may be subclinical, routine laboratory tests include TSH and thyroxine level determinations.

MANAGEMENT.   Treatment of abnormal thyroid function, once identified, often results in a decrease in the size of goiter. In patients with normal thyroid function, the clinician's goals are to prevent future growth of the goiter and to monitor for the development of hypothyroidism or symptoms. Asymptomatic patients with small goiters may be observed and periodically reevaluated. The value of suppressing the growth of the goiter with thyroid hormone is much debated, because few goiters actually shrink with therapy and because thyroid hormone treatment without documented hypothyroidism raises concerns about accelerating osteopenia and cardiac problems. Thyroid hormone suppression is most useful in patients whose goiters recently grew diffusely or who have autoimmune thyroiditis (suggested by the presence of serum antimicrosomal antibodies). Thyroid suppression in patients with autoimmune thyroiditis is reasonable not only because it often reduces the size of the goiter, but because it prevents the future development of hypothyroidism, a common outcome in these patients.

FOLLOW-UP.   Patients with goiters that grow during observation should receive a trial of thyroid hormone suppression. Goiters that grow during thyroid hormone therapy should be reevaluated, and surgical removal considered. After thyroidectomy, patients should be maintained on thyroid hormone to prevent regrowth of the goiter.

SOLITARY THYROID NODULES

EPIDEMIOLOGY/ETIOLOGY.   Solitary palpable thyroid nodules, which affect 2% of individuals in their 20s and 6% to 7% of those over the age of 60, may result from benign neoplasm, cysts, malignancies, or focal thyroiditis.

Although a thyroid nodule raises the concern of cancer, only 7% to 10% of palpable nodules are malignant. Malignancies are usually slow growing and have a good prognosis when properly managed. Malignancies are more common in large nodules (>3 cm), in younger patients, and in males.

SYMPTOMS AND SIGNS.   Nodules are usually asymptomatic and are found incidentally or during routine physical examination.

CLINICAL APPROACH.   Fine-needle aspiration biopsy by an experienced practitioner has largely replaced radionuclide scintigraphy and ultrasound (US) as the best initial approach. In patients with equivocal cytology, radionuclide scintigraphy is a helpful adjunctive test because autonomous or hot nodules are rarely malignant. Interpretation of radionuclide scans without cytologic results is inappropriate, however, because a few hot nodules reveal malignancy. Although US discriminates cystic from solid nodules and may reveal other nodules not found on examination, the results usually do not affect management because malignant nodules may have cystic components and multiple small nodules are found by US in 40% of the adult population.

When the patient has a small nodule that is smooth, round, and incidentally noted on physical examination, the clinician may follow it for signs of progression or suppress it with thyroid hormone. Patients with larger nodules (>1.5 cm) should undergo fine-needle aspiration biopsy.

MANAGEMENT.   If cytology reveals malignancy, the patient should be referred for surgical near-total thyroidectomy. Patients with benign cytologic findings should be followed or, if the nodule bothers the patient, treated with thyroid hormone suppression.

If the cytologic findings are nondiagnostic but suspicious or reveal follicular neoplasia, well-differentiated follicular carcinoma is still possible and can only be diagnosed after surgical removal by demonstrating capsular or vascular invasion. Radionuclide scintigraphy will help in the interpretation of equivocal cytology results. Young patients (<25 years) who have large (>3 cm) nodules with follicular neoplasia or suspicious findings on cytology should be evaluated by a specialist for consideration of surgical removal of the nodule. Patients with smaller lesions should be placed on thyroid hormone suppression for 6 to 12 months. If the nodule does not shrink in size, surgical removal should be considered.

FOLLOW-UP. Patients with nodules should be reexamined approximately every 3 months for the first year, whether or not suppression therapy is used. If the nodule is smaller or unchanged, yearly appointments are usually adequate.

HYPERTHYROIDISM

EPIDEMIOLOGY/ETIOLOGY. Causes of hyperthyroidism include Graves' disease (autoimmune stimulation) in 70%, toxic nodular goiter (autonomous nodule, single or multiple) in 15% to 20%, and thyroiditis (either subacute or "silent") in 5% to 10%. Thyrotoxicosis may also result from ingestion of oral thyroid hormone. Subacute thyroiditis probably results from viral inflammation and the release of stored thyroxine from thyroid follicles. Silent thyroiditis is most commonly seen 3 to 6 months post partum.

SYMPTOMS AND SIGNS. Heat intolerance and weight loss are common symptoms of excessive metabolism due to thyroid hormone. Increased adrenergic sensitivity due to hyperthyroidism causes palpitation, tachycardia, sweating, and tremors. Subacute thyroiditis also causes thyroid tenderness and pain and occasionally fever. Silent thyroiditis cannot be distinguished clinically from mild Graves' disease.

CLINICAL APPROACH. TSH levels of less than 0.1 mU/liter and elevated thyroid hormone levels confirm hyperthyroidism. The causes of hyperthyroidism are distinguished by thyroid palpation (in general, diffuse enlargement is associated with Graves' disease and thyroiditis, nodularity with toxic nodular goiter, tenderness with thyroiditis, and a normal examination with exogenous ingestion) and by measurement of radioactive iodine uptake (increased in Graves' disease and toxic nodular goiter, decreased in thyroiditis and exogenous hormone ingestion).

MANAGEMENT. The hyperthyroidism of subacute thyroiditis is self-limited; pain and tenderness respond to nonsteroidal anti-inflammatory medications, although the fever and severe pain of some patients may require corticosteroids. Silent thyroiditis is also a self-limited condition. The adrenergic symptoms of both silent and subacute thyroiditis respond to beta blockers (e.g., propranolol, 20 mg PO q.8h.).

Graves' disease and toxic nodular goiter may be treated effectively with antithyroid drugs, radioactive iodine, and surgery. Opinions differ, but in general most authorities choose ^{131}I for patients who are reliable and who understand they must be seen regularly to monitor for the development of hypothyroidism; pregnancy is an absolute contraindication to ^{131}I therapy. Antithyroid drugs are indicated for hyperthyroidism in pregnancy (see Section 212), in patients with small thyroids and mild hyperthyroidism (who may ultimately enter a remission, see below), or when preparing patients with severe symptoms for ^{131}I therapy or surgery. Surgery is an option in patients who have possible associated cancer or very large multinodular thyroid glands, or in patients who do not wish to be treated by radiation.

Treatment with β-adrenergic antagonists controls adrenergic symptoms. Antithyroid medications (initially, propothiouricil, 100 mg three times a day, or methimazole, 10 mg twice daily) require 4 to 6 weeks to achieve euthyroidism. Side effects include urticaria (4.0%) and granulocytopenia (0.4%). The white blood cell (WBC) count should be determined before and after 3 to 6 weeks of therapy. Patients should be warned to stop the medication if they develop severe pharyngitis or fever.

Iodine 131 has been used to treat hyperthyroidism for more than 40 years without evidence of increased leukemia, neoplasm, or genetic disorders. Radioiodine requires 8 to 12 weeks for full effect. Doses can be calculated to totally ablate thyroid function or to render the patient euthyroid, although late hypothyroidism develops at a rate of 2% to 3% per year in the latter patients.

FOLLOW-UP.   Patients on antithyroid drugs should be followed every 3 to 4 weeks with thyroxine levels until they become euthyroid. Following patients with the TSH determinations is inappropriate, because levels remain low until the patient is euthyroid and will not reflect therapeutic effect. When patients become euthyroid, the beta blockers are stopped and the antithyroid drug dose is reduced, usually by half. Medications are usually stopped after 6 to 12 months to determine whether a remission has occurred. About 20% to 40% of patients with mild hyperthyroidism and small thyroid glands enter a remission.

Iodine 131 has its maximum effect about 10 weeks after administration. After treatment with ^{131}I, patients should be followed every 1 to 2 months for several months, and thereafter yearly with TSH levels to detect hypothyroidism. Patients who become hypothyroid require thyroid replacement, with the dose increased until the TSH level returns to normal. The TSH level should be checked every 1 to 2 years in patients on replacement therapy. Thyroid requirements in patients older than 60 years may decrease to 50 to 125 μg/day.

HYPOTHYROIDISM

EPIDEMIOLOGY.   Clinical hypothyroidism is found in 1% to 5% of the female population. It is most frequent in the elderly. Most hypothyroidism is due to autoimmune thyroid disease or previous treatment of hyperthyroidism with radioiodine or surgery.

SYMPTOMS AND SIGNS.   Lethargy, weakness, slow speech, cold intolerance, and unexplained weight gain are among the common but nonspecific symptoms of hypothyroidism. The thyroid gland may be enlarged or normal.

CLINICAL APPROACH.   Primary hypothyroidism is confirmed by the findings of a low free thyroxine index and an elevated TSH level. Most hypothyroidism is permanent and requires life-long replacement with thyroid hormone. Transient hypothyroidism may occur during recovery from thyroiditis and shortly after radioiodine treatment of Graves' disease and surgery.

MANAGEMENT.   Older individuals and those with long-standing hypothyroidism require gradual replacement starting with 25 to 50 μg/day and increasing by 25 to 50 μg of thyroxine daily every 4 to 6 weeks until the TSH level falls to within the normal range. The usual replacement dose is approximately 1.7 μg/kg/day but varies slightly because of individual differences in absorption.

THYROID PAIN

CLINICAL APPROACH.   Thyroid pain is unusual, but may be caused by subacute thyroiditis (usually bilateral) or hemorrhage in a thyroid nodule. Hemorrhage is frequently absorbed within 4 to 6 weeks. Palpable abnormalities that persist beyond this time require needle aspiration. Patients with persistent pain may have a malignancy and should also undergo fine-needle aspiration biopsy.

Cross-references: Hyperlipidemia (Section 155), Management of Depression (Section 192), Thyroid Disorders in Pregnancy (Section 212), Preoperative Endocrine Problems (Section 219).

REFERENCES

1. Griffin JE. Southwestern Internal Medicine Conference: Management of thyroid nodules. Am J Med Sci 1988;296:336–347.
    Comprehensive review of management of thyroid nodules with recommendations and algorithm for evaluation and therapy.

2. Helfand M, Crapo LM. Testing for suspected thyroid disease. In Sox HC, Ed. Common Diagnostic Tests, 2nd ed. American College of Physicians, Philadelphia, 1990, pp. 148–182.
    Excellent review of thyroid testing for primary care physicians. Stresses the cost-effective use of testing in different clinical situations.

3. Surks MI, Chopra IJ, Mariash CN, Nicoloff JT, Solomon DH. American Thyroid Association guidelines for use of laboratory tests in thyroid disorders. JAMA 1990;263:1529–1532.
    Timely review of a complex and changing field.

4. Van Herle AJ, Rich P, Ljung BEL, Ashcraft MW, Solomon DH, Keeler EB. The thyroid nodule. UCLA Conference. Ann Intern Med 1982;96:221–232.
    Often quoted review of sensitivity and specificity of diagnostic procedures. Fine-needle aspiration biopsy in experienced hands is clearly superior.

157 DIABETES MELLITUS

Problem

ROGER E. PECORARO*

EPIDEMIOLOGY/ETIOLOGY.   Diabetes mellitus is one of the most common chronic diseases in the United States. More than 2% of the population have diagnosed non-insulin-dependent diabetes (NIDDM), and an additional 3% are believed to have undiagnosed NIDDM. Including the 10% of all diabetics who are insulin dependent, the prevalence of diabetes in the general population is 5% to 6% and rises with advancing age.

The classification of diabetes type, even though imprecise, provides a logical basis for selecting treatment. Diabetes mellitus is recognized clinically by the effects of abnormal carbohydrate metabolism, but the abnormality may result from a variety of different underlying etiologies. Because no specific markers are currently available, the type of diabetes is determined primarily from clinical criteria, such as history of the clinical presentation, the relative body mass, and family history.

Insulin-dependent diabetes mellitus (IDDM) is used synonymously with "type I" to describe patients whose endogenous insulin secretion is insufficient to prevent diabetic ketoacidosis. IDDM typically occurs in lean rather than obese individuals, often with no family history of diabetes. Half of cases occur before age 20 years, and presentation is rare after age 40. Accumulating scientific evidence suggests that autoimmune pancreatic destruction is the major cause of IDDM, although it is unlikely that all cases will be explained by the same combination of genetic and environmental factors.

Non-insulin-dependent diabetes mellitus has been used synonymously with "type II." In contrast to IDDM, NIDDM is associated with preservation of pancreatic insulin secretion that, although substantial in many instances, is insufficient to maintain euglycemia. Hyperglycemia in NIDDM is accompanied by peripheral insulin resistance and a secondary increase in the hepatic output of glucose. Type II diabetes usually occurs in people over age 30 who are overweight and have a family history of diabetes among first-degree relatives. Other categories of diabetes, predominantly within the non-insulin-dependent phenotype, include gestational diabetes and malnutrition-related diabetes mellitus.

SYMPTOMS AND SIGNS.   IDDM typically presents with sudden illness, usually precipitated by an identifiable physiologic stress such as bacterial infec-

---

*Deceased.

476

tion. Acute abdominal pain, nausea, vomiting, extreme thirst, polyuria, and mental confusion may progress rapidly to obtundation or coma. Hyperpnea, hypotension, and a characteristic breath of acetone are confirmatory signs. Laboratory abnormalities include hyperglycemia, metabolic acidosis with an increased anion gap and respiratory compensation, and hyperkalemia. Less frequently, IDDM occurs without acute illness, but rather with significant persistent polyuria, polydipsia, malaise, and progressive weight loss despite hyperphagia.

The symptoms of NIDDM are often indolent and include the subtle onset of polyuria, polydipsia, and malaise. However, NIDDM may persist without any symptoms for years and be diagnosed only when an elevated blood glucose level is found on routine testing. Less frequently, the initial presentation may be weight loss, neuropathy, or retinopathy. Ketoacidosis is rare in NIDDM but may occur in association with an acute severe illness.

Hyperosmolar obtundation or coma is an unusual but life-threatening presentation of NIDDM that follows prolonged neglect of symptoms such as polyuria. Usually seen in elderly people who are socially isolated and without regular medical care, hyperosmolar coma occurs when intervening illnesses prevent adequate oral fluid intake. This leads to osmotic diuresis, serum hyperosmolarity, hypovolemia, circulatory insufficiency, confusion, and eventually coma.

CLINICAL APPROACH.   Determination of the patient's present and past weights is important. Current symptoms and presence of complications, such as retinal abnormalities, hypertension, or foot lesions, should be documented. Laboratory testing includes blood glucose, glycated hemoglobin, creatinine, electrolytes, fasting lipids or lipoproteins, and urinalysis.

MANAGEMENT.   For NIDDM the initial choice of therapy depends on the extent of insulin deficiency as assessed by the clinician and on patient preferences and abilities. Obese patients with NIDDM probably have predominantly insulin resistance, not deficiency. Optimal therapy includes caloric restriction, gradual weight loss, and regular exercise, which unfortunately only the minority of patients achieve and maintain. Important principles of the diabetic diet include consistent caloric intake to maintain or gradually decrease weight, appropriate meal timing, restriction of saturated fat content, and avoidance of excessive amounts of free sugars, which can result in rapid excursions of blood glucose. There are no universal standards for the prescription of oral hypoglycemic agents or insulin, although medical therapy is indicated when symptoms persist despite sincere efforts to establish dietary and other behavioral treatments. Indications for medical treatment based solely on blood glucose criteria in NIDDM are arbitrary, and, in the absence of definitive results from prospective clinical research, opinions vary widely among practitioners.

The lean adult patient who presents with marked hyperglycemia and secondary symptoms, particularly weight loss, is unlikely to respond to oral hypoglycemic agents. Residual endogenous insulin secretion may be sufficient to inhibit lipolysis and therefore prevent ketoacidosis, but is unlikely to forestall net catabolism. These patients are best treated by insulin replacement, and any therapeutic trial with oral agents should be monitored closely and promptly abandoned if the response is marginal.

Patients with IDDM require insulin treatment, by definition. Among the variety of regimens proposed, the most common are split doses of intermediate-acting insulin that may be mixed with supplements of short-acting insulin, or a basal dose of intermediate-acting insulin supplemented with mealtime doses of short-acting insulin. Elective institution of insulin therapy in NIDDM is usually accomplished in the outpatient setting, with the help of the diabetes nurse educator when possible. For the typical mildly obese patient, a conservative starting dose of intermediate-acting insulin, e.g., 20 units of NPH, is appropriate. With the self-monitored blood glucose measurements used as a guide, the insulin dose is increased in 2- to 5-unit increments at 3- to 5-day intervals until the glycemic goal is approached. The regimen should be selected to optimize metabolic control while minimizing the risk of hypoglycemia, taking into account the patient's motivation and capabilities. The dose of insulin should be increased when hyperglycemic symptoms persist, in the presence of infection, and during pregnancy. The dose of insulin should be decreased promptly after any hypoglycemic reaction involving impaired consciousness that is not adequately explained by circumstances of diet or exercise.

Although it is widely believed that tight glucose control reduces the incidence of neurovascular complications, direct clinical studies are lacking. To date studies have shown only that aggressive glucose control slows the development of microalbuminuria, a marker for subsequent diabetic renal disease, and retards microscopic abnormalities of the skin that correlate with neurovascular complications. Such studies have involved patients with IDDM almost exclusively; even these limited data, therefore, should not be extrapolated to elderly patients with NIDDM. Multicenter randomized prospective clinical trials currently underway may clarify the effects of different levels of metabolic control in patients with IDDM and NIDDM.

Table 157–1 summarizes currently available oral hypoglycemic agents; Table 157–2 summarizes insulin formulations. First-generation oral agents are significantly less potent than second-generation agents on a weight basis but are similarly effective at comparable therapeutic doses. Chlorpropamide should be used cautiously in the elderly because of its long half-life and primary clearance by the kidney. There appears to be an increased secondary failure rate to oral hypoglycemics with increasing duration of NIDDM, associated with diminished pancreatic reserve. Therefore, insulin should be initiated in symptomatic patients unresponsive to glyburide or chlorpropamide.

Promoting patient responsibility and involvement is a cornerstone of diabetic management. Metabolic control should be evaluated jointly by the clinician and patient, focusing on symptoms of hyper- and hypoglycemia and the patient's diary of daily preprandial self-monitored blood glucose measurements, serial weights, and any symptoms suggestive of hypoglycemia, such as tremulous-

TABLE 157–1.   AVAILABLE ORAL HYPOGLYCEMIC AGENTS

Agent	Dosage Range (mg)	Duration of Action (hr)	Cost ($)[1]
First-generation Compounds			
Tolbutamide	500–3000	6–12	0.04 (500 mg, generic) 0.21 (500 mg, Orinase)
Chlorpropamide	100–500	60	0.03 (100 mg, generic) 0.27 (100 mg, Diabinese)
Tolazamide	100–750	12–14	0.08 (100 mg, generic) 0.21 (100 mg, Tolinase)
Acetohexamide	500–1500	12–18	0.30 (500 mg, generic) 0.37 (500 mg, Dymelor)
Second-generation Compounds			
Glyburide	2.5–20	Up to 24	0.45 (5 mg, DiaBeta) 0.46 (5 mg, Micronase)
Glipizide	2.5–45	Up to 24	0.27 (5 mg, Glucotrol)

[1]Average wholesale cost, 1991 *Drug Topics Red Book*.

ness, palpitations, impaired ability to concentrate, or frequent morning headaches. Laboratory tests of metabolic control should be used judiciously. A major goal of self-monitoring is to promote patients' understanding of their disease and the relationship between blood glucose levels and diet on therapy. Isolated fasting blood glucose levels are inadequate to assess average control in IDDM but may be reliable in most individuals with NIDDM, since the basal blood glucose level is typically stable. The glycated hemoglobin level (e.g. hemoglobin A_1C) estimates the mean overall glycemic control during the preceding 4 to 8 weeks but gives no indication of short-term glucose variability and therefore is an inappropriate test used alone to direct specific changes in medical therapy. The extremes of within-day glycemic excursions may differ widely among individuals with similar levels of glycated hemoglobin.

FOLLOW-UP.   In general, stable insulin-treated patients should be scheduled at least quarterly, and those receiving other treatments at least semiannually.

TABLE 157–2.   INSULIN FORMULATIONS AND PHARMACOKINETICS

Type	Action	Onset (hr)	Peak (hr)	Duration (hr)	Cost ($)[1]
Regular	Rapid	1	2–4	5–7	11.94–19.51
NPH	Intermediate	2	6–12	24–28	11.94–19.51
Protamine zinc	Prolonged	4	14–24	36+	11.94–19.51
Semilente	Rapid	1	2–4	12–16	11.94–19.51
Lente	Intermediate	2	6–12	24–28	11.94–19.51
Ultralente	Prolonged	4	18–24	36+	11.94–19.51

[1]Average wholesale cost, 1991 *Drug Topics Red Book*, 10 ml (100 units/ml).

Unstable glycemic control, recent changes in treatment regimen, and the presence of degenerative complications often mandate more frequent follow-up, as do common concurrent medical conditions such as hypertension, coronary and peripheral vascular disease, and hyperlipoproteinemia. All patients should be encouraged to contact the clinician for symptoms of acute illness, changes in vision, infections, foot ulcers, or unexplained or persistent changes in level of glucose control.

Practical guidelines provided by the American Diabetes Association for surveillance of specific complications include annual evaluation for retinopathy or other visual abnormalities, renal disorders, cardiovascular risk factors, peripheral sensory neuropathy, and other risk factors for foot ulceration. The feet should be examined for lesions at every visit. Selective referral to other health care professionals may be beneficial, including physician specialists, the nutritionist, podiatrist, and professional diabetes educator. Several special circumstances or problems are best managed by specialists, including IDDM in children and adolescents, diabetes during pregnancy, diabetic retinopathy, advanced renal insufficiency, and erectile dysfunction. Instruction by a diabetes nurse specialist or professional diabetes educator is often a valuable adjunct to the clinician's routine care.

Cross-references: Obesity (Section 15), Weight Loss (Section 17), Diabetic Retinopathy (Section 44), Ophthalmoscopy (Section 46), Diarrhea (Section 92), Constipation (Section 94), Ankle and Foot Pain (Section 113), Diabetic Foot Care Education (Section 125), Leg Ulcers (Section 134), Local Care of Diabetic Foot Lesions (Section 135), Peripheral Neuropathy (Section 149), Impotence (Section 171), Chronic Renal Failure (Section 181), Proteinuria (Section 183), Diabetes Mellitus in Pregnancy (Section 213), Gestational Diabetes Mellitus (Section 214), Preoperative Endocrine Problems (Section 219).

REFERENCES

1. American Diabetes Association. Clinical practice recommendations, American Diabetes Association, 1990–1991. Diabetes Care 1991;14(suppl 2):1–79.

    Position statements, technical reviews, and consensus statements that address specific clinical issues such as insulin administration, self-monitoring of blood glucose levels, and general standards of medical care for people with diabetes; to be updated annually.

2. American Diabetes Association. Physican's Guide to Insulin-Dependent (Type I) Diabetes: Diagnosis and Treatment. American Diabetes Association, Alexandria, Va, 1988.

    An excellent guide to routine management and special problems in the care of insulin-dependent diabetic patients.

3. Baynes JW, Bunn HF, Goldstein D, et al. National Diabetes Data Group: Report of the Expert Committee on Glucosylated Hemoglobin. Diabetes Care 1984;7:602–608.

    A summary of the nomenclature, methods for measurement, and clinical application of glycated hemoglobin levels.

4. Gries FA, Alberti KGMM. Management of noninsulin-dependent diabetes mellitus in Europe: A consensus statement. IDF Bull 1987;32:169–174.

A consensus of clinical experts regarding the objectives and clinical approach for care of patients with NIDDM.

5. National Diabetes Data Group. Diabetes in America. Government Printing Office, Washington, D.C., 1985.
    A compilation and assessment of useful data on diabetes and its complications.

158 FEMALE INFERTILITY

Problem

VICTOR Y. FUJIMOTO

EPIDEMIOLOGY/ETIOLOGY. Infertility, defined as 1 year of unprotected coitus without conception, has a prevalence of 10% to 15% among U.S. couples. The risk of infertility increases with maternal age, exceeding 20% and 25% when the female partner is between ages 35 to 39 and between ages 40 to 44, respectively. Primary infertility refers to couples who have never conceived; secondary infertility denotes that the female partner has previously been pregnant. Several potential causes of infertility may be simultaneously present in a given couple. Reasons for infertility in women include ovulatory deficiencies (40%), fallopian tube obstruction (30%–50%), cervical mucous problems (10%–20%), and endometriosis (25%). Problems in the male occur in up to 40% of couples. Some 5% to 10% of couples have idiopathic infertility.

SYMPTOMS AND SIGNS. The clinician should consider both the male's and the female's contribution to the problem. The potential causes of infertility are multiple. Important information to be obtained from the female partner includes her menstrual history (oligomenorrhea/amenorrhea), any prior pregnancy history (spontaneous or induced abortions, ectopic pregnancies), any history of abdominal or pelvic operations, previous gynecologic infections, previous intrauterine device use, and the frequency of coitus. The patient should be examined for galactorrhea, hirsutism, thyroid enlargement, and obesity. During the pelvic examination, the clinician should carefully search for uterine or adnexal masses and uterosacral nodularity.

CLINICAL APPROACH. Five clinical tests, each progressively more expensive and invasive, are commonly used to investigate infertility: assessment of ovulation, semen analysis, postcoital test, hysterosalpingography, and laparoscopy. The presence or absence of ovulation can be assessed with (1) basal body temperature (BBT) charts that reveal a sustained temperature rise of 0.6°C or (2) a midluteal serum progesterone level above 0.3 ng/ml or (3) secretory phase endometrium sampling (endometrial biopsy). A BBT chart is completed by obtaining a daily first morning oral temperature reading. A midluteal serum progesterone level should be drawn between 4 and 11 days prior to the expected next menses. An endometrial biopsy should be performed 2 to 4 days prior to the expected next menstrual period. Detection of more subtle ovulation problems such as luteal phase deficiency—a quantitative decrease in progesterone secretion after ovulation—is best left to infertility specialists. Serum prolactin levels and thyroid function tests are unnecessary unless there is anovulation, galactorrhea, or thyroid symptomatology.

The male partner should be initially assessed with a complete semen analysis. If sperm concentration is low ($<20 \times 10^6$/ml), if there is poor motility ($<50\%$ motility 2 hours after ejaculation), or if morphology is abnormal ($>40\%$ abnormal forms), there is likely a defect in spermatogenesis. Abnormalities should be confirmed by a second semen analysis (see Section 159).

If the semen analysis is normal and ovulation is occurring, the problem is tentatively classified as idiopathic infertility. At this point it is reasonable to discuss referral to a gynecologist or infertility specialist for further testing, which may include (1) a human sperm/hamster egg penetration test to assess the ability of his sperm to fertilize an oocyte; (2) a postcoital test to examine for the presence of motile sperm in cervical mucus obtained near the anticipated day of ovulation and shortly after intercourse; (3) hysterosalpingography, to diagnose tubal obstruction and uterine filling defects; and (4) diagnostic laparoscopy, to confirm tubal obstruction or the diagnosis of pelvic adhesions or endometriosis. The cause(s) of infertility are apparent in 90% of couples after completion of the entire evaluation.

MANAGEMENT. Idiopathic anovulation or oligo-ovulation is usually treated initially with clomiphene citrate. Hyperprolactinemia requires concomitant use of bromocriptine to lower serum prolactin levels. Hypothyroidism is reversed with thyroid replacement. When persistent anovulation that is unresponsive to clomiphene is present, the patient may be referred to a specialist for human menopausal gonadotropin (hMG) or pulsatile gonadotropin-releasing hormone (GnRH) therapy.

Surgery is often necessary for intrauterine defects (lysed during hysteroscopy) and pelvic adhesions or tubal obstruction (laparoscopy or microsurgical laparotomy).

When cervical abnormalities are present, treatment may include antibiotics for cervicitis, low-dose follicular phase estrogen to enhance cervical mucus, or bypass of the cervix via intrauterine inseminations. The pregnancy success rate for various treatments of infertility is given in Table 158–1.

Various therapies may be effective for male factor infertility: antibiotic therapy for pyospermia; high spermatic vein ligation for varicocele; low-dose clomiphene citrate therapy or seminal fluid washing with intrauterine insemination for idiopathic oligospermia; and donor insemination for severe oligospermia or azoospermia (see Section 159, Male Infertility).

TABLE 158–1.   **INFERTILITY AND PREGNANCY RATES**

Type of Infertility	Treatment	Pregnancy Rate[1]	Recommended Interval[2]
Tubal Factor			
Reversal of ligation	Tubal anastomosis	60%–80%	2 yr
	Fimbrioplasty	15%–20%	2 yr
Pelvic adhesions	Adhesiolysis	40%–60%	2 yr
Anovulation	Clomiphene	40%–60% overall 10%/cycle	6 mo
	Human menopausal gonadotropin (Pergonal)	25%/cycle	6 mo
Male factor	See Section 159, Male Infertility	20%–50%	2 yr
Endometriosis	Medical/surgical		
Mild		60%	18 mo
Moderate		40%	18 mo
Severe		20%	18 mo
Cervical Factor			
Cervicitis	Antibiotics	50%	6 mo
Unexplained	Clomiphene/ intrauterine insemination	10%/cycle	6 mo

[1]Pregnancy rates represent single factor infertility only.
[2]Interval prior to adjusting treatment.

Several new and expensive technologies are available (e.g., in-vitro fertilization [IVF], gamete intrafallopian tube transfer [GIFT], donor oocyte program [DOP]), but these should be reserved for selected couples who have not responded to conventional therapy. IVF is most often used for persistent tubal disease. GIFT or IVF may benefit couples with idiopathic infertility, endometriosis, and cervical factor infertility. For women with absent ovaries or premature menopause, IVF or GIFT using donor oocytes is available.

Finally, the emotional commitment of infertile couples to the process of becoming pregnant is substantial. Clinicians should provide couples with information on infertility support resources such as RESOLVE, and should discuss adoption as an alternative during the infertility workup and prior to any therapeutic attempt at pregnancy.

Cross-references: Male Infertility (Section 159), Impotence (Section 171).

REFERENCES

1. Corfman RS, Grainger DA. Endometriosis-associated infertility: Treatment options. J Reprod Med 1989;34(2):135–141.
    A comprehensive review of treatment modalities available for endometriosis-associated infertility.

2. deKretser DM. The management of the infertile male. Clin Obstet Gynecol 1974;1:409.
    Comprehensive review of male infertility.

3. Hammond MG, Halme JK, Talbert LM. Factors affecting the pregnancy rate in clomiphene citrate induction of ovulation. Obstet Gynecol 1983;62:196–202.
    Demonstrates the importance of confounding factors in the pregnancy success rate of clomiphene citrate treatment.

4. Medical Research International and Society for ART, American Fertility Society: In vitro fertilization-embryo transfer in the United States: 1988 results from IVF-ET Registry. Fertil Steril 1990;53:13–20.
    Description of 1988 results of 135 clinics practicing assisted reproductive technology in the United States.

5. Serafini P, Batzofin J. Diagnosis of female infertility: A comprehensive approach. J Reprod Med 1989;34(1):29–40.
    A thorough review of the diagnostic workup of the infertile female patient.

159 MALE INFERTILITY

Problem

RICHARD E. BERGER

EPIDEMIOLOGY/ETIOLOGY.   Infertility is usually defined as lack of conception within a 1-year period of unprotected intercourse. Some 10% to 15% of the population are infertile or unable to have as many children as desired. Of these couples, approximately 30% to 50% are believed to have a male factor contributing to the infertility. In one large series of patients with male infertility, the most common final diagnostic categories were varicocele (37% of patients) and idiopathic (25%).

SYMPTOMS AND SIGNS.   A man with infertility usually will have no symptoms other than inability to conceive. Lack of masculine secondary characteristics (e.g., decreased body hair) reflects severe hypogonadism. There may be a history of testicular trauma (from cryptorchidism, direct trauma, epididymitis, genital surgery), exposure to testicular toxins (e.g., chemotherapeutic agents), irradiation of the gonads, or exposure to pesticides or lead. A history of prior fertility indicates a better prognosis.

Physical examination may demonstrate the small testes of either primary or secondary hypogonadism (normal volume is 25 cc). Varicoceles are often associated with a small ipsilateral testicle (see Section 185, Scrotal Mass).

CLINICAL APPROACH.   Because both male and female factors must be taken into account in developing treatment options for the couple, close collaboration between male and female infertility specialists is required. Patients may have azoospermia (no sperm on semen analysis), oligospermia (<20 million sperm per ml on semen analysis), or a normal semen analysis. About half of infertile men have oligospermia and half have a normal sperm analysis; only about 2% of men have azoospermia. Evaluation of azoospermia, which reflects either lack of testicular production of sperm or obstruction in the ducts that carry the sperm from testicles to the urethra, includes measurements of semen fructose, FSH, LH, and testosterone levels and, in some cases, testicular biopsy. Patients with oligospermia require careful physical examination for varicoceles as well as measurements of gonadotropins and testosterone. Those with nor-

TABLE 159–1.   TREATABLE CAUSES OF MALE INFERTILITY

Cause	Clinical Findings	Treatment
Azoospermia		
Vasal obstruction	FHS normal, LH normal, T normal	Vasovasostomy
Epididymal obstruction	FSH normal, LH normal, T normal	Vasoepididymostomy
Ejaculatory duct obstruction	FSH normal, absent fructose in semen[1], noncoagulation of semen	Ejaculatory duct evacuation
Hypogonadotropic hypogonadism	FSH *normal,* LH normal, T decreased	Replace gonadotropic hormones[2]
Retrograde ejaculation	Low or zero sperm count, FSH normal, less than 1 cc semen	Sperm retrieval
Anejaculation	Previous spinal cord injury or retroperitoneal surgery	Electroejaculation
Oligospermia		
Varicocele	Varicocele on examination	Varicocelectomy or vein embolization
Hypogonadotropic hypogonadism	FSH normal, LH normal, T decreased	Replace gonadotropic hormones[2]
Idiopathic	FSH normal or increased, LH normal, T normal	hMG (?)[3], hCG (?), clomiphene citrate (?), in vitro fertilization (?)
Normospermia		
Sperm autoimmunity	Positive sperm antibody tests	Steroids (?), in vitro fertilization
Pyospermia	Increased leukocytes in semen, usually not infectious	Antibiotics (?)
Prostatitis	Positive semen culture for usual uropathogens (enteric gram-negative rods, enterococci)	Antibiotics (?)

Abbreviations: FSH = follicle-stimulating hormone, LH = luteinizing hormone, T = testosterone, hMG = human menopausal gonadotropin, hCG = human chorionic gonadotropin.
[1] Semen fructose originates in the seminal vesicles.
[2] Should evaluate the pituitary gland.
[3] ? = of unproven benefit.

mospermia may have disordered sperm function and should be considered for semen culture, blood and semen sperm antibody tests, and more sophisticated tests (e.g., hamster oocyte penetration test).

MANAGEMENT.   Treatment should be based on the etiology (Table 159–1). Treatable causes include asymptomatic bacterial prostatitis, varicocele, ductal obstruction, and hypogonadotropic hypogonadism and toxic exposures. If possible, the clinician should discontinue drugs that may affect spermatogenesis (e.g., cimetidine, metronidazole, nitrofurantoin, tetracycline, sulfa drugs, androgens, and cytotoxic drugs). Idiopathic oligospermia may respond to gonadotropic agents such as clomiphene citrate or hCG injections, but efficacy is unproven. Some poorly understood sperm disorders may benefit from in vitro fertilization. Untreatable male factor infertility may benefit from therapeutic donor insemination. All patients should receive counseling about adoption and therapeutic donor insemination. Psychological and marital counseling may be necessary, as infertility often causes personal and relationship problems.

Cross-references: Female Infertility (Section 158), Impotence (Section 171), Scrotal Mass (Section 185).

REFERENCES

1. Close CD, Roberts PL, Berger RE. Cigarettes, alcohol and marijuana are related to pyospermia in infertile men. J Urol 1990;144:900–903.

    Study of 164 men from infertile couples that suggests association between these exposures and pyospermia, unrelated to past or present genitourinary infection. Whether pyospermia definitely causes infertility is under study.

2. Fuchs EF, Alexander NJ. Immunologic considerations before and after vasovasostomy. Fertil Steril 1983;40:497–499.

    The presence of antisperm antibodies may have adverse effects on the return to fertility after vasectomy reversal.

3. Urry RL, Middleton RG. Modern concepts in the diagnosis and treatment of male infertility. Urol Clin North Am 1986;13:455–463.

    Excellent overview.

XIV CHAPTER
WOMEN'S HEALTH

160 CERVICAL CANCER

Screening

ANNE W. MOULTON

EPIDEMIOLOGY. Each year in the United States, there are approximately 13,000 new cases of cervical cancer and 7000 resulting deaths. An average woman has a lifetime risk of 0.7% for developing invasive cervical cancer and 2% for developing carcinoma in situ. During the last decade cervical cancer mortality has increased in younger women: 27% of deaths occur in women under the age of 50. This increase has been attributed to beginning sexual activity at an earlier age. Twenty-five percent of cervical cancer occurs in women over the age of 65, most of whom have not had regular screening. Cervical cancer rates are approximately two times higher for black, Hispanic, and native American women. Although most cervical cancer is squamous cell carcinoma, 5% to 10% of cases are adenocarcinoma, which has a significantly worse prognosis.

The two most important factors affecting risk of cervical cancer are early age at first intercourse (relative risk [RR] = 2–3) and a greater number of sexual partners (RR = 10–14 for more than six partners). Several studies also suggest a relationship between smoking and cervical cancer. Human papillomavirus (HPV) infections (especially with types 16 and 18) are important in the pathogenesis of squamous cell carcinoma of the cervix and probably adenocarcinoma as well.

RATIONALE. The natural history of cervical cancer (with a long preinvasive stage) and the availability of a simple, relatively inexpensive test make cervical cancer ideal for screening. Evidence for the efficacy of screening comes from many large screening programs in Scandinavia, Canada, and the United States. In the United States the number of cervical cancer cases has declined by more than 35% since the advent of screening programs. The majority of the clinically significant neoplasia arises from the squamocolumnar junction, the most important anatomic area of the cervix to screen. A sample from the endocervical canal, combined with a cervical scraping, provides the lowest false-negative rate. The probability that a Papanicolaou test will fail to detect a significant lesion ranges widely, from less than 5% to above 50%, because of a variety of factors, including technical issues such as sampling and slide preparation, accuracy in diagnosis and reporting, and different definitions of the false-negative rate. Use of the cervical brush is an effective method to optimize retrieval of endocervical cells. False-positive smears occur much less frequently (approximately 1%–9%) and primarily reflect errors in laboratory reporting.

STRATEGY. Screening should begin at age 18 or when the patient becomes sexually active. After three or more satisfactory normal annual examinations, the Papanicolaou test may be performed less frequently, although this is controversial. The Canadian Task Force recommends annual Papanicolaou testing only until age 35, followed by rescreening every 5 years until age 60. Cost-effectiveness models indicate that testing at 3-year intervals, beginning in the early 20s and continuing until age 65, reduces the effectiveness less than 5% compared to traditional recommendations.

Despite lack of clear recommendations, there is general agreement that testing can be stopped at age 65 if the patient has been regularly screened and always had normal Papanicolaou tests. Also subject to debate is routine screening following hysterectomy in women of any age. If the hysterectomy was performed for cervical cancer, there is a 2% to 12% risk of recurrence, and regular testing is indicated. If the surgery was for a benign condition, however, regular testing is unnecessary. Despite good technique, the Papanicolaou test lacks endocervical cells in 2% to 4% of smears, especially in postmenopausal women, in whom the squamocolumnar junction migrates up the endocervical canal. A repeat test in 3 to 6 months is indicated in all patients with an inadequate endocervical sample.

The original classification system for cervical smears (classes I to IV), while still in use in some laboratories, does not reflect the current understanding of cervical neoplasia (Table 160–1). The CIN system improves classification of precancerous lesions. In 1988, the Bethesda Classification System was developed to facilitate standardized reporting. An update of this classification system is expected in 1992. Depending on the laboratory, Papanicolaou test reports may contain information from one or all of the classification systems.

ACTION. Any patient with a suspicious cervical lesion should be referred for further evaluation if the Papanicolaou test is negative. In patients with atypia and no evidence of infection, some experts believe initial referral should be made for colposcopy, but this is controversial. Patients with atypia on Papanicolaou smears with evidence of infection should be treated for cervicitis (*Chlamydia* may be a cause in approximately 30%; see Section 178, Sexually Transmitted Diseases) and be retested in 3 months. If the atypia persists, referral for colposcopy is necessary. Patients with dysplasia (CIN 1–3, carcinoma in situ, both grades of SIL) should be referred directly for biopsy if a lesion is visible on the cervix or colposcopy. Additional diagnostic studies and treatment depend on the findings. Patients who have evidence of invasive carcinoma on

TABLE 160–1. CLASSIFICATION AND COMPARATIVE NOMENCLATURE OF CERVICAL SMEARS

	Original Classification	CIN System	Bethesda System
Class I:	Normal smear; No abnormal cells		
Class II:	Atypical cells present below the level of cervical neoplasia		Atypical squamous cell of undetermined significance
Class III:	Smear contains abnormal cells consistent with dysplasia	Mild dysplasia = CIN 1 Moderate dysplasia = CIN 2	Low-grade SIL (Changes associated with HPV and CIN 1) High-grade SIL (CIN 2, CIN 3, and carcinoma in situ)
Class IV:	Smear contains abnormal cells consistent with carcinoma in situ	Severe dysplasia and carcinoma in situ = CIN 3	
Class V:	Smear contains abnormal cells consistent with carcinoma of squamous cell origin		Squamous cell carcinoma

Abbreviations: CIN = cervical intraepithelial neoplasia, SIL = squamous intraepithelial lesion (Bethesda System, 1988).

cervical smear should be referred immediately for evaluation (biopsy or colposcopy) and definitive treatment. After treatment of dysplasia or carcinoma, follow-up Papanicolaou tests should be performed every 3 months for the first year and every 6 months subsequently.

Cross-references: Periodic Health Assessment (Section 7), Abnormal Uterine Bleeding (Section 162), Vaginitis (Section 166), Contraception (Section 167), Sexually Transmitted Diseases (Section 178).

REFERENCES

1. Campion MJ, Reid R. Screening for gynecologic cancer. Obstet Gynecol Clin North Am 1990;17:695–627.
    Excellent overview.

2. Eddy DM. Screening for cervical cancer. Ann Intern Med 1990;113:214–226.
    Superb review of the literature; includes mathematical models that address the ideal frequency of screening.

3. Koss LG. The papanicolaou test for cervical cancer detection: A triumph and a tragedy. JAMA 1989;261:737–743.
    Good discussion by a pathologist of the limitations of the Pap test.

4. Nelson JH, Averette HE, Richart RM. Cervical intraepithelial neoplasia (dysplasia and carcinoma in situ) and early invasive cancer. CA 1989;39:157–178.
    Excellent review of diagnosis and treatment. Includes flow charts for diagnostic response to abnormal cervical smears.

5. U.S. Preventive Services Task Force. Screening for cervical cancer. In: Guide to Clinical Preventive Services: An assessment of the Effectiveness of 169 Interventions. Report of the U.S. Preventive Services Task Force. Williams & Wilkins, Baltimore, 1989.
    Succinct review of screening recommendations.

161 BREAST CANCER SCREENING

Screening

ALVIN I. MUSHLIN

EPIDEMIOLOGY.   Breast cancer is the most common serious malignancy in women. The risk of breast cancer occurring sometime during a woman's life is on the order of 10%. By the ages of 30 to 49 years, about 400 women per 100,000 will have developed breast cancer, and the prevalence increases almost tenfold in older women (i.e., >70 years old). Similarly, only 20% of cancer deaths occur before age 55. The natural history of these tumors also varies by age: it is generally more rapidly progressive among very young women and less so in the middle-age ranges. In the elderly, the reported survival rates are also poor, but this may be confounded by less aggressive treatment choices. Breast malignancies are believed to have a latent period during which they are confined to the breast. In fact, some may never extend beyond the breast or threaten the individual's health (such "minimal" breast cancer may not uniformly behave as a malignancy). It is clear that the cure rate varies with the stage of the disease at the time of detection. These factors have direct implications for screening.

RATIONALE. Mammography has evolved into a very good screening test for early breast cancer. In specialized centers, it is now at least 75% sensitive and 90% to 95% specific. This degree of accuracy has been achieved despite progressively lower doses of ionizing radiation. At present a full examination requires less than 0.5 rad, a level believed to be safe in terms of inducing breast cancer. In actual community practice, however, the accuracy and safety of screening mammography may be lower. In addition to variability in the dosage of radiation and the quality of imaging itself, the sensitivity and specificity vary depending on the thresholds set by radiologists for detecting an abnormality. More cautious radiologists produce higher false-positive rates than those reported in the literature from specialized centers or clinical trials. Mammography is also less sensitive for malignancies in younger persons with denser breast tissue. Moreover, it may be less specific in younger women, because of the increased prevalence of benign breast disease.

Screening for breast cancer has been evaluated more extensively than any modern screening procedure. The findings from several randomized controlled trials in North America and Europe have resulted in general agreement that regular screening is associated with a survival benefit from breast cancer of approximately 20% to 30% in women over 50 years of age. Whether screening is beneficial in women under 50 is still being debated. However, many questions remain about the feasibility and cost implications of screening, and about whether and how frequently routine mammography is warranted from a cost-effectiveness standpoint. Even less clear is the value and cost-effectiveness of breast self-examination and routine breast palpation by a physician as part of a routine health maintenance examination.

STRATEGY. Women over 50 years of age should be offered yearly mammography at least until the age of 64. After the age of 65 the periodic frequency of mammography is an issue, because the tumors in this age group may have a longer latency period. Annual screening is recommended somewhat arbitrarily, as the randomized trials employed this interval, rather than because of evidence proving that longer intervals are less beneficial. The higher incidence of breast cancer in the elderly, however, argues that continued screening at some regular interval is warranted, although it may be less cost-effective than in younger individuals.

It is best to base decisions for screening women under age 50 on risk factors and patient preferences. Screening should be started at a younger age in women with a family history of premenopausal breast cancer in a close (first-degree) relative and in those who make an informed choice for screening. They should be advised that screening very young women may be less effective in preventing breast cancer mortality than in those over 50. Mammography in younger persons (because of a lower prevalence of malignancy and less than perfect specificity) may also lead to a greater chance that follow-up tests and or biopsies will be needed for false-positive mammography results. Teaching about breast self-examination should be provided to all women, but without reassurance that it alone will suffice for screening purposes.

ACTION.   Patients with a positive screening mammogram should undergo a careful physical examination and full diagnostic mammography to confirm the abnormality detected on the screening examination. If the findings suggest a cyst, fine-needle aspiration may provide reassurance and obviate the need for an excisional biopsy if the cytology is negative (see Section 165, Breast Masses and Breast Pain). Otherwise the patient should be referred to a surgeon for an open biopsy. Undue reassurance should not be given to those with a negative screening mammogram because interval masses may appear that require prompt attention by the patient and her clinician.

Cross-references: Periodic Health Assessment (Section 7), Breast Masses and Breast Pain (Section 165), Mammography (Section 169).

REFERENCES

1.   Boring CC, Squires TS, Tong T. Cancer statistics, 1991. CA 1991;41:19–36.
       Good quantitative overview of cancer statistics. Includes information about the risk of breast cancer over time, compared to other malignancies.

2.   Eddy DM. Screening for breast cancer. Ann Intern Med 1989;111:389–399.
       Reviews the various studies of the effectiveness of screening and includes a cost-effectiveness analysis of breast cancer screening at different age groups.

3.   Fisher M, Ed: Screening for Breast Cancer. Guide to Clinical Preventive Services. An Assessment of the Effectiveness of 169 Interventions. Williams & Wilkins, Baltimore, 1989.
       In addition to the U.S. PHSTF guidelines, this chapter includes an excellent review of the evidence for and against screening.

4.   Host H, Lund E. Age as prognostic factor in breast cancer. Cancer 1986;57:2217–2221.
       The use of a tumor registry and vital statistics to study breast cancer survival in young women compared to older age groups.

5.   Mushlin AI. Diagnostic tests in breast cancer: Clinical strategies based on diagnostic probabilities. Ann Intern Med 1985;103:79–85.
       Review of information about the accuracy of diagnostic tests and procedures, including screening mammography. Demonstrates how the probabilities of malignancy will vary depending on sensitivity, specificity, and disease prevalence.

162 ABNORMAL UTERINE BLEEDING

Symptom

DONALD E. MOORE

EPIDEMIOLOGY/ETIOLOGY. Abnormal uterine bleeding is one of the most common problems that affect women. Although bleeding may result from organic causes (e.g., pregnancy related, uterine myoma, endometrial cancer), most cases are hormone related and collectively referred to as "dysfunctional uterine bleeding." About 85% of dysfunctional uterine bleeding is anovulatory and 15% ovulatory. Most organic bleeding (except that related to pregnancy) is associated with ovulation. Table 162–1 lists the important organic causes of bleeding according to the patient's age. Most cases of anovulatory bleeding are idiopathic, although some result from polycystic ovarian disease, weight loss, extreme exercise, obesity, chronic illness (e.g., renal failure), drug addiction, or the changes that occur during or after menopause.

The average blood loss per menstrual cycle is 35 ml; loss of 80 ml or more per cycle is considered excessive because it often results in anemia. The duration of menstrual flow ranges from 3 to 7 days; 80% of the blood loss occurs during the first 2 days. Table 162–2 defines the terminology used to describe various uterine bleeding patterns.

CLINICAL APPROACH. The clinician should first establish that the bleeding is uterine and not from the rectum, urethra, bladder, or vagina. Nonuterine bleeding may originate from benign or malignant tumors, infections, trauma, and foreign bodies.

The patient interview should identify whether there was previous unprotected intercourse (suggesting pregnancy-related bleeding), easy bruising (suggesting coagulation disorder), history of an intrauterine device (IUD) (suggesting pelvic inflammatory disease or IUD complication), recent change in contraceptives (suggesting contraceptive complication), or abdominal pain (e.g., cramping dysmenorrhea of intrauterine myoma, sudden severe pain of ectopic pregnancy, or bilateral pelvic pain and spotting of pelvic inflammatory disease). Sore breasts and subtle changes in appetite or nausea are often found during early pregnancy. Symptoms that support ovulatory bleeding are bleeding between regular cycles that may be associated with breast tenderness, weight gain, bloating, or dysmenorrhea. Most anovulatory bleeding is oligomenorrheic, usually occurring every 2 to 6 months (see Table 162–2). Because the actual amount of blood loss often correlates poorly with the patient's report

TABLE 162–1. ORGANIC CAUSES OF UTERINE BLEEDING

Age Group	Most Common	Diagnostic Test	Uncommon	Diagnostic Test
Adolescents	Coagulation defects[1] (ITP, von Willebrand's disease, leukemia)	CBC with differential, coagulation panel	Hypothyroidism	T_4, TSH
Young adults (15–35 years)	Pregnancy (spontaneous abortion, ectopic pregnancy)	Serum hCG	Trophoblastic disease	Serum hCG
	Endometritis[2]	Endometrial biopsy	Endometriosis	History (dysmenorrhea plus dyspareunia)
	Contraceptive side effect (IUD, oral contraceptives)	History	Adenomyosis	History (dysmenorrhea plus enlarged uterus on pelvic examination)
			Endometrial cancer	Endometrial biopsy
Middle years (35–45 years)	Same as young adults			
	Large myoma	Pelvic examination		
	Submucous myoma or polyp	Hysterosalpingography and/or hysteroscopy		
Peri- and postmenopausal (45 years and older)	Endometrial cancer	Endometrial biopsy	Ovarian cancer	Pelvic examination, vaginal ultrasound

[1]Accounts for 20% of menorrhagia in adolescents.
[2]May occur without salpingitis (i.e., no pelvic pain).

TABLE 162–2. PATTERNS OF ABNORMAL UTERINE BLEEDING

Amenorrhea   No menses for 6 months or more if preceded by normal cycles; 12 months or more if preceded by oligomenorrhea.

Dysfunctional uterine bleeding (DUB)   Abnormal uterine bleeding unrelated to organic causes. Usually preceded by oligomenorrhea, occasionally by normal cycles.

Hypomenorrhea   Light regular ovulatory menstrual periods.

Intermenstrual bleeding   Bleeding or spotting between regular ovulatory menstrual periods.

Menometrorrhagia   Heavy and/or prolonged irregular and frequent uterine bleeding; may be ovulatory.

Menorrhagia (hypermenorrhea)   Heavy and/or prolonged regular menstrual periods (every 24–32 days), usually ovulatory.

Metrorrhagia   Bleeding or spotting irregularly, usually anovulatory.

Midcycle spotting   Usually related to the midcycle decrease in serum levels of estradiol; microscopic amounts of midcycle spotting are identified in 90% of women.

Oligomenorrhea   Menstrual interval greater than 40 days; if anovulatory, menstrual cycles typically occur every 2 to 6 months.

Polymenorrhea   Menstrual interval less than 22 days; usually associated with shortened follicular or luteal phase (i.e., is ovulatory).

(e.g., pads used), a complete blood count (CBC) is indicated when reported blood loss is significant.

The clinician should also determine whether the patient desires pregnancy, because some hormonal manipulations of dysfunctional bleeding inhibit ovulation and prevent pregnancy (see Management).

An organic etiology of uterine bleeding is particularly likely if the bleeding is ovulatory (i.e., occurs between regular menstrual cycles). In sexually active women of reproductive age, bleeding complications of pregnancy or contraceptives are common; a serum human chorionic gonadotropin (hCG) determination is usually indicated. If the patient is over 35 years of age, the clinician should refer the patient for endometrial sampling or biopsy to rule out endometrial cancer. In women in their 30s or 40s, submucous myomas or endometrial polyps are common, particularly if the bleeding is heavy, and are often difficult to diagnose without hysterosalpingography. Table 162–1 reviews the diagnostic tests necessary to identify the most important organic causes.

After organic causes of uterine bleeding are excluded, the clinician should focus on dysfunctional uterine bleeding, which is marked usually by oligomenorrhea, metrorrhagia, or menometrorrhagia and is responsive to hormonal therapy. Minimal ovulatory bleeding such as intermenstrual bleeding requires no evaluation or treatment other than patient reassurance and follow-up. If the precise bleeding pattern is difficult to identify (i.e., anovulatory vs. ovulatory), the basal body temperature (BBT), recorded daily over 1 to 2 months, can be helpful, though this is not necessary before treatment. The characteristic laboratory finding of polycystic ovarian disease is an elevated serum luteinizing hormone–follicle stimulating hormone (LH/FSH) ratio, usually greater than 3; other findings may include elevated levels of testosterone, free testosterone, or dehydroepiandrosterone. Women with suspected polycystic ovarian disease should probably undergo endometrial biopsy, because long-standing unopposed estrogen stimulation of the endometrium increases the risk of endometrial cancer.

MANAGEMENT. Treatment of organic bleeding depends on the specific cause. The treatment of dysfunctional bleeding, regardless of the etiology, depends on the bleeding pattern and amount.

Treatment of polymenorrhea is usually unnecessary unless fertility is desired. If the BBT reveals a short follicular (preovulatory) phase, ethinyl estradiol (20 μg/day) may be beneficial; if it reveals a short luteal (postovulatory) phase, progesterone (25 mg vaginally every 12 hours during the luteal phase) may be beneficial. Light bleeding associated with oligomenorrhea or anovulation may be treated monthly with 10 days of daily Provera (10 mg) to induce systematic shedding of the endometrium if the patient is not sexually active, oral contraceptives if she is sexually active, or clomiphene citrate if she desires pregnancy. The initial treatment of heavy bleeding associated with oligomenorrhea or anovulation is intensive oral contraceptives (Table 162–3), followed by the same treatment recommended above for light bleeding.

Heavy bleeding associated with ovulatory cycles may not respond to the above regimens, though oral contraceptives or ibuprofen (800 mg every 8 hours) are often beneficial. Refractory cases may respond to Depo-Provera or a gonadotropin-releasing hormone (GnRH) agonist (Lupron Depot), both of which induce an atrophic endometrium. Both of these treatments, however, should be reserved for bleeding unresponsive to other approaches, because both inhibit ovulation and prevent pregnancy. Depo-Provera continues to exert

TABLE 162–3.   TREATMENTS OF DYSFUNCTIONAL UTERINE BLEEDING[1]

Medication	Dose	Cost ($)[3]
Ovral ("intensive" oral contraceptive treatment)	3 PO q.d. × 7 days, followed by 1 q.d. × 21 days, followed by a 7-day pill-free interval, followed by two more 21/28 cycles[2]	102.48 for 3 months
Provera	10 mg PO q.d. × 10–13 days per month	5.10 for 10 days
Ibuprofen	800 mg PO q.8h. × 1–2 days	1.20 for 2 days
Premarin (intensive estrogen treatment for severe uterine hemorrhage)	25 mg PO t.i.d. × 1–2 days	4.38 for 2 days
Clomiphene citrate	50 mg PO q.d., days 5–9 of menstrual cycle	23.05 for 5 days
Depo-Provera	100 mg IM weekly × 4 weeks, followed by 100 mg every other week × 2 weeks, followed by 100 mg monthly (generally a total of 6 months is adequate)	6.68 per 100 mg
Lupron Depot	3.75 mg IM once monthly	315.00 per 3.75 mg

[1]Before initiating therapy, the clinician should confirm that the patient is not pregnant, either by documenting 3 days of low BBTs (<98°F) or by a negative serum hCG.

[2]21/28 cycle = 1 pill per day × 21 days, followed by 7 days of no medication.

[3]Average whosesale price, 1991 *Drug Topics Red Book*.

effects 9 months after the last injection, and Depo-Lupron is associated with hypoestrogenic effects and loss of bone density. Patients with persistent bleeding should be referred to a specialist for consideration of ablation of the endometrium by cautery or laser (a relatively new treatment that shows some promise) or, in extreme cases, hysterectomy.

Acute, severe uterine hemorrhage requires immediate treatment, usually with 25 mg Premarin by mouth every 8 hours for 1 to 2 days. An anti-emetic may have to be administered one-half hour prior to the Premarin. Once the bleeding is controlled, intensive oral contraceptive therapy can follow.

FOLLOW-UP.   Most patients with organic causes require referral to and follow-up with a specialist. Management of dysfunctional uterine bleeding requires careful monitoring of both the medication's efficacy and side effects. Patients should be seen 1 to 4 weeks after the initial evaluation for reassurance, adjustment of the prescribed medication (if necessary), changes to other medications (if the first is poorly tolerated), and evaluation of whether or not further investigation of organic causes is necessary.

Since the fundamental causes of abnormal uterine bleeding are usually chronic conditions, most patients need long-term follow-up and treatment, sometimes for years. Patients treated with intensive oral contraceptive therapy, Depo-Provera, Lupron Depot, or high-dose Premarin probably benefit from standard oral contraceptives or monthly progestogen withdrawal. In addition, because recommendations in this field are rapidly changing, yearly or biyearly contact with the patient allows modifications in therapy as new information evolves.

Cross-references: Abdominal Pain (Section 95), Female Infertility (Section 158), Contraception (Section 167), Bleeding (Section 197), Anemia (Section 201), Diagnosis of Pregnancy (Section 209).

REFERENCES

1. DeVore GR, Owens O, Kase N. Use of intravenous PremarinR in the treatment of dysfunctional uterine bleeding: A double-blind randomized control study. Obstet Gynecol 1982;59:285–291.
    Demonstrates the efficacy of PremarinR versus placebo in dysfunctional uterine bleeding.

2. Droegemueller W, Herbst AL, Mischell DR, Stenchever MA, Eds. Comprehensive Gynecology. C.V. Mosby, St. Louis, 1987, pp. 953–964.

3. March CM, Hoffman DI, Lobo RA. Dysfunctional uterine bleeding. In Mishell DR, Davajan V, Eds. Infertility, Contraception and Reproductive Endocrinology, 2nd ed. Medical Economics Books, Oradell, NJ, 1986, pp. 337–351.
    References 2 and 3 are good reviews of clinical features and medical and surgical treatment.

4. Speroff L, Glass RH, Kase NG, Eds. Clinical Gynecologic Endocrinology and Infertility, 4th ed. Williams & Wilkins, Baltimore, 1989, pp. 265–282.
    Good review of basic science and medical therapy.

163 PELVIC PAIN IN WOMEN

Symptom

JOHN F. STEEGE

EPIDEMIOLOGY. Acute pelvic pain primarily affects patients in the reproductive age group. Chronic pain usually affects those between the ages of 25 and 40 years. Postmenopausal pelvic pain usually results from abnormal pelvic support and is usually less severe.

ETIOLOGY. **Acute pelvic pain** may be caused by pelvic bacterial infection (most commonly gonorrhea or *Chlamydia*), a ruptured or bleeding ovarian cyst, severe constipation, ectopic pregnancy, torsion of an adnexa from ovary enlargement, or acute impairment of bowel function from chronic adhesions. Although rare, acute pain may also result from a ruptured or bleeding endometrioma. Nongynecologic causes of acute pain include urinary tract infection (probably the most common cause of overall pelvic pain) and appendicitis. **Chronic pain** is almost always due to either endometriosis or adhesions (postinfectious, postsurgical, or from endometriosis). Enlarging fibroids uncommonly cause acute or chronic pain. Gynecologic malignances rarely produce pain unless the disease is far advanced.

CLINICAL APPROACH. The approach to the patient with acute pelvic pain appears in Section 168 (Pelvic Inflammatory Disease) and will be briefly reviewed here.

In patients with acute symptoms, the location of the pain often correlates well with the location of abnormalities on pelvic examination. Unilateral acute pain may be due to appendicitis, hemorrhage into or from an ovarian cyst, torsion of the ovary caused by a cyst, or, more rarely, unilateral pelvic inflammatory disease. Ovarian cysts cause well-localized, sharp and constant discomfort, which may be accompanied by menstrual irregularity. Torsion of the adnexa causes extreme pain and exquisite tenderness of the ovary on examination. Pelvic inflammatory disease, in contrast to other etiologies, often produces bilateral pain and findings.

Because ectopic pregnancy is always a possibility, a sensitive serum pregnancy test is the most important laboratory test in patients with acute pain. Patients with positive test results should be referred to a specialist.

A complete blood count (CBC), erythrocyte sedimentation rate (ESR), cervical Gram stain, and cultures for gonorrhea and *Chlamydia* should be performed when infection is suspected. Ultrasound (US) distinguishes cystic from solid ovarian masses and detects significant peritoneal fluid or blood from cyst rupture, but is often unreliable in patients with previous pelvic surgeries. The clinical diagnosis of pelvic infection is inaccurate in up to 30% of cases. Gynecologic consultation should be obtained when any uncertainty exists. Laparoscopic examination is sometimes warranted.

Pelvic examination is insensitive in the diagnosis of both endometriosis and adhesions, the main causes of chronic pain. Laparoscopy is therefore liberally used to establish an accurate diagnosis of chronic pain, especially before initiating treatments that involve significant side effects or time commitment (e.g., long-term suppression of endometriosis with medroxyprogesterone).

If pain has been present for 6 months or longer, consideration of the chronic pain syndrome is appropriate (see Section 13, Chronic Pain Syndrome). The hallmarks of this syndrome include incomplete relief by previous treatments, significant change in physical activities, vegetative signs of depression (especially sleep disturbance), and altered relationships with family members. A patient having these characteristics may benefit from simultaneous mental health and gynecologic evaluation.

MANAGEMENT.   Section 168 reviews the management of suspected pelvic inflammatory disease. As long as a significant hemoperitoneum is not suspected, patients with ovarian cysts are usually managed as outpatients with analgesic medications (e.g., ibuprofen or codeine) and suppression of ovulation with oral contraceptives. Patients with any ovarian mass that fails to disappear after one cycle should be referred to a specialist. Torsion of an adnexa is a surgical emergency.

In women with chronic pelvic pain, the physician should treat contributing factors such as poor bowel habit, recurrent urinary tract infections, or bladder spasms. If adhesions or endometriosis are suspected, the patient should be referred to a gynecologist. Laser and operative laparoscopy are effective diagnostic and therapeutic tools and help guide further therapy. Laparoscopic adhesiolysis relieves pain in 50% to 85% of cases, the degree of success depending on concomitant psychological factors. Analgesia for chronic pain should be limited to nonnarcotic medications.

FOLLOW-UP.   Patients with acute pain should be reexamined within 2 days. Patients with chronic pain often benefit from a schedule of relatively frequent return visits (e.g., 2–4 weeks) so that various aspects of an often complicated medical and psychosocial situation can be systematically approached.

Cross-references: Chronic Pain Syndrome (Section 13), Abdominal Pain (Section 95), Abnormal Uterine Bleeding (Section 162), Pelvic Inflammatory Disease (Section 168), Urinary Tract Infections in Women (Section 177), Sexually Transmitted Diseases (Section 178), Somatization (Section 191), Diagnosis of Pregnancy (Section 209).

REFERENCES

1. Goldstein DP. Acute and chronic pelvic pain. Pediatr Clin North Am 1989;36:573–580.
    Good general review of the differential diagnosis and treatment of pelvic pain in reproductive-age women.
2. Steege JF, Stout AL, Somkuti SG. Chronic pelvic pain: Toward an integrative model. J Psychosom Obstet Gynecol 1991, in press.
    Reviews the evaluation and treatment of physical and psychological factors involved in chronic pelvic pain.

164 MENOPAUSAL SYMPTOMS

Symptom

MICHELE G. CYR
KAREN L. NIGUT

EPIDEMIOLOGY.   Menopause, defined as the permanent cessation of menstruation from loss of ovarian function, typically occurs between the ages of 48 and 55, with a median age of 51. Given a life expectancy of 81 years, most women in the United States, live nearly one-third of their lives after menopause. Approximately 40 million women in the United States are postmenopausal, making the treatment of related conditions a major public health concern.

About 50% to 60% of postmenopausal women seek medical attention for symptoms directly related to menopause, including menstrual flow or cycle changes, vasomotor symptoms (hot flashes/flushes), atrophic conditions, and the consequences of osteoporosis. Vasomotor symptoms occur in 75% to 85% of post-menopausal women and typically recur over a 1- to 2-year period, although they may persist longer than 5 years in 25% to 50% of women. Atrophy of estrogen-sensitive tissue, including the vaginal epithelium, urethra, base of the bladder, pelvic ligamentous supports, and dermal collagen, affects nearly all women within 5 years after menopause. For 25% of women the symptoms of atrophy will be severe enough to prompt them to seek medical attention.

Osteoporosis is present in 25% of all postmenopausal women and accounts for 1.3 million fractures per year in the United States. The rate of bone loss is accelerated for 3 to 6 years after menopause and declines by the age of 65 in untreated women.

SIGNS AND SYMPTOMS.   Menopausal symptoms are the result of systemic and end-organ responses to decreased estrogen. As estrogen levels decrease in the premenopausal years, symptoms may begin even prior to the actual cessation of menses. The climacteric refers to this period during which diminished reproductive potential becomes evident.

Vasomotor symptoms (hot flashes) often begin with a prodromal sensation of heat followed by reddening of skin over the head, neck and chest ("hot flushes"). Tachycardia and diaphoresis may also be present. Flushes typically last seconds to minutes, but can persist for up to an hour. Attacks may occur as often as every 10 minutes, increasing during periods of stress. Episodes are often most severe and frequent at night and can cause significant sleep disturbance.

Atrophy of the estrogen-responsive tissue can cause atrophic vaginitis and urethritis, recurrent vaginal infections, and dyspareunia. On physical examination, mucosal thinning and loss of vaginal rugae may be evident. Weakened pelvic ligamentous supports can lead to cystocele, rectocele, or uterine prolapse. Generalized loss of dermal collagen can cause decreased skin elasticity and lead to wrinkling, thinning, and increased fragility.

Osteoporosis may be asymptomatic or cause symptoms related to specific fractures. Vertebral compression fractures can present as decreased height, dowager's hump (thoracic kyphosis), back pain, or reduced mobility. Fractures can also occur in other susceptible parts of the skeleton, including the humerus, upper femur, ribs, and distal radius.

Although psychological symptoms such as anxiety, depression, irritability, tearfulness, and memory changes frequently appear during menopause, the relative etiologic roles of estrogen deficiency versus social circumstances are controversial. Some symptoms may respond to estrogen replacement, others may be manifestations of depression and should be treated with specific antidepressant therapy (progestin therapy may accentuate depressive symptoms). Depressed patients are more likely to complain about menopausal symptoms. Other nonspecific symptoms associated with menopause include headaches, insomnia, myalgias, fatigue, palpitations, dizziness, voice changes, and hirsutism. Decreased libido and dyspareunia may be due to estrogen deficiency or depression and can lead to significant sexual dysfunction.

CLINICAL APPROACH.   The diagnosis of menopause can be made retrospectively after 6 to 12 months of amenorrhea in a woman over 45 years of age. It may be desirable to document menopause earlier with an estradiol level less than 20 pg/ml or an FSH level greater than 40 mIU/ml. A medroxyprogesterone challenge can also be used to diagnose menopause. If no withdrawal bleeding occurs after a 10-day challenge with medroxyprogesterone, the patient is considered menopausal.

Vasomotor symptoms alone may cause enough discomfort to warrant treatment, but hormone replacement therapy should be considered for all of its potential benefits, including symptom control and prophylaxis for the short and long term. Any patient who experiences postmenopausal bleeding in the absence of hormone replacement therapy should undergo a complete pelvic examination and multiple-specimen endometrial aspiration biopsy to rule out carcinoma.

MANAGEMENT.   The decision to treat postmenopausal women with hormone replacement therapy is based on patient preference in the context of individualized risk-benefit analyses. Estrogen replacement therapy is effective in controlling many postmenopausal symptoms, including vasomotor flushes and atrophic conditions. Estrogen significantly reduces the risk of osteoporosis and may also relieve some psychological symptoms. Estrogen replacement must be continued indefinitely, however, to prevent recurrent atrophy of estrogen-dependent tissues and osteoporotic bone loss. Estrogen has been shown to be cardioprotective, probably through its beneficial effect on lipid profile (increased HDL and decreased LDL). In fact, women on estrogen replacement therapy have a relative risk of cardiovascular disease and stroke one-half that of women who are untreated.

Estrogen therapy is associated with an increased risk of endometrial cancer. Prior to the initiation of estrogen replacement, endometrial biopsy is recommended by some to rule out endometrial hyperplasia or carcinoma. Although hotly debated, most authorities now believe that estrogen therapy increases the risk of breast cancer negligibly if at all. Because preexisting breast cancer may be estrogen responsive, mammography is indicated in all women before hormone replacement is begun.

The absolute contraindications to estrogen therapy are active liver disease or thromboembolic disease, a history of breast or endometrial cancer, and undiagnosed vaginal bleeding. Relative contraindications to estrogen therapy variably include gallbladder disease, leiomyoma, poorly controlled hypertension, past thromboembolic events, and chronic liver dysfunction. In women with contraindications to estrogen therapy, medroxyprogesterone acetate (Depo-Provera, 150 mg IM per month, or Provera, 20 mg/day) may effectively control menopausal symptoms; alternatively, α-adrenergic agonists (e.g., clonidine) may be used, but are associated with a high incidence of side effects.

As a general rule, the lowest effective dose of estrogen is recommended. The vasomotor and atrophic symptoms usually respond to conjugated oral estrogen in a dose of 0.625 to 1.25 mg/day. Because the effects of treatment may be slow to appear, 3 to 4 weeks of observation is necessary before advancing to a higher dose. If a decision to discontinue estrogen therapy is made, it should be done gradually to prevent exacerbation of postmenopausal symptoms.

Transdermal estrogen preparations effectively prevent menopausal symptoms and osteoporosis, although they are not approved for the latter use. Although initially there were concerns that the absence of first-pass hepatic metabolism with transdermal preparations might eliminate all of their cardioprotective effect, these have not been supported by recent studies, which show preservation of some beneficial effects on the lipid profile. Vaginal estrogens have been used in the control of atrophic symptoms but have erratic systemic absorption.

Treatment with unopposed estrogen is associated with a tenfold increase in the risk for endometrial cancer. The addition of progestin for 10 to 13 days per month (Table 164–1) reduces the risk of endometrial cancer to baseline and eliminates endometrial hyperplasia when added for 12 days. The dose of progesterone is adjusted upward, based on the timing of withdrawal bleeding; if bleeding occurs on or before day 11, the dose should be increased (from medroxyprogesterone 5 mg to 10 mg) until bleeding occurs on day 12 or thereafter. Although this regimen reduces the cancer risk, many women find withdrawal bleeding unacceptable. An alternative is continuous combined therapy with estrogen and progesterone. Daily doses of 2.5 mg medroxyprogesterone acetate and estrogen effectively control postmenopausal symptoms. Although associated with a high incidence of irregular bleeding in the first 3 months of therapy, this regimen generally induces amenorrhea after the first year of treatment.

Although many regimens are being investigated, the most widely accepted for women with intact uteri is a schedule of oral conjugated estrogens continuously or for days 1 through 25, with medroxyprogesterone added for 12 days of the month. If the estrogen is cycled, then progesterone is given for days 14 through 25 (see Table 164–1). The usual dose of estrogen is 0.625 mg/day, and for medroxyprogesterone it is 5 to 10 mg/day. Women who have had hysterectomies can receive continuous estrogen therapy alone.

To maximally reduce the risk of osteoporosis, estrogen replacement should be started as early as possible after menopause. Adequate calcium intake (1500 mg elemental calcium per day) in the diet or as supplements improves the ef-

TABLE 164–1.   SUGGESTED HORMONE REPLACEMENT REGIMENS

Regimen	Drug	Dose	Route	Days of Month	Average Daily Cost ($)[1]
Cyclic/ combined	Estrogen *plus*	0.625 mg	PO	All	0.31 (0.625 mg, Premarin)
	Medroxy-progesterone	5–10 mg	PO	1–12	0.20 (10 mg, generic) 0.27 (2.5 mg, Provera) 0.41 (5 mg, Provera) 0.51 (10 mg, Provera)
Cyclic/ combined	Estrogen *plus*	0.625 mg	PO	1–25	
	Medroxy-progesterone	5–10 mg	PO	14–25	
Continuous/ combined	Estrogen *plus*	0.625 mg	PO	All	
	Medroxy-progesterone	2.5 mg	PO	All	

[1]Average wholesale price, 1991 *Drug Topics Red Book.*

fectiveness of estrogen at lower doses. Exercise increases bone mass and muscle mass, and improves joint function in the treatment of osteoporosis.

FOLLOW-UP.   All postmenopausal women on hormone replacement therapy should have an annual breast and pelvic examination, Papanicolaou smear, and mammography. The indications for endometrial biopsy during hormone replacement therapy are controversial and depend on the regimen. Women with intact uteri who are taking estrogen alone should undergo endometrial biopsies before treatment and yearly thereafter. Women treated with cyclic estrogen and progesterone may not need pretreatment biopsies but should undergo endometrial biopsy if bleeding occurs at unexpected times (before day 12 of cyclic progestins) or if bleeding is heavy and prolonged. While some authorities also recommend biopsy after 3 months of cyclic/combined therapy and every 2 to 3 years thereafter, others recommend no routine biopsies. Until more data are available, annual endometrial biopsy probably is prudent for women on continuous combined therapy.

Cross-references: Periodic Health Assessment (Section 7), Osteoporosis (Section 117), Breast Cancer Screening (Section 161), Abnormal Uterine Bleeding (Section 162), Mammography (Section 169), Dysuria (Section 172), Screening for Depression (Section 187).

REFERENCES

1. Hahn RG. Compliance considerations with estrogen replacement: Withdrawal bleeding and other factors. Am J Obstet Gynecol 1989;161:1854–1858.
    Review of factors that limit patient compliance with and physician acceptance of hormone replacement therapy. Strategies to overcome these factors are presented.

2. Notelovitz M. Estrogen replacement therapy: Indications, contraindications, and agent selection. Am J Obstet Gynecol 1989;161:1832–1841.
    Excellent review of symptoms associated with menopause and risks and benefits of hormone replacement with information regarding specific estrogen preparations.

3. Sitruk-Ware R. Estrogen therapy during menopause: Practical treatment recommendations. Drugs 1990;39:203–217.
    Review of literature regarding risks of estrogen replacement. Guidelines for cycling and dosing are presented.

4. Utian WH. Biosynthesis and physiologic effects of estrogen and pathophysiologic effects of estrogen deficiency: A review. Am J Obstet Gynecol 1989;161:1828–1831.
    Effects of estrogen depletion systemically and on estrogen receptive tissue are presented.

5. Whitehead MI, Hillard TC, Crook D. The role and use of progestogens. Obstet Gynecol 1990;75:59S–76S.
    Comprehensive review of hormone replacement regimens, with recommendations for endometrial biopsy.

165 BREAST MASSES AND BREAST PAIN

Problem

ROGER E. MOE

EPIDEMIOLOGY/ETIOLOGY.   A **breast mass** is an abnormal thickening or induration of breast tissue that is palpable, particularly when compared to the contralateral, mirror-image quadrant during simultaneous bilateral palpation. Breast masses are the most frequent reason for referral to surgical clinics. In one series of over a 1000 surgical outpatients referred for problems related to the breast, about 30% had a solid breast mass, 30% had mammographically demonstrated abnormalities, 15% had macrocysts, and 15% had breast pain. Seven percent were found to have breast cancer.

Breast cancer affects women of all ages (range, 16–92 years in one series), with as many as 20% of cases occurring before the age of 40. In patients younger than 35, 90% of breast cancers are discovered because of a palpable mass. Many of these are already metastatic.

Cyclic breast pain and tenderness are common in women of reproductive age, often unilateral, and usually of several days' duration, beginning before and disappearing after their menses. Cyclic pain, especially when severe and prolonged, may result from an inadequate luteal phase and low progesterone levels, leaving the effects of estrogen on the breast unopposed. This pain is often attributed to cysts. However, documented macrocysts (palpable cysts greater than 3 mm in diameter) are painful in only 50% of patients, and many patients with breast pain have never had cysts. Similarly, the term "fibrocystic disease" should be abandoned because has no precise definition.

Breast abscesses usually result from inoculation of central ducts through the nipple with oral or cutaneous flora including both aerobic (e.g., staphylococcal) and anaerobic (e.g., peptostreptococcal) species.

SYMPTOMS AND SIGNS.   Although some breast masses are associated with soreness, many are asymptomatic and discovered incidentally on breast self-examination, mammography, or clinical examination. No finding on physical examination reliably excludes cancer and confirms benign disease; hence, all breast masses require further evaluation.

One in six breast cancers are associated with breast discomfort, sometimes as seemingly trivial as breast itching, localized burning, or the sensation of tightening inside the breast. The findings of dimpling or thickening (*peau d'orange*) of the overlying skin, a visible lump, or axillary lymphadenopathy suggest the diagnosis of cancer, but these are all uncommon findings, seen in late disease. Bloody discharge from one nipple suggests proliferative disease, either benign or, less often, malignant.

Cyclic breast pain lasting a few days is normal. Many women experience more severe pain that is of longer duration or continuous. Affected patients may not be able to tolerate any pressure on their breasts or participate in athletic activities. Many are concerned that they may have cancer.

Breast infections cause acute breast pain, usually severe and throbbing, associated with exquisite tenderness and erythema that extends outward from the areola but is *localized* to a sector of the breast. Deep to this, there is induration extending under the areola toward the central ducts of the nipple. A visible swelling suggests an abscess. **Inflammatory cancer** of the breast may also cause erythema, tenderness and pain, but there are important differences: (1) the erythema of inflammatory cancer may completely surround the areola; because this finding never occurs in breast infections, patients should be presumed to have cancer until proven otherwise; (2) the pain and tenderness of inflammatory carcinoma may be less severe than in breast abscess, and the erythema may less bright and even faint pink or violet in color. Less severe pain and erythema may occur as a result of nonbacterial mastitis in postmenopausal women, but this condition must be differentiated from cancer.

CLINICAL APPROACH. Any breast mass or localized thickening requires a definitive diagnosis, usually by needle aspiration of fluid, needle biopsy, or open biopsy. Mammography is indicated in patients older than 25 years who have breast masses, but only to define other abnormalities in the breasts that require evaluation or, in the patient with cancer, to define the extent of disease. Because the sensitivity of mammography for breast cancer is only 85%, mammography should never replace or delay definitive diagnostic procedures.

The most efficient and inexpensive initial test for breast lumps in adults is needle aspiration. Ultrasound demonstrates fluid-filled cysts with a sensitivity of 80% to 90%, but needle aspiration of fluid is quick and unambiguous. A 21-gauge needle and a 20-ml syringe are used with an aspirating pistol grip. The aspirates are placed on microscope slides and placed in alcohol fixative (ethanol 95%, methanol 5%) for Papanicolaou staining. If aspiration recovers nonbloody fluid and the mass resolves, no further tests other than careful follow-up are necessary. If the mass is solid and does not resolve with aspiration, or if the aspirated fluid contains dark blood, the patient should be referred to a surgeon for open biopsy.

In teenagers, 95% of the round, rubbery, discrete masses found are fibroadenomas. Cysts and cancer are rare. Because fibroadenomas do not resolve and may enlarge, most authorities recommend needle aspiration cytology and referral of the patient to a surgeon for removal of the lump, usually during a school vacation.

Some breast masses are followed without initial biopsy. This is only appropriate when (1) the patient is followed by a clinician experienced with breast disorders and (2) the mass is decreasing in size, as documented by serial diagrams with actual measurements.

Evaluation of patients with breast pain includes a thorough gynecologic and breast examination, and mammography. Any identified breast mass should be evaluated as described above.

Patients with suspected infection should undergo sterile soft tissue aspiration for both aerobic and anaerobic cultures. The aspirating needle should be inserted through the erythema near the areola and slanted toward the deep central ducts. If purulent fluid is obtained, the patient should be referred to a surgeon for open drainage under general anesthesia. All patients with suspected infection should receive antibiotic therapy (see below).

MANAGEMENT.   Appropriate antibiotic therapy for acute breast infection includes 2 weeks or longer of amoxicillin-clavulanate (500 mg PO t.i.d.). Clindamycin (300 mg PO q.i.d.) is an alternative agent.

Although the presence of breast cancer can never be completely excluded, patients with cyclic breast pain and normal examinations should be reassured that these are not symptoms of breast cancer. Restriction of dietary methylxanthines (e.g., coffee, cola) and therapy with vitamin E is often recommended for cyclic breast pain, despite the absence of convincing data supporting efficacy. Treatment with medroxyprogesterone acetate or danazol (Table 165–1) effectively reduces breast pain but is associated with frequent side effects, including weight gain, depression, and mild hair loss. Nonsteroidal anti-inflammatory agents are generally ineffective.

FOLLOW-UP.   Any breast mass that was not biopsied but has not decreased in size at 1 to 2 months of follow-up should be removed. The biopsy report of all breast masses should be carefully studied for features of florid or atypical proliferation. Some of these features of benign biopsy specimens identify patients at increased risk for subsequent breast cancer.[2] More frequent surveillance of these patients may be indicated.

Patients with acute infections should be seen weekly until all inflammatory signs resolve. Patients with abscesses are usually followed by the surgeon, who leaves a Penrose drain in place until the cavity fills in.

TABLE 165–1.   AGENTS USED FOR BREAST PAIN

Agent	Dose	Cost ($)/Month[1]
Vitamin E	600 IU/day	1.50
Medroxyprogesterone acetate[2]	10 mg/day on days 15–25 of menstrual cycle	1.80
Danazol[2]	200 mg b.i.d. × 1 month, then 100 mg b.i.d.; begin treatment during menstruation	103.80

[1]Average wholesale price, 1991 *Drug Topics Red Book.*
[2]Frequent side effects; see text and *Physicians' Desk Reference.*

Cross-references: Breast Cancer Screening (Section 161), Mammography (Section 169).

REFERENCES

1. Barth V. Atlas of Diseases of the Breast. Year Book Medical Publishers, Chicago, 1979.
   Excellent illustrations of anatomy, pathology, and mammography; recommended for nonsurgical clinicians.

2. Dupont WD, Page DL. Risk factors for breast cancer in women with proliferative breast disease. N Engl J Med 1985;312:146–151.
   Analysis of 10,366 benign breast biopsies. Thirty percent of patients had "proliferative" findings and were at increased risk for future breast cancer. The combination of proliferative disease and a positive family history posed the greatest risk.

3. Frable JF. Needle aspiration of the breast. Cancer 1984;53:671–676.
   Useful instructions for needle aspiration, which had a sensitivity of 0.89 and specificity of 0.97 in the detection of breast cancer.

4. Love SM, Schnitt SJ, Connolly JL, Shirley RL. Treatment of benign breast symptoms. In Haris JR, Hellman S, Henderson IC, Kinne DW, Eds. Breast Disease. J.B. Lippincott, Philadelphia, 1987, pp. 26–30.
   Concise, critical survey of methods for treating breast pain and tenderness.

5. Walker AP, Edmiston CE, Krepel CJ, Condon RE. A prospective study of the microflora of nonpuerperal breast abscess. Arch Surg 1988;123:908–911.
   Best study showing how to obtain cultures to detect anaerobes, a major component of the mixed flora found.

166 VAGINITIS

Problem

JANE SCHWEBKE

EPIDEMIOLOGY/ETIOLOGY. Vaginal infections account for half of all patient visits to private gynecologists and 28% of visits by women to sexually transmitted disease (STD) clinics.

The three main causes of vaginitis in order of frequency of occurrence are bacterial vaginosis, candidiasis, and trichomoniasis. Of these, only *Trichomonas* infection is proven to be sexually transmitted.

SYMPTOMS AND SIGNS. The symptoms and signs of each of the three types of vaginitis appear in Table 166–1.

TABLE 166–1. CLINICAL AND LABORATORY FEATURES OF VAGINITIS

	Candida	Trichomonas	Bacterial Vaginosis
Symptoms	Vulvar pruritus; discharge	Pruritis; discharge	Fishy odor, especially after intercourse; discharge
Signs			
Discharge	White, "cottage cheese"	Yellow, thick, occasionally frothy	White-gray homogenous
Vulvar dermatitis	Common (erythema, fissures)	Occasional	Rare
Laboratory			
pH of discharge[1]	< 4.5	> 4.5	> 4.5
Amine odor with 10% KOH	Negative	Positive	Positive
Wet prep, saline, or 10% KOH[3]	Leukocytes; budding yeast and pseudohyphae	Leukocytes; motile trichomonads; ± clue cells[2]	Clue cells[2]
Gram stain	Leukocytes; yeast and pseudohyphae	Leukocytes; may see fixed trichomonads; ± clue cells[2]	Clue cells[2]; decreased numbers of lactobacilli; increased gram-variable rods, gram-positive cocci, and gram-variable curved rods (*Mobiluncus*)

[1]Not reliable during menses.
[2]Clue cells are squamous epithelial cells with large numbers of adherent bacteria.
[3]KOH useful in this setting only for detection of fungi.

CLINICAL APPROACH.   A speculum examination is necessary to determine whether the discharge in the vaginal vault is the result of vaginitis or cervicitis. A diagnosis based on a clinical impression of the characteristics of the vaginal discharge is frequently in error; microscopic diagnosis is required.

A thorough diagnostic approach includes determining the pH of the vaginal fluid, performing a "whiff test" (the addition of 10% potassium hydroxide [KOH] to the vaginal fluid produces a fishy odor if amines are present), and microscopic examination of a saline preparation (wet prep) for fungal elements, clue cells, motile trichomonads, and polymorphonuclear leukocytes. Examination of a KOH preparation and Gram-stained specimen may also be helpful. In general, cultures for yeast should not be performed, since many women normally harbor small numbers of yeast in the vagina. Culturing for *Trichomonas* may increase the sensitivity of laboratory diagnosis by up to 25%. Because bacterial vaginosis is a mixed infection composed of increased numbers of anaerobic bacteria, *Gardnerella,* and *Mycoplasma,* culture of the vagina is not recommended. Table 166–1 provides further details on laboratory diagnosis.

TABLE 166–2.   TREATMENT OF VAGINITIS

	Primary	Alternatives	Cost ($)[1]
Candida	Clotrimazole		12.42 (45 g cream)
			13.14 (7 supp)
	Miconazole		18.50 (45 g cream)
			20.15 (7 supp)
	Butaconazole		15.84 (28 g cream)
	Teraconazole		17.75 (45 g cream)
	suppositories or		17.75 (3 supp)
	cream q.h.s. × *3–7*		
	days		
Trichomonas	Metronidazole, 2 g PO		0.40
	in a single dose[2]		
		Metronidazole, 500 mg	1.40
		PO b.i.d. × 7 days[3]	
Bacterial Vaginosis	Metronidazole, 500		1.40
	mg PO b.i.d. × 7		
	days[3]		
		Clindamycin, 300 mg	26.88
		PO b.i.d. × 7 days	
		Amoxicillin–	43.47
		clavulanate, 500 mg	
		PO t.i.d. × 7 days	
		Clindamycin 2% cream	
		intravaginally, b.i.d.	
		× 7 days[4]	

[1]Average wholesale price, 1991 *Drug Topics Red Book.*

[2]Contraindicated in pregnancy; however, patients with severe symptoms may be treated after the first trimester with single-dose therapy.

[3]Contraindicated in pregnancy; use alternative regimen.

[4]Not commercially available; must be prepared by pharmacists.

MANAGEMENT.   Appropriate therapy for each infection is outlined in Table 166–2. Women with *Trichomonas* or bacterial vaginosis should be also screened for *Chlamydia* infection and gonorrhea, because they are at risk for multiple sexually transmitted infections. Treatment of partners is generally limited to those patients with *Trichomonas*. The partner should be examined prior to treatment to search for other STDs. Occasionally, partners of women with bacterial vaginosis are treated if the couple is monogamous and bacterial vaginosis is recurring frequently. To date, however, there are no definite data to support a reservoir for bacterial vaginosis in the male.

FOLLOW-UP.   Follow-up of vaginal infections is generally not required unless symptoms do not resolve.

Cross-references: Dysuria (Section 172), Sexually Transmitted Diseases (Section 178).

REFERENCES

1.   Centers for Disease Control. 1989 sexually transmitted diseases treatment guidelines. MMWR 1989;38(S-8):34–37.
     Current treatment options are outlined.

2.   Fleury FJ. Adult vaginitis. Clin Obstet Gynecol 1981;24:407–438.
     A general review, with emphasis on bedside diagnosis and treatment.

3.   Krohn MA, Hillier SL, Eschenbach DA. Comparison of methods for diagnosing bacterial vaginosis among pregnant women. J Clin Microbiol 1989;27:1266–1271.
     An up-to-date review of bacterial vaginosis.

4.   Rein MF, Holmes KK. "Nonspecific vaginitis," vulvovaginal candidiasis, and trichomoniasis: Clinical features, diagnosis, and management. Curr Clin Topics Infect Dis 1983;4:281–315.
     A general review.

5.   Sweet RL. Importance of differential diagnosis in acute vaginitis. Am J Obstet Gynecol 1985;152:921–923.
     Emphasizes the importance of an accurate diagnosis.

167 CONTRACEPTION

Problem

KIRK K. SHY

EPIDEMIOLOGY.   The National Survey of Family Growth (1988) indicated that 78% of women of reproductive age (15–44 years) had had intercourse in the preceding 3 months (43% of women aged 15–19 years). At first intercourse, 35% of women do not use contraception. This percentage is high regardless of race (white, non-Hispanic = 31%) and economic status (>200% federal poverty definition = 31%). In this survey, 28% of all births were mistimed, an additional 12% were unwanted. Less than 4% of women of reproductive age actively seek pregnancy. Among all sexually active women (15–44 years), the choice of contraceptive is as follows: sterilization, 33% (male = 19%, female = 14%); oral contraceptives, 32%; condoms, 17%; withdrawal, 6%; and periodic abstinence, 4%. The remainder use other barrier methods. As for oral contraceptives, 60% of prescriptions are for monophasic preparations and 40% for multiphasics.

CLINICAL APPROACH.   Clinicians should discuss the ranges of contraceptive effectiveness, side effects, and user satisfaction for all contraceptive methods, particularly for the newer methods (e.g., cervical cap, Norplant, etc.) that may be unknown to the patient. Reported here (Table 167–1) are failure rates in married women, 25 years or older, who were followed for several years (other sources of contraceptive failure data typically overestimate failure with barrier methods). The patient interview should focus on prior contraceptive use, frequency of intercourse, and the patient's viewpoint regarding management of an unplanned pregnancy.

MANAGEMENT.   Because latex **condoms** are associated with significant reductions in transmission of STDs, latex condoms should be used for all sexual relationships that are new or not assuredly mutually monogamous. Natural membrane, or skin condoms, do not prevent transmission of hepatitis B virus, or possibly human immunodeficiency virus (HIV). Because of superior contraceptive effectiveness, only condoms with a reservoir tip should be used. "Dry" silicon-based lubricants are most popular. Others use water-based surgical jelly. Oil-based lubricants should be avoided because they weaken condoms and increase breakage. Although contraceptive foam (a vehicle for spermicides: nonoxynol-9 or octoxynol) increases the effectiveness of condoms, the principal contraceptive effect is from the condom itself. Couples should not decide against condoms because the addition of foam is too much effort. Alone, foam, contraceptive suppositories, and contraceptive sponge are considerably

TABLE 167–1.   CONTRACEPTIVE EFFECTIVENESS*

Method	Failure Rate (per 100 Woman-Years)
Condom	3.6
Diaphragm	1.9
IUD (Paragard [TCu-380A] [Copper])	<0.8
Norplant (subdermal norgestrel implant)	<0.6
Oral contraceptive	
Combination (<50 μg estrogen)	0.27
Progestin only	1.2
Rhythm	15.5
Spermicides	11.9
Sterilization	
Female	0.13
Male	0.02
Withdrawal	6.7

*These data are from married women, 25 years or older, who were followed for an average of 9½ years at British family planning clinics. Data are from Vessey M, Lawless M, Yates D. Efficacy of different contraceptive methods. Lancet 1982;1:841–842, except for data concerning the Copper-TCu380A (from Trussel J, Hatcher RA, Cates W, et al. Contraceptive failure in the United States: An update. Studies Fam Plann 1990;21:51–54), and Norplant (from Shoupe D, Mishell DR. Norplant: Subdermal implant system for long-term contraception. Am J Obstet Gynecol 1989;160:1286–1292).

less effective than condoms. Many women choose to use both condoms (to diminish the risk of STDs) and oral contraceptives (to diminish the risk of pregnancy).

Clinician training is necessary to properly fit the **cervical cap** or **diaphragm**. The largest diaphragm ring that is comfortable and not distorted by the vagina is best. Almost all women can be fitted for a diaphragm and taught to insert it correctly, but a significant minority of women cannot be fitted for a cervical cap. Contraceptive jelly must be included between the cervix and diaphragm or cervical cap. The diaphragm should remain in place for at least 6 to 8 hours after intercourse, and it should be removed within 24 hours. The cervical cap can remain in place and is effective for 48 hours.

Oral contraceptives have a few absolute contraindications: thromboembolic disease (or a history of), cerebrovascular accident (or a history of), coronary artery disease (or history of), impaired liver function, hepatic cancer/adenoma (or history of), breast cancer (or history of), estrogen-dependent neoplasia (or history of), pregnancy, and previous cholestasis during pregnancy. Strong relative contraindications include vascular headaches, hypertension, forced immobility, and heavy smoking at ages 35 years or more. Relative contraindications to oral contraceptives must be considered in the context of the feasibility of alternative contraception and the patient's ability to respond to unplanned pregnancy.

The clinician should initially choose a pill with a daily dosage of 35 μg of estrogen (Table 167.2). Lower dosages are associated with higher rates of trou-

TABLE 167–2. ORAL CONTRACEPTIVES

Clinical Setting	Oral Contraceptive Agent	Estrogen Dosage	Progestin Dosage	Monthly Cost ($)[1]
Initial choice	Norinyl 1/35	EE 35 µg	NE 1.0 mg	18.28
Initial choice	Ortho-Novum 1/35	EE 35 µg	NE 1.0 mg	17.20
Initial choice	Brevicon	EE 35 µg	NE 0.5 mg	18.28
Initial choice	Modicon	EE 35 µg	NE 0.5 mg	19.30
Initial choice	Ortho-Novum 7/7/7[2]	EE 35 µg	NE 0.5/0.75/1.0 mg	17.95
Initial choice	Tri-Levlen[2]	EE 30 µg	NG 0.05/0.075/0.125 mg	15.23
Initial choice	Tri-Norinyl[2]	EE 35 µg	NE 0.5/0.75/1.0 mg	17.57
Initial choice	Triphasil[2]	EE 30/40 µg	NG 0.05/0.075/0.125 mg	17.40
History of estrogen side effect[3]	Loestrin 21 1/20	EE 20 µg	NA 1.5 mg	15.92
History of estrogen side effect[3]	Micronor[4]	None	NE 0.35 mg	22.20
History of estrogen side effect[3]	Nor-Q-D[4]	None	NE 0.35 mg	22.52
History of estrogen side effects[3]	Ovrette[4]	None	NG 0.075 mg	19.52
History of OC failure	Norinyl 1/50	EE 50 µg	NE 1.0 mg	18.28
History of OC failure	Ortho-Novum 1/50	EE 50 µg	NE 1.0 mg	17.20
Postcoital contraception[5]	Ovral	EE 50 µg	NG 0.5 mg	25.62

Abbreviations: OC = oral contraceptive, EE = ethinyl estradiol, NE = norethindrone, NG = norgestrel, NA = norethindrone acetate.

[1]Based on average wholesale price listing in 1991 *Drug Topics Red Book*.

[2]Triphasic oral contraceptive with weekly variation in progestin dosage.

[3]Estrogen-related side effects include breast tenderness, nausea, and cyclic weight gain.

[4]Progestin-only oral contraceptives are taken daily without a medication-free week. Pregnancy rates are somewhat greater with progestin-only oral contraceptives compared to monophasic products.

[5]Administration is two Ovral tablets within 72 hours of intercourse, followed by two additional tablets 12 hours later.

blesome endometrial bleeding, which may affect continuation rates. Higher dosages should be reserved for women with contraceptive failure at 35 μg. Progestin dosage should be 1 mg or less of norethindrone, or 0.15 mg or less of norgestrel. Triphasic oral contraceptives (Ortho-Novum 7/7/7, Tri-Norinyl, Triphasil) offer the theoretical advantage of lower complication rates because of lower steroid dosage. However, compared to standard monophasic oral contraceptives (Ortho-Novum 1/35, Norinyl 1/35, Modicon), the dosage reduction is small. **Progestin-only** oral contraceptives may be useful for breastfeeding women (estrogen inhibits lactation) or for women with estrogen-related side effects (e.g., breast tenderness, nausea, cyclic weight gain, etc.) or estrogen-related risk factors (e.g., history of thrombophlebitis).

There are several options for timing the beginning of oral contraceptives. They may be started (1) immediately (may cause unwanted vaginal bleeding), (2) 5 days after the next period, (3) on the first day of next period, or (4) on the first Sunday after the onset of the next menstrual period, which generally results in menstruation-free weekends. Except for the first option, effective contraception begins immediately.

Side effects of oral contraceptives include the following: (1) Intermenstrual bleeding, which generally resolves spontaneously in 3 months. (2) Nausea, which declines during the first 3 months of use. If persistent, nausea may improve with an oral contraceptive with 20 μg of estrogen (Loestrin 21 1/20) or a progestin-only pill. (3) Light periods (or amenorrhea), which affect most patients but do not adversely affect health. (4) Weight gain (unusual). (5) Chloasma (increased facial pigmentation), which is an indication for stopping oral contraceptives.

Depo-Provera and **Norplant** are effective long-acting hormonal contraceptives. The contraceptive effect of both begins immediately, and failure rates approach those of sterilization. The absolute contraindications (acute liver disease, history of liver tumor, acute thrombophlebitis, history of breast cancer, unexplained vaginal bleeding) for both are fewer in number than for oral contraceptives. Depo-Provera (medroxyprogesterone acetate in oil) is administered 150 mg IM every 3 months. Menstrual disturbance (initially metrorrhagia and later amenorrhea) occurs for most women. Weight gain averages 1 to 5 kg during the first year of use. Despite lack of FDA approval for contraceptive indication, Depo-Provera is widely used for contraception in the United States and throughout the world.

Norplant consists of six hollow Silastic rods filled with the progestin levonorgestrel and designed for subdermal implantation in the medial aspect of the upper arm. Insertion is simple and largely painless, but some instruction in technique is necessary. Removal is technically difficult but is necessary after 5 years, when the implants lose effectiveness. The major side effect is irregular uterine bleeding, which for some women is continuous throughout use of the implant. Charges for the device (~$350), insertion (~$150), and removal (~$200) vary.

The principal **intrauterine device** (IUD) is the Paragard (TCu-380A), a T-shaped, copper-covered, polyethylene IUD with a 6-year effectiveness. Pregnancy rates are similar to those with oral contraceptives. Pelvic inflammatory disease is substantially less common with this IUD than with its predecessors; nonetheless, because of this problem, IUDs should only be used by women in mutually monogamous relationships. Contraindications include a history of menorrhagia or dysmenorrhea, immunosuppression, valvular heart disease, or previous pelvic inflammatory disease. Insertion should be by trained practitioners. Charges for the IUD (~$150) and insertion (~$125) vary.

Postcoital contraception is effective with IUD insertion within 5 days after intercourse, or with oral contraceptives within 72 hours after intercourse (Ovral, two tablets initially, followed in 12 hours by two additional tablets). Before treating, however, the clinician should consider the possibility of a preexisting early pregnancy from another recent episode of unprotected intercourse.

FOLLOW-UP.   To assure compliance, most patients with prescription contraception should have a return appointment in 4 weeks. The clinician should monitor oral contraceptive users for increased blood pressure. IUD users should be examined for evidence of pelvic inflammatory disease and for string lengthening or shortening, which indicates potential improper IUD placement.

Cross-references: AIDS (Section 14), Abnormal Uterine Bleeding (Section 162), Pelvic Inflammatory Disease (Section 168), Urinary Tract Infections in Women (Section 177), Sexually Transmitted Diseases (Section 178), Diagnosis of Pregnancy (Section 209).

REFERENCES

1. Forrest JD, Fordyce RR. U.S. women's contraceptive attitudes and practice: How have they changed in the 1980's? Fam Plann Perspect 1988;20:112–118.
    This properly designed survey demonstrated the increasing acceptance of condoms and the continuing large number of couples who have unprotected intercourse.

2. Mishell DR. Contraception. N Engl J Med 1989;320:777–787.
    A general review.

3. Sivin I. International experience with Norplant and Norplant-2 contraceptives. Studies Fam Plann 1988;19:81–94.
    A balanced review of the new subdermal implant for contraception.

4. Wharton C, Blackburn R. Lower-dose pills. Pop Rep 1988;A(7):1–31.
    A practical guide to prescribing oral contraceptives.

168 PELVIC INFLAMMATORY DISEASE

Problem

PÅL WÖLNER-HANSSEN

EPIDEMIOLOGY/ETIOLOGY. Pelvic inflammatory disease (PID) is an acute infection of the upper genital tract in women. Estimates from the 1970s suggest that PID affects over 800,000 women annually. Risk factors for PID include young age, black race, single or divorced marital status, new sexual partner, previous PID, and possibly IUD use. Monogamous women and those using oral contraceptives are less susceptible to PID. *Neisseria gonorrhoeae* and *Chlamydia trachomatis* are the most important organisms that cause PID, followed by anaerobic bacteria (e.g., *Bacteroides, Peptococcus*) and gram-negative Enterobacteriaceae (e.g., *Escherichia coli*).

SYMPTOMS AND SIGNS. Continuous lower abdominal pain is the principal symptom of PID. The pain is typically dull with crampy exacerbations, usually bilateral, and varies in intensity from excruciating (common in women with perihepatitis) to no pain at all ("silent PID"). Associated symptoms, all nonspecific, include complaints referable to the gastrointestinal tract (nausea, vomiting, diarrhea, constipation, tenesmus), the urinary tract (dysuria, frequency, urgency), and/or the genital tract (increased discharge, abnormal odor from the vagina, abnormal bleeding).

On pelvic examination, adnexal tenderness, uterine tenderness, and cervical motion tenderness are typical though nonspecific signs of PID. Less than 20% of women with PID have fever.

CLINICAL APPROACH. The clinical diagnosis of PID is unreliable because the associated symptoms and signs are nonspecific. PID is often confused with ectopic pregnancy, appendicitis, ovarian cysts, and urinary tract infection. The history should thoroughly investigate the location, duration, character, and pattern of abdominal pain. Unilateral pain suggests appendicitis (if right-sided), ruptured ovarian cyst, twisted adnexa, or ectopic pregnancy. An abrupt onset of unilateral pain during intercourse is typical of ruptured ovarian cyst. A gradual onset of pain over several hours with migration from the epigastrium to the right lower quadrant suggests appendicitis. Slowly increasing pain in the right and/or left lower abdominal quadrants is more typical of PID. It is important to inquire about risk factors, including previous PID, a symptomatic and/or new sexual partner, or a recently introduced IUD. To differentiate between infection and pregnancy, a thorough menstrual history is helpful.

A complete abdominal and pelvic examination detects peritonitis and may help localize the disease process. A purulent cervical discharge indicates cervicitis and, together with lower abdominal pain and adnexal tenderness, is suggestive of PID. Lack of cervical discharge does not rule out PID. On bimanual pelvic examination, bilateral tenderness suggests PID, while palpable adnexal masses may reflect pelvic abscesses or ovarian cysts.

A rapid and sensitive pregnancy test is the most important laboratory test and should be performed in all young women with acute abdominal pain to determine whether the problem is related to pregnancy. An elevated WBC count or ESR suggests infection; normal findings do not exclude PID, however. In obese women and in those with a rigid abdomen due to peritonitis, ultrasound may help detect tubo-ovarian abscesses. In other patients, diagnostic ultrasound is less useful because uniform criteria for acute salpingitis do not exist.

MANAGEMENT.   Criteria for hospital admission include the following: (1) the diagnosis is uncertain (appendicitis or ectopic pregnancy cannot be excluded), (2) a pelvic mass is present (possible abscess), (3) right upper abdominal pain (possible perihepatitis) is present, (4) outpatient therapy will not be tolerated (nausea and vomiting, fever, peritonitis, severe abdominal pain), (5) there is no improvement after 48 hours of outpatient treatment follow-up, (6) the patient is unreliable, or (7) the patient is pregnant.

Table 168–1 lists the antibiotics for outpatient therapy currently recommended by the Centers for Disease Control. In the event of allergy to tetracycline, clindamycin should be substituted. The sexual partner(s) will require treatment and should be referred for evaluation.

FOLLOW-UP.   The patients should be evaluated after 48 hours of treatment. Patients unable to comply with therapy recommendations or whose conditions have deteriorated should be admitted. Patients should be evaluated again just after completion of oral therapy. Those who failed to respond or who have new pelvic masses should be referred to a specialist.

Cross-references: AIDS (Section 14), Abdominal Pain (Section 95), Female Infertility (Section 158), Abnormal Uterine Bleeding (Section 162), Pelvic Pain in Women (Section 163), Contraception (Section 167), Dysuria (Section

TABLE 168–1.   OUTPATIENT TREATMENT OF PELVIC INFLAMMATORY DISEASE

Antimicrobial Agent/Administration	Cost ($)[1]
Cefoxitin, 2 g IM, plus probenecid, 1 g PO	17.16
or	
Ceftriaxone, 250 mg IM	3.55
plus	
Doxycycline, 100 mg PO b.i.d. for 10–14 days	4.48
or	
Tetracycline, 500 mg PO q.i.d. for 10–14 days	3.92

[1]Average wholesale price, for course listed; 1991 *Drug Topics Red Book.*

172), Sexually Transmitted Diseases (Section 178), Diagnosis of Pregnancy (Section 209).

REFERENCES

1. Centers for Disease Control. 1989 Sexually transmitted diseases treatment guidelines. MMWR 1989;38(suppl 8):1S.

2. Eschenbach DA, Buchanan TM, Pollock HM, et al. Polymicrobial etiology of acute pelvic inflammatory disease. N Engl J Med 1975;293:166–171.
   Illustrates the importance of gonococci and mixed anaerobic-aerobic infections.

3. Jacobsson L, Westrom L. Objectivized diagnosis of pelvic inflammatory disease. Am J Obstet Gynecol 1969;105:1088–1098.
   The classic signs and symptoms of PID are insensitive and nonspecific.

4. Wolner-Hanssen P, Mardh P, Svensson L, Westrom L. Laparoscopy in women with chlamydial infection and pelvic pain: A comparison of patients with and without salpingitis. Obstet Gynecol 1983;61:299–303.
   In patients with chlamydial infection and pelvic pain, clinical criteria poorly distinguished those with salpingitis from those without; only irregular menstrual bleeding and an elevated ESR favored salpingitis.

169 MAMMOGRAPHY

Procedure

ALVIN I. MUSHLIN

INDICATIONS/CONTRAINDICATIONS.   Mammography is used to screen for occult breast neoplasms or to help in the evaluation of breast masses or other breast abnormalities. Although the technology used for both purposes is basically the same, there are important differences in the techniques and the required dose of radiation. Because screening mammography discloses possible abnormalities without characterizing them diagnostically and is used repetitively in individuals, it requires only a very low dose of radiation. The indications for screening mammography are covered in Section 161 (Breast Cancer Screening).

Diagnostic mammography should be performed in those with an abnormality on a screening examination in order to determine whether a malignancy is likely. If it is negative or has the characteristics of a benign abnormality, it may reduce the probability of breast cancer enough that close clinical follow-up is an acceptable option to the clinician and the patient. Mammography is also very helpful in the evaluation of breast masses detected by women during self-examination or by clinicians as part of routine breast palpation. It is useful in the evaluation of other breast symptoms such as pain, changes in the skin overlying the breast tissue, and for discharge from or inversions of the nipples. As with other diagnostic tests, the extent to which it can provide definitive information (posttest probability) is dependent on a quantitative assessment by the physician about the likelihood of a malignancy (pretest probability) and on the accuracy (sensitivity and specificity) of the procedure (see Section 12, Principles of Screening).

RATIONALE. Radiographs can be used to detect breast malignancy because normal and abnormal breast tissue differentially absorb x-rays and thereby produce images that are characteristic of each. Screening mammography is approximately 75% sensitive and more than 95% specific. Studies of the accuracy of mammography in distinguishing benign from malignant neoplasms report a sensitivity of around 80% and a specificity of 90%.

METHODS. Two types of radiologic procedures are available. Both require the use of a radiographic unit dedicated solely to mammography. The most widely used procedure is screen-film mammography. This uses a molybdenum rather than the usual tungsten target to produce x-rays that heighten the contrast between fat, parenchymal tissue, and calcifications. Less common is xeromammography, which uses a photoconductive plate of selenium-coated aluminum as the image receptor in place of x-ray film. Microcalcifications and spiculations are easily visualized, but poorly defined masses are less well visualized than with screen-film mammography. Low levels of radiation are required for both examinations: approximately 0.8 rad for xeromammography and 0.4 rad for screen-film mammography. Technical advances continue to lower these doses. Overall, the accuracy of both techniques is comparable, and the choice depends more on the radiologist's skill and familiarity with the technique. Mammography requires the patient to sit or stand for the procedure. Two views of the breast are taken and a moderate compression of the breast is needed to avoid motion and enhance visualization.

COSTS/COMPLICATIONS. Because cost is a significant barrier to screening women in the age groups in which screening has been shown to be beneficial, a major effort is being launched to decrease the costs of screening mammography. At present the cost to the patient of screening mammography varies from approximately $50 to $150. The charge for a diagnostic study will be toward the higher end of this range or more if specialized techniques such as ductography are required. Although some patients may complain of discomfort associated with breast compression, there are no direct complications of this procedure (other than through the additional tests or biopsies required to evaluate any false-positive results). The radiation dose is minimal.

Cross-references: Principles of Screening (Section 12), Breast Cancer Screening (Section 161), Breast Masses and Breast Pain (Section 165).

REFERENCES

1. American Cancer Society, Proceedings of the Workshop on Strategies to Lower the Costs of Screening Mammography—1986. Cancer Suppl 1987;60:1669–1702.

    Report of a recent conference that explored ways to reduce the cost of screening and to provide third-party coverage for appropriate age groups.

2. Baines CJ, McFarlane DV, Miller AB, et al. Sensitivity and specificity of film screen mammography in 15 NBSS centres. J Can Assoc Radiol 1988;39:273–276.

    Study of the accuracy of mammography in a large randomized controlled trial of screening for breast cancer.

3. Kopans DB, Meyer JE, Sadowsky N. Breast imaging. N Engl J Med 1984;310:960–967.

    Reviews the various modalities available for breast imaging.

4. Moskovic E, Sinnett HD, Parsons CA. The accuracy of mammographic diagnosis in surgically occult breast lesions. Clin Radiol 1990;41:344–346.

    Study of the accuracy of mammography in screening situations.

5. Mushlin AI. Diagnostic tests in breast cancer: Clinical strategies based on diagnostic probabilities. Ann Intern Med 1985;103:79–85.

    Reviews information on the accuracy of tests, including screening mammography. The probabilities of malignancy will vary, depending on sensitivity, specificity, and disease prevalence.

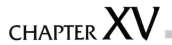
GENITOURINARY AND RENAL DISORDERS

170 CANCER OF THE GENITOURINARY SYSTEM

Screening

MICHAEL K. BRAWER

One-third of cancers occur in the genitourinary tract. At the time of presentation, 35% of testis, 65% of renal, 43% of bladder, and 32% of prostate carcinomas are metastatic. Despite investigations of numerous diagnostic tests, screening for genitourinary neoplasms has not improved patient survival.

CARCINOMA OF THE TESTIS

EPIDEMIOLOGY. Testicular cancer is the most common solid malignancy in men between age 27 years and age 35 years. The fact that this tumor represents one of the most curable of all malignancies underscores the need for early detection, despite its relatively low incidence (in 1989 there were 5700 new cases diagnosed and 350 deaths). One identified risk factor is a history of cryptorchidism.

RATIONALE. Potential screening tests include physical examination, transscrotal ultrasound, and serum tumor markers (human chorionic gonadotropin and alpha fetoprotein). The very low prevalence of these neoplasms makes transscrotal ultrasound (a sensitive test with low specificity) and serum tumor markers (specific tests but with low sensitivity) impractical.

Patients learn testicular self-examination easily. Most testicular tumors are palpable prior to metastasis. Because most patients present at an advanced stage (e.g., several months after the first appearance of the scrotal mass), many

522

physicians believe that patient education and self-examination programs would be beneficial, though no studies have proved this.

STRATEGY.   All clinicians should encourage their male patients, especially those with a history of cryptorchidism, to perform testicular self-examination.

ACTION.   Any man with an intratesticular mass should be urgently referred to a urologist.

BLADDER CARCINOMA

EPIDEMIOLOGY.   Bladder cancer represents the second most common genitourinary neoplasm, with an annual incidence of 47,000 cases and 10,200 deaths. The peak incidence occurs between ages 50 and 70 years, affecting men three times as often as women. Risk factors include cigarette smoking and exposure to industrial toxins, such as the aniline dyes beta-naphthylamine and benzidine.

RATIONALE.   The most commonly employed screening test for bladder cancer is urinalysis to detect the presence of hematuria.

Urinary cytology is a more specific test for early detection of transitional cell carcinoma of the bladder, with few false-positive results. The overall sensitivity of cytology correlates with the grade of cancer: most high-grade lesions are detected, but up to 50% of grade I carcinomas are not. Low-grade tumors, however, rarely become invasive or clinically important. Disadvantages with cytology include the need for a skilled pathologist and difficulties encountered with specimen transport and handling.

Urinary flow cytometry may have sensitivities as high as 91% but is not routinely available.

STRATEGY.   The relatively low prevalence of bladder cancer in the general population precludes mass screening. Some patients, perhaps those with a heavy cigarette smoking history or with significant industrial exposure, may benefit from screening urinalysis or urinary cytology, but studies supporting clinical benefit are unavailable.

ACTION.   Section 182 reviews the diagnostic approach to hematuria.

PROSTATE CARCINOMA

EPIDEMIOLOGY.   Prostatic carcinoma represents the most common neoplasm in men and the second most common cause of cancer death. In 1990 there were an estimated 100,000 new cases of prostate cancer diagnosed and 30,000 cancer-related deaths. Most diagnosed prostate cancer has already spread beyond the confines of the gland and is incurable.

RATIONALE.   Options for early diagnosis include digital rectal examination, serum markers (acid phosphatase and prostate-specific antigen), and transrectal ultrasound.

Digital rectal examination remains the traditional method by which most prostatic carcinomas are diagnosed. Its sensitivity for detecting disease confined to the prostate, however, is questionable; as many as 50% of patients staged to have locally confined disease by digital examination are classified at higher stages after radical prostatectomy. The positive predictive value of digital examination is also low, with only 6% to 30% of abnormalities revealing carcinoma. In most early detection studies, digital examination identified carcinoma in 1% to 2% of patients screened, but evidence supporting clinical benefit to the patients is unavailable.

The sensitivity of prostatic acid phosphatase (PAP) for localized disease is too low (.25–.40) to serve as a useful screening test. The glycoprotein prostate-specific antigen (PSA) is found only in normal hyperplastic or malignant prostatic epithelium and has never been demonstrated in nonprostatic primary or metastatic tumors. Some investigators question the specificity of PSA, reporting elevated levels in men with simple benign prostatic hyperplasia. Other investigators, however, find elevated PSA levels only when acute inflammation, prostatic intraepithelial neoplasia (a putative premalignant prostatic change), or carcinoma is present. Further study is necessary. The sensitivity of PSA for detection of carcinoma is poor, with a significant percentage of patients in most large radical prostatectomy series having normal PSA levels. In a patient with a prostate nodule on digital rectal examination, however, a PSA level greater than 4 ng/ml strongly suggests malignancy. Further investigation is necessary before PSA can be recommended as a general screening test.

Transrectal ultrasound represents the best method for imaging of the prostate gland. The most common sonographic appearance of carcinoma is a hypoechoic lesion in the peripheral (posterior) portion of the prostate. In self-referred screening populations, cancer detection rates of 2% to 3% have been achieved. Problems with transrectal ultrasound relate to cost, sensitivity (a significant number of carcinomas occur in regions of the prostate not imaged by ultrasound, and many cancers are not hypoechoic), and low positive predictive value (only approximately one-third of hypoechoic peripheral zone lesions reveal carcinoma on biopsy).

STRATEGY.   Despite the significant morbidity and mortality associated with prostate cancer and the fact that most carcinomas are detected with advanced local or metastatic disease, it remains to be proved whether screening by any modality will significantly diminish the mortality rate. Until large, randomized, prospective controlled studies compare unscreened to screened populations, there is insufficient evidence to recommend mass screening with any of these techniques.

Cross-references: Periodic Health Assessment (Section 7), Principles of Screening (Section 12), Prostate Cancer (Section 175), Hematuria (Section 182), Benign Prostatic Hyperplasia (Section 186).

REFERENCES

1. Brawer MK. Laboratory studies for the detection of carcinoma of the prostate. Urol Clin North Am 1990;17:759–768.
   A summary of the major studies utilizing serum markers for prostate cancer detection.

2. Hernandez AD, Smith JA. Transrectal ultrasonography for the early detection and staging of prostate cancer. Urol Clin North Am 1990; 17:745–757.
   Reviews the role of ultrasound in prostate cancer detection.

3. Scardino PT. Early detection of prostate cancer. Urol Clin North Am 1989;16:635–655.
   Perhaps the best-written review.

4. Thompson IM. The early detection of genitourinary neoplasms. AUA Update Series 1987; 6;26:1–8
   An excellent brief review on the current status of screening for genitourinary neoplasms.

171 IMPOTENCE

Symptom

RICHARD E. BERGER

EPIDEMIOLOGY.   Impotence is the inability to attain or maintain an erection necessary for intercourse. The prevalence increases with age; by age 60 years, 20% of men are impotent. Risk factors reflect conditions that damage penile blood vessels and nerves and include central and peripheral neurologic disorders, hypertension, atherosclerosis, smoking, and diabetes. Diabetic men tend to have impotence at an earlier age than nondiabetic men.

TABLE 171–1.   CAUSES OF IMPOTENCE

Cause	Percentage of Patients
Multifactorial	30.3
Vascular	21.1
Diabetic neuropathy	17.1
Nondiabetic neuropathy	10.5
Psychogenic	9.2
Drug effects	3.9
Hypogonadism	2.6
Peyronie's disease	1.3
Idiopathic	3.9

Source: Adapted from Mulligan T, Katz PG. Why aged men become impotent. Arch Intern Med 1989;149:1365–1366.

TABLE 171–2. TREATMENTS FOR ERECTILE PROBLEMS

Treatment	Advantages	Disadvantages	Tests Usually Needed before Therapy[1]
Sex therapy	No physical risks May improve sexual relationship May restore "normal" erections Does not preclude other options	Requires cooperative partner Cannot restore erections in men with organic causes of impotence	Basic tests
Suction device	Few physical risks if used correctly Relatively inexpensive Does not preclude other options	Mechanical device interrupts spontaneous sexual activity Not concealable	Basic tests
Vascular restoration (arterial reconstruction and/or venous leak surgery)	Restores "normal" erections If does not work, suction device or implant still possible	Applicable only to men with healthy vascular systems Modest success rates Requires surgery and hospitalization Relatively expensive	Basic tests, plus: arteriography, cavernosography, duplex Doppler

Penile shots	Relatively low cost If does not work, suction device or implant still possible	Risk of priapism, penile scarring, and penile bruising Can make physical problem worse or create new one Slightly painful Long-term side effects unknown at this time Requires giving oneself shot in penis and using external paraphernalia	Basic tests, plus diagnostic office injection
Penile implants	No external mechanical apparatus required No preparation required	Relatively expensive (some insurance and Medicare coverage) Carries risks of surgery If requires removal (rare), can be treated only by another implant or suction device	Basic tests

[1]Basic tests include history and physical examination, nocturnal penile tumescence, blood tests (see text), and psychological tests and interview.

527

ETIOLOGY.   Normal erections follow relaxation of the penile smooth muscle, which allows accumulation of blood in the penis. Impotence may result from lack of desire due to hypogonadism or hyperprolactinemia, psychogenic factors caused by performance anxiety, neurologic diseases that prevent transmission of neurologic messages to the blood vessels of the penis (peripheral neuropathy, spinal cord injury), decreased arterial flow into the penis (atherosclerosis), or failure to reduce penile venous flow. Impotence is a common side effect of medications and drugs; the most common offenders are alcohol, nicotine, and psychotropic, antihypertensive, diuretic, and cardiovascular medications. Table 171–1 lists the diagnoses found in one group of elderly men.

CLINICAL APPROACH.   The patient interview should review the patient's medications, alcohol intake, symptoms of stress or psychiatric disease, and relationship with his partner. If possible, the partner should be consulted during diagnosis and management. Physical examination focuses on the genital (testicular size), nervous, and vascular systems. Some clinicians use a biothesiometer, an instrument that provides graded vibratory stimuli, to measure penile sensory function. The serum testosterone should be measured in all patients; if it is low, gonadotropin and prolactin levels should be determined.

Although all antihypertensive drugs cause impotence by reducing penile blood pressure, the calcium channel blockers and angiotensin-converting enzyme inhibitors cause the least problems. Offending medications should be stopped or substituted, if possible, before the patient undergoes extensive testing.

No single test or piece of historical information distinguishes psychologic from physical impotence. In general, organic impotence is slow in onset and continuous, although it may be intermittent early on. The presence of nighttime erections by nocturnal penile tumescence testing does not exclude minor degrees of arterial, venous, or neurologic impotence. Absence of nighttime erections, assuming the patient is sleeping well, is highly suggestive of organic disease.

Patients should be referred to a urologist for further evaluation of the arterial and venous systems if they are candidates for vascular reconstruction (i.e., they desire reconstruction, are younger than age 65 years, and are without diabetes and severe systemic vascular disease). Such physical testing often helps to educate the patient about his problem and establishes realistic treatment goals. The best tests of arterial function are a cavernosal artery blood pressure or duplex Doppler scan of the deep penile arterial flow. Measurement of the blood pressure of the dorsal artery in the flaccid penis is a poor screening test because blood flow required for erection derives from the deep arteries. Infusion cavernosometry and cavernosography after injection of intracavernosal vasodilators are the best tests of venous function.

MANAGEMENT.   Therapeutic decisions depend on the acceptability to both partners of the various treatment alternatives, the etiology of the impotence, and, often, the cost of treatment. The patient should learn about all treatment alternatives (Table 171–2).

Treatment of primary hypogonadism is replacement with testosterone, 200 mg intramuscular (IM) every 2 weeks. Empiric use of testosterone without documented hypogonadism is inappropriate. Psychologic counseling and sex therapy may benefit not only patients with psychologic impotence but also those with organic impotence. Success rates of 80% are probable in appropriately selected men.

Suction constriction devices treat almost any cause of impotence and are effective in approximately 90% of men. These devices consist of a plastic tube and vacuum pump, which pulls blood into the penis, and a strong rubber ring, which is applied at the penile base to maintain the erection. They are very safe and can be prescribed by any physician. Penile injection therapy using vasodilating agents (papaverine or prostaglandin E_1) is appropriate for those with neurogenic impotence and mild arterial and venogenic impotence, but they may cause penile scarring and priapism and should be prescribed only by physicians experienced with their use. Venous and arterial reconstructive procedures may be performed in selected patients, but the success rate is only about 50%. Penile implant surgery is effective in 90% to 95% of patients and applicable to almost any cause of impotence but is irreversible and should only follow the failure of less invasive methods.

Cross-references: Diagnosis and Management of Alcoholism (Section 9), Smoking Cessation (Section 11), Essential Hypertension (Section 86), Peripheral Arterial Disease (Section 133), Peripheral Neuropathy (Section 149), Diabetes Mellitus (Section 157), Screening for Depression (Section 187), Generalized Anxiety (Section 188).

REFERENCES

1. Baskin HJ. Endocrinologic evaluation of impotence. South Med J 1989;82:446–449.
    Evaluation of 600 impotent men that identified androgen deficiency, thyroid deficiency, or hyperprolactinemia in 32% of subjects.

2. Freidenberg DH, Berger RE, Chou DE, et al. Quantitation of corporeal venous outflow resistance in men by corporeal pressure flow evaluation. J Urol 1987;138:533-538.
    Describes a technique that measures the degree of venous sinusoidal incompetence, a major cause of impotence.

3. Krane RJ, Goldstein I, de Tejada IS. Impotence. New Engl J Med 1989;321:1648–1659.
    Excellent review.

4. Lue TF, Tanagho EA. Physiology of erection and pharmacological management of impotence. J Urol 1987;137:829–836.
    Summarizes a practical approach from the urologist's perspective; reviews functional evaluation of penile arteries and veins.

5. Mulligan T, Katz PG. Why aged men become impotent. Arch Intern Med 1989;149:1365–1366.
    Study of 121 impotent men, age 60 to 85 years; 15% of cases were due to potentially reversible medical disorders (drug reactions, psychopathology, hypogonadism).

172 DYSURIA

Symptom

STEPHAN D. FIHN

Epidemiology/Etiology.   Dysuria is one of the fifteen most frequent reasons for visits to primary care physicians by women. In 70% to 90% of women with dysuria, the cause is urinary tract infection (UTI). Approximately one-half of these infections are characterized by growth of between 10^2 and 10^5 bacteria/ml in a midstream culture. The onset of symptoms due to UTI is typically sudden and accompanied by urgency, frequency, and occasionally suprapubic pain and gross hematuria. In women who use a diaphragm, UTI should be suspected. In 10% to 20% of women, the cause of dysuria is vaginitis, most often bacterial vaginosis due to anaerobes (nonspecific vaginitis). These patients frequently also complain of vaginal discharge, "external" dysuria, and vulvar pruritus. In sexually active young women, chlamydial cervicitis or urethritis is the cause of dysuria in 2% to 5% of cases; gonococcal infection occurs much less frequently. These entities should be suspected when the onset of symptoms is gradual, when the patient has had a recent change in sexual partners, and when the urinalysis demonstrates pyuria but is negative for bacteria. Uncommon causes of acute dysuria include herpetic infection and allergic reactions. In up to 10% of cases, no pyuria is present, and the cause of symptoms is obscure.

Women who have chronic dysuria without evidence of infection may have a poorly characterized syndrome of interstitial cystitis. There are no standard criteria for this diagnosis and no proved beneficial therapy.

Dysuria is less common among males. In younger, sexually active men, the most common cause is urethritis. Gonococcal urethritis is frequent among homosexual men and those with a history of prior gonorrhea. Nongonococcal urethritis is due to *Chlamydia trachomatis* in 30% to 50% of cases and *Ureaplasma urealyticum* in 15% to 20% of cases; in the remaining cases, a definite pathogen is not isolated. Nongonococcal urethritis is several times more common than gonococcal infection among most general heterosexual populations, although 25% of men with Chlamydia are coinfected with *Neisseria gonorrhoeae*.

In older men, dysuria often signifies UTI. However, in as many as half of men with dysuria or other irritative symptoms such as frequency and urgency, the cause may be conditions other than infection, including benign prostatic hypertrophy.

Clinical Approach.   In many instances, the history alone may be sufficient to make a diagnosis of UTI with a high degree of confidence. Women who have had prior UTIs are more than 90% accurate in identifying recurrences. Lacking an unequivocal history, proper diagnosis depends on laboratory studies. Ideally a quantitative urinary leukocyte count should be performed using a hemocytometer counting chamber along with a microscopic examination of uncentrifuged urine (Table 172–1). If pyuria (≥ 10 leukocytes per mm^3 or more than 10 per high power field) and bacteria are present, the likelihood of a UTI is approximately 90%, particularly if the patient uses a diaphragm. If facilities for microscopic examination of urine are unavailable, dipstick tests for leukocyte esterase, bacterially generated nitrate, or a combination of the two are a reasonable substitute. The performance of these tests is slightly poorer than direct microscopy. Like microscopy, these tests are most accurate in detecting UTIs characterized by colony counts exceeding 10^4 bacteria/ml and are less useful for detecting infections with lesser degrees of bacteriuria.

If pyuria is present without bacteriuria, a pelvic examination should be performed, if appropriate, to detect mucopurulent cervicitis and obtain cultures for Chlamydia and gonorrhea, as well as rapid diagnostic tests for Chlamydia when available. A pelvic examination is warranted if symptoms suggest vaginitis.

Young men with dysuria should be closely questioned about sexual exposures. The clinician should determine whether a urethral discharge is present. In gonococcal urethritis, the discharge is often copious and purulent, while that from Chlamydia is more often scant and mucoid. Symptoms may be more pronounced in the morning, especially with chlamydial infection. A specimen of urethral discharge should be obtained from all patients with suspected urethritis by milking the urethra or by swab, as described in Section 178 (Sexually Transmitted Diseases).

TABLE 172–1. PERFORMANCE CHARACTERISTICS OF TESTS FOR URINARY TRACT INFECTION IN WOMEN WITH DYSURIA

Laboratory Finding	Sensitivity	Specificity	Predictive Value	
			Positive	*Negative*
Midstream Culture				
Any coliforms	1.00	0.71	0.79	1.00
$\geq 10^2$ coliforms/ml	.95	.85	.88	.94
$\geq 10^5$ coliforms/ml	.51	.59	.98	.65
Microscopy				
≥ 8 leukocytes/mm³	.91	.50	.67	.83
≥ 20 leukocytes/mm³ and visible bacteria	.50	.95	.94	.54
Rapid Tests				
Leukocyte esterase strips	.75–.90	.95	.50	.92
Nitrite dipsticks	.35–.85	.95	.96	.27–.70
Leukocyte esterase/nitrite strips	.75–.90	.70	.75–.93	.41–.95

Older men with dysuria should be questioned about signs or symptoms of prostatism. In most cases a urine culture should be performed. Presence of 10^3 bacteria/ml or more indicates infection.

MANAGEMENT.   Management of patients with UTI, vaginitis, and urethritis is accomplished as described in Sections 177 and 179, 166, and 178, respectively.

Cross-references: Abdominal Pain (Section 95), Pelvic Pain in Women (Section 163), Vaginitis (Section 166), Pelvic Inflammatory Disease (Section 168), Urinary Tract Infections in Women (Section 177), Sexually Transmitted Diseases (Section 178), Urinary Tract Infections in Men (Section 179), Bacteriuria in the Elderly (Section 180), Hematuria (Section 182), Benign Prostatic Hyperplasia (Section 186), Bacteriuria in Pregnancy (Section 210).

REFERENCES

1. Berg AO, Heidrich FE, Fihn SD, et al. Establishing the cause of genitourinary symptoms in women in a family practice. Comparison of clinical examination and comprehensive microbiology. JAMA 1984;251:620–625.

    In a prospective study of women coming to a family medicine clinic with a variety of genitourinary symptoms, a diagnosis was made in 34% using simple tests and in 66% using sophisticated tests. The positive predictive value of dysuria for UTI was 67%.

2. Komaroff AL. Acute dysuria in women. New Engl J Med 1984;310:368–376.

    A thoughtful review of the causes of dysuria and a reasonable diagnostic approach.

3. Lipsky BA, Ireton RC, Fihn SD, et al. Diagnosis of bacteriuria in men: Specimen collection and culture interpretation. J Infect Dis 1987;155:847–854.

    Demonstrates that voided specimens from adult men are highly accurate, and the best diagnostic criterion for bacteriuria is 10^3/ml or more. Irritative symptoms often indicated bladder infections but occurred in several men who did not have infection.

4. Stamm WE, Wagner KF, Amsel R, et al. Causes of the acute urethral syndrome in women. N Engl J Med 1980;303:409–412.

    The earliest study to demonstrate the importance of sexually transmitted diseases, especially Chlamydia, as causes of dysuria and of pyuria as an important indicator of bladder or urethral infection.

5. Wathne B, Hovelius B, Mardh PA. Causes of frequency and dysuria in women. Scand J Infect Dis 1987;19:223–229.

    In a community-based prospective study, over 80% of women presenting with dysuria and urinary frequency were found to have UTI. Chlamydial infection was diagnosed in 10% of women without bacteriuria, 93% of whom had pyuria.

173 SCROTAL PAIN

Symptom

STEVEN R. McGEE

EPIDEMIOLOGY. Testicular torsion and testicular cancer affect men between ages 15 and 35 years. The incidence of testicular torsion peaks during puberty. Epididymitis affects men of all ages.

ETIOLOGY. Table 173–1 lists the important causes of scrotal pain. In men over age 20 years presenting with an acutely inflamed scrotum, epididymitis is the most common diagnosis, outranking torsion 10 to 1.

Testicular torsion occurs when the testis, lacking the normal fixation to the posterior scrotal wall, freely twists on the spermatic cord. If it is left untreated, necrosis of the testicle occurs in 10% to 20% of patients after 6 hours of symptoms and in more than 90% after 24 hours. **Epididymitis** results from bacterial infection of the epididymis. Heterosexual men under age 35 years usually have associated urethritis from *Chlamydia trachomatis* or *Neisseria gonorrhoeae*. In heterosexual men over age 35 years and in all homosexual men, epididymitis is associated with bacteriuria, usually from Enterobacteriaceae. Most men over age 35 years also have associated urinary tract abnormalities, typically benign prostatic hypertrophy. **Orchitis** is usually due to viral infections, especially mumps.

Additionally, scrotal pain may result from diseases distant to the scrotum, either along the course of the genitofemoral nerve in the retroperitoneum (abdominal aortic aneurysm, ureterolithiasis, retrocecal appendicitis) or along the posterior scrotal nerves (prostatic pain).

TABLE 173–1. CAUSES OF SCROTAL PAIN

Disease within Scrotum
Torsion of spermatic cord or testicular appendage
Epididymitis
Orchitis
Testicular tumor
Polyarteritis nodosa
Drugs: desipramine, mazindol, amiodarone

Disease Distant to Scrotum
Abdominal aortic aneurysm
Renal pain
Radicular pain
Prostatic pain: prostatitis, prostatodynia

Source: Adapted from McGee SR. Diagnosis of scrotal pain. Med Rounds 1988;1:280–289.

CLINICAL APPROACH.   Although testicular tenderness may occur in both local and distant disorders, the finding of scrotal redness, swelling, or mass always indicates an intrascrotal condition (Table 173–1). Routine laboratory tests include a urinalysis, urine culture, and, in sexually active patients, urethral Gram stain and culture.

In patients with acute scrotal pain, redness, and swelling ("acute scrotum"), radionuclide scanning of the testis accurately distinguishes torsion from epididymitis. Preliminary data suggest that color Doppler ultrasound may be as accurate. Real-time ultrasound, however, is inappropriate because it does not reliably discriminate between epididymitis and torsion.

In patients younger than age 40 years with an acute scrotum, the evaluation must be prompt to distinguish testicular torsion, a surgical condition in which delay increases the chances of necrosis, from epididymitis, a nonsurgical condition. Patients with any three of the following six findings should receive treatment for presumptive epididymitis: (1) gradual onset (days) of pain, (2) dysuria, urethral discharge, recent cystoscopy, urethral catheter, (3) fever (>38.3°C), (4) previous UTIs, (5) induration localized to the epididymis, and (6) pyuria (> 10 WBCs/hpf)[2]. In patients with fewer than three of these findings, the approach depends on the duration of the patient's pain. In those with less than 24 hours of pain, testicular salvage is possible, and nothing, including radionuclide scanning, should delay urologic consultation. If the pain has persisted beyond 24 hours, testicular radionuclide scanning is reasonable; even if torsion is diagnosed, surgery is less urgent because its only purpose is to remove the necrotic testicle and fix the contralateral one.

Renal colic begins gradually, is continuous (not colicky), and rarely lasts longer than 24 hours. In all men over age 50 years who have unexplained testicular pain or have suspected renal colic, the clinician should consider the diagnosis of abdominal aortic aneurysm.

MANAGEMENT.   The antibiotic management of epididymitis is based on the likely organism as described above and the results of Gram stains of the urethra or urine (see Section 178 [Sexually Transmitted Diseases], and Section 179 [Urinary Tract Infections in Men]). Referral to a urologist is mandatory for all patients with epididymitis that fails to respond to treatment; surgical exploration may reveal unsuspected tumors, abscesses, vasculitis, or tuberculosis. Up to 50% of documented testicular tumors are initially misdiagnosed as epididymitis.

Cross-references: Abdominal Pain (Section 95), Peripheral Arterial Disease (Section 133), Cancer of the Genitourinary System (Section 170), Dysuria (Section 172), Nephrolithiasis (Section 176), Sexually Transmitted Diseases (Section 178), Urinary Tract Infections in Men (Section 179).

REFERENCES

1. Berger RE, Alexander ER, Harnisch JP, et al. Etiology, manifestation and therapy of acute epididymitis: Prospective study of 50 cases. J Urol 1979;121:750–754.

   Defines the bacterial causes of epididymitis, based on the age of the patient.

2. Knight PJ, Vassy LE. The diagnosis and treatment of the acute scrotum in children and adolescents. Ann Surg 1984;200:664–673.

   The best study of clinical features that distinguish epididymitis from torsion (395 patients), although it includes only patients ages 17 years or younger.

3. McGee SR. Diagnosis of scrotal pain. Med Rounds 1988;1:280–289.

   Encyclopedic overview of all causes of scrotal pain, divided into disorders within the scrotum and those distant to the scrotum.

4. Sharer WC. Acute scrotal pathology. Surg Clin North Am 1982;62:955–970.

   Excellent review of testicular torsion, epididymitis, and other less common causes of the acutely inflamed scrotum.

174 URINARY INCONTINENCE

Symptom

SUBBARAO V. YALLA

MOHAMED ABDEL-AZIN

EPIDEMIOLOGY. Recognized urinary incontinence, sufficient to cause patients to seek medical attention, affects about 1% of the population (0.1% of men and 0.2% of women under age 65 years, 1.3% of men and 2.5% of women over age 65 years). Unrecognized incontinence is more common, affecting 2% of men and 8% of women under age 65 years and 6% of men and 12% of women over age 65 years.

ETIOLOGY. **Functional incontinence** is usually seen in elderly patients, who because of impaired cognition or mobility are unable to urinate hygienically.

Incontinence related to **bladder dysfunction** may reflect hyperreflexia, hypocompliance, or hypersensitivity of the detrusor muscle. **Detrusor hyperreflexia** (discrete involuntary contractions of the detrusor during bladder filling) occurs in neurologic diseases such as stroke, multiple sclerosis, Parkinson's disease, and suprasacral spinal cord injuries. "Detrusor instability" refers to involuntary detrusor contractions that occur without identifiable neurologic disease or bladder pathology. **Poor bladder compliance** (tonic increase in intravesical pressure during bladder filling) may be neurogenic (sympathetic and parasympathetic denervation) or due to bladder wall fibrosis. **Bladder hypersensitivity,** which occurs in acute cystitis, interstitial cystitis, and bladder cancer, causes incontinence because of the uncontrollable desire to rid oneself of painful bladder sensations that occur during bladder filling.

Outlet-related incontinence ("stress incontinence") indicates reduced sphincter function. In women, it typically occurs when pelvic floor muscles fail to maintain the proximal urethra in the retropubic intra-abdominal position. In men, outlet-related incontinence usually follows surgical injury to the sphincter mechanism (e.g., after prostatectomy). Neurologic disease may cause outlet incompetence in men and women.

Overflow incontinence results from bladder overdistension and high intravesical pressures that overcome the urethral pressure. The most common causes, sometimes seen in combination, are urethral obstruction (e.g., prostatic enlargement) and a hypoactive detrusor muscle.

CLINICAL APPROACH.   The clinician should initially exclude reversible causes of incontinence, such as UTI, atrophic vaginitis, urinary retention, adverse drug effects (e.g., cold remedies with anticholinergic or alpha-adrenergic activity, loop diuretics, sedatives), and acute conditions that cause delirium or restricted mobility.

The patient interview should focus on defining the mechanism of urinary loss. Stress incontinence occurs with increases in intra-abdominal pressure (e.g., coughing, laughing, or lifting objects), usually when the patient is upright. In severe cases, urinary loss may follow minimal exertion, even in the supine position. Patients with urge incontinence experience the desire to void and have insufficient control to prevent bladder emptying. This type of incontinence usually suggests intrinsic bladder pathology, neurologic disease, or outlet obstruction (e.g., benign prostatic hypertrophy). Patients who have lost the sensory bladder component have no sensation of urgency preceding voiding (e.g., sensory neurogenic bladder). Patients with total incontinence experience constant leakage and wetness without associated urgency, although normal voiding may be possible. This type of incontinence usually reflects outlet incompetence.

Symptoms of hesitancy, poor caliber and strength of the urinary stream, straining to void, and a feeling of incomplete emptying indicate a hypotonic or areflexic bladder, an outlet obstruction, or both. Irritative bladder symptoms such as frequency, urgency, and nocturia usually indicate bladder instability. Other causes of irritative bladder symptoms, usually associated with suprapubic pain and dysuria, include cystitis, interstitial cystitis, or bladder carcinoma in situ. Patients with neurologic disease may also complain of ejaculatory dysfunction, impotence, and, because of the similar innervation of the bladder and rectum, frequent bowel movements.

In men, the penis is examined for phimosis, meatal stenosis, or other abnormalities that may produce obstruction. Examination of the prostate identifies the size and any other prostatic abnormalities, although an enlarged prostate gland has no meaning in itself unless associated with obstructive symptoms and signs (see Section 186). Rectal examination must be performed to detect fecal impaction in elderly patients. (Fecal impaction may produce large postvoid residuals and occasional overflow incontinence.) In women, a vaginal examination focuses on the urethral meatus and any signs of atrophic vaginitis. The posterior vaginal retractor facilitates evaluation of the anterior vaginal wall in order to locate fistulas, urethral diverticula, and cystoceles. Simple procedures like the "stress test" may help establish the diagnosis of stress incontinence: when the patient increases intra-abdominal pressure, posterior movement of the urethra and bladder base as detected by the examiner's fingers next to the anterior vaginal wall, associated with a brief spurt of urine from the urethra, is diagnostic. Leakage of urine in the absence of such movement suggests a severely impaired urethral sphincter, a fistula, or a stress-related inappropriate detrusor contraction.

Neurologic examination should include the bulbocavernosus reflex (reflex contractions of the perineal muscles with stimulation of glans or clitoris), anal wink (perianal muscle contraction with anal stimulation), and perineal sensation. Decreased anal sphincter tone suggests paralysis of the anal sphincter, previous anal sphincter surgery, or chronic overstretching from constipation. Voluntary contraction of the anal sphincter tests the same pathways that voluntarily control bladder and urethral function.

Laboratory evaluation should include urinalysis, urine culture, and urine cytology to exclude UTI and other causes of bladder hypersensitivity, such as carcinoma in situ. To exclude polyuria as the cause for incontinence, the serum calcium (hypercalcemia), glucose (diabetes mellitus), and electrolytes should be measured.

Uroflowmetry provides information about the integrated function of the detrusor and bladder outlet. The normal maximum flow rate ranges from 12 ml/sec to 30 ml/sec. Normal voiding time varies from 10 seconds to 20 seconds for a voided volume of 100 ml, to 25 seconds to 35 seconds for a voided volume of 400 ml. Visual inspection of the flow curve is important for diagnosing whether the patient is applying stress maneuvers, experiencing detrusor hyperreflexia, or having striated sphincter dyssynergia (inappropriate involuntary contractions of striated sphincter during voiding). Determination of postvoid residual urine volume by ultrasound or postvoid catheterization, when combined with the uroflowmetry, furnishes important information and helps identify overflow incontinence. A residual volume is abnormally large when two or more measurements exceed one-third of the bladder capacity (e.g., for a normal bladder capacity of 300–400 ml, a residual volume exceeding 100 ml is abnormal).

MANAGEMENT.   Patients with functional incontinence due to dementia or restricted mobility may improve on a program of scheduled toileting, together with medication that inhibits bladder muscle contractions. Examples of bladder muscle suppressants are anticholinergics, smooth muscle relaxants, calcium channel blockers, beta-adrenergic stimulants, and tricyclic antidepressants (e.g., imipramine). Oxybutynin, propantheline, and flavoxate hydrochloride are most popular (Table 174–1). Terodilene, a calcium channel blocker with

TABLE 174–1. DRUG TREATMENT OF INCONTINENCE

Drug	Initial Dose	Indication	Adverse Effects	Cost ($)[1]
Alpha-agonists				
Phenylpropanolamine (e.g., Propagest, Dexatrim, max. strength)	25 mg b.i.d.	Stress incontinence (outlet-related)	Hypertension, anxiety, insomnia, headache, tremors, arrhythmias	0.14
Anticholinergic[2]				
Propantheline	7.5 mg b.i.d.	Urge incontinence (bladder-related incontinence)	Dry mouth, blurred vision, tachycardia, constipation	0.12
Oxybutynin	2.5 mg t.i.d.			0.30
Imipramine[3]	25 mg q.d.			0.02

[1]Average wholesale daily cost, initial dose listed, 1991 *Drug Topics Red Book*.
[2]Contraindicated if narrow-angle glaucoma, outlet obstruction.
[3]Contraindicated if on monoamine oxidase (MAO) inhibitors; other adverse effects include rash, abnormal liver function tests, and agranulocytosis.

anticholinergic and local anesthetic properties, appears promising and is being investigated for its efficacy. External collecting devices and indwelling catheters may be necessary for intractable cases. A urinary fistula requires surgical correction.

Mild forms of stress incontinence usually respond to pelvic floor exercises, sometimes in combination with pharmacologic therapy (alpha-agonists) (Table 174–1). If conservative therapy fails, surgical alternatives include bladder neck suspension and fascial sling operations (in women) and artificial sphincter implantation.

The treatment of urge incontinence begins with pharmacologic therapy (Table 174–1). Although anticholinergic agents increase the volume to the first involuntary contraction, decrease the amplitude of contractions, and increase the total bladder capacity, they do not increase the warning time between the feeling of an urge to void and actual voiding and therefore must be combined with toilet programs that schedule voiding before the urge appears. Oxybutynin chloride, in addition to its anticholinergic actions, is a powerful smooth muscle relaxant and local anesthetic that has been shown to reduce detrusor hyperreflexia successfully. If urge incontinence persists despite medications, surgery that increases bladder capacity (e.g., bladder denervation or augmentation cystoplasty) may be necessary.

Patients with overflow incontinence may benefit from surgical procedures intended to reduce outlet resistance, such as bladder neck incision, bladder neck resection, or transurethral resection of the prostate. In those with poor bladder contractility and high postvoid residuals despite successful outlet surgery, clean intermittent catheterization or the placement of an indwelling catheter may be the only options.

FOLLOW-UP.   Patients should be referred to a urologist if they (1) have intractable incontinence not easily managed by empirical therapy such as anticholinergic medications (i.e., patients may require urodynamics), (2) are candidates for surgery (i.e., outlet obstruction or refractory stress incontinence), or (3) have positive urine cytologies or hematuria (i.e., require cystoscopy).

Cross-references: Muscular Weakness (Section 139), Peripheral Neuropathy (Section 149), Diabetes Mellitus (Section 157), Dysuria (Section 172), Urinary Tract Infections in Women (Section 177), Urinary Tract Infections in Men (Section 179), Bacteriuria in the Elderly (Section 180), Benign Prostatic Hyperplasia (Section 186), Back Pain in the Cancer Patient (Section 208).

REFERENCES

1. McGuire EJ. The neuropathic urethra. In Mundy AR, Stephenson TP, Wein AJ, Eds. Urodynamics: Practice and Application. Churchill Livingstone, Edinburgh, 1984.
    Reviews urethral instability.

2. Resnick NM. Voiding dysfunction in the elderly. In Yalla SV, McGuire EJ, Elbadawi A, Blaivas JG, Eds. Neurourology and Urodynamics: Principles and Practice. Macmillan, New York, 1988.

Excellent review on urinary incontinence that includes the use of medications in the elderly and important side effects.

3. Resnick NM, Yalla SV. Management of urinary incontinence in the elderly. N Engl J Med 1985;313:800–805.
    Reviews the etiology and classification of urinary incontinence.

4. Wein AJ. Clinical neuropharmacology of the lower urinary tract. In Yalla SV, McGuire EJ, Elbadawi A, Blaivas JG, Eds. Neurourology and Urodynamics: Principles and Practice. Macmillan, New York, 1988.
    Reviews the pharmacologic treatment of urinary incontinence.

5. Yalla SV, Kirsh L, Kearney G, et al. Post-prostatectomy incontinence: Urodynamic assessment. Neurourol Urodynamics 1982;1:77–87.
    Discusses the urodynamic evaluation of incontinence.

175 PROSTATE CANCER

Problem

MICHAEL K. BRAWER

EPIDEMIOLOGY.   In the United States, adenocarcinoma of the prostate is the most common malignancy in men and the second leading cause of cancer deaths. In 1990, there were an estimated 30,000 deaths and more than 100,000 new cases of prostate cancer. There are significantly more cases in North America and Europe than in Asia. American black men have the highest incidence of this disease in the world.

The cause of this neoplasm remains obscure. At least 30% of men over age 50 years have histologic evidence of prostate cancer (it is rare in young men). Because the histologic incidence of cancer far exceeds clinically evident disease, considerable controversy over the proper management of this tumor exists.

SYMPTOMS AND SIGNS.   The symptoms and signs reflect the stage of the disease (Table 175–1). Approximately 10% to 20% of men undergoing simple prostatectomy have carcinoma in the specimen (stage A).

In the majority of patients, carcinoma of the prostate is diagnosed as a result of an abnormal digital rectal examination. The normal prostate should feel like the contracted thenar eminence. Although carcinoma classically feels "stony hard" on digital rectal examination, this finding is not always present, prompting many urologists to investigate any induration or asymmetry.

TABLE 175–1. PROSTATE CANCER CLINICAL STAGING

Stage	Definition
A1	Less than 5% of prostatectomy specimen contains cancer (specimen obtained from surgery for benign disease)
A2	More than 5% of prostatectomy specimen contains cancer
B1	Cancer nodule 1 cm or less in size, confined to prostate
B2	Cancer nodule greater than 1 cm in size, confined to prostate
B3	Both lobes of gland involved, confined to prostate
C	Extension beyond the prostatic capsule
D1	Pelvic lymph node metastases
D2	Bone or visceral metastases

Many patients present with symptoms of urinary frequency, nocturia, hesitancy, decreased force of urinary stream, or dribbling. Spread of the cancer to the regional lymph nodes may cause ureteral obstruction with azotemia or unilateral lymphedema. D2 carcinoma may cause bone pain from skeletal metastasis, which most often involves the lumbar and sacral spine and pelvis. Rarely, metastasis to the lungs or liver may occur.

CLINICAL APPROACH.   A discussion of screening for prostatic carcinoma appears in Section 170. Any abnormality of the prostate, whether asymmetry, induration, or nodule, deserves evaluation by a urologist. Confirmed abnormalities require transrectal aspiration for cytology, transperineal biopsy, or transrectal needle biopsy. Most urologists prefer transrectal biopsies with either digital or transrectal ultrasonographic guidance. Ultrasound-guided procedures are simple, safe, quick, and relatively painless techniques, performed in the outpatient department without anesthesia. Ultrasound guidance also allows biopsy of other sites of the prostate, which may be useful in staging. This technique, however, requires further evaluation: as many as 15% of carcinomas occur in sonographically normal areas of the prostate, while only one-third of suspicious hypoechoic peripheral zone lesions actually reveal carcinoma.

Local staging of prostatic carcinoma remains based largely on the digital rectal examination. Computed tomography, magnetic resonance imaging, and transrectal ultrasound have been disappointing in their ability to access accurately extracapsular spread or pelvic lymph node involvement. Radionuclide bone scans are the most sensitive tests for bony metastasis.

Two tumor markers, prostatic acid phosphatase (PAP) and prostate-specific antigen (PSA), are frequently elevated in patients with advanced disease, but PAP is an insensitive measure of disease confined to the prostate. The performance characteristics for PSA in early detection are currently being assessed (see Section 170).

MANAGEMENT.   Selection of the therapeutic approach depends not only on the stage of the disease but on the patient's general health and associated illnesses. Patients with associated illness and life expectancy less than 10 years are unlikely to benefit from curative surgery or radiation, and for them no treatment is a reasonable choice. In patients with localized prostatic carcinoma (stage B), treatment options are no treatment, radical prostatectomy, or radiation therapy.

Radical prostatectomy, through either a retropubic or perineal approach, removes the prostate and seminal vesicles and reconstructs the bladder neck, attaching it to the membranous urethra. If the pathologist confirms organ-confined disease after radical prostatectomy, patients have a disease-free survival indistinguishable from age-matched controls without prostatic carcinoma. Complications of this major operation include thrombophlebitis, pulmonary embolism, lymphocele, wound infection, urethral stricture, urinary incontinence, and erectile dysfunction. Although recently improved surgical techniques maintain potency in up to 80% of men, many experts feel these techniques are appropriate only when disease is very localized.

Radiation therapy—by external beam, internal (brachytherapy), or a combination of approaches—is used to treat clinically localized prostatic carcinoma, as well as advanced local (stages C and even D1) disease. How radiation therapy compares to radical prostatectomy is unclear. The only prospective randomized study, which compared external beam radiation therapy to radical retropubic prostatectomy, favored the latter but has come under criticism; further study is necessary. Radiation therapy may injure the gastrointestinal and urinary systems and produce diarrhea, tenesmus, rectal pain, urinary frequency, urgency, and dysuria, although these side effects are usually controlled by medication. More severe complications include urethral stricture, urinary incontinence (1–2%), and erectile dysfunction (20–40%). Interstitial radiotherapy consists of seeds of iodine 131, gold 198, or, more recently, iridium 192, that are placed into the prostate gland. Early studies with iodine and gold failed to demonstrate long-term disease-free survival in most patients. Iridium produces higher local doses of radiation; studies utilizing ultrasound-guided placement of the iridium seeds are ongoing.

Endocrine therapy is based on the androgen dependence of most prostatic cells and on the observation that the withdrawal of androgens decreases mitosis and cell metabolism, causing cell death. In general, endocrine therapy is used in patients with metastatic prostatic carcinoma. Whether treatment should begin immediately after diagnosis or only after symptoms (e.g., bone pain) appear is unclear and under study. Although most patients respond to endocrine manipulation, the response is relatively short-lived: the median survival in stage D2 disease after androgen ablation is approximately 2 years.

Many approaches to endocrine manipulation exist. Orchiectomy, the simplest approach, may be complicated by psychological problems. Estrogens, which previously were widely used, inhibit the release of luteinizing hormone from the pituitary. Most clinicians now avoid estrogens because of complications of gynecomastia and, more important, significant cardiovascular disease. Antiandrogens (flutamide, anadron, and casodex) inhibit the uptake of circulating testosterone into prostatic cells and may block the binding of testosterone to receptors. The luteinizing hormone-releasing hormone analogs, leuprolide and goserelin, chronically stimulate the production of luteinizing hormone by the pituitary but eventually result in decreased receptor numbers and diminished testosterone levels. Recently, depot preparations have obviated the need for daily injections. Other uncommon approaches to androgen ablation therapy include progestins, prolactin inhibitors, antiestrogens, hypophysectomy, and adrenalectomy. Combination treatment is under study.

FOLLOW-UP. After radical prostatectomy, patients should be monitored with serial measurements of prostate-specific antigen, an exquisitely sensitive marker that should be undetectable because it is elaborated only by prostatic tissue.

The effect of radiation therapy on prostate-specific antigen levels is less clear. Although patients with a generally favorable course tend to have a significant drop in their PSA level, absolute conclusions cannot be made. Following endocrine manipulation, PSA levels usually fall, often dramatically; a climbing PSA level in a patient with known metastatic disease is usually an ominous sign. Monitoring patients with PSA levels has largely replaced the need for routine bone scans.

Cross-references: Cancer of the Genitourinary Tract (Section 170), Benign Prostatic Hyperplasia (Section 186), Back Pain in the Cancer Patient (Section 208).

REFERENCES

1. Bagshaw W, Cox RS, Ramback JE. Radiation therapy for localized prostate cancer: Justification by long-term follow-up. Urol Clin North Am 1990;17:787–802.
    Summarizes the authors' extensive experience.

2. Eggleston JC, Walsh PC. Radical prostatectomy with preservation of sexual function: Pathological findings in the first 100 cases. J Urol 1985;134:1146–1148.
    Potency-preserving radical prostatectomy.

3. Fukuda CS, Brawer MK. Update: Carcinoma of the prostate. Compr Ther 1990;16(11): 15–25.
    An overall review of prostate cancer written for general practitioners.

4. Stamey TA. Prostate cancer: Some basic clinical and morphometric observations. Monographs Urol 1989;10:79–91.
    An important monograph describing the relationship of prostate cancer grade, volume, and stage.

5. Whitmore WF. Natural history of low-stage prostatic cancer and the impact of early detection. Urol Clin North Am 1990;17:689–697.
    Addresses the importance of the natural history of prostate cancer.

176 NEPHROLITHIASIS

Problem

STEPHAN D. FIHN

EPIDEMIOLOGY/ETIOLOGY.   Kidney stones occur three to five times more often in men (approximately 124/100,000 male population per year) than in women (36/100,000 women per year). Over 50% of all stones are composed of a calcium salt, most commonly calcium oxalate and/or calcium phosphate. Forty percent of all stones and 50% of calcium stones occur in persons with hypercalciuria. Hyperuricosuria potentiates the precipitation of urinary calcium, and 80% of stones in persons with excessive uric acid excretion are composed mainly of calcium. Hyperuricosuria accounts for 25% of all calcium stones and occurs mainly in the elderly, who often have a defect in alkalinizing their urine. Hyperuricosuria and hypercalciuria coexist in 10% of stone formers. Less common causes of stones include hyperoxaluria (due to hyperabsorption following ileojejunostomy or Crohn's disease of the terminal ileum, excessive intake in the form of vitamin C or sorrel, or congenital); chronic UTI by urea splitting organisms such as *Proteus mirabilis,* causing magnesium ammonium phosphate (struvite) stones; citrate deficiency; or cystinuria, a rare disorder of amino acid transport transmitted as an autosomal dominant.

Forty percent of men who have one calcium stone will not have another. For the remainder, recurrence is maximal at 2 to 3 years and usually occurs within 5 to 10 years.

SYMPTOMS AND SIGNS.   Stones usually present with renal colic, a severe pain that has an abrupt onset, increasing in intensity over 1 hour or 2 hours and lasting up to 6 hours or longer. The pain may be centered in the flank, back, or lower abdominal quadrant. Shifting pain suggests passage of the stone across the pelvic brim or into the uterovesical junction. In males, pain may radiate into the ipsilateral testis. Gross hematuria is common.

CLINICAL APPROACH.   A renal stone should be suspected in the presence of characteristic pain and hematuria, gross or microscopic. For patients with a history of previous stones, the pain will be familiar. Patients should be questioned about excessive intake of ascorbic acid or sorrel tea and about family history of stones. The diagnosis is confirmed by excretory urography, if readily available, or ultrasonography. Both procedures also detect hydronephrosis, if present. All patients should have a serum calcium, phosphate, creatinine, and uric acid test plus a urinalysis to check for the presence of crystals. Analysis of the stone composition is not useful.

TABLE 176–1.   EVALUATION OF HYPERCALCIURIA (>200 mg/24 hr)

Characteristic	Idiopathic	Absorptive	Hyperparathyroidism
Serum Ca^{++}	Normal	Normal	>10.3
Serum PO$_4^-$	Normal	Low	<3.1
Parathyroid hormone (PTH)	Increased	Normal or decreased	Increased
Mechanism	Renal tubular leak of Ca^{++}	Increased gut absorption of Ca^{++}	Increased filtered load of Ca^{++}

Following a second episode of stone formation, investigation should be undertaken to determine the etiology. Repeat determinations of serum calcium, uric acid, phosphate, and creatinine should be obtained along with a spot urine sample for uric acid and a 24-hour urine collection for calcium and creatinine.

Hypercalciuria is defined as excretion of over 200 mg urinary calcium per 24 hours. The cause may be classified as renal (idiopathic, due to a renal tubular leak), absorptive (due to excessive gastrointestinal absorption as in sarcoidosis), or excessive filtered load (hyperparathyroidism) (Table 176–1).

Hyperuricosuria is defined as excretion of over 800 mg uric acid per 24 hours or by a spot determination demonstrating excretion of more than 0.6 mg/dl of glomerular filtration rate, computed by dividing the product of the urine urate concentration and the serum creatinine by the urine creatinine concentration.

Since excretion of calcium and uric acid may be variable, these determinations should be repeated several times if initially negative. If persistently negative, 24-hour urine specimens should be collected for citrate and oxalate.

MANAGEMENT.   Renal colic is usually controlled with narcotics, parenteral or oral, as required. Patients with obstruction, complicated urinary infection, or intractable pain should be referred to a urologist for consideration of stone removal cystoscopically or with lithotripsy.

For long-term prevention of stones due to hypercalciuria, thiazides are the treatment of choice unless hyperparathyroidism is the cause (Table 176–2). Calcium intake should be reduced if excessive, and adequate fluids should be consumed. In younger persons, stones due to hyperuricosuria should be treated with allopurinol; in the elderly, alkali plus an adequate fluid intake is recom-

TABLE 176–2.   PREVENTION OF RENAL STONES

Etiology	Treatment
Idiopathic hypercalciuria or absorptive hypercalciuria	Hydrochlorothiazide or chlorthalidone 25–50 mg q.d.
Hyperparathyroidism	Surgical removal of adenoma or hyperplastic gland
Hyperuricosuria	
Younger adult	Allopurinol 200–300 mg q.d.
Elderly	Fluids plus potassium citrate 20 mEq b.i.d. or t.i.d.

mended. Adoption of a low-sodium, low-protein diet may be helpful in some patients.

FOLLOW-UP.   In the average patient, no special follow-up is required. Patients who continue to form stones despite therapy should be referred to a specialist.

Cross-references: Gout/Hyperuricemia (Section 120), Scrotal Pain (Section 173), Hematuria (Section 182), Electrolyte Abnormalities (Section 184).

REFERENCES

1. Consensus Conference. Prevention and treatment of kidney stones. JAMA 1988;260:977–981.

    A succinct review that advocates the conservative approach to evaluation outlined in this section and emphasizes the importance of medical therapy to prevent recurrence.

2. Coe F, Parks J. Recurrent renal calculi: Causes and prevention. Hosp Pract 1986;21:49–57.

    Outlines a rather detailed strategy for outpatient evaluation of patients with recurrent stones.

3. Drach GW, Dretler S, Fair W, et al. Report of the United States cooperative study of extracorporeal shock wave lithotripsy. J Urol 1986;135:1127–1133.

    A relatively early but large report on the results of lithotripsy in over 2000 patients. In patients with small (<1 cm) stones, complications were infrequent; patients with larger or multiple stones more frequently experienced obstruction, increased pain, or need for urologic intervention.

4. Pak CYC, Ed. Renal Stone Disease: Pathogenesis, Prevention and Treatment. Martinus Nijhoff, Boston, 1987.

    An exhaustive review.

177 URINARY TRACT INFECTIONS IN WOMEN

Problem

STEPHAN D. FIHN

EPIDEMIOLOGY.   Approximately 20% of all women will have a UTI during their lifetime. The vast majority of these infections are uncomplicated. The incidence rises sharply with onset of sexual activity and increases slowly thereafter. Three-quarters of those having an initial UTI have sporadic recurrences, and about 3% to 5% have two to three reinfections each year. Use of diaphragm and spermicides raises the risk of UTI by twofold to threefold. Seventy percent to 80% of UTIs in young women are caused by *Escherichia coli* and 15% to 20% are due to *Staphylococcus saprophyticus*.

Twenty percent to 30% of women over age 65 years have bacteriuria, which may come and go, often without specific treatment. In elderly women, the incidence of bacteriuria is higher in those who are institutionalized or debilitated.

SYMPTOMS AND SIGNS. Dysuria is a cardinal symptom, but urgency and frequency may be more common. Gross hematuria and suprapubic pain or tenderness are highly specific for UTI but occur in only 10% to 20% of cases. Nausea, vomiting, fever, chills, and flank pain suggest pyelonephritis. Fever and flank tenderness are usually absent unless pyelonephritis is present. Elderly patients with UTI may lack some of these features and may present with more protean manifestations, such as mental status changes or nonspecific gastrointestinal or respiratory symptoms.

CLINICAL APPROACH. In a woman who presents with dysuria and describes her symptoms as identical to those occurring in prior documented UTIs, a diagnostic test is often unnecessary, and empirical treatment may be prescribed. If this history is lacking, microscopic evaluation of the urine is the most useful next step. Visible bacteria on Gram stain or direct microscopy is highly specific (>90%) for UTI but not sensitive (<50%). Pyuria (defined by the presence of 8 or more white blood cells per cubic millimeter [WBC/mm^3] on a quantitative leukocyte count of 5 WBC/high power field or more) is sensitive (about 90%) but has relatively low specificity (50–75%). Microscopically visible bacteria and pyuria are almost always present in acute pyelonephritis unless obstruction is present. Rapid tests for bacteria or pyuria are sensitive for UTIs associated with high levels of bacteriuria but insensitive for infections associated with lower colony counts.

In women with acute dysuria, a clean-catch midstream culture will yield 10^5 bacteria/ml or more in only 50% of those with proved infection. Using 10^2 or more as the criterion for infection is 95% sensitive and provides a positive predictive value of close to 90%. This lower definition of infection is more clinically relevant to the ambulatory setting. A culture is generally required only when urine microscopy is negative or there are complicating factors, including recent urinary tract instrumentation, childhood UTI, abnormality of the urinary tract, recent use of antibiotics, pregnancy, symptoms present for more than 1 week, diabetes, or immunosuppression.

MANAGEMENT. Short-course treatment (a single dose or over 2–3 days) is appropriate in an uncomplicated infection. Three-day treatment is probably optimal for most patients. In the presence of complicating factors, longer therapy is warranted (Table 177–1).

Women who experience recurrent UTIs should be counseled to void promptly after intercourse, and diaphragm users should be counseled about the possibility of using other contraceptive methods. Prophylactic antimicrobials given to women who have had three or more recurrences within a year is cost

TABLE 177–1. TREATMENT OF URINARY TRACT INFECTION (UTI) IN WOMEN[1]

Clinical Setting	Antimicrobial Agent[2]	Administration	Daily Cost ($)[3]
Acute UTI, uncomplicated	TMP-SMX (DS)	1 tab. b.i.d. for 2–3 days	0.24
	TMP-SMX (DS)	2 tabs, 1 dose	.24
	Trimethoprim	4 100 mg tabs, 1 dose	.56
	Trimethoprim	100 mg b.i.d. for 2–3 days	.28
	Nitrofurantoin	100 mg q.i.d. for 3 days	.48
	Ampicillin	500 mg q.i.d. for 3 days	.68
	Amoxicillin	500 mg b.i.d. for 3 days	.30
	Sulfisoxazole	500 mg q.i.d. for 3 days	.20
Acute UTI, complicated	TMP-SMX (DS)	1 tab b.i.d. for 7–10 days	.48
	Trimethoprim	100 mg b.i.d. for 7–10 days	.28
	Norfloxacin	400 mg b.i.d. for 7–10 days	4.04
	Ciprofloxacin	250 or 500 mg b.i.d. for 7–10 days	4.42/5.10
	Ofloxacin	400 mg b.i.d. for 7–10 days	6.36
	Amoxicillin-clavulanate 500	1 tab q.8h. for 7–10 days	6.21
Recurrent UTI (regimen to be initiated after therapy of acute infection)	TMP-SMX (SS)	½ tab q.h.s. or thrice weekly for 6 months	.06/.04
	Trimethoprim	100 mg q.h.s. for 6 months	.14
	Nitrofurantoin	50 or 100 mg q.h.s. for 6 months	.12
	First-generation cephalosporin	125 or 250 mg q.h.s. for 6 months	.14 (cephalexin)
	TMP-SMX (SS)	½ or 1 tab postcoitus	.23
	Nitrofurantoin	50 or 100 mg postcoitus	.12/dose
	Cephalexin	250 mg postcoitus	.14
	TMP-SMX (DS)	1 tab at onset of symptoms	.12
Acute pyelonephritis, mild symptoms	TMP-SMX (DS)	1 tab b.i.d. for 14 days	.24
	Trimethoprim	100 mg b.i.d. for 14 days	.28
	Norfloxacin	400 mg b.i.d. for 14 days	4.04
	Ciprofloxacin	250 or 500 mg b.i.d. for 14 days	4.42/5.10
	Ofloxacin	400 mg b.i.d. for 7–10 days	6.36
	Amoxicillin-clavulanate 500	1 tab q.8h. for 14 days	6.96

[1]Therapeutic options given in descending order of general preference. The choice of therapy in any individual patient must be guided by specific clinical factors and by antimicrobial sensitivities when available.

[2]Abbreviations: TMP-SMX = trimethoprim-sulfamethoxazole; DS = double-strength (TMP 160 mg + SMX 800 mg); SS = single strength (TMP 80 mg + SMX 400 mg).

[3]Average wholesale price, *1991 Drug Topics Red Book.* Prices for generic equivalents given as available.

effective and reduces morbidity. This should be initiated only after the urine has been sterilized. Prophylaxis may be given on a continuous basis or only after intercourse in women whose infections are clearly related to sexual activity. Most regimens of prophylaxis reduce the incidence of infection to less than an average of 0.4 infections per year. Responsible women with frequent recurrences may be given the option of taking single-dose treatment on their own early after the onset of symptoms.

Women with acute pyelonephritis who show signs of toxicity (high fever, nausea, and vomiting) should be admitted for parenteral therapy. Women with milder symptoms may be appropriately managed as outpatients under close supervision. Two-week therapy for pyelonephritis is as effective as that lasting 6 weeks. However, patients who relapse following a 2-week course should be given an additional 6 weeks of therapy.

Elderly women with symptomatic UTIs can usually be treated in the same fashion, although admission to the hospital for pyelonephritis is indicated more often than is the case with younger women. In general, asymptomatic bacteriuria in elderly women does not require treatment unless the patient is at higher than average risk of upper tract infection or sepsis (see Section 180).

FOLLOW-UP.   Follow-up of uncomplicated infections is generally not required unless symptoms persist or recur. Women with complicated infections should have a urine culture 2 weeks to 3 weeks after therapy. Recurrent infections after that time are usually reinfections and may be treated with short-course therapy if appropriate.

Women with recurrent UTI do not routinely require excretory urography or cystoscopy unless history, symptoms, or pattern of recurrences suggest structural abnormalities of the urinary tract.

Cross-references: Abdominal Pain (Section 95), Pelvic Pain in Women (Section 163), Dysuria (Section 172), Bacteriuria in the Elderly (Section 180), Hematuria (Section 182), Bacteriuria in Pregnancy (Section 210).

REFERENCES

1. Fihn SD, Latham RH, Roberts P, et al. Association between diaphragm use and urinary tract infection. JAMA 1985;254:240–245.

    One of the early studies demonstrating the clear relationship between diaphragm/spermicide use and UTI using both case control and cohort designs. Diaphragm users were frequently shown to have replacement of the normal vaginal flora by *E. coli.*

2. Hooten TM, Stamm WE. Management of acute uncomplicated urinary tract infections in adults. Med Clin North Am 1991;75:339–357.

    A good overview that advocates empiric 3-day treatment for most women with presumptive uncomplicated UTI without obtaining an initial culture. The authors also recommend that posttreatment cultures be omitted unless complicating factors or upper tract involvement are present.

3. Stamm WE, Counts GW, Running K, et al. Diagnosis of coliform infection in acutely dysuric women. N Engl J Med 1982;307:463–468.

    Provides the basis for using 10^2 bacteria/ml or more as the criterion to diagnose UTI.

4. Stamm WE, McKevitt M, Counts GW. Acute renal infection in women: Treatment with trimethoprim-sulfamethoxazole or ampicillin for two or six weeks. A randomized trial. Ann Int Med 1987;106:341.

> In patients with pyelonephritis who are not so ill they must be hospitalized, trimethoprim-sulfa is superior to amoxicillin, and 2-week therapy is preferable to 6-week treatment.

5. Stamm WE, Counts GW, Wagner KF, et al. Antimicrobial prophylaxis of recurrent UTIs: A double-blind, placebo-controlled trial. Ann Int Med 1980;92:770–775.

> Prophylactic antibiotics dramatically reduced the incidence of UTI with almost no adverse effects.

178 SEXUALLY TRANSMITTED DISEASES

Problem

THOMAS M. HOOTON

URETHRITIS

EPIDEMIOLOGY.   Urethritis is the most common sexually transmitted disease and afflicts several million men annually in the United States. Gonococcal urethritis is caused by *Neisseria gonorrhoeae* and is accompanied by infection with *Chlamydia trachomatis* in 20% to 30% of patients. Nongonococcal urethritis (NGU) is caused by *C. trachomatis* in 30% to 50% of patients, *Ureaplasma urealyticum* in 15% to 20% of cases, and miscellaneous bacteria or the protozoan *Trichomonas vaginalis* in a small proportion of cases. In as many as 20% to 30% of patients with NGU, no etiology can be determined. There is a high prevalence of infection with *N. gonorrhoeae* or *C. trachomatis* among female partners of men infected with these pathogens.

SYMPTOMS AND SIGNS.   Dysuria with or without urethral discharge is the main symptom of urethritis, and most men have objective evidence of urethral discharge. However, both *N. gonorrhoeae* and *C. trachomatis* may be present in men with no symptoms or signs of urethritis. Gonococcal urethritis tends to cause more abrupt symptoms, a shorter incubation period, and a more purulent discharge than NGU, but a clear distinction cannot be made in the individual patient without an examination. Symptoms and signs are most prominent in the morning before urinating, especially with NGU.

CLINICAL APPROACH.   A Gram stain of discharge (if present) or a urethral swab specimen should be examined for evidence of urethral inflammation and gram-negative diplococci. The hallmark of urethritis is the presence of five or more leukocytes per oil immersion (1000X) field in a urethral Gram-stained specimen or fifteen or more leukocytes per 400X field in the spun sediment of a first-voided urine specimen. In a symptomatic male, the urethral Gram stain is highly sensitive (95%) and specific (95%) in distinguishing gonococcal from nongonococcal urethritis. While specificity remains high in the asymptomatic patient, sensitivity is approximately 70%. A urethral culture or antigen test is necessary to determine whether *C. trachomatis* is present. Because *U. urealyticum* is commonly found in normal sexually active men and women, routine cultures for this organism are unnecessary.

MANAGEMENT. Gonococcal urethritis should be treated with a single IM injection of ceftriaxone 250 mg because this regimen is effective at all potentially infected sites (urethra, rectum, and pharynx). In the penicillin-allergic patient, spectinomycin 2 g IM in a single dose should be given. Alternative gonococcal treatment regimens are listed in Table 178–1. All patients with gonorrhea should also receive treatment for *C. trachomatis* because of the high rate of coinfection. Additionally, patients with gonorrhea should be offered testing for syphilis and human immunodeficiency virus (HIV). Patients with NGU should receive doxycycline 100 mg orally twice daily for 7 days or, in the patient who cannot take tetracycline, erythromycin base 500 mg orally four times daily for 7 days. Norfloxacin, ciprofloxacin, cephalosporins, and spectinomycin have inadequate activity against infection with *C. trachomatis*. Recent sexual partners of men with urethritis should be examined, cultured, and treated for gonorrhea or Chlamydia, as appropriate.

FOLLOW-UP. All men with persistent or recurrent symptoms should be reevaluated for evidence of urethritis. It is very unusual to have persistent infection with *N. gonorrhoeae* if ceftriaxone was used or *C. trachomatis* if doxycycline was used and if the patient was compliant in taking these antibiotics. Men with gonorrhea who were treated with ceftriaxone should return for reex-

TABLE 178–1.   TREATMENT REGIMENS FOR GONOCOCCAL URETHRITIS[1]

Drug	Dose	Duration	Cost ($)[2]
Ceftriaxone	250 mg IM	Once	10.24
Spectinomycin	2 g IM	Once	14.03
Cefixime	400 mg PO	Once	4.68
Ciprofloxacin[3]	500 mg PO	Once	2.55
Norfloxacin[3]	800 mg PO	Once	4.06
Ofloxacin[3]	300 mg PO	Once	3.181
Cefuroxime axetil	1 g PO	Once	4.98
plus probenecid	1 g PO	Once	
Cefotaxime	1 g IM	Once	11.45

[1]All regimens should be followed by doxycycline 100 mg PO twice daily or erythromycin 500 mg four times daily for 7 days to treat concomitant Chlamydia infection.

[2]Average wholesale price, Drug Topics Red Book.

[3]Ciprofloxacin, norfloxacin, and ofloxacin are contraindicated in children age 16 years or less.

amination 1 to 2 months after therapy for a test of cure and for detection of reinfection with this pathogen. Men with NGU require no follow-up if their symptoms resolve. Men with recurrent NGU in whom reinfection is likely should be retreated with doxycycline as already noted. If reinfection is unlikely (i.e., the patient has not resumed unprotected intercourse), the patient should be treated with erythromycin for 7 days. Continued persistence or recurrence of NGU should be retreated with several weeks of erythromycin. Routine evaluation of the prostate gland or cystourethroscopy is not routinely indicated in the patient with persistent or recurrent NGU.

GENITAL ULCERS

EPIDEMIOLOGY/ETIOLOGY.   In the United States, genital herpes is by far the most common cause of genital ulcer syndrome, followed by syphilis and chancroid. Chancroid is the most common etiology in many underdeveloped countries and is now endemic in several large U.S. cities. Lymphogranuloma venereum and donovanosis are uncommon in the United States. Traumatic ulcers are often confused with those of an infectious etiology. The incidence of genital ulcers in the United States is difficult to estimate because syphilis is the only reportable cause. Genital ulcers appear to place patients at greater risk for acquiring HIV infection.

SYMPTOMS AND SIGNS.   Genital ulcers may be painful or asymptomatic. The ulcers caused by herpes simplex virus (HSV) are typically small, multiple, shallow, tender, and relatively free of exudate but may coalesce or become large, tender, and indurated due to secondary infection. Such lesions may be easily mistaken for those caused by chancroid or syphilis. The lymphadenopathy that frequently accompanies genital herpes is usually bilateral, tender, and only rarely fluctuant.

The classical syphilitic chancre is a solitary, painless, indurated ulcer that is not purulent or undermined and develops and disappears slowly. Multiple ulcers or ulcers with an atypical appearance, however, are as common as the classic chancre in primary syphilis. Chancres are often accompanied by bilateral, nontender, and firm lymphadenopathy.

Chancroid causes one or more painful ulcers, which are usually deep, tender, and friable, with ragged, undermined edges. The ulcer base is usually purulent. Painful, tender, unilateral inguinal lymphadenopathy with fluctuant nodes is usually present.

CLINICAL APPROACH.   The diagnosis of genital ulceration is difficult due to the frequent atypical presentation of the different syndromes. Lesions of HSV, syphilis, and chancroid can appear identical. Every patient with a genital ulcer should be tested for syphilis because of its importance. Dark field microscopy is a sensitive and specific method for diagnosing primary syphilis when performed by trained personnel. Because the nontreponemal antibody tests

(VDRL and RPR) are positive in only 70% of patients with primary syphilis, repeat serological testing 4 weeks to 6 weeks later is usually warranted to document seroconversion. Treponemal antibody tests, such as the fluorescent treponemal antibody absorption test (FTA-ABS) or HATTS, are more specific and, if positive, exclude biologic false-positive nontreponemal antibody tests.

Culture is the most sensitive diagnostic method for HSV but has a sensitivity of less than 60% during the ulcerated stage of the disease. In the setting of a dark field-negative ulcer, a culture or antigen detection test for HSV is warranted, even if characteristic vesicles are absent.

Haemophilius ducreyi is a fastidious gram-negative organism that requires a selective medium for isolation. Gram stain evaluation of ulcers is neither sensitive nor specific in diagnosis.

MANAGEMENT.   Effective treatment regimens for these genital syndromes are listed in Table 178–2. Treatment for recurrent HSV is generally ineffective unless started early in the course of the recurrence. Topical acyclovir is less effective than oral acyclovir. Patients should keep involved areas dry and avoid occlusive underwear.

The proper treatment of primary, secondary, and early latent (less than 1 year) syphilis is benzathine penicillin 2.4 million units IM once. Patients with syphilis of longer duration or unknown duration without evidence of neurologic involvement should receive benzathine penicillin 2.4 million units IM every week for 3 weeks. Neurosyphilis documented by cerebrospinal fluid (CSF) findings warrants extended high-dose penicillin therapy. Some authorities recommend evaluation of the CSF for evidence of neurosyphilis in any patient with syphilis of more than 1 year's duration or with HIV infection. Patients treated for syphilis at any stage should be warned about the possibility of an acute febrile reaction (Jarisch-Herxheimer reaction). Expert advice should be sought for treatment of penicillin-allergic patients. All patients with syphilis should be tested for HIV infection.

FOLLOW-UP.   Patients with genital herpes do not require routine follow-up. Patients treated for syphilis should be reexamined at 3 months and 6 months and more frequently if they are HIV positive. The VDRL titer should decrease at least fourfold within 3 months of treatment for primary and secondary syphilis and within 6 months for early latent syphilis. Unless reinfection is likely, failure of the VDRL titer to fall or persistence of signs or symptoms indicates treatment failure; the patient should undergo examination of the CSF and be retreated appropriately. The VDRL reponse seen with syphilis of longer duration is more variable.

Chancroid ulcers generally improve within 7 days after institution of therapy, whereas the lymphadenopathy may resolve more slowly. Patients should be observed until the ulcer is completely healed. Poor response to therapy in the compliant patient suggests misdiagnosis, antimicrobial-resistant *H. ducreyi,* or coinfection with another STD. Coinfection with HIV may also result in a poorer response to treatment.

TABLE 178–2. TREATMENT REGIMENS FOR GENITAL ULCER SYNDROMES

Syndrome	Drug	Dose	Duration	Cost ($)[1]
Primary HSV	Acyclovir	200 mg PO 5 × daily	7–10 days	31.90 (7 days)
	Acyclovir	400 mg PO 3 × daily	7–10 days	38.48 (7 days)
Recurrent HSV	Acyclovir	200 mg PO 5 × daily	5 days	23.50
	Acyclovir	400 mg PO 3 × daily	5 days	28.20
Syphilis <1 yr	Benzathine penicillin G	2.4 million units IM	Once	19.24
Syphilis >1 yr or unknown duration	Benzathine penicillin G	2.4 million units IM	Weekly for 3 weeks	57.72
Neurosyphilis	Aqueous Crystalline penicillin G	2.4 million units IV q.4h.	10–14 days[2]	96.86 (10 days)
	Procaine penicillin G	2–4 million units IM once daily, plus probenecid 500 mg 4 × daily	10–14 days[2]	97.30 (10 days)
Chancroid	Erythromycin base	500 mg PO 4 × daily	7 days	7.28
	Ceftriaxone	250 mg IM	Once	10.24
	Ciprofloxacin	500 mg PO 2 × daily	3 days	15.30

[1] Average wholesale price for regimens listed, 1991 *Drug Topics Red Book.*
[2] Follow with benzathine PCN G weekly for 3 weeks.

CERVICITIS

EPIDEMIOLOGY.   Cervicitis is caused by *Neisseria gonorrhoeae, Chlamydia trachomatis,* or HSV. The incidence of cervicitis in the United States is unknown because nongonococcal causes of cervicitis are not reportable. Pelvic inflammatory disease and its serious sequelae, discussed in Section 168, may result from spread of pathogens from the cervix into the upper genital tract.

SYMPTOMS AND SIGNS.   Compared with urethritis in men, cervicitis is more often asymptomatic, and the diagnostic criteria are less well defined. The patient may complain of vaginal discharge, dyspareunia, or vaginal odor. Cervicitis causes a purulent endocervical discharge, friability of the endocervix, and edematous cervical ectopy or some combination thereof. Vesicles or ulcerations on the ectocervix suggest the diagnosis of HSV infection. Fever, lower abdominal pain or tenderness, or a pelvic mass suggests pelvic inflammatory disease (PID).

CLINICAL APPROACH.   An endocervical Gram stain should be performed to look for evidence of inflammation (>30 leukocytes per 1000X field on a cervical Gram stain) and for gram-negative diplococci. Although highly specific, the Gram stain is insensitive for detecting infection with *N. gonorrhoeae,* and a cervical culture is necessary. A cervical culture for *C. trachomatis* should also be obtained. Both *N. gonorrhoeae* and *C. trachomatis* may be present in the cervix of a woman who has no symptoms or signs of cervicitis.

MANAGEMENT.   Cervical gonorrhea should be treated with ceftriaxone 250 mg IM as a single dose. Alternative regimens for treatment of *N. gonorrhoeae* are the same as for gonococcal urethritis in males (see Table 178–1). The quinolones are contraindicated during pregnancy and in children age 16 years or less. Nongonococcal cervicitis should be treated with doxycycline 100 mg twice daily for 7 days or with alternative regimens as recommended for NGU in a male (see "Urethritis" in this section). Patients with gonorrhea should also receive treatment for chlamydia. Patients with signs of pelvic inflammatory disease should be treated accordingly (see Section 168). Male sexual partners should be examined, cultured, and treated for gonorrhea or Chlamydia as appropriate.

FOLLOW-UP.   Patients with gonococcal cervicitis should be followed in the same manner as men who have gonococcal urethritis. Patients with nongonococcal cervicitis should be reexamined after 2 weeks to 3 weeks and, if cervicitis is persistent, re-treated as outlined for men with persistent or recurrent NGU. A follow-up culture for *N. gonorrhoeae* in women should always include a culture of the rectum, even if this site was not initially infected, because many women will have persistence of the organism at this site only.

Cross-references: AIDS (Section 14), General Approach to Arthritic Symptoms (Section 107), Pelvic Pain (Section 163), Pelvic Inflammatory Disease (Section 168).

REFERENCES

1. Bowie WR. Urethritis in males. In Holmes KK, Mardh P-A, Sparling F, et al., Eds. Sexually Transmitted Diseases, 2d ed. McGraw-Hill, New York, 1989, pp. 627–639.
   General review.

2. Centers for Disease Control. 1989 STD treatment guidelines. MMWR 1989;38(suppl 8): 1–43.
   Succinct treatment guidelines and rationale.

3. Holmes KK. Lower genital tract infections in women: Cystitis, urethritis, vulvovaginitis, and cervicitis. In Holmes KK, Mardh P-A, Sparling PF, et al., Eds. Sexually Transmitted Diseases, 2d ed. McGraw-Hill, New York, 1989, pp. 533–554.
   General review.

4. Hooton TM, Wong ES, Barnes RC, Roberts PL, Stamm WE. Erythromycin for persistent or recurrent nongonococcal urethritis: A randomized, placebo-controlled trial. Ann Intern Med 1990;113:21–26.
   Erythromycin significantly decreased pyuria in men with persistent or recurrent NGU, especially in those with evidence of prostatic inflammation.

5. Piot P, Plummer, FA. Genital ulcer adenopathy syndrome. In Holmes KK, March P-A, Sparling PF, et al., Eds. Sexually Transmitted Diseases, 2d ed. New York: McGraw-Hill, 1989, pp. 711–716.
   General review.

6. Stamm WE, Koutsky LA, Benedetti JK, et al. *Chlamydia trachomatis* urethral infections in men: Prevalence, risk factors, and clinical manifestations. Ann Intern Med 1984;100: 47–51.
   Demonstrated the high prevalence of asymptomatic infection with *C. trachomatis*.

179 URINARY TRACT INFECTIONS IN MEN

Problem

BENJAMIN A. LIPSKY

EPIDEMIOLOGY/ETIOLOGY.   In community surveys, bacteriuria occurs rarely in young men (prevalence $\leq 0.1\%$), in about 5% of those age 65 to 85 years (one-third the rate in women), and in about 15% of those over age 85 years (two-thirds the rate in women).[2] Bacteriuria is found in about 5% of adult male outpatients and over 25% of elderly hospitalized or institutionalized men. The major factor contributing to UTIs in older men is prostatic hypertrophy, resulting in bladder outlet obstruction. This predisposes to infection directly by creating a residual of urine in the bladder after voiding and indirectly by leading to genitourinary instrumentation.

Gram-negative bacilli cause about 75% of UTIs in men. As opposed to women, *Escherichia coli* is responsible for only 25% to 50% of the infections, while *Proteus* and *Providencia* species cause most of the rest. UTIs in men are occasionally caused by other gram-negative bacilli, streptococci (especially enterococci), staphylococci (both coagulase-positive and negative), or, rarely, fastidious organisms such as *Gardnerella vaginalis* or *Haemophilus influenzae*.[2,4,5] Men who are institutionalized, require a urinary catheter, or have received recent courses of antibiotics are likely to have uropathogens that are resistant to commonly prescribed antibiotics.

SYMPTOMS AND SIGNS. Genitourinary symptoms of a UTI are usually primarily irritative (i.e., dysuria, frequency, urgency, strangury) but may also be obstructive (i.e., hesitancy, nocturia, slow stream, and dribbling). Systemic symptoms (e.g., fever, malaise) usually suggest involvement of the epididymis, prostate, or kidney. Infection in these sites can often be detected by physical examination. A urethral discharge usually indicates urethritis rather than a UTI.

CLINICAL APPROACH. A urine culture should be obtained in all men with symptoms suggesting a UTI and in men in whom bacteriuria must be excluded (e.g., before genitourinary instrumentation). A voided specimen is highly accurate for men. Several studies have shown that circumcision status, meatal cleansing, and midstream sampling have little effect on the accuracy of urine cultures, making the clean-catch midstream void technique unnecessary for most men.[2,3,5] The best laboratory criterion for diagnosing true (i.e., bladder) bacteriuria in men is growth of 10^3 colony-forming units (CFU) per milliliter or more of a single or predominant species. In one study this criterion had a sensitivity and specificity of 0.97. Defining bacteriuria as $\geq 10^5$ CFU/ml missed about a third of bacteriuric men.[3]

When a bladder specimen is needed, suprapubic aspiration is generally easier, more accurate, and less painful than urethral catheterization.[3] Specimens from a man wearing a condom catheter should be obtained by collecting the first 10 cc to 20 cc of urine produced after applying a clean catheter and collection bag; bacteriuria of 10^5 CFU/ml or more has a positive predictive value of over 90% if the same organism is found on two consecutive specimens.

Localizing the site of infection in bacteriuric men is usually unnecessary. Pyelonephritis is generally diagnosed clinically, and it is only rarely necessary to know which kidney is infected. Acute bacterial prostatitis presents as an acute febrile illness with an exquisitely tender prostate. Determining when chronic prostatic infection is present is more difficult; clinical diagnosis is inaccurate, the recommended four-cup test is a cumbersome and rarely used procedure, and immunologic methods are not routinely available.[2]

MANAGEMENT. All symptomatic men with bacteriuria should receive antibiotic treatment, but the appropriate duration of therapy is debated. Single-dose or short-course therapy probably has no role in treating bacteriuric men. Available data suggest that 7 days to 10 days of treatment with various antibiotics cures uncomplicated cystitis in most men. For those with a UTI complicated by pyelonephritis, prostatism, or another anatomic or functional genitourinary problem, more prolonged treatment (2–3 weeks) may be necessary. Men with recurrent bacteriuria, most of whom probably have a prostatic focus of infection, require at least 6 weeks of antibiotic therapy. When prostatic infection is believed to be present, an agent that penetrates the prostate—trimethoprim, erythromycin, doxycycline or a quinolone—is needed. When recurrent UTIs are frequent or severe, they can be effectively suppressed by daily antibiotic treatment, for example, with cotrimoxazole (1 regular-strength tablet a day).

FOLLOW-UP.   For patients in whom it is important to eradicate bacteriuria, a follow-up urine culture should be obtained 2 weeks to 3 weeks after treatment. Earlier recurrences are usually relapses; later ones are reinfections. The indications for a urologic diagnostic evaluation in a man with bacteriuria are not well defined. While genitourinary abnormalities are frequent in bacteriuric men, the clinical and prognostic significance of most of these findings is undetermined. Certainly men presenting with evidence of urinary tract obstruction or those with recurrent infections, progressive renal dysfunction, or other complicating features should be evaluated. The workup may include renal ultrasonography, excretory urography, cystoscopy, or urodynamic studies.[1,2]

Cross-references: Dysuria (Section 172), Scrotal Pain (Section 173), Urinary Tract Infections in Women (Section 177), Bacteriuria in the Elderly (Section 180).

REFERENCES

1.   Gower PE. Urinary tract infections in men. Investigate at all ages. Br Med J 1989;298:1595–1596.

    An editorial that succinctly summarizes several key issues and argues for urogenital diagnostic investigations in bacteriuric males of all ages.

2.   Lipsky BA. Urinary tract infections in men. Epidemiology, pathophysiology, diagnosis, and treatment. Ann Intern Med 1989;110:138–150.

    A thorough review with diagnosis and treatment algorithms and 107 references.

3.   Lipsky BA, Ireton RC, Fihn SD, et al. Diagnosis of bacteriuria in men: Specimen collection and culture interpretation. J Infect Dis 1987;155:847–854.

    Presents data from 76 comprehensive evaluations of 66 bacteriuric and nonbacteriuric men demonstrating that voided specimens are highly accurate, and the best diagnostic criterion for bacteriuria is $\geq 10^3$ CFU/ml.

4.   Maskell R. Urinary Tract Infection in General Practice. Edward Arnold, London, 1988.

    A summary of the author's approach to UTIs in men formulated from laboratory-based research.

5.   Sugarman ID, Pead LJ, Payne SR, et al. Bacteriological state of the urine in symptom-free adult males. Br J Urol 1990;66:148–151.

    Voided specimens from 120 asymptomatic men yielded no aerobic organisms in pure growth; 26% had fastidious organisms but none in counts of $\geq 10^4$ CFU/ml.

180 BACTERIURIA IN THE ELDERLY

Problem

BENJAMIN A. LIPSKY

EPIDEMIOLOGY/ETIOLOGY.   The prevalence of bacteriuria increases with age and debility (Table 180–1). Rates of infection are highest in hospitalized or institutionalized patients. Factors contributing to bacteriuria in the elderly include: (1) in men, prostatic hypertrophy and age-related decrements in prostatic secretion antimicrobial activity; (2) in women, fecal incontinence and age-related changes in vaginal secretions and bladder function; and (3) in both sexes, bladder catheterization and other coexisting diseases (especially those interfering with bladder emptying). Bacteriuria is often intermittent (even without therapy), and the infecting organism may change over time. Among patients with asymptomatic bacteriuria, repeat cultures 1 to 5 years later are negative in about 80% of men and 50% of women. Among those with sterile cultures, about 10% of men and 20% of women will develop bacteriuria.

Although *Escherichia coli* is the most frequent cause of UTIs in the elderly, other gram-negative bacilli, such as *Proteus, Providencia, Klebsiella, Enterobacter, Pseudomonas,* and *Serratia* species, are isolated more often than in younger patients. Polymicrobial infections are also more common in the elderly. Uropathogens from institutionalized, instrumented, or recurrently infected patients are often resistant to antibiotics.

SYMPTOMS AND SIGNS.   Most elderly bacteriuric subjects have no urinary or systemic symptoms. With an acute UTI, most elderly patients have typical irritative genitourinary symptoms of dysuria, frequency, urgency, or incontin-

TABLE 180–1. APPROXIMATE PREVALENCE OF BACTERIURIA IN ELDERLY SUBJECTS (%)

Population	Men	Women
Community based		
Ages 65–85 years	5	15
Age > 85 years	13	25
Patient based		
Inpatients age < 70 years	8	30
Inpatients age > 70 years	25	30
Institutionalized	>30	>30

ence. Diagnosing a UTI in the elderly is made more difficult by the fact that some patients present with only urinary incontinence or generalized symptoms (e.g., a change in mental status, anorexia, malaise), and many nonbacteriuric elderly patients have irritative urinary symptoms. If symptoms are of recent onset or are accompanied by dysuria, a UTI should be considered.

Low-level pyuria is frequently unrelated to bacteruria in elderly ambulatory women, although its absence strongly suggests a sterile culture. Among elderly institutionalized women, however, the finding of a quantitative urine leukocyte count of $20/mm^3$ or more has a positive and negative predictive value of about 80% for upper tract infection.

CLINICAL APPROACH.   In asymptomatic patients, bacteriuria is defined as growth of $\geq 10^5$ CFU/ml from a voided specimen on two separate cultures. Because overlap exists, genitourinary symptoms should not be automatically attributed to bacteriuria; other causes, such as prostatic hypertrophy or vaginitis, should be looked for. A urine culture is indicated only if there is an intent to treat bacteriuria once detected.

Bacteriuria, whether symptomatic or not, may reflect more than uncomplicated cystitis; half or more of elderly bacteriuric women have upper tract infections, and about half of bacteriuric elderly men have prostatic infections. Twenty percent of cases of acute pyelonephritis are initially misdiagnosed in elderly patients because attention is focused on nonurinary symptoms. Bacteremia and shock are more frequent with pyelonephritis in elderly patients than in younger patients.

MANAGEMENT.   Because UTIs are the most frequent cause of sepsis in the elderly, all symptomatic patients with bacteriuria should receive antibiotic treatment. Because single-dose or short-course therapy has an unacceptably high failure rate in elderly patients, 1 to 2 weeks of therapy are recommended (see the recommendations in Sections 177 and 179). Patients with indwelling bladder catheters invariably develop bacteriuria but do not require treatment unless they develop urinary symptoms or fever. Elderly patients with acute pyelonephritis should be hospitalized to exclude bacteremia, to identify the etiologic organism, and to monitor the initial response to therapy.

A major issue in elderly patients is whether to treat asymptomatic bacteriuria. Despite earlier studies to the contrary, asymptomatic bacteriuria per se is probably not associated with premature mortality but is simply a marker for other serious medical problems, particularly dementia. In the absence of obstruction, treatment of asymptomatic bacteriuria appears to provide no improvement in survival or reduction in the rate of symptomatic UTIs. In view of the expense of detection and treatment, the potential for adverse reactions to antimicrobials (which occur in up to a quarter of elderly patients), and its frequent spontaneous disappearance, routine treatment of asymptomatic bacteriuria is not warranted. Treatment should be considered for patients who are immunologically compromised or will be undergoing genitourinary instrumentation or placement of prosthetic devices. Studies in hospitalized patients have shown that recurrence rates of asymptomatic bacteriuria after antimicrobial treatment are high.

FOLLOW-UP.   The indications for diagnostic evaluation of the urinary tract are discussed in Sections 177 (for women) and 179 (for men).

Cross-references: Fever (Section 16), Urinary Tract Infections in Women (Section 177), Urinary Tract Infections in Men (Section 179).

REFERENCES

1. Boscia JA, Abrutyn E, Kaye D. Asymptomatic bacteriuria in elderly persons: Treat or do not treat? Ann Intern Med 1987;106:764–765.

    This editorial presents the available data pertaining to this issue, as well as a summary of the authors' extensive experience in the epidemiology and treatment of bacteriuria in the elderly.

2. Boscia JA, Abrutyn E, Levison ME, et al. Pyuria and asymptomatic bacteriuria in elderly ambulatory women. Ann Intern Med 1989;110:404–405.

    Cultures and urinary leukocyte counts of voided urine specimens from 317 asymptomatic women revealed a positive predictive value for bacteriuria of pyuria of 39% and a negative predictive value for no pyuria of 96%.

3. Mulholland SG. Urinary tract infection. Clin Geriatr Med 1990;6 (Urologic Care in the Elderly):43–53.

    An excellent up-to-date overview of the available information in this area, with 47 references.

4. Nicolle LE, Mayhew WJ, Bryan L. Prospective randomized comparison of therapy and no therapy for asymptomatic bacteriuria in women. Am J Med 1987;83:27–33.

    Among fifty women, no differences in genitourinary morbidity or mortality were observed between the treatment and nontreatment groups, and antimicrobial therapy was associated with an increased incidence of reinfection, adverse antimicrobial effects, and antimicrobial resistance.

5. Nicolle LE, Muir P, Harding GKM, et al. Localization of urinary tract infection in elderly, institutionalized women with asymptomatic bacteriuria. J Infect Dis 1988;157:65–70.

    In fifty-one women with asymptomatic bacteriuria, bladder washout localized the infection to the kidney in two-thirds of patients. The positive and negative predictive values of the antibody-coated bacteria test were 82% and 43%, respectively, and the quantitative leukocyte count of 20/mm^3 or more, 80% and 88%, respectively.

181 CHRONIC RENAL FAILURE

Problem

MEREDITH MATHEWS

EPIDEMIOLOGY/ETIOLOGY. Chronic renal failure is a slowly progressive, irreversible loss of kidney function. It typically develops over months to years from ongoing nephron loss due to toxic injury, systemic disease, or primary renal disease. A subset of patients with chronic renal failure progress to end-stage renal failure, requiring chronic dialysis or transplantation to survive. The incidence of end-stage renal failure is 82 per 1 million population. The incidence is three times higher in blacks than whites, is 30% to 40% higher in men than women, and increases steeply with age (ages 0–14 years, 7 per 1 million; ages 65–74 years, 241 per 1 million). The three leading causes of end-stage renal disease are hypertension (23% of cases), diabetes (22%), and glomerulonephritis (20%).

SYMPTOMS AND SIGNS. Patients usually experience no symptoms until they lose 75% of renal function. Signs and symptoms, which follow a predictable pattern as nephrons are progressively lost, reflect the accumulation of substances normally excreted by the kidney or the failure of the kidney to produce key substances required for normal metabolic processes (e.g., erythropoietin and vitamin D) (Table 181–1).

CLINICAL APPROACH. The clinician should (1) quantify the degree of renal failure by measuring the creatinine clearance, (2) identify any potential reversible disorders, and (3) identify aggravating conditions that may promote renal failure.

The clinician should search for reversible causes of worsening renal function, including volume depletion, congestive heart failure, urinary obstruction (especially if associated with infection), nephrotoxic agents (nonsteroidal anti-inflammatory agents, aminoglycosides, radiocontrast dyes), and hypercalcemia. On ultrasound examination, small kidneys signify irreversible loss of functioning nephrons.

Hypertension is present in up to 80% of patients with a glomerular filtration rate (GFR) less than 30 ml/min. Because hypertension accelerates the progression of all types of renal disease, appropriate control is essential.

Many authorities recommend protein restriction as a method to retard the progression of renal failure, although during the early stages of renal failure, its role is controversial. With the help of a dietitian, the clinician can restrict the diet to 0.6 g/kg daily, with at least 0.35 g/kg daily of the dietary protein allotment consisting of high biologic-value protein (essential amino acids). Restric-

562

tion of protein below this level should be done only by an experienced nephrologist because of the risk of protein-calorie malnutrition. In patients with a GFR below 25 ml/min, protein restriction also helps control serum phosphate levels.

MANAGEMENT. Appropriate treatment usually focuses on the following areas.

Osmolality. The kidney in chronic renal failure excretes an isosmotic urine and cannot concentrate or dilute the urine. Hypo- or hypernatremia occur only if patients drink more or less water than they lose through the urinary tract, the gastrointestinal tract, or sweat and respiration, and can be avoided by advising the patient to drink only when thirsty.

Saline Excess/Depletion. With declining renal function, sodium excretion becomes fixed, putting the patient at risk for saline (i.e., extracellular space fluid) excess or depletion. When the GFR is below 25 ml/min, modest sodium restriction (3 g/day) may prevent saline excess. If mild sodium restriction is insufficient, a loop diuretic (furosemide) should be used. During periods when the patient has an intercurrent illness, the clinician should carefully monitor the patient's body weight and supplement fluid intake to prevent volume depletion.

Hypertension. Treatment begins with dietary sodium restriction (3 g/day), since hypertension in most azotemic patients is sodium dependent. If this is insufficient, the addition of diuretics is helpful. At a GFR of less than 25 ml/min, thiazide diuretics are usually ineffective, and loop diuretics (e.g., furosemide) are necessary. When diuretics are insufficient, therapeutic options include calcium channel blockers (nifedipine has the most potent antihypertensive effect), beta-blockers, and vasodilators (e.g., hydralazine, minoxidil). Angiotensin II–converting enzyme inhibitors (e.g., captopril, enalapril, lisinopril) are effective but require close monitoring because they may lead to accelerated renal failure or hyperkalemia.

Acidosis. The most frequent type of acidosis in patients with renal failure results from the accumulation of the breakdown products of protein metabolism. Treatment with sodium bicarbonate or sodium citrate (1 mEq/kg/day) is indicated if the serum bicarbonate drops below 16 mEq/liter. Hyperchloremic acidosis (type IV, associated with hyperkalemia) occurs in the elderly, diabetics, or other patients with tubulo-interstitial disease. In most cases, the hyperkalemia can be adequately treated with small doses of furosemide, although a small number of cases require a mineralocorticoid (e.g., fludrocortisone).

Secondary Hyperparathyroidism. To prevent hyperparathyroidism, the clinician should restrict dietary phosphate to less than 1000 mg/day when the GFR reaches 25 ml/min. This is usually accomplished by eliminating dairy products in the patient's diet. If dietary restrictions do not maintain the serum phosphate below 6 mg/dl, phosphate binding antacids (calcium carbonate or calcium acetate) should be given with meals. Serum calcium should be maintained in the normal range. If these steps are ineffective, calcitriol (1,25 (OH)2 vitamin D) should be added. The clinician should carefully monitor the serum creatinine (particularly when calcitriol is used), calcium, and phosphate. Hypercalcemia

TABLE 181–1. LOSS OF RENAL FUNCTION: CLINICAL FINDINGS

Category (GFR)	Finding	Cause	Therapy
Decreased renal reserve (25–50 cc/min)	Anemia (mild)	Decreased erythropoietin	
	Prolonged half-life of drugs	Decreased sodium handling	Adjust medications as appropriate
		Decreased renal mass	
Renal insufficiency (10–25 cc/min)	Nocturia	Concentrating defect	
	Morning anorexia, nausea, vomiting	Nocturnal dehydration	Decrease sodium in diet to 3 g/day; adequate fluid replacement; drink water at night while up
	Poor response to salt load/depletion; hypertension	Decreased ability to excrete sodium; expanded extracellular fluid space	Loop diuretics
	Decreased concentration/calculating ability	Uremic metabolites	Avoid sedatives and hypnotics
	Poor response to potassium-sparing diuretics	Decreased renal mass	Avoid use of spironolactone, triamterene
	Hyperphosphatemia	Decreased phosphate clearance	Dietary phosphate restriction (1000 mg/day); phosphate binders; calcium supplementation; 1,25 dihydroxycholecalcitrol (Rocaltrol)
	Acidosis	Decreased acid clearance	If bicarbonate <15 mEq/L, use sodium citrate or sodium bicarbonate
	Hyperkalemia	Decreased renal clearance of potassium	Avoid salt substitutes or potassium supplements

Uremia (<10 cc/min)		
Hyperkalemia	Decreased renal mass	Dialysis
Bleeding tendency	Decreased platelet aggregation	Avoid aspirin
Increased susceptibility to infection	Decreased CD4 function	Treat infections promptly
Neuropathy; asterixis; confusion; seizure; hiccups; vomiting; pericarditis	Uremic metabolites	Dialysis
Increased risk of drug toxicity	Altered protein binding, poor clearance	Adjust medications as appropriate
Pruritus	Calcium phosphate in skin	—
Pathologic fractures	Osteodystrophy	Avoid falls
Impotence, decreased sperm count; cessation of menstruation	Uremic metabolites in testes; decreased hypothalamic responsiveness	—

or a high calcium × phosphate product (>60) has been shown to accelerate renal deterioration.

Anemia.   The hematocrit begins to decrease when the GFR reaches 30 ml/min, due to the loss of the kidney's ability to produce erythropoietin. Treatment of the anemia with erythropoietin may be necessary in the occasional patient with very severe anemia or cardiac decompensation. Since many patients with chronic renal failure have other reasons for anemia, the clinician should always consider the possibility of nutritional deficiency or blood loss.

Modification of Drug Doses.   Standard tables of drug dosing guidelines for patients who have renal failure are available.[1] Below a GFR of 25 ml/min, several drugs are contraindicated, including potassium-sparing diuretics, nitrofurantoin, acetohexamide, and phenformin.

Uremia.   The definitive treatment of uremic symptoms is with dialysis or transplantation. Protein restriction can ameliorate some uremic symptoms if dialysis is not readily available or if definitive methods are not appropriate for the patient.

FOLLOW-UP.   Patients with chronic renal failure should be vaccinated against influenza. The frequency of follow-up depends on the stage of the renal failure and the severity of the patient's symptoms. When the creatinine clearance drops to 15 ml/min, the patient should be referred to a nephrologist to discuss the treatment options and, if appropriate, establish access for dialysis.

Cross-references: Anorexia (Section 18), Fatigue (Section 21), Pruritis (Section 23), Diabetes Mellitus (Section 157), Proteinuria (Section 183), Electrolyte Abnormalities (Section 184), Benign Prostatic Hyperplasia (Section 186).

REFERENCES

1.   Bennett W, Galper TA. Drug therapy in renal disease. In Rubenstein E, Federman D, Eds. Scientific American Medicine. WH Freeman, New York, 1988.

2.   Eschbach JW, Adamson JW. Guidelines for recombinant human erythropoietin therapy. Am J Kid Dis 1989;14(2)(suppl 1):2–8.
     Practical review of indications, dosages, and complications.

3.   Heyka RJ, Vidt DG. Control of hypertension in patients with chronic renal failure. Cleve Clin J Med 1989;56:65–76.
     Overview of pathophysiology and treatment.

4.   May RC, Mitch WE. Chronic renal failure. In Branch WT, Jr, Ed. The Office Practice of Medicine, 2d ed. W.B. Saunders Co., Philadelphia, 1987, pp. 608–634).
     A thorough review.

182 HEMATURIA

Problem

MEREDITH MATHEWS

EPIDEMIOLOGY. Hematuria, defined as more than 3 red blood cells per high power field (RBC/hpf) on urinalysis, is common and occurs in 13% to 24% of the population.

ETIOLOGY. Hematuria results from many important genitourinary disorders, including cancer, UTIs, trauma, tuberculosis, polycystic kidney disease, immunologic disorders (glomerulonephritis and vasculitis), and kidney stones. Malignant lesions are more common in those over age 50 years, men, smokers, and those with severe hematuria. Although symptomatic patients often have identifiable underlying disease, asymptomatic patients do not; population-based studies of patients with asymptomatic microscopic hematuria document clinically significant urologic disease in 2% to 3% and renal or bladder cancer in only 0.5%.

CLINICAL APPROACH. The patient interview should focus on symptoms suggestive of infection (urgency, frequency, dysuria, fever), nephrolithiasis (unilateral flank pain), malignancy (weight loss), glomerulonephritis (rash, recent respiratory tract infection), and whether there is associated trauma (urinary catheter, exercise, contact sports), menstruation (suggesting a false-positive urinalysis), or family history of polycystic kidney disease or sickle cell disease. Important physical findings include flank mass (polycystic kidney disease, cancer), prostate nodule or tenderness, heart murmurs or arrhythmias (renal artery embolism), new rash or hypertension (immunologic disorder), or abnormalities of the external genitalia. Important initial laboratory data include a blood urea, creatinine, complete blood count, and urine culture and sediment examination.

Patients with active gross hematuria require prompt referral to a urologist for early cystoscopy and identification of the bleeding site. Patients with other symptoms (e.g., flank pain, fever, dysuria, weight loss) also require evaluation. The more common clinical problem, however, is whether to evaluate patients who are asymptomatic (i.e., intermittent gross hematuria or microscopic hematuria). Because the probability of significant disease is low, many authorities recommend that one of the following criteria be present before beginning an evaluation: (1) more than 3 RBC/hpf or a positive dipstick on two of three urine samples, (2) one episode of gross hematuria, or (3) one episode of high-grade hematuria (>100 RBC/hpf). Figure 182–1 presents one logical diagnostic approach in these patients.

567

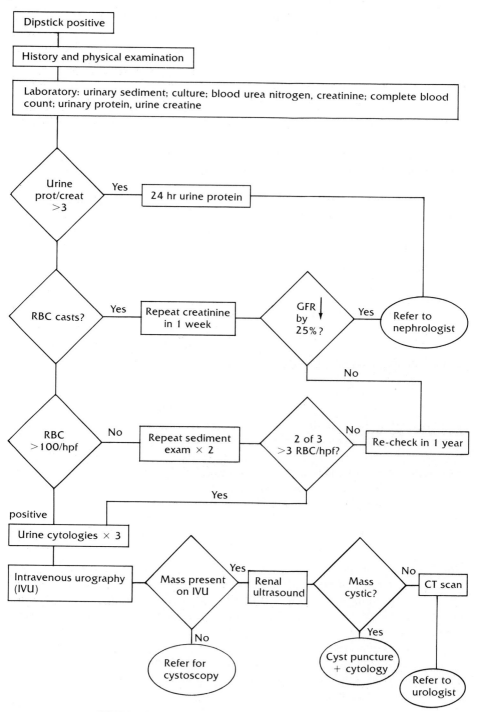

FIGURE 182–1. Approach to asymptomatic hematuria.

The dipstick test of the urine is 97% sensitive and 84% specific in detecting significant hematuria (>3 RBC/hpf). False-positive tests (e.g., hemoglobinuria or myoglobinuria) or false-negative tests (ascorbic acid in the urine) may occur. Findings in the urine sediment that suggest a glomerular source include significant proteinuria (>1 g/day) or red cell casts. Cytology has an overall sensitivity of 67% and specificity of 96% and is more sensitive for detecting poorly differentiated, sessile, or in situ lesions than for well-differentiated carcinomas or papillary carcinomas. The latter lesions tend to be visible and are more easily discovered with cystoscopy.

MANAGEMENT.   Sections 177 and 179 review the management of urinary tract infections (in women and men, respectively); and nephrolithiasis is covered in Section 176. Patients should be immediately referred to a specialist if they have gross hematuria (actively bleeding), acute deterioration of renal function, or nephrotic range proteinuria (>3 g/24 hours/1.73 M^2).

FOLLOW-UP.   If the initial workup is negative, the patient should be followed for at least 3 years. The follow-up program includes urinalysis every 6 months with intravenous urography and cystoscopy at 2 years if hematuria persists. Cytology could also be repeated at 2 years. If findings remain negative (other than hematuria), further workup is unnecessary.

Cross-references: Cancer of the Genitourinary System (Section 170), Dysuria (Section 172), Prostate Cancer (Section 175), Nephrolithiasis (Section 176), Urinary Tract Infections in Women (Section 177), Urinary Tract Infections in Men (Section 179), Bacteriuria in the Elderly (Section 180).

REFERENCES

1. Jones DJ, Langstaff RJ, Holt SD. The value of cystourethroscopy in the investigation of microscopic haematuria in adult males under age 40 years. Br J Urol 1988;62:541–545.
    Concludes that cystourethroscopy is of minimal diagnostic value in young men with microscopic hematuria.

2. Mariani AJ, Mariani MC, Macchioni C. The significance of adult hematuria evaluations including a risk-benefit and cost-effectiveness analysis. J Urol 1989;141:350–355.
    In 1000 consecutive adults with asymptomatic gross or microscopic hematuria, life-threatening lesions were found in 9% and lesions requiring at least observation in 23%.

3. Paola AS. Hematuria: Essentials of diagnosis. Hosp Pract (November) 1990:144–152.
    Concise clinical review.

4. Restrepo NC, Carey PO. Evaluating hematuria in adults. Am Fam Phys 1989;40:149–156.
    Excellent overview.

5. Sutton JM. Evaluation of hematuria in adults. JAMA 1990;263:2475–2480.
    State-of-the-art review with an algorithm.

183 PROTEINURIA

Problem

MEREDITH MATHEWS

Epidemiology/Etiology. Proteinuria is defined as the excretion of greater than 150 mg of protein in the urine over a 24-hour period. The prevalence of proteinuria in adult populations is variably reported as 0.6% to 8.8%. Table 183–1 lists common causes.

Signs and Symptoms. There are three classifications of proteinuria:

1. *Functional proteinuria:* Small amounts of protein (<1.0 g/day) are excreted intermittently and associated with normal renal function.

2. *Orthostatic proteinuria:* Small amounts of protein (<1.0 g/day) are excreted only in the upright position. This condition is present in 15% to 20% of young men but is seen also during recovery from pyelonephritis or glomerulonephritis.

3. *Fixed (constant) proteinuria.*

TABLE 183–1. CAUSES OF PROTEINURIA

Functional proteinuria (transient or intermittent)
Fever
Exercise
Exposure to cold
Congestive heart failure

Orthostatic proteinuria

Fixed proteinuria
Renal disease secondary to systemic disease
  Glomerulonephritis
    Postinfectious
    Diabetes mellitus
    Tumors
    Drugs (nonsteroidal anti-inflammatory drugs)
  Tubulointerstitial diseases
    Drugs (antibiotics, nonsteroidal anti-inflammatory drugs)
    Diabetes mellitus

Primary renal disease
  Glomerular disease
    Focal glomerular sclerosis
    Minimal change lesion
    Membranous glomerulonephritis
    Membranoproliferative glomerulonephritis
    Proliferative glomerulonephritis
    Tubulointerstitial disease (hereditary nephritis)

The prognosis of functional and orthostatic proteinuria is excellent, with few, if any, patients developing renal insufficiency during follow-up. In patients with orthostatic proteinuria, proteinuria is absent in 15% after 5 years and in 50% after 10 years.

Some patients with fixed proteinuria ultimately develop chronic renal failure. Patients older than age 50 years are more likely to have a poor prognosis than younger patients. When the protein loss exceeds 2.5 g per day, patients may develop the nephrotic syndrome, characterized by hypoalbuminemia and edema. With more severe nephrotic syndrome, malnutrition, increased susceptibility to infection, and hyperlipidemia are seen.

CLINICAL APPROACH.   The patient interview should focus on the patient's medications, symptoms of systemic disease (fever, rash, arthritis), family history of kidney disease, or history of diabetes. The physical findings of hypertension or rash may suggest glomerulonephritis or vasculitis.

The two methods commonly used to measure protein in the urine are the dipstick and sulfosalicylic acid method. Urinalysis (by dipstick) detects proteinuria with a sensitivity of 70% and specificity of 92%. False-positive tests occur with alkaline urine and gross hematuria, and false-negative tests occur with nonalbumin proteinuria (e.g., urinary immunoglobulin of multiple myeloma) or with a dilute urine. The sulfosalicylic acid test will detect nonalbumin proteinuria. Because both tests measure concentration and not quantity, they should always be compared to the specific gravity measurement (i.e., when comparing two qualitative urine proteins from the same patient taken at separate times, the specific gravity should be used as a reference point).

The evaluation of proteinuria is not recommended unless urinalyses are consistently positive (fixed proteinuria). Figure 183–1 reviews one approach that identifies a group of patients who are most likely to have diseases for which early therapeutic intervention would be of benefit, thus justifying extensive and sometimes invasive diagnostic tests and procedures.

In the patient who requires evaluation, routine laboratory tests include a urine sediment examination (to identify red cell, white cell, or renal tubular epithelial cell casts), serum glucose, blood urea, creatinine, albumin, and a spot urine protein/creatinine ratio. The protein/creatinine ratio is highly recommended in the ambulatory setting and correlates well with the 24-hour excretion; a spot ratio of less than 0.2 correlates with normal 24-hour protein excretion (<200 mg/24 hr); a ratio of more than 3 correlates well with nephrotic range proteinuria (>3.0 g/24 hr).

In patients with an abnormal ratio, a 24-hour collection should be performed at least once to quantitate the proteinuria. Measurement of the amount of creatinine in the sample confirms that the 24-hour collection was adequate. (Males excrete 16–26 mg/kg of creatinine per day, females 16–20 mg/kg/day, elderly or cachectic patients as little as 9–11 mg/kg/day.) In patients older than age 50 years, especially if nonalbumin proteinuria is suspected (i.e., negative dipstick and positive sulfosalicylic acid test), a urine protein electrophoresis is indi-

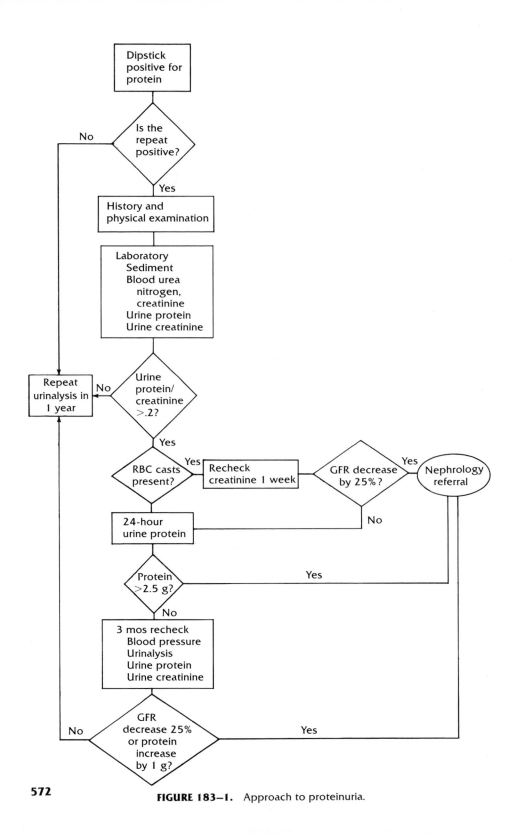

FIGURE 183–1. Approach to proteinuria.

cated. There are no clear indications for intravenous urography or cystoscopy in the workup of proteinuria.

MANAGEMENT. Specific therapy depends on the underlying cause. Proteinuria per se requires no specific treatment. Patients with nephrotic syndrome may require a diet high in protein (1 g/kg/day with high biologic value protein), dietary salt restriction, institution of diuretics, and treatment for hypercholesterolemia (see Section 155). Pneumococcal immunization is recommended.

FOLLOW-UP. Transient proteinuria requires no follow-up. Patients with intermittent or fixed proteinuria, especially in the older age group, should have annual visits to monitor the blood pressure, urinalysis, blood urea, and creatinine until proteinuria disappears completely. Patients should be referred to a nephrologist for further evaluation if they have nephrotic range proteinuria, rapidly advancing azotemia (decrease of renal function by >25% in less than 1 year), or increasing proteinuria (increases > 1 g/24h/year).

Cross-references: Osteoporosis (Section 117), Hyperlipidemia (Section 155), Chronic Renal Failure (Section 181), Pregnancy and Hypertension (Section 215).

REFERENCES

1. Abuelo JG. Proteinuria: Diagnostic principles and procedures. Ann Int Med 1983;98:186–191.
   Thorough review with emphasis on mild to moderate proteinuria.

2. Morrin PAF. Urine sediment in the interpretation of proteinuria. Ann Int Med 1983;98:254–255.
   Urinary sediment findings in 100 patients with renal biopsies are reviewed, confirming the role of urine sediment examination in the workup of proteinuria.

3. Papper S. Asymptomatic proteinuria. Postgraduate Med 1977;62:125–130.
   Excellent review of diagnosis and management of patients with 150 mg to 2500 mg of proteinuria and no symptoms.

4. Schwab SJ. Quantitation of proteinuria by the use of protein-to-creatinine ratios in single urine sample. Arch Int Med 1987;147:943–944.
   Protein/creatinine ratio is compared to 24-hour collection in inpatients and outpatients. The overall correlation between the two tests was .96.

5. Stewart DW, Gordon JA, Schoolwerth AC. Evaluation of proteinuria. Am Fam Physician 1984;29:218–225.
   A very good review addressing the value of the dipstick. Includes diagnostic recommendations.

184 ELECTROLYTE ABNORMALITIES

Problem

MEREDITH MATHEWS

POTASSIUM PROBLEMS

Hypokalemia

EPIDEMIOLOGY/ETIOLOGY. Hypokalemia, defined as a serum potassium less than 3.5 mEq/liter, is the most common electrolyte abnormality encountered in ambulatory medicine. It usually occurs because of renal losses of potassium (e.g., diuretics, renal tubular acidosis, hypomagnesemia, hyperaldosteronism) or gastrointestinal losses (vomiting, diarrhea).

SYMPTOMS AND SIGNS. Hypokalemia is usually asymptomatic until the potassium concentration falls below 3 mEq/liter. The earliest clinical findings are cardiac arrhythmias, particularly in patients receiving digitalis treatment. As hypokalemia becomes more severe, a variety of signs and symptoms appear, including constipation, muscle weakness, glucose intolerance, polyuria, and polydipsia. Renal failure from rhabdomyolysis and acute respiratory failure may rarely occur.

CLINICAL APPROACH. Patients with symptoms or arrhythmias should be admitted to the hospital for intravenous potassium replacement.

If the cause is not obvious from the initial interview (i.e., diuretic use, gastrointestinal losses), important laboratory studies include serum bicarbonate, urea nitrogen, creatinine, magnesium, and urine studies (potassium, creatinine, sodium). In rare cases, measurement of the plasma renin and aldosterone may be necessary to identify the cause of renal potassium losses. Gastrointestinal loss of potassium is likely when there is a history of excessive vomiting, diarrhea, or surreptitious use of laxatives and is characterized by urinary excretion of less than 20 mEq/day (or a spot K^+/creatinine ratio of less than 20.4 mEq K^+/g of creatinine). The most common cause of renal loss (suggested by absence of gastrointestinal symptoms and a urinary potassium exceeding 20 mEq/day) is diuretic use (suggested by the patient interview), followed by hyperaldosteronism (suggested by the combination of alkalosis, hypertension, and hypokalemia) and distal renal tubular acidosis (suggested by association of acidosis and hypokalemia). The combination of hypokalemia with hypocalcemia or hypophosphatemia suggests associated hypomagnesemia from renal wasting, usually due to alcohol abuse.

MANAGEMENT. Symptomatic patients require emergent inpatient intravenous replacement of potassium, administered at rates up to 10 mEq/h. More rapid correction mandates continuous electrocardiograph (ECG) monitoring in an intensive care unit.

Asymptomatic patients with only mild potassium depletion can be corrected with oral supplements at 40 mEq/day to 80 mEq/day or, if conventional diuretics are the cause, with the addition of potassium-sparing diuretics. Of these, amiloride is preferred because it has fewer side effects than spironolactone or triamterene.

Hyperkalemia

EPIDEMIOLOGY/ETIOLOGY.   Defined as a potassium greater than 5 mEq/liter, hyperkalemia is an uncommon outpatient problem, usually associated with acute renal failure. Other causes include mineralocorticoid deficiency, type 4 renal tubular acidosis, and medications (angiotensin-converting enzyme inhibitors, nonsteroidal anti-inflammatory agents). Conditions that artifactually elevate the potassium measurement are hemolysis, leukocytosis (>100,000), thrombocytosis (>1 million), or prolonged tourniquet placement during phlebotomy.

SYMPTOMS AND SIGNS.   With severe hyperkalemia, life-threatening arrhythmias (e.g., ventricular fibrillation) and severe muscle weakness may occur.

CLINICAL APPROACH.   The clinician should confirm that significant potassium elevation exists, usually by obtaining an ECG. Typical ECG features of hyperkalemia are peaked symmetric T waves (the earliest sign), loss of the P wave, and prolongation of QRS; if these features are absent, the serum potassium should be rechecked. Next, the clinician should exclude an exogenous source of potassium (e.g., salt substitute), exclude drugs that cause hyperkalemia (e.g., angiotensin-converting enzyme inhibitors, potassium-sparing diuretics), and consider type IV renal tubular acidosis.

MANAGEMENT.   Patients with ECG changes or muscle weakness require emergent hospitalization and therapy with a combination of intravenous calcium, bicarbonate, glucose and insulin, sodium polystyrene sulfonate resin (Kayexalate), and/or dialysis.

In patients with less severe hyperkalemia, the clinician should remove or treat the specific cause (e.g., exogenous potassium, offending drugs) and consider a low-potassium diet (<60 mEq/day). Patients with type 4 renal tubular acidosis may respond to fludrocortisone acetate (0.2–1.0 mg/day).

CALCIUM PROBLEMS

Hypocalcemia

ETIOLOGY.   Hypocalcemia is defined as a total calcium less than 8.5 mg/dl (assuming a normal pH and serum albumin) or an ionized calcium of less than

4.0 mg/dl (independent of pH and albumin). The most common causes of hypocalcemia are hypoparathyroidism, hypomagnesemia, vitamin D deficiency (malabsorption, phenytoin), hyperphosphatemia (ingestion of phosphate, leukemia, lymphoma), pseudohypoparathyroidism, and chronic renal failure. A low total calcium may result from hypoalbuminemia, although the ionized calcium in these patients is normal.

SYMPTOMS AND SIGNS.   The patient's presentation depends not only on the severity of hypocalcemia but also on how quickly it develops. Depression, intellectual impairment, cramps, and tetany may occur. Positive Chvostek's and Trousseau's signs (classic physical findings of tetany) are rarely found. With increasing severity, patients may develop seizures, myopathy, and cardiac arrhythmias (hypocalcemia enhances digitalis toxicity). Prolonged hypocalcemia leads to cataracts and basal ganglion calcification.

CLINICAL APPROACH.   The clinician should first verify hypocalcemia by documenting a low ionized calcium or by correcting the total calcium for the serum albumin (a decrease in the albumin of 1 gm/dl% results in a decrease in total calcium of about 0.8 mg/dl%). If the initial interview does not reveal chronic renal failure, malabsorption, or prior thyroidectomy (a common cause of hypoparathyroidism), the clinician should exclude hypomagnesemia, hypoparathyroidism (i.e., measure the intact PTH hormone), and vitamin D deficiency.

MANAGEMENT.   Patients with severe, symptomatic hypocalcemia are at risk for laryngospasm and seizures and require urgent hospitalization and intravenous replacement. In patients without symptoms, outpatient management may include calcium supplementation (2–4 g/day), given as calcium gluconate (90 mg/1gm tab) or calcium carbonate (260 mg/650 mg tab), or vitamin D (5000–10,000 U/day), which is usually added if calcium supplements alone are ineffective. Some patients with hypoparathyroidism or with advanced renal failure require 1,25 OH 2D3 (calcitriol). A third possibility is hydrochlorthiazide (50 mg/day), which may decrease the dosage requirement for calcium and vitamin D by enhancing renal tubular reabsorption of calcium.

FOLLOW-UP.   The patient's calcium should be checked every 2 weeks until stable and then every 6 months. The 24-hour urine calcium excretion should be monitored monthly until stable and should not exceed 300 mg/24 hours. The major risks of therapy are the induction of hypercalcemia or hypercalciuria.

Hypercalcemia

EPIDEMIOLOGY/ETIOLOGY.   Hypercalcemia, defined as a total calcium more than 10.5 mg/dl or ionized calcium more than 5.5 mg/dl, is relatively common. Malignancy and hyperparathyroidism account for 70% to 90% of cases. Other causes are granulomatous disease (sarcoidosis, tuberculosis, berylliosis), vitamin D intoxication, prolonged immobilization (especially with Paget's disease), thiazide diuretics, and lithium therapy.

SYMPTOMS AND SIGNS.   The clinical presentation usually reflects the underlying disease (e.g., malignancy), the severity of hypercalcemia, and how quickly it develops. Nausea, vomiting, polyuria, polydipsia, and hypertension may be followed by lethargy, stupor, and renal failure. With slowly progressive or stable, mild hypercalcemia, renal stones may occur without other symptoms of hypercalcemia.

CLINICAL APPROACH.   The patient interview should identify common drugs that cause hypercalcemia (e.g., lithium, thiazide diuretics, vitamin A, vitamin D, calcium-containing antacids). The physical examination adds little except to document the severity of hypercalcemia (e.g., stupor) or occasionally reveal the underlying disease (e.g., malignancy). Important laboratory studies include an intact PTH assay (elevated in hyperparathyroidism), 25 OH vitamin D level (elevated with excess vitamin D intake), 1,25 (OH) vitamin D levels (elevated in granulomatous disease), and PTH-related peptide (PTHrp, a polypeptide released by most cancers that cause hypercalcemia). If hypercalcemia is asymptomatic and stable, these tests may be sequenced, with the intact PTH assay usually being the initial test. Otherwise, all of the tests should be obtained as soon as possible so specific treatment can be initiated quickly. If these studies are unavailing, an occult tumor that does not release PTHrp but directly invades bone is most likely; chest radiography, mammography, stool occult blood, liver function tests, serum protein electrophoresis, and bone scans may be necessary for diagnosis.

MANAGEMENT.   In patients with advanced malignancy and severe hypercalcemia, the clinician should initially decide whether any therapy is appropriate. Therapy that focuses only on patient comfort may be more appropriate for patients with less than 6 months to live.

If the clinician decides to treat the hypercalcemia, correction of volume depletion, followed by brisk diuresis with furosemide, is very effective. In most patients, initial therapy requires hospitalization, parenteral fluids and diuretics, and parenteral replacement of the measured water and electrolytes lost in the diuresis (other than calcium). These measures alone usually lower the calcium to a safe range (<13.5 mg% for total or 8.0 mg% for ionized calcium). Other measures that act rapidly include aminohydroxypropilidene (APD, a newly released bisphophonate that suppresses bone resorption), corticosteroids, and calcitonin. The response to mithramycin is somewhat slower. When patients do not respond promptly to these measures and do not appear to have a malignancy, the clinician should expedite the PTH assay and consider referral for emergency parathyroidectomy.

FOLLOW-UP.   Although follow-up depends on the underlying disease, most patients who require ongoing therapy are seen frequently (weekly to monthly) to measure the calcium level.

PHOSPHATE PROBLEMS

Hypophosphatemia

EPIDEMIOLOGY/ETIOLOGY.   Hypophosphatemia is defined as a serum phosphate less than 3 mg/dl. Causes include gastrointestinal losses (antacids, malabsorption, vitamin D deficiency), renal losses (hyperparathyroidism, proximal renal tubular acidosis, glycosuria, acetazolamide or metolazone therapy, corticosteroids, hypomagnesemia, hypokalemia), or redistribution (insulin or glucose administration). In the outpatient setting, the most common causes are malabsorption and antacid use. Risk factors for hypophosphatemia include alcoholism, diabetes, and tumors (especially of mesenchymal origin).

SYMPTOMS AND SIGNS.   Severe hypophosphatemia (<1.0 mg/dl) is necessary to produce symptoms, which include muscle weakness, irritability, paresthesias, confusion, osteomalacia, and a reversible hemolytic anemia. A reversible, dilated cardiomyopathy has also been described.

CLINICAL APPROACH.   Patients with severe symptoms require immediate replacement therapy (see "Management") before further evaluation. The best initial diagnostic test is measurement of the 24-hour urinary excretion of phosphate. If the urine phosphate exceeds 100 mg/day, renal phosphate wasting is confirmed. Subsequent tests include serum PTH, bicarbonate, potassium, and magnesium. Urine phosphate measurements less than 100 mg/day suggest gastrointestinal loss.

MANAGEMENT.   For patients with serious symptoms or severe hypophosphatemia (<1.0 mg/dl), intravenous replacement should be initiated. In less severe cases, oral phosphate replacement may include skim or low-fat milk (1 quart = 1 g) or phosphosoda (100 cc = 16.4 g). Replacement should not exceed 2 g/day and is stopped when the phosphate level reaches 2.5 mg/dl.

FOLLOW-UP.   Periodic monitoring is necessary since many of the conditions causing phosphate depletion are not reversible.

Hyperphosphatemia

EPIDEMIOLOGY/ETIOLOGY.   Hyperphosphatemia, defined as a serum phosphate more than 6.0 mg/dl, is uncommon in the outpatient setting but may occur in chronic renal failure, primary hypoparathyroidism, or rarely as a consequence of thyrotoxicosis, acromegaly, or treatment with diphosphonates.

SYMPTOMS AND SIGNS.   The clinical presentation usually reflects the hypocalcemia that accompanies hyperphosphatemia (see "Hypocalcemia"). In the patient with renal failure, metastatic calcifications can occur.

CLINICAL APPROACH.   Routine laboratory tests include serum creatinine.

MANAGEMENT.   Discussion of the management of chronic renal failure appears in Section 181. Most patients require a low-phosphate diet (<1000 mg/day) and phosphate binders (calcium acetate, 5–6 g/day, with meals).

FOLLOW-UP.   The clinician should periodically evaluate the calcium phosphate product, which equals the serum calcium × serum phosphate (units of both in mg/dl). This product should not exceed 60.

MAGNESIUM PROBLEMS

Hypomagnesemia

EPIDEMIOLOGY/ETIOLOGY.   Hypomagnesemia is defined as a serum magnesium of less than 1.5 mEq/liter. The prevalence in a mixed ambulatory and hospitalized population is 9% to 12%. The principal causes are inadequate intake (normal intake = 250–350 mg/day), gastrointestinal losses (malabsorption, alcoholism), and renal losses (loop diuretics, hyperaldosteronism, hypercalcemia, idiopathic hypercalciuria, inappropriate antidiuretic hormone syndrome, phosphate depletion, alcoholism, renal tubular acidosis, aminoglycosides, cisplatin, and amphotericin). Alcoholism and malabsorption, or both, are the most common causes.

Hypomagnesemia may lead to hypocalcemia, hypokalemia, and/or hypophosphatemia. If any one of these other electrolyte disorders is present, the likelihood of coexistent hypomagnesemia is 30%; if two are present, the likelihood of hypomagnesemia increases to more than 60%.

SYMPTOMS AND SIGNS.   The symptoms of hypomagnesemia are nonspecific and include weakness, anorexia, nausea, vomiting, muscle cramps, and refractory arrhythmias.

CLINICAL APPROACH.   The clinician should separate inadequate intake or gastrointestinal loss from renal wasting of magnesium by determining the 24-hour urinary excretion of magnesium. If urine magnesium is less than 2.0 mEq per 24 hours, inadequate intake or gastrointestinal losses from laxative abuse, steatorrhea, alcoholism, or pancreatitis are likely. If the 24-hour excretion exceeds 4.0 mEq, renal tubular wasting is the cause.

MANAGEMENT.   Treatment with 50 mg to 100 mg of magnesium three or four times daily for 3 days to 4 days will treat the usual deficit seen in symptomatic individuals. Choices of replacement are magnesium gluconate (500 mg tab has 27 mg magnesium), magnesium carbonate (250 mg tab has 60 mg magnesium), and chelated magnesium (500 mg has 100 mg magnesium).

FOLLOW-UP.   In patients who consume a normal diet, follow-up is usually unnecessary.

Hypermagnesemia

EPIDEMIOLOGY/ETIOLOGY.   Hypermagnesemia, defined by a serum magnesium greater than 3.0 mEq/liter, is rare in the ambulatory setting. Hypermagnesemia requires the combination of decreased renal function and an increased intake of magnesium. Elderly patients who may have reduced renal function and a tendency to abuse laxatives are at greatest risk, followed by patients with renal failure using magnesium-containing antacids.

SYMPTOMS AND SIGNS.   When the magnesium level exceeds 4 mEq/liter, though this is rarely observed, symptoms occur, including depressed consciousness, hypotension, and cardiac arrest.

MANAGEMENT.   The clinician should discontinue any exogenous magnesium compounds. If symptoms are present, hospitalization and consideration of dialysis are indicated.

Cross-references: Diagnosis and Management of Alcoholism (Section 9), Essential Hypertension (Section 86), Diarrhea (Section 92), Osteoporosis (Section 117), Muscular Weakness (Section 139), Seizures (Section 141), Dementia (Section 142), Chronic Renal Failure (Section 181), Changes in Mentation in the Patient with Cancer (Section 205).

REFERENCES

1. Brautbar N, Kleeman CR. Hypophosphatemia and hyperphosphatemia: Clinical and pathophysiologic aspects. In Nachman B, Massry SG, Eds. Clinical Disorders of Fluid and Electrolyte Metabolism, 4th ed. McGraw-Hill, New York, 1987, pp. 789–830.

2. Brautbar N, Massry SG. Hypomagnesemia and hypermagnesemia in Clinical Disorders of Fluid and Electrolyte Metabolism, 4th ed. McGraw-Hill, New York, 1987, pp. 831–49.

3. Nardone DA, McDonald WJ, Girard DE. Mechanisms of hypokalemia. Medicine 1978;57:435–446.

4. Narins RG, Heifets M, Tannen RL. The patient with hypokalemia or hyperkalemia. In Schrier RW. Manual of Nephrology, 3d ed. Little, Brown, Boston, 1990, pp. 37–54.

5. Raymond KH, Kunau RT. Hypokalemic states. In Nachman B, Massry SG, Eds. Clinical Disorders of Fluid and Electrolyte Metabolism, 4th ed. McGraw-Hill, New York, 1987, pp. 519–546.

185 SCROTAL MASS

Problem

STEVEN R. McGEE

EPIDEMIOLOGY. Varicoceles and testicular cancer occur most often between ages 15 and 35 years; hydroceles and spermatoceles usually affect men over age 30 years. Varicoceles are found in 9.5% of young healthy men, though most of these masses are small and asymptomatic.

ETIOLOGY. **Hydroceles** result from accumulation of fluid between the two layers of the tunica vaginalis, the remnant of peritoneum that descends during fetal development into the scrotum with the testes. Most hydroceles are idiopathic, although some are due to trauma, inguinal surgery, epididymitis, or a testicular tumor. Bilateral hydroceles are common in patients with anasarca (e.g., uncontrolled congestive heart failure, nephrotic syndrome). **Spermatoceles** are sperm-containing cysts on top of the testis that presumably occur because of blockage in the efferent ductules of the rete testis. **Varicoceles,** associated in many studies with abnormal sperm counts, are dilated veins in the pampiniform plexus of the spermatic cord. Seventy-eight percent to 93% of varicoceles appear in the left hemiscrotum; the remainder are bilateral. Most **testicular tumors** are malignant and originate from germ cells.

In surveys of men referred for ultrasound because of nontender scrotal swellings (inguinal hernias excluded), hydroceles are found in 33% to 56% of cases, spermatoceles in 9% to 29%, cancer in 5% to 18%, varicoceles in 4% to 16%, and miscellaneous diagnoses (e.g., cysts, nontesticular tumors, chronic epididymitis) in 14% to 18%.

CLINICAL APPROACH. The approach to the acutely painful and inflamed scrotum appears in Section 173. In those with nontender scrotal swellings, the examination should include bimanual scrotal palpation with the patient standing and supine, and transillumination (Table 185–1). The length of the normal adult testis is 3.5 cm to 5.0 cm.

Any intratesticular mass found on examination should be regarded as testicular cancer until proved otherwise. These patients should be promptly referred to a urologist; ultrasound may provide additional information but should not delay consultation. All other patients with nontender scrotal swellings—unless inguinal hernia is suspected—require a ultrasound examination to confirm the diagnosis, for two reasons. First, ultrasound is more accurate than clinical examination; up to 28% of cancers identified in some ultrasound surveys were found in patients referred with benign diagnoses. Second, some patients have more than one diagnosis; 10% of testicular tumors, for example, present with hydroceles that prevent adequate palpation of the testis.

TABLE 185–1. NONTENDER SCROTAL MASSES: CLINICAL EXAMINATION

Condition	Findings	Transilluminates?	Supine versus Standing
Inguinal hernia	Mass *extends* into inguinal region Unable to get fingers above mass Mass increases with Valsalva Bowel sounds in mass Sometimes reducible	No	Often smaller supine
Hydrocele	Large, pear-shaped anterior mass Skin stretched, shiny, red Penis appears shortened Obscures testis in 90%	Yes[1]	No change
Spermatocele	Discrete cystic mass on superior testis Usually < 2 cm diameter May be multiple	Yes	No change
Varicocele	Bluish discoloration "Bag of worms" Involves cord May increase with Valsalva	No	Collapses or disappears in supine position
Tumor	Firm intratesticular mass	No	No change
Sebaceous cyst	Round (size of marble), firm, yellow Confined within scrotal skin	No	No change

[1]In chronic hydroceles, thickened wall may prevent transillumination.

The acute appearance of symptomatic varicoceles in elderly men suggests obstruction of the spermatic veins by retroperitoneal disorders, frequently renal tumors. Right varicoceles are associated with total situs inversus.

MANAGEMENT. Patients with inguinal hernias should be referred to a surgeon. Most hydroceles and spermatoceles require no treatment, but if they become large, uncomfortable, or embarrassing, referral to a urologist for excision is appropriate. Aspiration of hydroceles is a reasonable alternative for the symptomatic patient with contraindications to surgery, but fluid usually appears again within weeks to months. Whether varicocele repair improves abnormal sperm counts is controversial.

Cross-references: Male Infertility (Section 159), Cancer of the Genitourinary System (Section 170), Scrotal Pain (Section 173).

REFERENCES

1. Fowler RC, Chennells PM, Ewing R. Scrotal ultrasonography: A clinical evaluation. Br J Radiol 1987;60:649–654.
   Ultrasound is diagnostically superior to physical examination.

2. Kromann-Andersen B, Hansen LB, Larsen PN, et al. Clinical versus ultrasonographic evaluation of scrotal disorders. Br J Urol 1988;61:350–353.
   In 104 consecutive patients with scrotal abnormalities, the sensitivity/specificity of physical diagnosis, compared to the surgical diagnosis as the gold standard, was 0.9/0.81 for cancer, 0.89/0.96 for hydrocele, 0.74/0.94 for spermatocele, and 0.93/1.0 for varicocele.

3. Macksood MJ, James RE. The scrotal mass: Cause and diagnosis. Am J Surg 1983;145:297–299.
   Retrospective survey of 278 patients; includes a recommended approach.

4. Spittel JA, DeWeerd JH, Shick RM. Acute varicocele: A vascular clue to renal tumor. Mayo Clin Proc 1959;34:134–137.
   The initial presentation of left hypernephroma in three men, age 46 to 58 years, was acute symptomatic left varicocele.

5. Zornow DH, Landes RR. Scrotal palpation. Am Fam Physician 1981;23:150–154.
   Excellent review of normal and abnormal examination.

186 BENIGN PROSTATIC HYPERPLASIA

Problem

JOHN B. STIMSON

EPIDEMIOLOGY. Eighty-five percent of men over age 80 years have histologic evidence of benign prostatic hyperplasia (BPH). Prostatectomy to treat clinically significant BPH is the most common surgery performed in men over age 65 years. The cause is not known, but the process is clearly androgen dependent.

SYMPTOMS AND SIGNS. Obstructive symptoms of BPH include decreased force of urine stream, hesitancy, intermittent stream, and postvoid dribbling. Nocturia, urgency, and frequency are also symptoms seen in BPH but are termed "irritative" because they are felt to reflect detrusor muscle instability rather than a direct effect of obstruction. Irritative symptoms are less likely to abate with surgical treatment. Although acute urinary retention can complicate BPH, it is not necessarily related to the severity of preexisting symptoms and is generally precipitated by medications or spontaneous infarction of hyperplastic prostatic tissue. Rarely, patients with unsuspected renal failure from severe bladder outlet obstruction present with uremic symptoms despite minimal symptoms of BPH.

Few useful physical signs exist. Prostate size on rectal examination correlates poorly with symptom severity, although rectal examination is performed to detect prostate cancer or prostatitis. The bladder may be palpable in the lower abdomen if it decompensates and becomes distended.

CLINICAL APPROACH. Symptoms suggesting BPH can be caused by a number of other conditions. Intrinsic renal disease, glycosuria, and diuretic therapy cause frequency and nocturia and exacerbate symptoms in those with mild prostatism. Sympathomimetic and anticholinergic medications often worsen the obstructive symptoms of BPH. UTI can cause obstructive as well as irritative symptoms. Neurologic diseases affecting bladder function (e.g., stroke, autonomic neuropathy, multiple sclerosis, Parkinson's disease) may be difficult to differentiate from BPH. A careful medication and neurologic history, neurologic examination, and urinalysis, with culture if necessary, will identify these conditions. Serum blood urea and creatinine should be obtained, and, if elevated, hydronephrosis from severe bladder outlet obstruction should be excluded by ultrasound. If confirmed, prostatectomy is best postponed until bladder drainage by catheter stabilizes renal function.

MANAGEMENT. Patients with normal renal function and tolerable symptoms can be reassured and followed yearly. Symptoms can be minimized by avoidance of diuretics, caffeine, alcohol, sympathomimetics, and anticholinergics. Those with intolerable symptoms warrant further evaluation to confirm that BPH is the cause. Maximum urine flow rate is an easily performed test that helps confirm the presence of obstruction. If more than 150 ml is voided, maximum flow rates less than 10 ml/min indicate either significant obstruction to urine flow or detrusor muscle weakness. Cystourethroscopy visually confirms the presence of obstructing prostatic tissue and rules out a urethral stricture but is not routinely necessary prior to therapy.

Although surgery is the treatment of choice for patients with significant symptoms, the alpha-blockers prazosin (up to 2 mg b.i.d.) or terazosin (2–10 mg q.d.), modestly improve symptoms and offer an option for those who decline surgery or are too ill to withstand the procedure.

Transurethral resection of the prostate is the most common surgical approach used, with open prostatectomy reserved for large prostates that would take too long to resect transurethrally. Transurethral incision of the prostate is appropriate for small glands because full resection in this circumstance carries an unacceptably high risk of bladder neck contracture. Recent reviews of claims data suggest that open prostatectomy is associated with fewer reoperations for recurrent obstruction, but this has not been confirmed by a randomized trial.[2]

Risks of surgery include death (0.2–4.2%), late postoperative bleeding (1.1–7.5%), urge incontinence (1.5–6%), total incontinence (<1%), urethral stricture (7.8–9.5%), bladder neck contracture (highly variable), impotence (5–34%), UTI (15–30%), and epididymitis (0–6%). The re-operation rate for recurrent obstruction is 0.6% to 2.5% per year.

Hormonal therapy with luteinizing hormone-releasing hormone agonists reduces prostatic size and improves symptoms in many patients but also renders them impotent. Oral 5-alpha reductase inhibitors are under investigation and appear to have similar effects on the prostate without altering sexual function, offering a promising nonsurgical treatment for many patients.

Cross-references: Cancer of the Genitourinary System (Section 170), Dysuria (Section 172), Prostate Cancer (Section 175), Urinary Tract Infections in Men (Section 179), Bacteriuria in the Elderly (Section 180), Chronic Renal Failure (Section 181).

REFERENCES

1. Barry MJ, Mulley AG, Fowler FJ, et al. Watchful waiting vs. immediate transurethral resection for symptomatic prostatism: The importance of patients' preferences. JAMA 1988; 259:3010–3017.
    Decision analysis in symptomatic patients without chronic retention demonstrates that patient preferences are the most important factor in the decision to recommend prostatectomy.

2. Roos NP, Wennberg JE, Malenka DJ, et al. Mortality and re-operation after open and transurethral resection of the prostate for benign prostatic hyperplasia. N Engl J Med 1989;320:1120–1124.

When compared with open prostatectomy, re-operation was 2.7 times to 6.7 times more likely after transurethral resection of the prostate. Mortality was 10% to 45% higher, despite adjustments for co-morbidity. Raises questions about current surgical practice and provides support for a head-to-head randomized trial.

3. Stimson JB, Fihn SD. Benign prostatic hyperplasia and its treatment. J Gen Intern Med 1990;5:153–165.

Recent review summarizes literature on natural history and treatment of BPH.

XVI CHAPTER

PSYCHIATRIC AND PSYCHOSOMATIC DISORDERS

187 SCREENING FOR DEPRESSION

Screening

GREGORY E. SIMON

EPIDEMIOLOGY. Major depression has a prevalence of 2% to 3% among the U.S. population, with prevalence among medical outpatients of 20% to 40%. Depression is an episodic illness with first onset in adolescence or early adulthood, peak prevalence in middle age, and declining prevalence in later years. Prevalence rates for females are approximately twice those for males in clinical and population samples. Most treatment of depression in the United States is delivered by primary care medical providers. Less than one-third of community residents with recent major depression report use of specialty mental health services.

RATIONALE. Major depression carries a burden of morbidity and disability equivalent to serious chronic medical illness. Depression also increases mortality through both an increase in suicide rates and a generalized increase in all-cause mortality. Patients with depression accompanying other medical conditions report more severe symptoms and poorer functional outcomes. Depression is associated with increased use of outpatient medical services. Treatment of depression is effective in approximately 65% of cases, and early treatment appears to reduce the risk of chronicity. In typical primary care practices, though, only 50% of patients with major depression are recognized, and a smaller portion receive effective treatment.

STRATEGY. Routine new-patient questionnaires should include screening questions for depression—either standard self-report instruments [Beck Depression Inventory, Hopkins Symptom Checklist Depression Scale, or Center for Epidemiologic Studies Depression Scale (CES-D)] or new items added to the usual review of systems checklist inquiring about sad or depressed mood, loss of interest or energy, crying spells, and suicidal ideation. These standard screening questionnaires typically achieve sensitivities of over 80% with specificities of over 50% when compared with structured psychiatric interview as the gold standard. Positive responses to screening questions should be followed up with specific questions covering diagnostic criteria for major depression described in Section 192. This examination typically takes less than 10 minutes. Patients who have positive screening tests but do not meet diagnostic criteria for current major depression should be reexamined at their next visit. Specific examination for depression should also be triggered by clinical problems strongly associated with depression in primary care (e.g., chronic pain, insomnia, multiple unexplained physical symptoms, and high use of medical services) or by medical conditions frequently complicated by depression (e.g., stroke, Parkinson's disease, and systemic lupus erythematosus).

ACTION.   See Section 192 (Management of Depression).

Cross-references: Periodic Health Assessment (Section 7), Somatization (Section 191), Management of Depression (Section 192).

REFERENCES

1.   Katon W, Sullivan MD. Depression and chronic medical illness. J Clin Psychiatry 1990;51(suppl 6):3–11.

Reviews comorbidity of depression with medical illness, lack of recognition of depression in primary care, and evidence for efficacy of treatment.

2.   Schurman RA, Kramer PD, Mitchell JB. The hidden mental health network. Arch Gen Psychiatry 1985;42:89–94.

Demonstrates the primary role of medical providers in managing depression, especially among the elderly.

188 GENERALIZED ANXIETY

Symptom

GREGORY E. SIMON

EPIDEMIOLOGY. Clinically significant anxiety affects 2% to 5% of the U.S. general population and approximately 20% of patients in a medical clinic population. Anxiety disorders typically begin in early adulthood and affect women approximately twice as often as men.

ETIOLOGY. Anxiety may be a nonspecific response to various biological, psychological, and social factors. Although anxiety in primary care medical patients may result from undiagnosed medical illness, clinicians should avoid exhaustive efforts to exclude all potential medical causes, no matter how rare. Metabolic states associated with anxiety include withdrawal syndromes, medication side effects and intoxication, hyperthyroidism, hypoglycemia, and hypoxia. Specific psychiatric disorders accompanied by anxiety include alcohol or drug abuse or dependence, panic disorder, phobia, and depression. Nonspecific generalized anxiety refers to the heterogeneous group remaining once these more specific syndromes have been excluded.

CLINICAL APPROACH. After a reasonable medical evaluation (including review of prescription and nonprescription medication), evaluation should focus on symptoms of depression, panic attacks, and alcohol or drug use. Phobic anxiety occurs in specific feared situations (e.g., bridges, heights, crowds, open spaces), while generalized anxiety is more pervasive although often heightened by social stresses.

MANAGEMENT. Treatment should first focus on any specific medical or psychiatric disorder that may contribute to anxiety. Alcohol and drug abuse or dependence take precedence over other diagnoses, and no separate diagnosis of anxiety disorder should be considered until after weeks of abstinence. All patients with generalized anxiety (even those with no pattern of substance abuse) should be advised to avoid all caffeine and alcohol. The short-term anxiolytic effects of alcohol are often followed by withdrawal anxiety. Generalized anxiety associated with depression or panic disorder typically responds well to treatment of those specific problems. For patients with nonspecific anxiety, cognitive and behavioral approaches should be the primary treatments. Good self-help manuals to guide patients through these treatments are available (see References).

Cognitive approaches to anxiety focus on the half-conscious, often unreasonable thoughts associated with anxiety. Patients are asked to focus on the specific thoughts occurring during times of greatest distress. By learning to

589

examine the irrational fears associated with anxiety, patients gain a sense of calm and self-control. For example, a patient reporting disabling symptoms of fear, ruminative worry, nausea, and tension headaches after starting a new job would be asked to examine out loud the thoughts associated with these anxiety symptoms. After describing fears of failing at work leading to being fired, losing his or her apartment, and being left penniless, the patient is asked to separate reasonable concerns (increased work pressures) from exaggerated ones (bankruptcy and homelessness). Performing this exercise, initially with the help of a calm and concerned clinician, will help him or her to master subsequent anxious thoughts. Practice at home and reinforcement during later visits are critical to building confidence. Anxiety following specific life stresses often responds to such an approach.

Behavioral approaches to anxiety use relaxation exercises to relieve associated physical symptoms. Typical exercises begin with rhythmic deep breathing followed by visualization of relaxing images and progressive muscle relaxation. Systematically tensing and relaxing specific muscle groups helps patients to focus on relaxation while avoiding distracting fearful thoughts. After initial instruction during an office visit, patients should practice two to three times a day at home to build skill and self-confidence. Exercises focusing on muscle relaxation are especially useful to patients suffering from tension-related physical complaints (headache, muscle stiffness, dyspnea).

Phobic anxiety also calls for strategies to overcome situational fears. Avoidance of feared situations reinforces anxiety and leads to a cycle of increasing anxiety and withdrawal. Clinicians should assist patients in developing a plan for gradually increasing their exposure to feared situations. For example, a patient with intense fear of shopping in crowded stores is first told to go to the supermarket at an uncrowded time in the company of a friend. Although this may produce some anxiety, he or she should remain until the initial wave of fear passes. This exercise should be repeated until it no longer provokes any anxiety. Then the patient should gradually increase the level of exposure (e.g., going into the store alone while a friend remains in view outside). Using this incremental technique, he or she should increase the level of exposure after tolerating the lower exposure level without difficulty. With this approach, most phobic patients can confront previously intolerable situations with a manageable level of anxiety.

Benzodiazepine anxiolytics, although useful for management of short-term situational anxiety, should be avoided for management of chronic anxiety states. As-needed use of anxiolytics for generalized anxiety should be confined to periods of 1 month or less and avoided completely for patients with histories of alcohol or sedative abuse. Accumulation of benzodiazepines in the elderly carries risks of oversedation, cognitive impairment, and injury due to falls. Shorter half-life medications carry less risk of tolerance, dependence, and accumulation. Less lipophilic drugs have more gradual onset and thus less reinforcement for frequent use. Lorazepam and oxazepam satisfy both of these criteria (Table 188–1).

TABLE 188–1.   SELECTED ANXIOLYTIC DRUGS

Drug	Starting Dose	Speed of Onset[1]	Half-life (hr)[2]	Daily Cost ($)[3]
Diazepam	5 mg b.i.d. PRN	+ + + +	20–100	0.05
Chlordiazepoxide	10 mg b.i.d. PRN	+ +	10–30	0.05
Lorazepam	0.5 mg t.i.d. PRN	+ +	5–20	0.15
Oxazepam	15 mg t.i.d. PRN	+	5–15	0.60
Alprazolam	0.25 mg t.i.d. PRN	+ + +	8–12	1.32
Buspirone	5 mg b.i.d.	0	20–100	0.96

[1]+ + + +, rapid onset; 0, very slow onset.
[2]May be greatly prolonged in the elderly.
[3]Average wholesale cost for starting dose listed, 1991 *Drug Topics Red Book*.

Buspirone, a new nonbenzodiazepine anxiolytic, appears to have little potential for abuse and does not provoke tolerance or dependence. Although quite effective in some patients with generalized anxiety, it appears less universally efficacious than benzodiazepines and provokes agitation in a significant minority. It must be dosed regularly for 1 week to 2 weeks to achieve therapeutic effect and is thus not suitable for PRN use. Patients with histories of alcohol or benzodiazepine abuse (the population for whom this drug might be most useful) appear to respond less often to buspirone.

FOLLOW-UP.   Cognitive and behavioral techniques require both continued practice by patients and reinforcement by clinicians to remain effective. Group programs offering instruction in cognitive and behavioral techniques may be helpful. Psychiatric consultation may be necessary in cases of significant generalized anxiety persisting over 1 month and unresponsive to nonpharmacologic interventions. Both patients and clinicians must realize that complete relief of chronic generalized anxiety is an unrealistic goal. Management should focus on relief of symptoms and reduction of functional disability.

Cross-references: Diagnosis and Management of Drug Abuse (Section 8), Diagnosis and Management of Alcoholism (Section 9), Dyspnea (Section 19), Fatigue (Section 21), Chest Pain (Section 74), Palpitations (Section 76), Tremor (Section 138), Screening for Thyroid Disease (Section 153), Insomnia (Section 189), Hyperventilation Syndrome (Section 190), Panic Disorder (Section 194).

REFERENCES

1. Burns DD. The Feeling Good Handbook. Plume Press, New York, 1979.
    Good, practical guide to cognitive treatment of anxiety.

2. Rosenbaum JF. The drug treatment of anxiety. New Engl J Med 1982;306:401–404.
    Reviews evaluation and treatment of anxiety, with focus on benzodiazepines.

3. Weekes C. Peace from Nervous Suffering. Bantam Books, New York, 1972.
    Brief, practical, and supportive guide to self-treatment of anxiety and phobias, with focus on relief of physical symptoms.

189 INSOMNIA

Symptom

SUE ANNE WIEDENFELD

EPIDEMIOLOGY.   Insomnia refers to a group of problems characterized by difficulty initiating and maintaining sleep. Thirteen percent to 30% of the general population experience insomnia in any given year, and half of them rate their problem as severe. Fifty percent of psychiatric patients report a sleep complaint. Insomnia is twice as common among women as men and becomes more common with advanced age.

ETIOLOGY.   Insomnia may be transient (situational) or chronic. Transient insomnia results from temporary medical conditions (especially those associated with pain, discomfort, anxiety, or depression), use of pharmacologic agents (e.g., amphetamines, beta-blockers, steroids), or temporary emotional stress.

Chronic insomnia is often associated with chronic medical conditions (cardiac, respiratory, or renal disease), other chronic physiologic conditions (nocturnal myoclonus, sleep apnea, sleep-wake cycle disturbance), psychiatric conditions (especially depression and anxiety disorders), chronic drug use (alcohol, caffeine, nicotine, and sedatives), environmental factors, and poor sleep habits. Chronic use of sedative-hypnotic medication (especially in the elderly, who are already at higher risk for sleep disturbance) interferes with normal sleep patterns by suppressing the dream phase of sleep.

CLINICAL APPROACH.   The clinician should determine whether the insomnia is of recent onset or chronic, and carefully consider each of the possible causes. The evaluation should focus on the patient's sleep habits, underlying medical or psychiatric conditions, emotional stress, use of medication, alcohol, and caffeine, and symptoms that appear at night (e.g., nocturia, dyspnea). Marked daytime drowsiness may suggest sleep apnea or narcolepsy.

MANAGEMENT.   Treatment of the primary medical condition or substance abuse may alleviate insomnia. Review of optimal sleep conditions (Table 189–1) with the patient is helpful. Psychotherapy or biofeedback may decrease stress and reduce arousal during the night. Suspected physiologic conditions (sleep apnea, narcolepsy, nocturnal myoclonus, and circadian rhythm dysfunction) are best referred to a center experienced in sleep disorders.

Sleeping pills are prescribed in the lowest dose for the shortest time possible—a few weeks at most—and are appropriate during temporary conditions such as a short hospitalization or a death in the family. Benzodiazepines are usually recommended but are contraindicated for sleep apnea patients, sub-

TABLE 189–1.   OPTIMAL SLEEP CONDITIONS

Behavioral Changes
Eliminate daytime naps.
Maintain a fixed schedule of waking times, regardless of sleep.
Exercise early in the day.
Limit intake of caffeine or alcohol.
Go to another room if you can't sleep and return when tired.
Plan relaxing activities in the evening.
Avoid eating in bed or eating large quantities late in the day.
Restrict liquids late in the day.
Use relaxation exercises before sleep.
Use general daytime stress management strategies.
Use cognitive coping strategies.

Environmental Changes
Use a quiet room reserved for sleeping.
Place the clock out of sight.
Use dark shades.
Soundproof the room if necessary.
Minimize clutter and distractions.
Keep the room at a comfortable temperature.

stance abusers, and pregnant women. Tolerance to hypnotic medication may result in rebound insomnia after withdrawal of the drug. Changing sleep habits are always preferable to sedative medication. The amino acid L-tryptophan should not be used because it has been associated with eosinophilic myositis and fascitis.

FOLLOW-UP.   Patients with refractory insomnia should be referred to a sleep clinic.

Cross-references: Chronic Pain Syndrome (Section 13), Fatigue (Section 21), Sleep Apnea Syndrome (Section 64), Restless Legs Syndrome (Section 114), Fibromyalgia (Section 122), Screening for Depression (Section 187), Generalized Anxiety (Section 188), Management of Depression (Section 192).

REFERENCES

1.   Fredrickson P. The relevance of sleep disorders: medicine to psychiatric practice. Psychiatr Ann, 1987;17:2,91–100.
     Describes epidemiology and treatment of insomnia and discusses other sleep disorders such as excessive somnolence, sleep-wake disorders, and parasomnias.

2.   Gillian J, Byerley W. The diagnosis and management of insomnia. N Engl J Med 1990;322:239–248.
     Describes etiologic factors and management issues in short- and long-term insomnia, with extensive discussion of specific sleeping pills and their clinical usefulness.

3.   Hauri P, Esther M. Insomnia. Mayo Clin Proc 1990;65:869–882.
     Describes diagnostic assessment in insomnia and provides in-depth discussion of treatment strategies.

4. Kales A, Soldatos CR, Kales JD. Sleep disorders: Insomnia, sleepwalking, night terrors, nightmares, and enuresis. Ann Intern Med 1987;106:582–592.
   In-depth review of diagnosis and treatment of five sleep disorders.

5. Prinz P, Vitiello M, Rasking M, et al. Geriatrics: Sleep disorders and aging. N Engl J Med 1990;323:520–526. .
   Reviews common causes of sleep disturbance in the elderly and the use of sedative hypnotic agents in this population.

190 HYPERVENTILATION SYNDROME

Problem

ERIKA GOLDSTEIN

EPIDEMIOLOGY. **Hyperventilation syndrome** describes symptoms produced by ventilation in excess of metabolic requirements, and excludes physiologic causes of hyperventilation (e.g., pneumonia, heart failure, metabolic acidosis). The incidence of hyperventilation syndrome in the general population reportedly varies between 6% and 11%, although in studies conducted in general medical clinics, up to 30% to 40% of patients have symptoms attributable to it. Most cases occur between ages 20 and 40 years, but hyperventilation syndrome can occur at any age and may be more common in women. The diagnosis of hyperventilation syndrome overlaps considerably with anxiety disorders, and their precise relationship is controversial.

SIGNS AND SYMPTOMS. Acute hyperventilation syndrome is rare (1% of cases) and is characterized by dramatic hyperpnea, anxiety, tetany, and carpopedal spasm. The chronic form is vastly more common (99% of cases) and is often misdiagnosed because the presenting symptoms may be referable to any organ system (Table 190–1). The breathing pattern often appears normal. Signs and symptoms result from metabolic derangements induced by hyperventilation and from anxiety. Most patients present with cardiovascular (52%) or neurologic symptoms (23%) rather than respiratory complaints (6%).

CLINICAL APPROACH. The diagnosis of hyperventilation syndrome relies on the exclusion of organic disease by history and physical examination and is confirmed by performing a hyperventilation provocation test. A positive test is defined by reproduction of the patient's symptoms within 5 minutes while breathing deeply and rapidly (30–40/min). The test should be discontinued after 5 minutes or when the patient complains of dizziness. A blood gas determina-

TABLE 190–1.   HYPERVENTILATION SYNDROME: ASSOCIATED SYMPTOMS

General	Cardiovascular
Irritability	Palpations
Weakness	Chest pain
Exhaustion	Tachycardia
Fatigue	
	Neurologic
Respiratory	Headache
Sighing and yawning	Dizziness
Shortness of breath	Lightheadedness
Air hunger	Numbness and tingling
	Unsteadiness
Musculoskeletal	Impaired memory/concentration
Arthralgia	Giddiness
Tremors	Visual disturbances
Myalgia	
Carpopedal spasm	**Gastrointestinal**
Tetany	Belching
	Flatulence
Psychogenic	Dysphagia
Apprehension	Dry mouth
Anxiety/panic	Bloating
Nervousness	Globus sensation
Tension	Abdominal distress
Sweating	Anorexia and/or nausea

Source: Brashear RE. Hyperventilation syndrome. Lung 1983;161:257–273.

tion to confirm hypocapnia is probably unnecessary. Once symptoms appear, rebreathing into a paper bag will terminate symptoms. Provocative testing is contraindicated in patients with chronic obstructive pulmonary disease, chronic hypercapnia, sickle cell anemia, or history of seizures or strokes. In patients with coronary artery disease or spasm, continuous electrocardiogram (ECG) monitoring should accompany the test.

MANAGEMENT.   Seventy percent of patients improve dramatically after the relationship between symptoms and the metabolic derangements induced by hyperventilation is demonstrated by provocative testing and explained by the provider. Although rebreathing terminates symptoms acutely, it is not adequate long-term therapy. More effective are psychotherapy, behavior therapy, physical training to correct "bad breathing habits," and drug therapy. Pharmacologic therapies, in order of preference, include imipramine (25–150 mg q.d.) or other antidepressants, beta-blockers (propranolol, 80 mg q.d.), monoamine oxidase inhibitors (phenelzine, 45–90 mg q.d. in 3 divided doses), and benzodiazepines (to be used only for limited periods of time).

FOLLOW-UP.   If symptoms resolve after provocative testing and patient education alone, no further follow-up is needed. Psychiatric consultation may be necessary when there is a coexistent anxiety disorder or when psychotherapy, behavior therapy, or assistance with pharmacologic management is required.

Cross-references: Dyspnea (Section 19), Dizziness (Section 20), Pleuritic Chest Pain (Section 74), Syncope (Section 75), Palpitations (Section 76),

Headache (Section 140), Screening for Depression (Section 187), Generalized Anxiety (Section 188), Panic Disorder (Section 194).

REFERENCES

1. Brashear RE. Hyperventilation syndrome. Lung 1983;161:257–273.
   Excellent review of etiology, presentation, diagnosis, and treatment.

2. Cowley DS, Roy-Byrne PP. Hyperventilation and panic disorder. Am J Med 1987;83:929–937.
   Discusses the relationship of these disorders.

3. Gardner WN, Bass C. Hyperventilation in clinical practice. Br J Hosp Med 1989;41:73–81.
   Contains an interesting discussion of the physiology of the syndrome.

4. King JC. Hyperventilation—a therapist's point of view: Discussion paper. J Roy Soc Med 1988;81:532–536.
   An intriguing and unconventional approach to the etiology of hyperventilation.

5. Magarian GJ. Hyperventilation syndromes: Infrequently recognized common expressions of anxiety and stress. Medicine 1982;61:219–236.
   An excellent review with a particularly good discussion of management issues.

191 SOMATIZATION

Problem

GEOFFREY H. GORDON

EPIDEMIOLOGY.   Somatization is broadly defined as the experience and expression of emotional distress as physical symptoms. Patients who chronically somatize make frequent or intense requests for medical care, with many unscheduled visits, multiple providers, and repetitive but unrevealing workups ("much doctoring, little curing"). Somatization can occur in the presence of physical illness, with symptoms unrelated or out of proportion to objective findings. The severity of somatization varies from transient amplification of minor physical concerns during times of stress to adoption of illness as a pervasive and disabling life-style.

Somatization is an important clinical problem. Half of all patients given psychiatric diagnoses are seen solely by nonpsychiatrists, and three-quarters of them present with physical symptoms related to emotional distress. Physical symptoms due to psychosocial distress account for an estimated 25% to 75% of visits to primary care providers.

CLINICAL APPROACH.   An obscure or persistent physical symptom can represent an unspoken fear of disability or hidden request for reassurance, information, tests, treatments of disability. It is useful to ask patients what they believe is wrong (or what concerns them the most) and what they think should be done (or how they hope their physician can help). Translators for non–English speaking patients should explain cultural beliefs about the meaning of the illness in addition to providing literal translations.

Certain psychiatric disorders are particularly prevalent among somatizing patients, but classification of individual patients using the current psychiatric *Diagnostic and Statistical Manual* (DSM-IIIR) can be difficult. In one study, nearly 50% of 100 consecutive somatizing outpatients had major depression. In addition to cognitive and affective symptoms, depressed patients may report somatic symptoms such as headache, dizziness, or abdominal pain. Panic disorder, a type of anxiety disorder, occurs in approximately 6% of primary care patients and presents with clusters of severe episodic cardiac, gastrointestinal, and neurologic symptoms that are often misdiagnosed. Depression and anxiety often coexist and are usually overlooked as patients (and their providers) focus on the physical symptoms and dismiss the mood disturbance as a secondary or nonpathological condition. Alcoholism and substance abuse can cause a variety of physical symptoms or conceal underlying psychiatric disorders.

Four "somatoform disorders" present with physical symptoms that cannot be explained by the presence or severity of a physical disorder. The most reliable of these diagnostic entities, **somatization disorder,** is characterized by multiple symptoms in multiple organ systems starting before the age of 30 years. Current diagnostic criteria require the presence of 13 of a possible 35 medically unexplained symptoms of sufficient severity to lead the patient to take medicine, see a doctor, or change life-style; however, patients with fewer symptoms ("abridged" criteria) may follow a similar course. The prevalence of somatization disorder is 2% in the general population and up to 6% in medical clinics. Most patients with somatization disorder are women. Besides multiple symptoms, workups, procedures, medications, and surgeries, they often have chaotic relationships and occupational histories and suffer from depression, anxiety, substance abuse, or personality disorders. **Conversion** symptoms are medically unexplainable losses or changes in body function (e.g., nonanatomic paralysis). The symptoms may follow a pattern suggested by the patient's past experiences with illness (e.g., unexplained chest pain on the anniversary of the loss of a parent from heart disease). Conversion symptoms are produced unconsciously and are usually transient but may recur. Most occur in the presence of another psychiatric disorder, especially somatization disorder. **Hypochondriasis** is characterized by excessive fear of disease, preoccupation with bodily function, and frequent conviction of the presence of serious illness. Hypochondriacal patients have many symptoms and describe them in boring detail (hence the term "organ recital") and are often demanding and critical of their physicians. Hypochondriasis accompanies up to 5% of all medical and psychiatric illnesses. Patients with **somatoform pain disorder** are preoccupied with pain that has lasted for at least 6 months with little relation to objective findings. The relationship of this disorder to chronic pain syndrome is poorly defined. The clinical features of the four somatoform disorders overlap with each other and with those of anxiety and depression; this diagnostic category will probably be revised in the next version of the DSM.

MANAGEMENT.   Somatizing patients are not reassured by a "negative workup" and may experience the news that "nothing is wrong" as an accusation of lying ("I'm not making it up, doc"), being crazy ("You think it's all in my head!"), or threat of abandonment ("Where are you going to send me this time?"). Thus, an important early step in treatment is to legitimize the presence of the symptoms ("I can see this pain is really a problem for you"), the frustration with multiple attempts to "find it and fix it" ("It must be really frustrating for you to have all these doctors and tests and still not get help for your symptoms"), and to express continued interest and hope ("I'd like to work with you on these problems").

Convincing yourself and the patient that no physical disease is present is rarely possible or useful. However, it is important to establish that there is no immediate danger or need for further testing. Reaching this level of certainty may be difficult in some circumstances (e.g., functional chest pain in a patient with known coronary disease). Familiarity with the patient over time through a continuing primary care relationship is very useful. Periodic evaluation of chronic symptoms and investigation of new ones should be conservative and logical. Descriptive diagnostic terms are preferable to misleading labels that are hard to prove or disprove and may lead to unnecessary testing and treatment. (For example, "chronic abdominal pain of unknown etiology" is preferable to "possible adhesions".) Somatizing patients are generally at greater risk for iatrogenic disease than from missed nonpsychiatric diagnoses.

The treatment plan should focus more on restoring and maintaining function than on removing, reducing, or explaining symptoms ("care, not cure"). Medication and other treatment trials should be time limited and linked to positive functional outcomes. (For example, "This medication will not relieve all of your symptoms, but it may help you do more of the activities you want to do, such as volunteer work. Let's try it for 8 weeks. We'll know whether the medicine is working by counting the days you were able to volunteer successfully.") Disability and compensation seeking should be discouraged as contrary to the goal of maximizing function.

Other reasonable treatment goals include fewer unscheduled, catastrophic, or disruptive calls and visits and less doctor shopping. Scheduling brief but regular office visits or telephone contacts reassures patients that they will not be abandoned and demonstrates that they do not have to have worsened symptoms in order to be seen. Successful functional improvement requires that both physicians and patients not expect a "quick fix." Improvement may be impressive, but often it is slow and may not be appreciated by students and residents who have not seen patients in long-term follow-up.

There are several useful techniques for addressing the psychosocial aspects of the illness. One is to listen carefully to the uninterrupted story of illness, taking note of the patient's spontaneous associations of symptoms with events, circumstances, or other people. Asking patients for details or clarification of their own stories is more effective than taking a stereotyped psychosocial history. Another technique is to "normalize" stress and ask about its effects in the individual ("Everyone has stress in their lives, and we know that stress aggravates most medical conditions. How does stress affect you?"). Still another strategy is to ask about the effect of the symptoms on psychosocial function ("What things have these symptoms kept you from doing?"). This can be presented in a way that broaches treatment options. For example, a physician who wants to elicit symptoms of depression and lay the foundation for biologic treatment might ask a patient, "Sometimes illness causes chemical changes in the nervous system that affect sleep, appetite, energy, or even the ability to enjoy things. Has that happened to you?"

Often the best strategy for dealing with chronic unexplained symptoms is to acknowledge the complexity of the condition and the importance of taking time to consider carefully all potential pieces of information, including biologic and psychosocial factors. Patients can help by keeping a symptom diary, rating the intensity of one or more symptoms on a scale from 1 to 10, and describing related circumstances (e.g., food, activity, other people) and perhaps their stress level, again on a numeric scale. These ratings can be done twice or three times a day for 1 to 2 weeks and brought in for discussion at the next office visit. Patients should share their diaries verbally, since further history (such as antecedents or consequences of symptoms) may be uncovered. Family members can be interviewed for their perceptions of the patient's illness.

A mental health consultant can help with diagnosis, medications, and treatment planning, although many somatizing patients refuse to see this person. Patients who agree to referral should be told that the purpose is to help understand the illness and to gather new information. They should be told whom they will see and what to expect. ("Dr. Baker is a psychologist who works with medically ill patients. He may be able to help us develop a treatment plan. He will talk with you for about 40 minutes and then call me.") They should be reassured of continuity of care. ("I'll schedule a visit with you soon afterward so we can discuss his ideas.") In addition to medications for depression and anxiety when indicated, somatizing patients may benefit from cognitive therapy (e.g., identifying and correcting catastrophic thinking), behavior therapy (e.g., monitoring and changing the antecedents and consequences of pain behavior), relaxation training, biofeedback, and group or family therapy.

FOLLOW-UP. In one study, treatment applying the principles outlined markedly reduced the health care utilization of a group of patients with somatization disorder. Physicians should be aware of their own personal reactions, strengths, and weaknesses in working with somatizing patients. Discussing a difficult patient with a colleague is one way to maintain perspective.

Cross-references: Effective Communication in the Ambulatory Setting (Section 3), Diagnosis and Management of Drug Abuse (Section 8), Diagnosis and Management of Alcoholism (Section 9), Chronic Pain Syndrome (Section 13), Fatigue (Section 21), Chest Pain (Section 74), Abdominal Pain (Section 95), Low Back Pain (Section 108), Fibromyalgia (Section 122), Headache (Section 140), Pelvic Pain in Women (Section 163), Screening for Depression (Section 187), Generalized Anxiety (Section 188), Management of Depression (Section 192), The Difficult Patient (Section 195).

REFERENCES

1. Kaplan C, Lipkin M Jr., Gordon GH. Somatization in primary care: Patients with unexplained and vexing medical complaints. J Gen Int Med 1988;3:177–190.
    A comprehensive review article.

2. Katon W, Lin E, Von Korff M, et al. Somatization: A spectrum of severity. Am J Psychiatry 1991;148:34–40.
    Somatization disorder is a spectrum with no clear threshold for diagnosis; the authors recommend revising the DSM.

3. Katon W, Ries RK, Kleinman A. A prospective DSM-III study of 100 consecutive somatization patients. Comprehensive Psychiatry 1984;25:305–314.
    Somatizing patients referred to a psychiatric consultation service had significantly more depression, panic, personality disorders, and psychophysiologic illness than a control group of nonsomatizing referral patients.

4. Quill TE. Somatization: One of medicine's blind spots. JAMA 1985;254:3075–3079.
    Captures the flavor of the clinical presentation and diagnosis of somatization disorder, reviews barriers to effective care, and outlines a treatment approach.

5. Smith GR, Monson RA, Ray DC. Psychiatric consultation in somatization disorder: A randomized controlled study. New Engl J Med 1986;314:1407–1413.
    Psychiatric consultation in conjunction with continuity primary care produced a 53% decrease in health care charges, compared with a 77% increase among the control group. After crossing over, the control group had a 49% decrease in charges, mainly due to decreased hospital use. There was no decline in patients' functional health or satisfaction with care.

192 MANAGEMENT OF DEPRESSION

Problem

GREGORY E. SIMON

EPIDEMIOLOGY. Depression is a common, disabling condition in primary care practice. (See Section 187, Screening for Depression.)

SYMPTOMS AND SIGNS. The hallmarks of depression are a pervasively sad mood, markedly diminished interest or pleasure in almost all activities, or both. These are typically accompanied by physical symptoms of depression (change in weight or appetite, increased or decreased sleep, motor agitation or retardation, and fatigue) and cognitive symptoms (feelings of guilt or worthlessness, impaired concentration, and thoughts of death or suicide). Current diagnostic criteria for major depression require a 2-week period of depressed mood, loss of interest, or both, accompanied by at least four of these associated symptoms. More severe depression may be accompanied by psychotic symptoms, including hallucinations and delusions.

Depression is typically an episodic illness, with onset in the teens or twenties. Episodes often recur, and each recurrence carries a progressively greater risk of chronicity. In bipolar disorder, episodes of depression are associated with one or more episodes of hypomania (elevated mood or irritability, increased energy, impulsivity) or mania (all of those associated with hypomania plus psychosis). Although some episodes of depression may appear to be related to stressful life events, classifying depression based on relation to life stresses ("reactive" versus "endogenous") does not reliably predict clinical course or treatment response.

CLINICAL APPROACH. Reports of depressed mood, crying spells, insomnia, fatigue, or loss of interest should prompt the provider to inquire specifically about depressive symptoms. Observations by family members, friends, or physicians might also prompt further examination. Straightforward inquiry about each of the symptoms listed is usually well received (e.g., "Have you noticed any change in your sleeping—either trouble sleeping or sleeping too much?" "Have you noticed trouble concentrating or feeling as if your thinking has slowed down?"). Questions about suicide should begin by determining the presence of any suicidal ideas ("Have you been thinking a lot about death or dying?" "Have you been feeling as if you might rather be dead?"), followed by specific questions to determine the level of risk ("Have you had thoughts about killing yourself?" "Have you made any plans for how to do it?" "Have you taken any steps toward doing it?" "Do you feel now as if you would want to kill yourself?" "Are you planning to?"). This diagnostic evaluation typically takes less than 10 minutes.

Four specific areas should always be addressed in evaluating patients with significant depression:

1. Substance abuse often causes or complicates depression. Alcohol is a potent depressant, and abstinence from cocaine can produce severe symptoms of depression. Substance abuse must be addressed initially, and consideration of independent depression should be postponed until after a few weeks of abstinence.

2. Depression may be accompanied by psychosis that requires specific treatment. Straightforward inquiry about psychotic symptoms is the best approach. ("Have you had any trouble with hearing voices or hearing things that might not be there?" "Have you been seeing visions or seeing things that might not be there?" "Have you had any unusual ideas that someone has been interfering with your mind?"). Psychotic depression often involves delusions of guilt or disease. Psychotic symptoms should prompt psychiatric consultation regarding need for antipsychotic medication or hospitalization.

3. Patients with current mixed (manic and depressive) symptoms or histories of mania may become manic when treated with conventional antidepressants. Ask specifically about a history of mania ("Have you ever had a period of a week or more when you felt unusually high or energetic, didn't sleep, acted on impulse, or a doctor said you were manic?") and about current manic symptoms (mood lability, irritability, impulsivity). Suspicion of mania should prompt psychiatric consultation regarding need for lithium or other pharmacotherapy.

4. Significant risk of suicide should prompt hospitalization. Patients who report any current intent or plan to attempt suicide should be offered voluntary hospitalization and be considered for involuntary treatment. Those reporting suicidal ideas with no current intent or plan do not require hospitalization if they can agree to contact the physician's office, hospital emergency room, or other community resources if suicidal urges appear.

Crisp separation of normal grief from depression is not possible. Grieving may involve all symptoms of major depression, and the distinction must be made according to duration and severity. Bereaved patients with disabling depressive symptoms that persist longer than 2 months or result in threats to health should be considered for the treatments outlined under "Management."

Patients with chronic pain or other "functional" physical symptoms may deny depressed mood and loss of interest while reporting other associated symptoms (such as insomnia, decreased energy, poor concentration, and anorexia). Because these patients may benefit from antidepressant medication, such syndromes have been labeled "masked depression." This relabeling, however, tends to irritate patients and focus attention away from the primary complaint. Instead, one should explain that the pharmacologic and nonpharmacologic techniques used in treatment of depression may also relieve a variety of chronic physical symptoms.

MANAGEMENT.   Effective treatment of depression should include both pharmacotherapy and psychotherapy, both of which are feasible and effective in primary care medical practice. Patients with depression severe enough to meet criteria for major depressive episode often benefit from antidepressant medication. For less severe depression, the benefit of medication is not established. Drugs used in the treatment of depression include conventional tricyclic antidepressants, newer antidepressants, monoamine oxidase inhibitors, and some unconventional agents (lithium, thyroid supplementation, anticonvulsants). Primary care physicians should understand the use of tricyclic antidepressants and newer related drugs. Treatment with unconventional agents should be deferred to specialists or the especially interested generalist.

Tricyclic antidepressants and newer agents are equally effective when used in comparable doses. Each is effective in 60% to 70% of patients with major depression, and over 80% of major depression will respond to at least one of them. Therapeutic effect is first evident in 1 week to 2 weeks, with full effect in 3 weeks to 6 weeks.

Antidepressants differ primarily in their side effects, which appear after the first dose (Table 192–1). These include sedation, anticholinergic effects (dry mouth, constipation, urinary retention, tachycardia), and postural hypotension. These effects are usually greater with earlier, tertiary amine tricyclics (amitriptyline, imipramine, doxepin) than with their secondary amine descendants (desipramine, nortriptyline). Newer nontricyclic antidepressant agents have different side effect profiles. Trazodone has minimal anticholinergic effect but is highly sedating and may rarely cause priapism (all males taking trazodone should be warned about this effect). Fluoxetine can cause nausea, headache, increased muscle tension, and feelings of agitation. Amoxapine has some neuroleptic activity and has caused extrapyramidal side effects (dystonia, parkinsonism, and tardive dyskinesia).

TABLE 192–1.   SELECTED ANTIDEPRESSANT DRUGS

Drug	Initial Dose[1] (mg)	Maintenance Dose (mg)	Sedative Effect[2]	Anticholinergic Effect[2]	Daily Cost ($)[3]
Amitriptyline	50 q.h.s.	150 q.h.s.	+ + + +	+ + + +	0.08
Imipramine	50 q.h.s.	150 q.h.s.	+ + +	+ + +	0.12
Doxepin	50 q.h.s.	150 q.h.s.	+ + + +	+ + +	0.30
Desipramine	50 q.d.	150 q.d.	+	+	0.75
Nortriptyline	25 q.h.s.	75 q.h.s.	+ +	+	1.77[4]
Trazodone	100 q.h.s	300 q.h.s.	+ + +	0	0.90
Amoxapine	50 q.d.	150 q.d.	+	+	1.95
Fluoxetine	20 q.o.d.	20 q.d.	0	0	1.67

[1]In elderly or chronically ill patients, use 50% of listed dose.
[2]+ + + + = most pronounced, 0 = absent.
[3]Average wholesale price for maintenance dose listed, *1991 Drug Topics Red Book*.
[4]Expected to decline when patent rights expire in 1992.

The cardiac effects of antidepressants have generated most concern among medical providers. Tricyclic antidepressants have quinidine-like effects on cardiac rhythm. They typically suppress ambient ventricular ectopy but may cause idiosyncratic increases in atrial and ventricular arrhythmias, as well as, during an overdose, refractory arrhythmias. Preexisting arrhythmias do not contraindicate use of tricyclics, but one must exercise the same caution one would use in starting treatment with quinidine. Tricyclics also may impair atrioventricular conduction and prolong the P-R interval or aggravate a preexisting conduction disturbance. In patients with first-degree atrioventricular or bundle-branch block, dosage increases should occur slowly and only after reevaluation of the ECG. Although tricyclics may depress ventricular function during an overdose, they do not in routine clinical use. Postural hypotension is usually the most important adverse cardiovascular effect of tricyclics in patients with heart disease. The newer antidepressants appear to have less effect on cardiac rhythm, conduction, and venous tone, but clinical experience remains limited, and the precise cardiac effects are not established.

The selection of an antidepressant should be guided initially by the patient's history of previous treatment. An antidepressant that previously yielded relief of depression without intolerable side effects should be used again. A drug that previously was ineffective (when given in therapeutic dose) or caused intolerable side effects should be avoided. Previous difficulty with oversedation or overstimulation argues for an antidepressant with the opposite effect. For patients with no prior history of antidepressant treatment, the choice of an initial agent depends on side effects. Patients with significant insomnia should initially receive a more sedating agent. Lethargy and decreased energy argue for less of a sedative effect. Older tricyclics (amitriptyline, imipramine, and doxepin) offer considerable cost savings at the price of greater sedative and anticholinergic side effects. These drugs may be acceptable to younger patients, but older or chronically ill patients often find these side effects intolerable. The newer tricyclics (nortriptyline and desipramine) offer a reasonable compromise of cost, side effects, and experience with use in ill and elderly patients.

Initiating treatment at low doses and building to therapeutic dose over 7 days to 10 days will minimize initial side effects. The doses listed in Table 192–1 represent averages for healthy young or middle-aged patients. Doses in elderly or chronically ill patients should initially be reduced by one-half, although some elderly patients ultimately may require the full dose. The maintenance doses listed lie in the lower range of therapeutic effect. In general, maintenance doses should be increased after 3 weeks to 4 weeks if side effects are tolerable but depression has not significantly improved. Side effects should be managed first by reducing either the dose or the rate of dose increase before changing medication. Tolerance to side effects often develops with time. A relationship between serum level and drug efficacy is well established for nortriptyline and somewhat established for desipramine. Serum levels for these drugs may be helpful in ill or elderly patients, patients with side effects at low doses, and patients unresponsive to usual doses. For other agents, serum levels are commercially available but of unproved value.

Cognitive-behavioral psychotherapy appears as effective as antidepressants in the treatment of mild and moderately severe depression. These techniques are applicable within the training and time constraints of primary care practice. This treatment builds on the premise that negative and pessimistic thought patterns are a major component of depression and that recognition and alteration of these thoughts can relieve depressed mood. Patients are asked to attend to the negative thoughts accompanying depressed mood and to learn to recognize the distortions or exaggerations that often underlie those thoughts. By learning to recognize and challenge negative thoughts during a physician visit, patients can eventually learn to deal effectively with depression as it arises. Self-help manuals (see References) provide clear guidance in these techniques.

FOLLOW-UP. Psychiatric consultation is indicated for depression that is unimproved after 4 weeks of appropriate treatment. Development of significant suicide risk, psychosis, or mania during treatment should also prompt referral. When effective, tricyclic antidepressants should be continued for 4 weeks to 6 months. Most patients can then taper medication over 2 weeks to 3 weeks, with a low probability of relapse. Recurrence of depression should prompt resumption of the antidepressant for another 2 months to 3 months before another attempted taper. Only rare patients require antidepressant treatment for over 8 months to 10 months. Cognitive-behavioral techniques are especially helpful in preventing relapse of depression. Continued practice is essential.

Cross-references: Diagnosis and Management of Drug Abuse (Section 8), Diagnosis and Management of Alcoholism (Section 9), Chronic Pain Syndrome (Section 13), Weight Loss (Section 17), Anorexia (Section 18), Fatigue (Section 21), Constipation (Section 94), Fibromyalgia (Section 122), Screening for Dementia (Section 137), Dementia (Section 142), Screening for Thyroid Disease (Section 153), Impotence (Section 171), Screening for Depression (Section 187), Insomnia (Section 189), Hyperventilation Syndrome (Section 190), Somatization (Section 191), Psychosis (Section 193).

REFERENCES

1. Burns DD. The Feeling Good Handbook. Plume Press, New York, 1989.
    Excellent guidebook (for patients and their doctors) to self-treatment of depression using cognitive techniques.

2. Katon W, Sullivan MD. Depression and chronic medical illness. J Clin Psychiatry 1990;51(6,suppl):3–11.
    Reviews relationship of depression to medical illness and somatization in primary care.

3. McGreevy JF, Franco K. Depression in the elderly: The role of the primary care physician in management. J Gen Int Med 1988;3:498–507.
    Reviews diagnosis and management, with good discussion of initial antidepressant choice.

193 PSYCHOSIS

Problem

GREGORY E. SIMON

EPIDEMIOLOGY. Schizophrenia and the affective psychoses (bipolar disorder and related disorders) have a combined prevalence in the community of 1% to 2%. Average prevalence among medical clinic patients is probably four to five times as high, but rates vary widely according to type of medical practice and are much higher in emergency rooms or clinics serving socioeconomically disadvantaged populations and lower among more privileged groups. Schizophrenia and related disorders are characterized by psychotic symptoms, impairment of overall function, chronicity, and absence of prominent fluctuations in mood. Affective psychoses typically present with episodes of depression and mania, which occur in varying patterns accompanied by varying levels of psychotic symptoms. In practice, the boundaries between schizophrenia and bipolar disorder (in presentation, course, and treatment response) are indistinct.

SYMPTOMS AND SIGNS. **Hallucinations** are false perceptions that are most often auditory but may affect any sensory mode. They range in complexity from simple noises to elaborate conversations involving an identifiable cast of characters. **Delusions** are fixed false beliefs that are inconsistent with the patient's cultural and social network. These are typically impervious to evidence and argument. Delusions often concern paranoid suspicions or bizarre communications (e.g., mind reading). **Disturbed affect** is expressed as emotions that are exaggerated or constricted or appear inappropriate to the situation (e.g., apparently lighthearted discussions of murder or suicide). In **thought disorders,** thought and speech may be accelerated or slowed. Connections between thoughts may be loosened, bizarre, or nonexistent.

CLINICAL APPROACH. Psychotic disorders are typically chronic, episodic illnesses; the history (from patient, records, or other contacts) is critical. Both "functional" psychotic disorders (schizophrenia and affective psychoses) and organic psychoses (e.g., intoxication, encephalitis) may have an acute clinical presentation. A prior history of psychosis makes an undiagnosed medical cause of psychotic symptoms less likely, but exacerbations of chronic psychosis may be precipitated by intercurrent medical illness or drug intoxication or withdrawal. In addition, patients with chronic psychotic disorders have high rates of undiagnosed medical illness because of their personal neglect, disorganized life-style, impaired communication, and concomitant substance abuse. Consequently, any psychotic presentation requires an evaluation for drug intoxication or withdrawal or precipitating medical illness.

The acute presentation of schizophrenia and bipolar disorder is also difficult to differentiate. This distinction, however, is more important to long-term management.

The initial evaluation should focus on the patient's level of threat to self or others and on his or her ability to provide for daily needs. The evaluation of potential danger includes questioning the patient directly about current urges to harm self or others, current plan or intent to do so, and previous history of violence. The evaluation of self-care includes observation of the patient's current state (hygiene, nutrition, etc.) and investigation of available family and community supports. Patients who are unable to care for themselves or who pose a significant threat of violence should be hospitalized. Laws regarding criteria for involuntary psychiatric treatment vary by state, but most apply a standard consistent with this approach.

MANAGEMENT. Dealing with psychotic patients can be quite frustrating. Delusions and hallucinations are by nature impervious to argument. Often it is best to "agree to disagree"—tell the patient that while you appreciate how firmly he or she believes what he or she thinks (sees, hears, etc.), you do not agree. Explain that you will continue to care for him or her as best you can despite this disagreement.

Antipsychotic medications are usually effective in reducing agitation, hallucinations, and delusions. They are somewhat less effective in reducing withdrawal, disorganization of thought, and disturbance of emotional expression. Available antipsychotics (except clozapine) appear equal in effectiveness when given in equivalent doses (Table 193–1). More potent drugs usually cause less sedation, postural hypotension, and anticholinergic effect at the expense of greater tendency for extrapyramidal side effects. Common extrapyramidal effects include acute dystonia (often involving tongue, neck, or face), drug-induced Parkinsonism, and akathisia (irresistible motor restlessness). Young

TABLE 193–1. SELECTED ANTIPSYCHOTIC DRUGS

Drug	Initial Dose	Maximum Dose[1]	Sedation[2]	Extrapyramidal Symptoms[2]	Cost ($)[3]
Haloperidol	5 mg b.i.d.	5 mg q.i.d.	+	+ + + +	0.40
Thiothixene	10 mg b.i.d.	10 mg b.i.d.	+	+ + +	0.60
Perphenazine	24 mg b.i.d.	24 mg q.i.d.	+ +	+ +	2.70
Prochlorperazine	25 mg t.i.d.	50 mg t.i.d.	+ + +	+ +	0.45
Chlorpromazine	200 mg b.i.d.	200 mg t.i.d.	+ + + +	+	0.20
Thioridazine	200 mg b.i.d.	200 mg t.i.d.	+ + + +	+	0.40

[1]Seek consultation if no response.
[2]+ + + + = most pronounced, + = least pronounced.
[3]Average wholesale daily cost, initial dose listed, 1991 *Drug Topics Red Book*.

males appear at highest risk for these complications. Use of prophylactic anti-Parkinsonian agents is controversial but is often unnecessary with less potent antipsychotics or with lower-risk patients (female or elderly patients). Typical anti-Parkinsonian regimens used prophylactically or therapeutically (following emergence of side effects) include benztropine (Cogentin) 0.5–1.0 mg b.i.d., trihexyphenidyl (Artane) 1–2 mg b.i.d., or amantadine (Symmetrel) 100 mg up to b.i.d. Acute treatment should begin with doses listed in Table 193–1 and should be increased after 24 hours to 48 hours if no improvement is apparent. Doses of less potent drugs may be limited by sedation and hypotension. Psychiatric consultation should be sought if response is not rapid.

Clozapine, a newly developed antipsychotic drug, appears to carry little risk of tardive dyskinesia and may be more effective against symptoms of disorganization and withdrawal. Because it carries significant expense and risk of hematologic side effects, it is not a first-line treatment.

FOLLOW-UP.   Continued use of antipsychotics raises questions about alternative maintenance treatments (lithium, antidepressants, etc.), as well as risks (especially tardive dyskinesia). Psychiatric consultation should be obtained soon after beginning acute treatment. The guiding principle for continued antipsychotic use is to seek the lowest effective dose.

Cross-references: Diagnosis and Management of Drug Abuse (Section 8), Diagnosis and Management of Alcoholism (Section 9), Dementia (Section 142), Alcohol Withdrawal (Section 144), Management of Depression (Section 192), The Difficult Patient (Section 195).

REFERENCES

1. Gelenberg AJ. Psychoses. In Bassuk EL, Schoonover SC, Gelenberg AJ, Eds. Practitioner's Guide to Psychoactive Drugs. Plenum, New York, 1984.
    Good guide to medication selection and side effects.

2. Hyman SE. Acute psychosis. In Hyman SE, Ed. Manual of Psychiatric Emergencies. Little, Brown, Boston, 1984.
    Concise discussion of emergency evaluation and management.

194 PANIC DISORDER

Problem

GREGORY E. SIMON

EPIDEMIOLOGY. Panic disorder has a point prevalence of 0.5% among community residents. Its prevalence peaks in early adulthood, is at least ten times higher in most medical clinics, and is two to three times higher in females. Because of associated physical symptoms, patients with panic disorder often present to emergency departments, as well as cardiology, neurology, and otolaryngology clinics. Panic disorder often follows an episodic course with symptomatic recurrences precipitated by periods of life stress.

SYMPTOMS AND SIGNS. Panic disorder presents with discrete, unprovoked attacks of fear or discomfort accompanied by various physical symptoms (dyspnea, palpitations, dizziness, tremors, sweating, choking, nausea, paresthesias, chest pain). Either fear or physical symptoms may be more prominent, but questioning usually reveals both. Some physical symptoms of panic (dyspnea, dizziness, palpitations) appear to be mediated by acute hyperventilation. The panic syndrome varies in severity from rare, isolated panic attacks to severe daily attacks with completely disabling phobic fear. Panic attacks are often accompanied by depression and phobic anxiety (especially phobias of crowds, open spaces, waiting in lines, and leaving home alone).

CLINICAL APPROACH. Because dramatic physical symptoms often focus attention (both patients' and doctors') on serious, urgent medical problems, the recognition of panic disorder is difficult and often delayed. Patients may persistently demand diagnostic testing. Symptoms of panic may resemble symptoms of almost any paroxysmal neurologic or cardiovascular event, including angina, pulmonary embolus, arrhythmia, transient ischemic attack, presyncope, or seizure. This does not imply that clinicians should exclude each of these disorders before considering the diagnosis of panic but that panic disorder should be considered when any of these medical diagnoses is entertained. Among young healthy patients (especially women), the prior probability of panic disorder far exceeds that of a malignant arrhythmia or angina. Alcohol withdrawal may also cause attacks of anxiety with associated physical symptoms. In these cases, the initial step should be treatment of the primary alcohol problem.

MANAGEMENT. The intense focus on physical symptoms and medical illness accompanying panic attacks often poses problems for medical providers. Recurrent panic symptoms can rapidly reverse the most careful reassurance and education. Relief of anxiety symptoms offers the best reassurance that no serious undiagnosed medical condition exists.

609

Cognitive and behavioral techniques (discussed in Section 188, Generalized Anxiety) can be effective in reducing panic symptoms and limiting phobic avoidance. Good self-help manuals are available (see References). Some panic patients paradoxically feel more anxious with breathing or relaxation exercises.

Both anxiolytic and antidepressant medication are effective in treatment of panic attacks. Anxiolytics offer more immediate relief but carry risks of tolerance and dependence. Patients with rare and uncomplicated attacks or patients unwilling to take scheduled daily medication may be treated with low-dose anxiolytics alone. Higher potency benzodiazepines may have greater efficacy against panic. Good choices are alprazolam 0.25 mg to 0.5 mg up to three times daily (faster onset but greater rebound anxiety) or clonazepam 0.5 mg to 1.0 mg twice daily (more steady effect but onset too slow for PRN use). Patients with panic accompanied by depression often respond poorly to anxiolytics alone. These patients with associated depression and others not responding to the anxiolytic doses may require antidepressant treatment. All tricyclic antidepressants appear equally effective, although newer agents are less well studied. Monoamine oxidase inhibitors may be more effective than tricyclics, but risk and inconvenience make these second-line agents in primary care. Initial dosing is similar to that for depression (see Section 192), but panic disorder may respond to lower doses. Some patients with panic disorder may experience transient increase in agitation or anxiety upon starting antidepressants. When this occurs, the usual dosing schedule should be reduced to allow accommodation, and patients should be reassured that this response usually indicates eventual benefit.

Ingrained phobic avoidance may persist even after panic attacks have resolved. These patients will benefit from the behavioral programs for phobia (described in Section 188 and described in available self-help manuals; see References).

FOLLOW-UP.   Psychiatric consultation should be arranged for patients unresponsive to the standard treatments noted in "Management." Patients who respond can usually taper antidepressant medication after 3 months to 4 months, although rarer cases may require longer-term treatment. Even for those who respond, panic disorder is often a chronic remitting and relapsing condition. Because cognitive and behavioral strategies provide some prophylactic benefit, the physician should encourage the patient to practice continually.

Cross-references: Diagnosis and Management of Drug Abuse (Section 8), Diagnosis and Management of Alcoholism (Section 9), 74spnea (Section 19), Dizziness (Section 20), Pleuritic Chest Pain (Section 74), Syncope (Section 75), Palpitations (Section 76), Dyspepsia (Section 96), Tremor (Section 138), Alcohol Withdrawal (Section 144), Screening for Thyroid Disease (Section 153), Generalized Anxiety (Section 188), Hyperventilation Syndrome (Section 190).

REFERENCES

1. Clancy J, Noyes R. Anxiety neurosis: A disease for the medical model. Psychosomatics 1976;17:90–93.
    Good description of extensive medical evaluations panic patients often undergo.

2. Grant B, Katon W, Beitman B. Panic disorder. J Fam Pract 1983;17:907–914.
    Practical discussion of diagnosis and management in primary care.

3. Sheehan DV. Panic attacks and phobias. New Engl J Med 1982;307:156–158.
    Brief and practical review.

4. Weekes C. Peace from Nervous Suffering. Bantam Books, New York, 1972.
    Excellent self-help manual for treatment of panic attacks and phobias.

195 THE DIFFICULT PATIENT

Problem

GREGORY E. SIMON

SYMPTOMS AND SIGNS.   Even the most caring and courteous clinicians experience troubling and unproductive doctor-patient relationships. Although the resulting conflict and disappointment often lead to accusations from both parties, these difficult situations are almost never the result of malice or bad intentions. Practitioners and patients usually come together with a shared purpose, mutual trust, and a desire for understanding. When attempts to form a working partnership fail, the clinician must draw on that original trust and goodwill.

Certain patients have difficulty with practically every provider they see and may experience similar problems in other important interpersonal relationships. These patients often suffer from chronic emotional distress and poor coping strategies that lead to interpersonal conflict. The hope and authority attached to health providers can make provider-patient relationships both more powerful and unsettling. For example, a seriously ill patient caught between fear of life-threatening complications and the desire to lead a normal life might try to relieve internal conflict by creating an external one. By acting irresponsibly, he or she might steer the physician into the role of guardian and disciplinarian, which, if left unchecked, may culminate in an angry conflict in which the patient complains of being treated like a child. The harried clinician must recall that these patients are usually just doing the best they can with a difficult situation.

Other doctor-patient difficulties are more idiosyncratic and reflect the conflicting styles of a particular doctor and patient. Most clinicians learn that certain types of patients may be personally difficult. Some physicians are irritated by patients' desiring a high level of authority and control, while others object to patients who ask for extra reassurance and support. These preferences do not indicate pathology or psychological difficulty; they simply represent the vagaries of human personality. Early recognition of these patterns can prevent personal conflict.

When the clinical relationship becomes difficult, both providers and patients often feel hurt. Discussion shifts from shared attempts at understanding and managing health problems to increasing conflict over authority and support. Clinicians find themselves more concerned with their personal adequacy than with medical diagnosis and management. Patients speak more of their dissatisfaction with care than the health concerns that brought them in. The initial complaint can be easily obscured by these recriminations. Physicians may be troubled by unusually strong personal reactions or find themselves straying into unusual patterns of practice (either overly solicitous or unreasonably withholding). This pattern of increasingly personalized interaction (focus on personal conflict, feelings of inadequacy, "special" types of care) should serve as an early warning of trouble.

CLINICAL APPROACH.   Breakdowns in doctor-patient relationships often result when patients' usual ways of coping are inadequate to manage personal distress. For some patients, this appears to be a chronic condition. For others, their coping mechanisms are temporarily overwhelmed when internal stress exceeds a manageable level or when personal resources are weakened. The clinician should try to identify life stresses that upset this balance, transforming a stressed patient into a difficult one. Because adequate cognitive function is required to manage emotional and interpersonal affairs, any cognitive impairment may precipitate a decompensation. Alcohol or drug intoxication may be the most striking example of transient impairment of interpersonal function. Dementing illness may first manifest as personality change and irritability. Medical illness may cause decompensation by increasing the level of stress and by impairing the ability to cope. Shifting the focus from personal conflict to the causes of coping failure may help restore mutual trust and cooperation.

MANAGEMENT.   Just as difficult doctor-patient relationships suffer from a high degree of personalization, rebuilding those relationships requires shifting attention away from personal conflict, blame, and feelings of inadequacy. The clinician must first decide that the patient is neither malicious nor defective and then proceed to examine the causes of the conflict. Following are a few practical suggestions.

An intellectual understanding of breakdowns in the doctor-patient relationship may be helpful to the clinician but is usually not helpful to the patient. For example, a provider may come to understand that a patient's angry demands for unnecessary diagnostic tests arise from a fear that his or her chest pain is not being taken seriously. A frightened and angry patient will find little comfort in this explanation, but this understanding will help the clinician to offer the right kind of reassurance. Instead of focusing on the expense, risk, and low yield of the requested diagnostic tests, the provider should express concern about the pain and discuss strategies to relieve it.

The clinician should try to recall a sense of shared purpose by returning to the patient's original concern. In the midst of a conflict in which the physician is portrayed as cruel and heartless and the patient as unreasonably demanding, the original goal of the visit may be lost. All encounters begin with a common purpose: to understand and relieve suffering. It may be helpful to say, "I am concerned that we haven't made much progress helping you with the pain that brought you here. Maybe we should go back and work on that again."

It is essential to clarify mutual expectations. Unreasonable expectations often fade when assurances of reasonable care are given. For example, a patient who angrily demands unlimited access may calm considerably when offered clear reassurance that calls will be returned and urgent problems handled appropriately. Conversely, a clinician may be less angry with a noncompliant patient after negotiating an agreement about managing at least part of a complex medical regimen.

Conflict over clinically unimportant issues should be avoided. Misplaced hostility can lead to escalating struggles over surprisingly insignificant questions. Disagreement is worthwhile for substantive questions (e.g., chronic use of anxiolytics in a patient with active alcohol abuse), but providers should avoid large struggles over small differences (e.g., a 3-week prescription for anxiolytics instead of only 2 weeks).

Increasing a patient's fear or anxiety is almost never helpful. For example, an emergency room patient with chest pain who adamantly refuses a necessary intensive care admission is probably too frightened to acknowledge the real threat. Emphasizing the risk of death is unlikely to win this person over. Instead, the provider should focus on how hospitalization would more rapidly relieve the patient's discomfort and speed recovery.

Setting limits is rarely effective when done in anger. For example, a patient taking narcotics for chronic pain who repeatedly reports losing the prescription and requests early refills may engender a sense of mistrust and irritation. After granting this request several times, a clinician might angrily refuse to prescribe any more narcotics, provoking a confrontation. This scenario might be avoided by setting explicit limits before mounting irritation prompts a sudden shift in care. After the first lost prescription, the patient should be given a refill and told that future prescriptions will have to last for their expected period without exception.

Clinicians should remember that idealization and devaluation are two sides of the same coin. A patient who lavishes unreasonable praise on a new physician while vilifying all previous ones will become dissatisfied soon enough. The clinician can best deal with this criticism of previous physicians by acknowledging the patient's disappointment and restating a commitment to providing good care.

On rare occasions, a doctor-patient relationship may fail. A provider and patient may be unable to negotiate a working agreement for continued care. Such a decision should be openly discussed and mutually agreed upon. Avoidance of open disagreement through referral or rejection only reinforces a pattern of disappointment and hostility.

FOLLOW-UP.   A busy primary care physician may regard energy spent on interpersonal negotiations as an unnecessary distraction, taking time away from issues of diagnosis and treatment that may seem more urgent. Effective care of distressed patients, however, requires a working doctor-patient relationship. Progress is slow but meaningful. A patient's long-term relationship with a calm and tolerant physician has great therapeutic power. Primary care physicians are uniquely suited to this task.

Cross-references: Determinants of Patient Satisfaction (Section 2), Effective Communication in the Ambulatory Setting (Section 3), Diagnosis and Management of Drug Abuse (Section 8), Diagnosis and Management of Alcoholism (Section 9), Chronic Pain Syndrome (Section 13), Fatigue (Section 21), Dementia (Section 142), Generalized Anxiety (Section 188), Somatization (Section 191), Psychosis (Section 193).

REFERENCES

1.   Groves JE. Taking care of the hateful patient. New Engl J Med 1978;298:883–887.
     A classic paper with much practical wisdom.

2.   Quill TE. Partnerships in patient care: A contractual approach. Ann Int Med 1983;98:228–234.
     Excellent model for building constructive relationships with trying patients.

3.   Stoudemire A, Thompson TL. The borderline personality in the medical setting. Ann Int Med 1982;96:76–79.
     Describes problems in the care of this difficult group and offers useful guidelines for inpatient and outpatient medical care.

196 PSYCHOLOGICAL ASSESSMENT

Procedure

SUE ANNE WIEDENFELD

INDICATIONS/CONTRAINDICATIONS. Psychological testing is indicated for the following reasons:

1. To evaluate cognitive, affective, and adaptive functioning in patients who have known or suspected organic brain dysfunction (e.g., cognitive disturbance following head injury or stroke).
2. To evaluate cognitive disturbances in those without identified cerebral disease (e.g., dementia, delirium, aphasia).
3. To discriminate between functional and organic cognitive disturbances (e.g., residual effects of drug and/or alcohol abuse versus psychosis).
4. To assess learning disability or residual abilities after injury or disease (e.g., degree of mental retardation, competence to handle financial affairs).
5. To monitor treatment outcomes (e.g., recovery from encephalitis).

Contraindications are acute psychotic state, severely altered state of consciousness, and acute drug toxicity (e.g., alcohol intoxication, overdose).

RATIONALE. The neuropsychological evaluation consists of a battery of comprehensive mental status examinations that evaluate cerebral functioning. Most neuropsychological tests have been standardized using both healthy persons and patients with brain damage. Because results from these evaluations are quantifiable, subtle changes in performance over time can be identified.

METHODS. Testing takes from 2 hours to 6 hours to complete and is administered and interpreted by a trained neuropsychologist. The test may measure any of the following: behavior, attention, and mood; intelligence (verbal, nonverbal); achievement (reading, spelling, arithmetic); memory (verbal/nonverbal, learning and retention); complex problem solving (abstract nonverbal reasoning, flexibility in thinking, manipulative problem solving), language (comprehension, expressive), sensory perceptual functioning (vision, hearing, tactile), motor and visual motor abilities, and personality and social functioning.

COST/COMPLICATIONS. Neuropsychologic batteries range in cost from $200 to $1200 and are free from complications.

Cross-references: Diagnosis and Management of Drug Abuse (Section 8), Diagnosis and Management of Alcoholism (Section 9), Dementia (Section 142), Cerebrovascular Disease (Section 148).

REFERENCES

1. Filskov S, Boll T. Handbook of Clinical Neuropsychology. Wiley & Sons, New York, 1986.
   General review that includes a chapter on neuropsychological findings in several specific medical disorders.

2. Jarvis PE, Barth JT. Halstead-Reitan Test Battery: An Interpretive Guide. Psychological Assessment Resources, 1984.
   Describes selected neuropsychological tests with case illustrations; an excellent basic discussion.

3. Lezak M. Neuropsychological Assessment. Oxford University Press, New York, 1983.
   Describes neuroanatomical correlates of behavior, reviews neuropsychological assessment and interpretation, and provides in-depth discussions of specific neuropsychological tests.

4. Strub R, Black F. Neurobehavioral disorders: A Clinical Approach. FA Davis, Philadelphia, 1981.
   A clinical discussion of the major behavioral syndromes associated with brain dysfunction.

XVII CHAPTER

HEMATOLOGIC DISORDERS

197 BLEEDING

Symptom

GERALD J. ROTH

EPIDEMIOLOGY. The symptom of bleeding may result from abnormalities of the hemostatic system or may occur following trauma or surgery in patients with normal hemostasis. This section deals with hemostatic disorders, which affect an estimated 30 to 50 patients per 100,000 of the general population.

ETIOLOGY. Hemostasis (*hemo,*"blood"; *stasis,*"stopping") involves the blood itself, blood flow, and blood vessels (Virchow's triad), but most bleeding problems involve the blood alone, specifically platelets, plasma coagulation, or both.

Platelets. Platelet disorders, either quantitative (thrombocytopenia) or qualitative defects, result in mucocutaneous bleeding: blood loss through the skin (bruising) or mucous membranes (epistaxis, menorrhagia). Thrombocytopenia (platelet count less than 150,000) commonly results from bone marrow and megakaryocyte suppression due to medications or malignancy (e.g., leukemia). It also occurs when the normal platelet life span (10 days) is shortened by premature destruction of circulating platelets, often due to antiplatelet antibodies (idiopathic thrombocytopenic purpura). Platelet function defects are caused by disorders such as von Willebrand's disease or aspirin ingestion and are marked by an inability of platelets to aggregate or secrete.

Plasma Coagulation. Both congenital (e.g., hemophilia) and acquired (e.g., ingestion of anticoagulants) disorders can affect the plasma coagulation system. The resultant bleeding is characteristically visceral (muscular) or within joints (hemarthrosis).

Disseminated Intravascular Coagulation. Serious systemic illness, particularly gram-negative sepsis, can activate the hemostatic system and lead to consumption of both platelets and plasma coagulation factors. The resultant bleed-

617

ing disorder includes features of thrombocytopenia and coagulation factor deficiency.

CLINICAL APPROACH.   The patient interview provides the most practical and direct assessment of the patient's hemostatic system and should focus on the patient's response to prior hemostatic challenges (surgery, trauma, tooth extraction), drug ingestion (particularly aspirin), family history, and associated diseases that could impair hemostasis (e.g., uremia or lupus erythematosus). The physical examination assesses the extent of bruising, the presence of petechiae, the presence of joint deformity, or evidence of associated diseases such as chronic liver disease. This initial assessment defines the severity of the defect and whether platelets or plasma coagulation factors are responsible (Table 197–1).

Simple, inexpensive laboratory tests should precede more specific tests. For example, if the history and physical examination suggest a platelet disorder, a platelet count should be obtained; if the count is normal, a bleeding time should be performed to assess platelet function. Subsequent workup may include platelet aggregometry to detect a defect in platelet aggregation or secretion. For plasma coagulation, the activated partial thromboplastin time (APTT) is used to assess the intrinsic system of coagulation (factors XII, XI, IX, VIII, X, V, II), and the prothrombin time (PT) screens the extrinsic factors (X, VII, V, II). Additional tests, such as specific factor assays, thrombin time, fibrinogen level, and tests for fibrin or fibrinogen degradation products, may be necessary for a more specific diagnosis.

MANAGEMENT.   Management of bleeding disorders requires an accurate diagnosis so that therapy can be directed to a specific abnormality. Examples are platelet transfusion for thrombocytopenia based on inadequate platelet production or specific factor replacement in hemophilia A (factor VIII deficiency) or Christmas disease (factor IX deficiency).

Cross-references: Epistaxis (Section 55), Hemoptysis (Section 62), Abnormal Uterine Bleeding (Section 162), Thrombocytopenia (Section 199), Transfusion Therapy (Section 204), Preoperative Hematologic Problems (Section 220).

TABLE 197–1.   BLEEDING DISORDERS: CLINICAL FEATURES

Clinical Feature	Platelet Disorders	Plasma Coagulation Disorders
Type of bleeding	Mucocutaneous	Visceral/joint
Onset of bleeding (after trauma or surgery)	Immediate	Delayed
Sex predominance	Females	Males
Family history	Often negative	Often positive

REFERENCES

1. Bachmann F. Diagnostic approach to mild bleeding disorders. Sem Hematol 1980;17:292–305.
    Reviews the epidemiology and etiology of mild bleeding disorders in a large population.

2. Karpatkin S. Autoimmune thrombocytopenic purpura. Sem Hematol 1985;22:260–288.
    An up-to-date, general review that addresses modern treatment in adults, particularly those with refractory disease.

3. Rapaport SI. Introduction to Hematology, 2d ed. Lippincott, Philadelphia, 1987; pp 432–577.
    A concise and up-to-date discussion of hemostatic mechanisms, common bleeding disorders, and an approach to an evaluation of the bleeding patient.

4. Rapaport SI. Preoperative hemostatic evaluation: Which tests if any? Blood 1983;61:229–231.
    An exceptionally practical and pointed discussion of how to evaluate the bleeding patient.

198 LYMPHADENOPATHY

Symptom

DAVID C. DALE

EPIDEMIOLOGY. "Lymphadenopathy" or "adenopathy" is a general term for any infectious, inflammatory, or malignant disease involving lymph nodes. Usually lymphadenopathy causes lymph node enlargement and is reactive, occurring because a person has been exposed to new antigens. Children have lymphadenopathy more often than adults, because of both the lack of previous exposures and the more rapid proliferative responses of lymphoid cells in young individuals. With a careful examination, almost all children less than age 12 years have palpable cervical, axillary, and inguinal lymph nodes. Cervical adenopathy can be detected in about 50% of persons between ages 20 and 50 years; it tends to decline thereafter. Prominent cervical, axillary, or inguinal adenopathy is uncommon in older adults in the absence of a significant underlying disease. However, mild bilateral inguinal adenopathy (i.e., a few discrete, nontender nodes in both groins) is common throughout life.

Individual lymph nodes normally vary in size from a few cubic millimeters to 1 cubic centimeter to 2 cubic centimeters. When lymphadenopathy occurs, it is often both the enlarged node and inflammation in surrounding tissues that is palpable.

ETIOLOGY.   Lymphadenopathy occurs worldwide; its etiologies follow somewhat distinctive geographic and age-specific patterns. Upper respiratory infections and oral and periodontal inflammation are the most common causes for cervical lymphadenopathy. In young adults, cervical lymphadenopathy with pharyngitis and constitutional symptoms suggests infectious mononucleosis. Prominent inguinal adenopathy prompts consideration of sexually transmitted diseases. Generalized lymphadenopathy in homosexual persons suggests human immunodeficiency (HIV) infection and syphilis. In areas with endemic parasitic infections (e.g., filariasis and trypanosomiasis), these causes should be considered. In older adults, enlarging lymph nodes suggest a malignant process.

The causes of lymphadenopathy are outlined in Table 198–1, including notations of the most frequent causes for a general medical practice in the United States. Frequently patients recognize their own lymphadenopathy, especially when it occurs acutely as with most infections, drug reactions, cutaneous in-

TABLE 198–1.   CAUSES OF LYMPHADENOPATHY

Infections
Bacterial: Group A and other streptococci,[1] *S. aureus,*[1] syphilis,[1,2] cat scratch disease,[1] oral/
   dental infections (anaerobic streptococci and other mouth anaerobes[1]), *Mycobacterium
   tuberculosis* and other mycobacteria,[2] brucellosis,[2] leptopirosis,[2] mellioidosis,[2] chancroid,
   plague, tularemia, rat bite fever
Viral: Adenovirus,[1] immunodeficiency virus (HIV),[1,2] infectious mononucleosis,[1,2] herpes
   simplex,[1] measles,[2] rubella,[2] cytomegalovirus,[2] hepatitis,[2] Kawasaki disease.
Mycotic: Sporotrichosis, histoplasmosis,[2] coccidiomycosis[2]
Rickettsial: Rocky Mountain spotted fever,[1,2] scrub typhus[2]
Chlamydial: Chlamydia trachomatis, lymphogranuloma venereum
Protozoan: Toxoplasmosis,[2] trypanosomiasis,[2] kala-azar[2]
Helminthic: Filariasis,[2] onchocerciasis

Immunologic
Stings and bites[1]
Drug reactions:[1,2] phenytoin, hydralazine
Serum sickness[1,2]
Collagen vascular diseases: Rheumatoid arthritis,[2] dermatomyositis,[2] angioimmunoblastic
   lymphadenopathy[2]

Malignancies
Hematologic: Hodgkin's disease,[1] acute leukemia,[2] chronic lymphocytic leukemia,[2] chronic
   myelogenous leukemia,[2] lymphoma,[2] myelofibrosis[2]
Other: Metastic carcinoma, sarcomas

Endocrine Diseases
Hyperthyroidism[2]

Histocytic Disorders
Lipid storage disease,[2] malignant histocytosis,[2] Langerhans' (eosinophilic) histocytosis

Miscellaneous
Sarcoidosis, amyloidosis,[2] chronic granulomatous disease, lymphomatoid granulomatosis,
   necrotizing lymphadenitis

[1]Most common causes in general practice in the United States.
[2]Usually cause generalized lymphadenopathy.

juries, bites, and stings. In the other disorders, when the onset is insidious and the nodes are nontender, the patient may not notice them.

CLINICAL APPROACH. Because there are so many causes of lymphadenopathy, the clinical evaluation should always be conducted in stages, tailoring the evaluation to the clinical and epidemiologic circumstances. The time of onset of lymph node enlargement, associated symptoms, and evidence for contiguous inflammation (pharyngitis, cutaneous abrasions, ulcers, lymphangitis, etc.) should be noted. Lymphadenopathy is usually attributable to regional viral or bacterial infection. When such a cause is not readily apparent, a more detailed history, including drug exposures, sexual activity, travel, work, and hobbies, is important.

With the initial examination, the clinician should carefully record the characteristics of the lymphadenopathy: location; size; tender or nontender; discrete or matted together; hard, soft, or fluctuant. Many soft, tender, discrete nodes suggest a reactive process. Predominantly regional or asymmetric enlargement suggests a localized inflammatory process, although this pattern is also the most frequent presentation of Hodgkin's disease. Very tender, enlarged, and fluctuant nodes may have central necrosis, a finding in some severe bacterial infections such as tularemia. Discrete rubbery lymph nodes are common in chronic lymphocytic leukemia and the lymphomas. Discrete, asymmetric, hard lymph nodes suggest a metastatic malignancy.

During the rest of the physical examination, particular attention should be paid to the skin (rashes, pustules, ulcers, or erythema nodosum), eyes (conjunctivitis, iritis), throat (redness, exudate), ears (otitis externa or media, mastoiditis), chest (rales, dullness), heart (murmurs), abdomen (hepatic or splenic enlargement, stool for occult blood), and extremities (bone tenderness, local swelling or pain). In obscure cases, the diagnosis is found only after repeated examinations.

When acute lymphadenopathy is easily attributed to pharyngitis or a skin infection, multiple laboratory tests and follow-up are generally unnecessary. In less clear-cut circumstances, an extensive laboratory investigation may be required. The three most useful initial tests are the complete blood count (CBC) with blood smear examination, bacterial cultures, and a chest radiograph. The CBC may show anemia (a sign of chronic inflammation), atypical or abnormal blood leukocytes, leukopenia, leukocytosis, or eosinophilia. Throat cultures for beta-hemolytic streptococci, skin cultures for *Stapylococcus aureus* or *Cornynebacterium diphtheriae* and cultures of any discrete lesions can be very helpful. The chest radiograph may show infiltrates or hilar adenopathy. In young adults with cervical or generalized adenopathy, a monospot is often useful. Jaundice, hepatomegaly, or right upper quadrant tenderness mandates liver function tests and hepatitis serologies. In a small proportion of cases, lymphadenopathy cannot be easily explained based on the history, physical examination, or basic laboratory tests. In these instances, and in a few special circumstances, lymph node aspiration or a surgical biopsy is indicated. Prior to a cervical node biopsy, thorough laryngeal examination (i.e., indirect or direct laryngoscopy) is warranted, particularly in older adults with a history of smoking. With very enlarged or fluctuant adenopathy and a high suspicion of a bacterial pathogen, aspiration and culture for *Francisella, Yersinia,* and other pathogens under careful laboratory conditions (the material can be very infectious) is justified. Tuberculosis may also be diagnosed in cases of scrofula from aspirated lymph node tissue but biopsies are preferable.

Ordinarily, lymph node biopsy is reserved until it is clear the lymphadenopathy is a manifestation of a serious illness that cannot be diagnosed by examination of the blood or by biopsy of other more accessible tissues. For instance, in patients with suspected granulomatous inflammation (e.g., sarcoidosis, tuberculosis, histoplasmosis), biopsies of the skin, liver, or bone marrow should be considered as alternatives. If a biopsy is necessary, it is better to biopsy a central rather than a peripheral node. It is always important to discuss the probable diagnoses with the surgeon and pathologist before the biopsy is obtained. It is not unusual to obtain nondiagnostic tissue from patients suspected to have a serious infiltrative or malignant disease. In these instances, it is wise to consider a second biopsy soon if the diagnosis remains obscure and the illness persists.

MANAGEMENT.   In most cases of lymphadenopathy, the focus is on making a precise diagnosis. It rarely takes more than a few weeks for the lymphadenopathy to resolve or a diagnosis to be made. Empiric therapy with antibiotics is justified when there is a strong suspicion that lymphadenopathy is due to a pyogenic infection; otherwise antibiotic trials are often confusing and unhelpful. Corticosteroids ameliorate severe lymphadenopathy in patients with infectious mononucleosis and other viral illnesses, but their use is generally not necessary or indicated. Radiation therapy will shrink enlarged nodes but should not be used without a precise indication.

FOLLOW-UP.   Acute lymphadenopathy due to infection or inflammation usually resolves within 1 week to 3 weeks. Serial physical examinations as well as laboratory evaluation as outlined under "Clinical Approach" should be done in all patients with lymphadenopathy persisting beyond 3 weeks.

Cross-references: AIDS (Section 14), Detection and Initial Management of Oral Cancer (Section 47), Pharyngitis (Section 54).

REFERENCES

1.   Brook I. The swollen neck: Cervical lymphadenitis, parotitis, thyroiditis, and infected cysts. Inf Dis Clin North Am 1988;2:221–236.
    Discusses diagnosis and treatment of common causes of neck swelling.

2.   Greenfield S, Jordan MC. The clinical investigation of lymphadenopathy in primary care practice. JAMA 1978;240:1388–1393.
    Includes useful algorithms.

3. Slap GB, Brooks JSJ, Schwartz JS. When to perform biopsies of enlarged peripheral lymph nodes in young patients. JAMA 1984;252:1321–1326.
    Describes a predictive model that correctly classified 97% of enlarged lymph nodes as benign or granulomatous/malignant. The model helps in the selection of patients for lymph node biopsy.

4. Williamson HA. Lymphadenopathy in a family practice: A descriptive study of 249 cases. J Fam Pract 1985;20:449–452.
    Serious disease was rare in asymptomatic patients, justifying a period of observation.

5. Winterbauer RH, Belic N, Moores KD. A clinical interpretation of bilateral hilar adenopathy. Ann Intern Med 1973;78:65–71.
    In patients with bilateral hilar adenopathy, the absence of symptoms or presence of erythema nodosum suggests sarcoidosis.

199 THROMBOCYTOPENIA

Problem

STEVEN H. PETERSDORF

EPIDEMIOLOGY/ETIOLOGY.   Thrombocytopenia is defined as a platelet count of less than 150,000/cu mm. The risk of serious bleeding increases when the platelet count is less than 50,000/cu mm, and spontaneous bleeding usually occurs only when the platelet count is less than 20,000/cu mm. Although many agents may cause thrombocytopenia, including drugs (e.g., thiazide diuretics, gold, heparin, quinine) and viruses (e.g., HIV, hepatitis B), most patients who are exposed to these agents do not develop this problem. Table 199–1 outlines the differential diagnosis of thrombocytopenia. Table 199–2 lists common medications associated with thrombocytopenia.

SYMPTOMS AND SIGNS.   The tendency to bleed is the primary clinical manifestation of thrombocytopenia. In mild cases, petechiae appear in dependent areas such as the feet or ankles or lining the buccal mucosa. Increasingly severe thrombocytopenia leads to more diffuse petechiae and epistaxis, gingival bleeding, ecchymoses, and increased menstrual bleeding. The severity of the bleeding depends on the platelet count, as well as other underlying hemostatic defects.

CLINICAL APPROACH.   Thrombocytopenia is caused by decreased production or increased destruction of platelets. The history (drug history, duration of bleeding), physical examination (location of bleeding, presence of splenomegaly), and laboratory studies (including a CBC, review of the peripheral smear, and bone marrow evaluation) are necessary parts of the evaluation.

TABLE 199–1.   DIFFERENTIAL DIAGNOSIS OF THROMBOCYTOPENIA

A. Thrombocytopenia secondary to decreased marrow production (decreased bone marrow megakaryocytes)
  1. Viral infection
  2. Alcohol
  3. Drugs (e.g., thiazide diuretics)
  4. Disorders associated with marrow invasion (e.g., leukemia, infection, metastatic carcinoma)
  5. Disorders associated with ineffective myelopoiesis (e.g., aplastic anemia, myelodysplasia, paroxysmal nocturnal hemoglobinuria)
B. Thrombocytopenia secondary to increased platelet destruction (normal to increased megakaryocytes in the bone marrow).
  1. Immune-mediated destruction
    a. Immune thrombocytopenic purpura (ITP)
    b. Posttransfusion purpura
    c. Infection (HIV)
    d. Drug-induced purpura (quinine, gold, heparin)
  2. Nonimmunologic destruction
    a. Hypersplenism
    b. Disseminated intravascular coagulation
    c. Thrombotic thrombocytopenic purpura (TTP)
    d. Hemolytic-uremic syndrome (HUS)

Thrombocytopenia due to decreased production may be associated with drug exposure (e.g., alcohol, thiazide diuretics) or a primary bone marrow problem such as marrow failure or infiltration. There will be decreased megakaryocytes in the bone marrow and possibly other abnormalities in the CBC, such as nucleated red blood cells or unusually small or large platelets.

Thrombocytopenia secondary to increased destruction may be associated with drug exposure (e.g., quinine, gold, heparin), a history of recent transfusion or pregnancy, infection with HIV, or other autoimmune phenomenon. The bleeding time is normal in immune thrombocytopenia (ITP) because the few platelets present are hyperfunctional. On bone marrow examination megakaryocytes are increased in all causes of thrombocytopenia caused by increased destruction. Fragmentation of red cells on the peripheral smear is associated with thrombocytopenia caused by thrombotic thrombocytopenic purpura (TTP) or disseminated intravascular coagulation (DIC). Finally, patients with splenic sequestration have splenomegaly on physical examination and normal to increased megakaryocytes in the bone marrow.

TABLE 199–2.   DRUGS COMMONLY ASSOCIATED WITH THROMBOCYTOPENIA

Alpha methyldopa (Aldomet)	Digoxin
Carbamazepine (Tegretol)	Phenytoin (Dilantin)
Cephalosporins	Heparin
Chlorothiazides	Quinine/quinidine
Cimetidine (Tagamet)	Sulfa drugs
Diazepam (Valium)	

MANAGEMENT.   Platelet transfusions, with either random donor pooled platelets or single donor pheresed platelets, are appropriate in patients with frank bleeding or a platelet count less than 20,000 if the thrombocytopenia is due to decreased production or increased destruction from a nonautoimmune phenomenon. Subsequent management requires removal of the offending agent or treatment of the underlying cause. For patients with ITP, transfused platelets have a very short survival and are not of benefit unless the patient has uncontrolled bleeding. Initial treatment of ITP includes prednisone at a dose of 2 mg/kg/day. If the thrombocytopenia has not resolved after 2 weeks, splenectomy is indicated. Approximately 10% to 20% of patients with ITP do not respond to any of these measures and require immunosuppressive therapy with cyclophosphamide, azathioprine, or vincristine. An alternate approach is therapy with intravenous immunoglobulin (400 mg/kg/day for 5 days).

FOLLOW-UP.   Thrombocytopenia secondary to decreased production from drugs should correct within 7 days to 14 days of removal of the offending agent. Recovery from exposure to quinine takes 3 days to 14 days, and the recovery after gold exposure may take slightly longer. The thrombocytopenia of adult patients with ITP or TTP may have a relapsing course.

Cross-references: AIDS (Section 14), Epistaxis (Section 55), Cirrhosis and Chronic Liver Failure (Section 100), General Approach to Arthritic Symptoms (Section 107), Abnormal Uterine Bleeding (Section 162), Anemia (Section 201), Transfusion Therapy (Section 204), Preoperative Hematologic Problems (Section 220).

REFERENCES

1. Berchtold P, McMillan R. Therapy of chronic idiopathic thrombocytopenic purpura in adults. Blood 1989;74:2309–2317.
    Review of the acute and long-term management of adults with ITP.

2. Hackett T, Kelton JG, Powers P. Drug-induced platelet destruction. Semin Thromb Hemost 1982;8:116–137.
    Comprehensive review of drug-associated thrombocytopenia.

3. Wilson JS, Neane PB, Kelton JG. Infection-induced thrombocytopenia. Semin Thromb Hemost 1982;8:217–233.
    Comprehensive review of thrombocytopenia caused by infection; does not mention HIV.

200 POLYCYTHEMIA

Problem

STEVEN H. PETERSDORF

EPIDEMIOLOGY/ETIOLOGY. Polycythemia refers to an increased red blood cell concentration. There are three types: (1) polycythemia vera (PV), a clonal stem cell disorder characterized by increased production of red cells, granulocytes, and platelets; (2) secondary polycythemia, which represents increased red blood cell mass due to increased erythropoietin production, high-affinity hemoglobin, or a chronic hypoxemic state; and (3) relative polycythemia, which occurs when the red cell mass is normal but the plasma volume is decreased.

Polycythemia vera is a rare disease. There are 5 to 17 cases per million people diagnosed each year in the United States. There is a slight male predominance (1.2:1). The median age at diagnosis is age 60 years, and the disease is rare below age 30 years. The incidence of secondary polycythemia is increased in smokers and patients with chronic obstructive lung disease who are persistently hypoxemic. The patients who develop relative polycythemia have an increased incidence of hypertension.

SYMPTOMS AND SIGNS. The clinical presentation of polycythemia is directly related to increased concentration of red blood cells, which leads to increased blood viscosity. Neurologic symptoms are most common and include headache, weakness, and dizziness. With severe hyperviscosity, confusion, paresthesias, pruritis, and impaired visual acuity are frequent. Clinical signs include a ruddy complexion, plethora of conjunctival blood vessels, and dilated veins noted on fundoscopic examination. Splenomegaly is found in 70% to 90% of patients with polycythemia vera.

CLINICAL APPROACH. If the hematocrit is greater than 60%, the red blood cell mass is almost certainly increased. If the hematocrit is between 55% and 60% and the patient has a normal Pao_2, the red blood cell mass should be determined by the 51-CR red blood cell assay. If the red cell mass is normal, the patient has relative polycythemia. If the mass is elevated, the patient should be evaluated for polycythemia vera or secondary polycythemia. The presence of associated leukocytosis, basophilia, thrombocytosis, splenomegaly, and trilinear hyperplasia of the bone marrow is consistent with polycythemia vera. The serum erythropoietin level is normal in polycythemia vera.

If the hematologic workup is normal, the patient should be evaluated for secondary polycythemia. Conditions associated with secondary polycythemia include chronic pulmonary disease with hypoxemia, smoking with elevated carboxyhemoglobin, hemoglobinopathies with increased oxygen affinity, and inappropriate erythropoietin secretion (usually associated with renal cysts or renal tumors). Consequently, evaluation should include arterial blood gases, measurement of the p50 to screen for impaired oxygen release (abnormal, <27 mm Hg), and an ultrasound evaluation of the kidneys to rule out a renal lesion. The serum erythropoietin level will usually be elevated in secondary polycythemia (>30 mU/ml).

MANAGEMENT.   Relative polycythemia can usually be corrected by cessation of smoking or controlling the hypertension that is usually present. Patients with secondary polycythemia from hypoxemia should have phlebotomy performed, with removal of 250 cc to 500 cc of blood every other day until the hematocrit reaches less than 45 in men and 43 in women. Patients with underlying cardiovascular and cerebrovascular disease should have phlebotomy with reduced volume (100–200 cc) and simultaneous replacement with volume expanders to correct hyperviscosity that may result. Although supplemental oxygen may benefit those with arterial Pao$_2$ less than than 60 mm Hg, red cell mass will not decrease unless smoking is stopped. Secondary polycythemia from hemoglobinopathy can be managed in the same way. Polycythemia from erythropoietin-secreting tumors or cysts can be managed with phlebotomy and removal of the lesion.

The hematocrit of patients with polycythemia vera should be maintained at less than 44 to prevent thrombotic complications. Younger patients (less than age 40 years) should be treated with phlebotomy. Since older patients have a much greater incidence of thrombotic complications, they should receive chemotherapy as well as phlebotomy. Options include phosphorus-32 intravenously every 3 months as necessary, busulfan (4–6 mg PO q.d. for 4–6 weeks), or hydroxyurea (500–1000 mg every day as blood counts permit). These drugs require consultation with a hematologist and close monitoring of blood counts to prevent marrow aplasia.

FOLLOW-UP.   Patients with relative polycythemia should be monitored for thromboembolic complications, which occur in 30% to 70% of patients. Follow-up of the patient with secondary polycythemia includes frequent hematocrit readings as well as correction of the underlying disorder.

The patient with polycythemia vera may suffer from thrombotic and hemorrhagic complications due to the hyperviscosity. In addition, acute leukemia evolves in 15% of patients with polycythemia vera, and 15% to 30% of patients develop myelofibrosis with myeloid metaplasia. The median survival of patients with polycythemia vera who have optimum therapy is 10 years to 15 years.

Cross-references: Smoking Cessation (Section 11), Pruritis (Section 23), Sleep Apnea Syndrome (Section 64), Asthma and Chronic Obstructive Pulmonary Disease (Section 68).

REFERENCES

1. Adamson JW. Polycythemias: Diagnosis and treatment. Hosp Pract 1983;18(12):49–57.
   Provides excellent algorithms for evaluating patients with polycythemia.

2. Berk PD, Goldberg JD, Donovan PB, et al. Therapeutic recommendation in polycythemia vera based on the Polycythemia Vera Study Group Protocols. Semin Hematol 1986;23:132–143.
   A useful review of 10 years of clinical trials in polycythemia vera.

3. Hocking WG, Golde DW. Polycythemia: Evaluation and management. Blood Rev 1989; 3:57–65.
   Provides excellent algorithms for evaluating patients with polycythemia.

201 ANEMIA

Problem

STEVEN H. PETERSDORF

Epidemiology/Etiology.   Anemia reflects an underlying pathologic process and is a common finding in a wide variety of acute and chronic diseases. Anemia is defined as a hemoglobin concentration less than 12 g/dl in women and 13.5 g/dl in men. The common causes of anemia are iron deficiency (25% of patients), acute blood loss (25%), anemia of chronic inflammatory disorders (25%), hemolysis (10%), megaloblastic anemia (10%), and bone marrow failure or replacement (<5%).

Symptoms and Signs.   The anemic patient may present with nonspecific complaints such as lethargy, fatigue, weakness, or palpitations. Symptoms are more pronounced with rapidly developing anemia, more severe anemia, and underlying cardiovascular disease.

Physical signs of anemia may include pallor, tachycardia, postural hypotension, and a systolic murmur, though all are nonspecific.[4] Other findings provide clues to the cause of the anemia, such as jaundice (hemolysis), lymphadenopathy (marrow infiltrative process), hepatosplenomegaly (hemolysis, marrow infiltration), ecchymoses (blood loss), hemocult positive stools (blood loss and/or iron deficiency), and neurologic findings (megaloblastic anemia).

Clinical Approach.   After anemia is diagnosed by measuring a decreased red cell mass, hemoglobin concentration, and hematocrit, the specific cause should be determined. Once acute blood loss is excluded by history and physical examination, the initial evaluation includes a reticulocyte index to determine whether the anemia is secondary to decreased production or increased destruction of red blood cells. If the corrected reticulocyte index is less than 2% to 3%, the anemia is secondary to decreased production (Table 201–1). Additional studies should include review of the peripheral smear and red cell indexes. Where appropriate, measurement of iron, total iron binding capacity, ferritin, folate, and B_{12} should be performed. If the reticulocyte count is greater than 3%, the patient should be evaluated for increased destruction of red cells. The peripheral smear should be examined for spherocytes (a sign of immuno-hemolytic anemia), fragmented cells (signifying microangiopathic anemia), and sickle cells. Bone marrow examination should be performed if there is an unexplained hypoproliferative anemia or if nucleated red blood cells or blasts are seen on the peripheral smear.

MANAGEMENT. Long-term correction of the anemia requires resolution of the underlying medical condition. The nutritional anemias (i.e., iron, folate, B_{12} deficiency) can be corrected by replacement. Iron deficiency can usually be corrected by administering 300 mg of ferrous sulfate three times a day orally, which provides 180 mg of elemental iron daily. The reticulocyte count will peak 5 days to 10 days after starting iron. The hemoglobin level should reach normal within 2 months, and therapy should be continued for 6 months to replace iron stores fully. Vitamin B_{12} deficiency can be corrected rapidly with 100 μg of intramuscular (IM) cobalamin per day for a week, followed by 100 μg twice a week for 6 weeks, and then 100 μg cobalamin IM monthly for life. Folate deficiency can be corrected with 1 mg of folate every day or twice daily for 1 month to 4 months.

Patients who are anemic secondary to chronic renal failure may benefit from the administration of recombinant human erythropoietin (rhEPO). The role of rhEPO in other chronic anemias is under study.

Transfusion of red cells should be performed when diminished tissue oxygenation is secondary to decreased red cell mass. Accepted indications include the presence of angina in a severely anemic patient or an acute blood loss of more than 750 cc to 1000 cc of blood (see Section 204, Transfusion Therapy).

FOLLOW-UP. The patient should be monitored for resolution of the underlying disorder. Unless the cause of blood loss is obvious (e.g., menorrhagia), patients with iron deficiency should be evaluated for gastrointestinal sources of blood loss (see Section 105). Long-term management of other types of anemia depends on the underlying cause.

Cross-references: Fatigue (Section 21), Angina (Section 78), Congestive Heart Failure (Section 79), Colorectal Cancer Screening (Section 91), Sigmoidoscopy and Colonoscopy (Section 105), General Approach to Arthritic Symptoms (Section 107), Peripheral Neuropathy (Section 149), Abnormal Uterine Bleeding (Section 162), Chronic Renal Failure (Section 181), Transfusion Therapy (Section 204), Dyspnea in the Cancer Patient (Section 207), Preoperative Hematologic Problems (Section 220).

TABLE 201–1. DIFFERENTIAL DIAGNOSIS OF ANEMIA

Diagnosis	Blood Smear	Diagnostic Test[1]
1. Anemia secondary to decreased production (corrected reticulocyte count <2%; no maturation abnormality)		
a. Iron deficiency	Hypochromic, microcytic	Fe decreased; TIBC increased; Fe/TIBC<15%
		Marrow iron stores absent
b. Sideroblastic anemia	Hypochromic, microcytic	Fe increased, Fe/TIBC 60–95%
	Basophilic stippling	(check lead level)
c. Anemia of chronic, renal, or endocrine diseases	Normochromic, normocytic	Fe and TIBC decreased
		Marrow iron present
d. Anemia secondary to marrow replacement or failure	Normochromic, normocytic	Marrow empty or replaced with leukemia or metastatic tumor
2. Anemia secondary to decreased production from maturation abnormality (corrected reticulocyte count < 2%)		
a. Megaloblastic anemia	Macrocytic, macroovalocytes, hypersegmented neutrophils	Vitamin B_{12} or serum/red cell folate decreased
b. Refractory anemia	Dimorphic with macro- and microcytes	Ringed sideroblasts or ineffective erythropoiesis in marrow
3. Anemia secondary to increased destruction (corrected reticulocyte count > 2%)		
a. Mechanical destruction	Red cell fragments	Increased bilirubin, LDH; decreased haptoglobin
b. Autoimmune hemolysis	Spherocytes	Positive Coombs test
c. Hereditary membrane defects	Spherocytes, elliptocytes	
d. Hemoglobinopathy	Sickle cells present	Hemoglobin electrophoresis

[1]Fe = iron; TIBC = total iron binding capacity; LDH = lactate dehydrogenase.

REFERENCES

1. Bessman JD, Gilmer PR Jr, Gardner FH. Improved classification of anemias by MCV and RDW. Am J Clin Pathol 1983;80:322–326.
    An attempt to correlate anemias with electronically obtained red cell indexes.

2. Hillman RS, Finch CA. The Red Cell Manual, 5th ed. FA Davis, Philadelphia, 1985.
    A complete review of normal and abnormal pathophysiology.

3. Lee GR. The anemia of chronic disease. Semin Hematol 1983;20:61–80.
    Excellent review of pathophysiology and clinical evaluation.

4. Nardone DA, Roth KM, Mazur DJ, et al. Usefulness of physical examination in detecting the presence or absence of anemia. Arch Intern Med 1990;150:201–204.
    Evaluates the utility of physical findings in determining the presence of anemia.

202 SICKLE CELL DISEASE

Problem

STEVEN H. PETERSDORF

EPIDEMIOLOGY/ETIOLOGY.   Sickle cell disease includes not only sickle cell anemia but also other disorders that result from interactions between hemoglobin S and other beta hemoglobin abnormalities such as thalassemia or hemoglobin C. In the United States, approximately 8% of blacks carry a gene for sickle cell (Hb S, sickle cell trait), and approximately 0.15% of black children have the disease (Hb SS). Other sickle cell syndromes such as Hb SC (1:2600 blacks) are less common. The relatively high incidence of sickle cell trait is due to the survival advantage of the heterozygote under the selective pressure of falciparum malaria infection.

SYMPTOMS AND SIGNS.   Patients with sickle cell trait (Hb AS) usually are asymptomatic, although some experience painless hematuria that is typically mild and self-limiting.

Patients with sickle cell disease develop hemolytic anemia within a few months after birth. Adults typically present with pain from a vasoocclusive crisis, the severity and frequency of which varies among patients. Pain occurs in 50% of patients, most often in the hips, shoulders, and long bones. Other acute presentations include priapism (40% of males), stroke, and a chest syndrome secondary to vasoocclusion in the lungs that may be difficult to distinguish from pneumonia (10–20% of adults). Patients may develop an aplastic crisis with severe anemia due to infection with parvovirus. Finally, patients have impaired splenic function and develop increased susceptibility to infections with encapsulated organisms (pneumococcus, *Haemophilus influenzae,* meningococcus). Osteomyelitis due to *Salmonella* spp. is relatively unique to sickle cell disease.

Physical examination may be notable for scleral icterus, cardiomegaly, hepatomegaly, and lower-extremity skin ulcers.

CLINICAL APPROACH.   The diagnosis of sickle cell disease is typically made in childhood. Evaluation of patients with sickle cell disease demonstrates a hemoglobin concentration of 7 to 9 g/dl, mild leukocytosis (12–15,000) reflecting splenic atrophy, and a peripheral blood smear with sickled and nucleated red blood cells. Hemoglobin electrophoresis reveals 75% to 95% of the total being hemoglobin S; the remainder is hemoglobin A2 and F.

All patients with painful crises should be evaluated for underlying infection, a common inciting event. The chest radiograph may show an infiltrate reflecting a chest crisis or underlying pneumonia. If the patient has persistent bone pain, aseptic necrosis or osteomyelitis must be excluded.

MANAGEMENT.   Sickle cell disease is a chronic condition. Although there is no treatment to prevent sickling, certain measures may reduce the frequency of crisis and complications, including good nutrition, folic acid supplementation, avoiding temperature extremes and dehydration, and immunizations.

Treatment of painful crisis includes intravenous fluids for rehydration and analgesics. Narcotics may be required to alleviate severe pain. Transfusions should be performed only during an aplastic crisis, because they may precipitate a crisis by increasing blood viscosity. Direct exchange transfusion, however, is indicated to break the cycle of recurring vascular occlusive events, to assist the healing of chronic leg ulcers, and to prevent complications during pregnancy or prior to surgery.

FOLLOW-UP.   Sickle cell disease is a chronic disease that may lead to deterioration of several organ systems. Aseptic necrosis of the hips and shoulders, proliferative retinopathy, and leg ulcers are common complications. Health care maintenance of these patients dictates evaluation of cerebral, hepatic, cardiac, renal, pulmonary, orthopedic, and ophthalmologic evaluation every 3 months to 6 months.

Prenatal diagnosis of the disease can be made with chorionic villus sampling or amniocentesis.

Cross-references: Adult Immunizations (Section 10), Abdominal Pain (Section 95), Leg Ulcers (Section 134), Anemia (Section 201).

REFERENCES

1. Embury SH. The clinical pathophysiology of sickle cell disease. Ann Rev Med. 1986; 37:361–376.
    Complete review of the pathophysiology and complications of sickle cell anemia.

2. Schecter AN, Bunn HF. What determines severity in sickle cell disease. N Engl J Med 1982;306:295–297.
    Useful discussion of factors that may exacerbate sickle cell anemia.

203 CHRONIC ANTICOAGULATION

Procedure

NANCY J. ROBEN

INDICATIONS/CONTRAINDICATIONS.   The decision to anticoagulate a patient chronically must balance the benefits with the risks of therapy. Table 203–1 lists the indications for warfarin anticoagulation.

Contraindications to warfarin anticoagulation include active bleeding, recent cerebrovascular hemorrhage, severe congenital or acquired defect of hemostasis, recent major surgery, especially of the central nervous system or eye, and pregnancy. (Warfarin crosses the placenta and may cause birth defects and fetal hemorrhage; optimal anticoagulation during pregnancy is controversial.)

Relative contraindications include severe hepatic or renal disease, chronic alcohol use, markedly elevated blood pressure (>200/105 mm Hg), requirements for intensive salicylate or nonsteroidal anti-inflammation agents, poor patient compliance, unstable gait, history of falling, and history of gastrointestinal, urologic, or intracranial hemorrhage.

RATIONALE.   Warfarin interferes with the synthesis of vitamin K–dependent coagulation factors. Although the half-life of warfarin is 24 hours to 48 hours, 2 weeks of therapy may be required to achieve a stable state of anticoagulation due to the half-lives of the previously synthesized K–dependent clotting factors (VII = 6 hr; IX = 24 hr; X = 40 hr; II = 60–100 hr).

Warfarin therapy is monitored with the prothrombin time (PT), which varies greatly according to the reagents used by the local aboratory. Many laboratories have standardized this test by using the International Normalized Ratio (INR), which enables providers to apply national recommendations and readily compare PT values obtained from different laboratories. Two levels of intensity of anticoagulation are recommended: a less-intensive range, defined as an INR 2.0 to 3.0 (approximating a PT ratio [patient's time in seconds divided by control time] of 1.3–1.5), and a higher-intensity INR of 3.0 to 4.5 (approximating a PT ratio of 1.6–2.0). The less-intensive range is recommended for all patients

TABLE 203–1. RECOMMENDED INDICATIONS, ANTICOAGULATION RANGES, AND DURATION FOR WARFARIN THERAPY

Warfarin Indication	Recommended INR Range	Duration of Therapy
Mechanical cardiac valves in any position	3.0–4.5	Lifetime
First systemic embolism from any source	3.0–4.5, then 2.0–3.0	1 year, then indefinitely
Recurrent systemic embolism from any source	3.0–4.5	Lifetime
Venous Thromboembolism		
Treatment of proximal vein thrombosis or pulmonary embolism	2.0–3.0	3–6 mo
Recurrent thrombosis or pulmonary embolus or continuing risk factors such as antithrombin-III or protein C or S deficiencies or malignancy	2.0–3.0	Long-term therapy unless risks outweigh benefit of therapy
Isolated symptomatic calf vein thrombosis[1]	2.0–3.0	3 mo
Prophylaxis for elective or fractured hip surgery	2.0–3.0	6 wk
Myocardial Infarction		
Anterior transmural infarcts	2.0–3.0	3 mo
With atrial fibrillation and congestive failure	2.0–3.0	3 mo
Valvular Heart Disease		
Rheumatic mitral valve with systemic embolism	3.0–4.5, then 2.0–3.0	1 year, then indefinitely
Rheumatic mitral valve with atrial fibrillation or sinus rhythm with left atrium >5.5 cm	2.0–3.0	Long term
Mitral valve prolapse or annular calcium with atrial fibrillation or systemic embolism	2.0–3.0	Long term
Bioprosthetic valves in mitral position with sinus rhythm	2.0–3.0	Long term
		Stop 3 mo after surgery
Atrial Fibrillation		
Chronic atrial fibrillation[2]	2.0–3.0	Long term
Cardioversion for atrial fibrillation	2.0–3.0	Therapeutic INR for 3 wk before and 4 wk after sinus rhythm established

Source: Adapted from ACCP and Roben NJ, Kent DL, Fihn SD. Management of warfarin anticoagulation. Med Rounds 1990;3:63–75, with permission.

[1]Many regard this indication controversial.

[2]Excluding patients with "lone" atrial fibrillation. See Section 83.

except those with mechanical prosthetic valves or recurrent systemic embolism (see Table 203–1).

METHODS.   In the outpatient setting, warfarin should be started at 2.5 mg to 5 mg daily; larger loading doses lead to excessive anticoagulation and subsequent wide fluctuations of the PT/INR. Patients who are elderly, medically unstable or taking drugs that potentiate warfarin should receive the 2.5-mg dose. The PT should be monitored every 5 days to 7 days in the same laboratory until it is stable. Dosage changes should generally be made in increments of 2.5 mg per week. Once stable, the PT/INR is monitored every 4 weeks to 6 weeks. Flow sheets that record warfarin dose and PT/INR results assist all who care for the patient.

The simplest warfarin regimens are based on days of the week and use a single tablet size and drug manufacturer. The patient should receive some warfarin every day, even when only small doses (1–2 mg) are required. For example, a patient may take 5 mg on Monday, Wednesday, and Friday and 7.5 mg on all other days; or 7.5 mg every Sunday and 5 mg all other days. Use of "even" and "odd" days leads to patient confusion and may result in unstable anticoagulation from week to week and during months with 31 days.

Patients vary widely in their warfarin requirements. Any change in the patient's disease process or medications may affect the PT/INR results (see Tables 203–2 and 203–3).

Warfarin is extensively protein bound and is susceptible to displacement by other more strongly bound drugs (Table 203–3). When any of these drugs is initiated, altered, or discontinued, the PT requires close monitoring. Drugs that affect platelet function (e.g., aspirin, sulfinpyrazone, certain antibiotics) or

TABLE 203–2.   QUESTIONS TO POSE WHEN UNEXPECTED PROTHROMBIN TIME OR INTERNATIONAL NORMALIZED RATIO VALUES ARE ENCOUNTERED

1. Is the recommended warfarin dosing regimen being followed?
2. Specifically, have any doses been missed in the past 5 to 7 days?
3. Is there confusion regarding tablet size of warfarin?
4. Have any medications been added, deleted, or altered? Any nonprescription medication use?
5. Are there any medications recently added or deleted known to influence warfarin pharmacokinetics?
6. Have there been any bruising or bleeding problems?
7. Has there been any acute illness in the past 10 days (e.g., diarrhea, fever)?
8. Are there any signs or symptoms to suggest that congestive heart failure, liver disease, hepatic congestion, or renal disease has developed or become more unstable at present?
9. Has thyroid disease, a malignancy, or a malabsorption syndrome recently been identified?
10. Have there been any changes in diet (e.g., increased leafy green vegetables, diet preparations, or formulas)?
11. Has there been any change in the patient's use of alcohol?
12. Is there a question about laboratory reliability? Could the abnormal PT (international normalized ratio) be an error?

Source: Adapted from Roben NJ, Kent DL, Fihn SD. Management of warfarin anticoagulation. Med Rounds 1990;3:63–75, with permission.

TABLE 203–3. DRUGS KNOWN TO INTERACT WITH WARFARIN*

Drugs Known to Increase INR and PT	Drugs Known to Decrease INR and PT	Drugs with Variable INR Effects on INR and PT
Allopurinol	Antacids	*Alcohol*
Amiodarone	Antihistamines	Chloral hydrate
Aspirin (high doses)	*Barbiturates*	Diuretics
Chlorpropamide	*Carbamazepine*	Phenytoin
Cimetidine	Chlordiazepoxide	Ranitidine
Clofibrate	Cholestyramine	
Disulfiram	Colestipol	
Ethacrynic acid	Griseofulvin	
Fenoprofen	Laxatives	
Gemfibrozil	Oral contraceptives	
Indomethacin	*Rifampin*	
Phenylbutazone	*Vitamin K*	
Piroxicam		
Quinidine		
Quinine		
Sulfonamides, long-acting		
Sulindac		
Thyroid drugs		
Tricyclic antidepressants		
Trimethoprim/ Sulfamethoxazole		
Quinolones		

Source: Adapted from Roben NJ, Kent DL, Fihn SD. Management of warfarin anticoagulation. Med Rounds 1990;3:63–75, with permission.

*This table does not represent a total list of known drug versus warfarin reactions. The drugs that are italicized often produce a dramatic effect. Each patient needs to be monitored carefully for individual differences.

damage gastric mucosa (aspirin and other nonsteroidal agents) are best avoided. When the PT/INR exceeds the therapeutic range, the clinician should withhold one dose, substitute a lower maintenance dose, and monitor the PT/INR every other week until stable. If the PT/INR becomes dangerously high, the patient should be hospitalized; those with active bleeding or an extremely high PT may require vitamin K or fresh-frozen plasma to reverse the anticoagulation.

Patients should repeatedly receive the information that appears in Table 203–4. The decision to anticoagulate a patient should be reevaluated every 6 months. When the warfarin is discontinued, no tapering is necessary.

COST/COMPLICATIONS. Warfarin is available as a 1-mg (pink), 2-mg (lavender), 2.5-mg (green), 5-mg (peach), or 10-mg (white) scored tablet. The retail cost of 100 tablets of warfarin 5 mg ranges from $20.00 (generic) to $50.00 (du Pont). The cost of a PT test ranges from $19.50 to $29.00, often with an additional $5.00 blood drawing or handling charge.

The main complication of anticoagulation therapy is bleeding. The overall risk of major hemorrhage is approximately 3 per 100 patient-years. The risk of death is approximately 1 per 100 patient-years in outpatients who start war-

TABLE 203—4.   ADVICE TO PATIENTS

1. Report bleeding and unusual or unexplained bruising.
2. Check for blood in urine and stool on a regular basis.
3. Report all medication changes within 3 days.
4. Limit alcohol use to occasional beer, wine, or 2 ounces of liquor.
5. Minimize injury in activities of daily living, including work or hobbies.
6. Avoid aspirin-containing drugs; substitute acetaminophen up to 2000 mg per day.
7. Take warfarin at the same time each day, and never take extra doses to compensate for missed doses.
8. If menses are delayed more than 3 or 4 days and pregnancy is a risk, contact the provider.
9. Review care and prevention techniques for stopping nose bleeding.
10. Avoid changes in diet.

farin. Independent risk factors for major bleeding include hypertension; intensity of anticoagulation; presence of underlying gastrointestinal, urologic, or intracranial lesion that may bleed; and duration of anticoagulation, with those just beginning anticoagulation at highest risk.

Warfarin-induced necrosis of the skin and subcutaneous tissue is rare; lesions appear, usually in women, on the lower half of the body within 3 days to 10 days of initiation of therapy. The "purple toe syndrome," also rare, occurs early during therapy and causes bilateral, painful purplish discoloration of the toes.

Cross-references: Aortic Stenosis (Section 80), Other Valvular Disease (Section 82), Atrial Fibrillation (Section 83), Cerebrovascular Disease (Section 148), Preoperative Hematologic Problems (Section 220).

REFERENCES

1. Dalen JE, Hirsh J, Eds. Chest 1989;95(2)(Feb suppl).
   Issue summarizes recommendations made by the Second American College of Chest Physicians Conference on Antithrombotic Therapy. Recommendations from the third conference are due out in 1992.

2. Landefield CS, Goldman L. Major bleeding in outpatients treated with warfarin: Incidence and prediction by factors known at the start of bleeding. Am J Med 1989;87:144–152.
   Study of 187 outpatients starting warfarin; five independent risk factors for major bleeding were identified.

3. Roben NJ, Kent DL, Fihn SD. Management of warfarin anticoagulation. Med Rounds 1990;3:63–75.
   Helpful in the clinical management of patients.

4. Stults BM, Dere WH, Caine TH. Long-term anticoagulation—indications and management. West J Med 1989;151:414–429.
   A thorough review of chronic anticoagulation.

204 TRANSFUSION THERAPY

Procedure

GERALD J. ROTH

INDICATIONS/CONTRAINDICATIONS. Blood banks fractionate donor blood into red cells, platelets, plasma, and plasma components (e.g., cryoprecipitate). Each fraction is used for specific indications, such as anemia or thrombocytopenia.

RATIONALE. Blood transfusion to prevent or treat shock from hemorrhage is a major indication for transfusion. For example, surgery or trauma can result in acute blood loss that requires both volume and red cell replacement. In these instances, a combination of saline and packed red blood cells (RBCs) is indicated, and whole blood may be useful. In the absence of acute blood loss, blood components are used.

Red Blood Cells. Packed (sedimented) RBC preparations, with a hematocrit of 60% to 70%, are customarily used. The most common indication for RBC transfusion is anemia (hemoglobin < 7 g%). Patients who are transfused for less severe anemia (hemoglobin > 7 g%) may not benefit from additional oxygen-carrying capacity, although those with cardiopulmonary disease may respond to RBCs with a reduction in symptoms such as angina or dyspnea. The use of RBCs in mild symptomatic anemia is individualized and based on the degree of anemia (hemoglobin, 7–10 g%) and benefit observed. Single unit RBC transfusions are rarely indicated.

Platelets. The degree of thrombocytopenia that warrants platelet transfusion lies in the range of 15,000/mm³ to 20,000/mm³, although many patients with platelet counts of 5000 to l0,000 do not experience severe bleeding. A unit of transfused platelet concentrate usually raises the circulating platelet count approximately 10,000/mm³; antiplatelet antibodies, fever, or infection frequently blunt this ideal response. Although thrombocytopenia secondary to decreased platelet production or increased platelet loss is a common indication for transfusion, platelet concentrates can also provide functional platelets in patients whose endogenous platelets are numerically normal but functionally abnormal.

Plasma and Cryoprecipitate. Fresh-frozen plasma is a convenient but dilute source of plasma coagulation factors. Cryoprecipitate is enriched in both fibrinogen and von Willebrand's factor (vWf) and therefore is used to replace fibrinogen in patients with disseminated intravascular coagulation (DIC) and to provide vWf in patients with von Willebrand's disease.

Granulocytes. Granulocyte transfusion is reserved for neutropenic patients (absolute neutrophil count < 500/mm³) with an identified microbial infection that is unresponsive to appropriate antibiotic therapy. Granulocyte colony stimulating factors (e.g., GMCSF, GCSF) may obviate the need for granulocyte transfusions.

METHODS.   Medical personnel administering blood products must ascertain that the product is indeed intended for the recipient. Most problems arise from inaccurate labeling or from inadvertent administration of a correctly labeled product to the wrong recipient. In handling a transfusion accident, the clinician should first discontinue the transfusion while obtaining new samples of blood and urine for laboratory testing. The original intravenous line is retained to facilitate later therapy.

COSTS/COMPLICATIONS.   Representative current costs for a single unit of an individual blood component are: whole blood, $68; packed RBCs, $68; platelets, $33; fresh-frozen plasma, $31; and cryoprecipitate, $14.

The hazards of RBC transfusion include volume overload in patients with cardiopulmonary disease, acute and delayed hemolytic transfusion reactions, febrile and pulmonary hypersensitivity reactions, and transmission of infectious contaminates. Platelet transfusions can also cause febrile responses. Blood products are screened for markers of viral disease (i.e., HIV, hepatitis); nevertheless, transmission of viral illness may occur despite these precautions.

Cross-references: Bleeding (Section 197), Thrombocytopenia (Section 199), Anemia (Section 201), Preoperative Hematologic Problems (Section 220).

REFERENCE

1. Masouredis SP, Nusbacher J, Murphy S, et al. Preservation and clinical use of blood and blood components. In Williams WJ, Beutler E, Erslev AJ, et al., Eds. Hematology, 4th ed. McGraw-Hill, New York, 1990, pp. 1628–1673.

    Provides a detailed discussion of the appropriate use and risk of blood components (erythrocytes, leukocytes, platelets, plasma, and plasma fractions).

CHAPTER XVIII

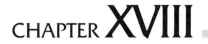

THE PATIENT WITH KNOWN CANCER

205 CHANGES IN MENTATION IN THE PATIENT WITH CANCER

Symptom

ANTHONY L. BACK

EPIDEMIOLOGY. Altered mental status is second only to pain as the most frequent neurologic problem patients with cancer experience. Although statistics for oncology outpatients are unavailable, altered mental status was the presenting complaint in 13% of patients requiring hospitalization at one solid tumor inpatient service.

ETIOLOGY. Altered mental status in cancer patients can result from direct invasion of the central nervous system (CNS) by tumor, indirect effects of the tumor on the CNS, or complications of therapy (Table 205–1). Brain metastases, narcotics, and metabolic derangements are by far the most frequent etiologies, followed by leptomeningeal metastases and infections. Hepatic encephalopathy secondary to hepatic metastases occurs only after replacement of the entire normal liver parenchyma. Hyperviscosity syndrome is restricted, except in rare instances, to patients with Waldenstrom's macroglobulinemia (IgM myeloma). Up to 30% of patients who have received brain irradiation, including prophylactic irradiation (e.g., small cell lung cancer), subsequently develop symptomatic cerebral dysfunction, presumably due to the radiation itself. CNS infections occur mostly in patients under treatment with chemotherapy who become neutropenic; unlike the situation in patients with acquired immunodeficiency syndrome (AIDS), CNS toxoplasmosis is rare in cancer patients. Paraneoplastic syndromes, nonbacterial thrombotic endocarditis, and hypercoagulable states are rare. Several chemotherapy drugs have been reported to cause encephalopathy, and intracarotid chemotherapy infusions have caused strokes. Failure to define an etiology for altered mental status in cancer patients is rare.

TABLE 205–1.   ALTERED MENTATION IN CANCER PATIENTS

Metastases
Brain metastases
Leptomeningeal metastases

Stroke Syndromes
Embolic: Nonbacterial thrombotic endocarditis
Thrombotic: Hypercoagulable states
Hemorrhagic: Metastasis related

Paraneoplastic Syndromes
Dementia
Multifocal leukoencephalopathy

Metabolic Derangements
Hypercalcemia
Hyponatremia (including syndrome of inappropriate antidiuretic hormone)
Hepatic encephalopathy
Uremia
Hyperviscosity syndrome

Infection
Sepsis
Meningitis, especially *Listeria* and *Cryptococcus*
Encephalitis, especially herpes

Depression

Therapy Related
Brain irradiation
Medications, especially narcotics

CLINICAL APPROACH.   History and physical examination usually indicate the diagnosis. Headache is relatively nonspecific. Focal neurologic signs suggest intracerebral metastases or a stroke syndrome. Isolated cranial nerve palsies usually indicate leptomeningeal metastases. Meningeal signs are seen with leptomeningeal metastases as well as meningitis. Diffuse alterations in level of consciousness suggest metabolic derangements, infection, medications, or rarely—as a diagnosis of exclusion—paraneoplastic dementia.

Diagnostic studies should include serum electrolytes, creatinine, calcium, liver function tests, complete blood count, absolute neutrophil count, prothrombin time, and activated partial thromboplastin time. Noncontrast computed tomograms (CT) should precede lumbar puncture to exclude midline shift because mass lesions sometimes present without focal findings. To detect intracerebral metastases, magnetic resonance (MR) scans are most sensitive, followed by contrast CT scans. Both multifocal leukoencephalopathy and herpes encephalitis have characteristic appearances on CT and MR studies. The sensitivity of cerebrospinal fluid (CSF) cytology for detecting leptomeningeal metastases is directly related to the volume of CSF collected; three CSF specimens of 10 cc each may be necessary. If the CSF is negative, MR may detect meningeal disease. Even when nonbacterial thrombotic endocarditis is suspected, echocardiograms are usually unrevealing because the valvular lesions are small (1–2 mm).

MANAGEMENT.   For patients with symptomatic brain metastases, corticosteroids often improve neurologic symptoms; the usual regimen is dexamethasone 4 mg every 6 hours. Phenytoin dilantin given prophylactically does not benefit patients with brain metastases who have not experienced a seizure. In selected patients with solitary brain metastases, surgical resection may be the therapy of choice; otherwise, brain radiation is the primary therapy. Approximately 60% of patients receiving radiotherapy experience some palliative benefit, but the median survival of patients with brain metastases is only 3 months to 6 months.

Patients with leptomeningeal metastases may receive intrathecal chemotherapy, but response rates are poor. Paraneoplastic neurologic syndromes respond poorly to chemotherapy. Hyperviscosity syndromes can respond dramatically to plasmapheresis.

Hypercalcemia may require admission for treatment with intravenous fluid and furosemide; further therapy may include gallium, mithramycin, diphosphonates, and corticosteroids.

Cross-references: Cirrhosis and Chronic Liver Failure (Section 100), Muscular Weakness (Section 139), Headache (Section 140), Seizures (Section 141), Dementia (Section 142), Electrolyte Abnormalities (Section 184), Management of Depression (Section 192).

REFERENCES

1. Cohen N, Strauss G, Lew R, Silver D, et al. Should prophylactic anticonvulsants be administered to patients with newly diagnosed cerebral metastases? J Clin Oncol 1988;6(10):1621–1624.
    The best recent review.

2. Gilbert MR, Grossman SA. Incidence and nature of neurologic problems in patients with solid tumors. Am J Med 1986;81(6):951–54.
    A compilation of neurologic complications encountered on an inpatient solid tumor service.

3. Patchell RA, Posner JB. Neurologic complications of systemic cancer. Neurol Clin 1985;3(4):729–50.
    A comprehensive review.

4. Weissman DE. Glucocorticoid treatment for brain metastases and epidural spinal cord compression: A review. J Clin Oncol 1988;6(3):543–551.
    An excellent review.

206 MANAGEMENT OF PAIN IN THE PATIENT WITH CANCER

Symptom

ANTHONY L. BACK

EPIDEMIOLOGY. Moderate to severe pain is reported by a third of cancer patients receiving active therapy and from 60% to 90% of patients with advanced cancer. Many cancer patients report that physicians undertreat their pain, which ranks high among patients' fears.

ETIOLOGY. Approximately two-thirds of pain syndromes in cancer outpatients result from direct tumor involvement (Table 206–1). Nerve infiltration or compression produce deafferentation pain, a severe, precisely localized burning or electric shock sensation. Metastatic bone lesions generally produce somatic pain, which is aching, deep, and well localized. Diffuse metastatic bone lesions and abdominal pain related to liver metastases, bowel involvement, or malignant ascites produce visceral pain, a poorly localized squeezing or pressing sensation; if acute, visceral pain may include autonomic symptoms of nausea, vomiting, and diaphoresis.

A second type of cancer-related pain is related to therapy (chemotherapy, radiation, or surgery). Common examples in outpatients include oral mucositis due to chemotherapy or radiotherapy, skin burns due to radiotherapy, aseptic

TABLE 206–1. TYPES OF CANCER-RELATED PAIN

Neurogenic Pain
Peripheral nerve compression or infiltration
Nerve root compression or infiltration
Spinal cord compression

Bone Pain
Bone metastases
Pathologic fractures

Abdominal Pain
Liver metastases
Bowel obstruction
Malignant ascites

Therapy Related
Mucositis
Radiation skin burns
Radiation fibrosis syndromes
Steroid osteonecrosis

necrosis of the femoral head due to corticosteroids, and radiation fibrosis involving nerves or soft tissues.

As many as 10% of cancer outpatients have pain that is unrelated to their cancer or cancer therapy.

CLINICAL APPROACH.   A careful pain history and directed physical examination are essential, with special attention to the neurologic examination. Use of a simple pain measurement scale helps measure the initial severity of pain and subsequent response to therapy ("Rate your pain on a scale of 1 to 10, where 1 is pain you can barely feel, and 10 is the worst pain imaginable"). The status of the patient's cancer will help determine whether specific cancer therapy will be useful in relieving the pain syndrome. These therapies include local radiation, hormonal manipulation, palliative surgical procedures, and palliative chemotherapy.

Certain pain complaints require prompt diagnostic evaluation. Back pain may warn of imminent spinal cord compression (see Section 208, Back Pain in the Cancer Patient). Bone pain in weight-bearing areas may require surgical stabilization and radiotherapy in order to prevent pathologic fracture. Headache should prompt evaluation for intracerebral metastases.

Because psychological distress may contribute to pain, evaluation by a psychiatrist, psychologist, or social worker may benefit the patient.

MANAGEMENT.   Oral analgesics provide relief to most patients and facilitate the workup, but severe pain may require immediate hospitalization and intravenous analgesics. Early consideration should be given to pain management techniques other than oral medications (for example, epidural nerve blocks in patients with metastatic disease involving the sacrum). Transdermal fentanyl may be useful in some patients who are unable to take oral narcotics.

For mild pain, nonsteroidal anti-inflammatory drugs (NSAIDs: aspirin, acetaminophen, ibuprofen, and others) are the drugs of choice. The gastrointestinal and hematologic side effects of these drugs may be dose limiting, especially in patients with platelet counts less than $100,000/mm^3$. If pain relief is not obtained or the pain presents at the moderate to severe level, opioid analgesics should be used.

For those with moderate to severe pain or pain unrelieved by NSAIDs, the second level of pain medication is the "weak" opioids, such as codeine and oxycodone (Table 206–2). These are most often prescribed in fixed-dose mixtures with NSAIDs (e.g., acetaminophen plus codeine) but can be given as single agents when NSAIDs are contraindicated.

The third level of pain medication is the "strong" opioids, such as morphine, methadone, and meperidine. In most patients, sustained-release morphine should be first the choice among agents in this class. Methadone can be difficult to manage because of its long half-life (average 24 hours) and because sedating side effects outlast its analgesic action. Meperidine (Demerol) is poorly absorbed when given orally and has a short half-life (3–4 hr); its metabolite normeperidine has a long half-life (12–16 hr) and causes seizures at high levels. Sublingual morphine dispensed for PRN use is helpful for breakthrough pain.

TABLE 206–2.   COMMONLY USED NARCOTIC ANALGESICS

	Starting Oral Dose Range	Cost ($)[1]
Codeine	15–30 mg q.3–4h.	0.20 (15 mg)
Oxycodone	5–10 mg q.3–4h.	0.12 (5 mg, generic[2])
		0.52 (5 mg, Percocet[2])
		0.52 (5 mg, Tylox[2])
		0.57 (4.5 mg, Percodan[3])
Morphine SR	30–60 mg q.8–12h. (for SR form)	0.90 (30 mg, MS Contin)
Methadone	5–10 mg q.6–12h.	0.05 (5 mg)

[1]Average wholesale price, per dose listed, 1991 *Drug Topics Red Book.*
[2]Contains acetaminophen.
[3]Contains aspirin.

Mixed agonist-antagonist drugs (e.g., pentazocine) are of limited use because of psychotomimetic side effects (e.g., hallucinations) that occur with dose escalation; these drugs also precipitate narcotic withdrawal in patients who are dependent on morphine agonists.

Combinations of narcotics and NSAIDs can often provide additive analgesia. The clinician should avoid combinations of narcotics with other drugs that increase sedation (e.g., narcotics and benzodiazepines).

For moderate and severe pain, patients should be instructed to take the analgesics regularly. Efficacy of a regimen should not be evaluated until steady-state drug levels have been achieved (usually four doses).

For neurologic deafferentation pain, a diverse group of medications, including phenytoin, carbamazepine, tricyclic antidepressants, and corticosteroids, has empirically proved useful.

When oral medications produce insufficient analgesia or excessive sedation, specialized techniques may be useful, including continuous subcutaneous infusion, epidural or intrathecal infusions, nerve blocks, and neurosurgical ablative procedures.

FOLLOW-UP.   Side effects of narcotics are common. Patients starting narcotics should receive stool softeners and be advised about cathartics. Sedation can be minimized by discontinuing other drugs that may interact (including cimetidine, barbiturates, and benzodiazepines), and administering smaller doses more frequently. Nausea and vomiting can be treated with antiemetics or trial of a different narcotic (most patients become tolerant to this side effect). Intentional overdose in cancer patients is rare, and when a patient on a stable drug regimen suddenly develops signs of overdose (excessive sedation and respiratory depression), the most common reason is medical deterioration and superimposed metabolic encephalopathy.

Tolerance develops in all patients chronically taking narcotics and usually becomes evident as a decrease in duration of analgesia provided by a given dose of a narcotic. Increases in dose and frequency of administration may be necessary.

Many cancer patients fear addiction, but these patients rarely become drug abusers. If their narcotics are abruptly discontinued, however, they develop narcotic withdrawal, with symptoms of anxiety, nervousness, and alternating chills and hot flashes. Signs of withdrawal include increased salivation, lacrimation, and diaphoresis, sometimes progressing to nausea, vomiting, abdominal cramps, and myoclonus. Withdrawal can be avoided by decreasing narcotic doses by 25% every 2 days until a total daily dose of 10 mg to 15 mg morphine is reached, when the drug can be discontinued.

Cross-references: Death of Clinic Patients (Section 6), Abdominal Pain (Section 95), Management of Depression (Section 192), Back Pain in the Cancer Patient (Section 208).

REFERENCES

1. American Pain Society. Principles of analgesic use in the treatment of acute pain and chronic cancer pain. Clin-Pharm 1990;9(8):601–612.
    A useful consensus statement.

2. Elliott K, Foley KM. Neurologic pain syndromes in patients with cancer. Crit Care Clin 1990;6(2):393–420.
    A comprehensive review reflecting the extensive clinical experience at Memorial Sloan-Kettering Cancer Center.

3. Inturrisi CE. Management of cancer pain. Pharmacology and principles of management. Cancer 1989;63(11 suppl):2308–2320.
    The basic principles underlying the management of pain medications.

207 DYSPNEA IN THE CANCER PATIENT

Symptom

ANTHONY L. BACK

EPIDEMIOLOGY.   Dyspnea is the subjective sensation of uncomfortable respiration—being "short of breath." In patients with known cancer, early recognition and treatment of pulmonary complications can avert respiratory failure, which carries a grim prognosis. For cancer patients with respiratory failure requiring mechanical ventilation, the overall mortality is at least 75%.

ETIOLOGY.   In adult primary care clinics, dyspnea most commonly results from congestive heart failure or chronic obstruction pulmonary disease (COPD) (see Section 19, Dyspnea). In patients with cancer, however, there are additional diagnostic considerations. Dyspnea can be caused directly by tumor. Bronchial obstruction is most often due to primary or metastatic lung cancer but can be produced by metastatic renal cell carcinoma. Lymphangiitic tumor commonly results from metastatic breast, lung, or head and neck carcinoma. Superior vena cava (SVC) syndrome is most often produced by lymphoma or lung cancer (small cell more often than nonsmall cell). Malignant pleural effusions and cardiac tamponade are frequent complications of lung and breast carcinoma.

Dyspnea can also represent a toxic effect of cancer therapy. Five percent to 15% of patients undergoing radiotherapy to the chest develop radiation pneumonitis, which is usually evident as an infiltrate in the shape of the radiotherapy port developing 6 weeks to 6 months after therapy has been completed. Less commonly, pulmonary toxicity is due to chemotherapy; bleomycin, methotrexate, and BCNU are most frequently implicated. Chemotherapy-induced pneumonitis can occur within hours of administration as a hypersensitivity-induced drug effect or can develop over weeks. Patients who have received large cumulative doses of anthracyclines (doxorubicin [adriamycin], daunomycin [daunorubicin]) most often for treatment of breast cancer or sarcomas, can develop congestive cardiomyopathy as a dose-dependent side effect. Clinically evident congestive heart failure is uncommon below a total doxorubicin dose of 400 mg/M^2.

Infectious pneumonitis most commonly presents as dyspnea. Patients receiving chemotherapy are at greatest risk, particularly if they become neutropenic (absolute neutrophil count < 1000/mm^3) and have indwelling catheters or subcutaneous ports used for chemotherapy administration.

CLINICAL APPROACH.   Review of recent treatment may suggest chemotherapy or radiation toxicity. Physical examination may disclose pulsus paradoxus (tamponade), unilateral wheezing (bronchial obstruction), dilated chest wall veins (superior vena cava syndrome), dullness to percussion (pleural effusion), S3 (congestive heart failure), elevated neck veins, or pathologic lymph nodes. Evaluation should be guided by clinical suspicion based on history, physical examination, and chest radiograph. A hematocrit, absolute neutrophil count, and platelet count are required for patients receiving chemotherapy or with advanced cancer. In diagnosing SVC syndrome, computed tomography (CT) of the chest with contrast is more useful than angiography. Echocardiography may support the diagnosis of tamponade in cases where physical signs are borderline. Pulmonary function tests may be helpful in suspected chemotherapy toxicity, which does not always present with abnormalities on chest radiograph. A radionuclide ejection fraction is useful in suspected anthracycline cardiotoxicity.

MANAGEMENT.   Patients with mild, slowly progressive dyspnea can often be managed as outpatients. Pulmonary toxicity secondary to radiation and chemotherapy is treated with corticosteroids, usually requiring a slow taper. Anthracycline cardiotoxicity is treated with diuretics, digoxin, and angiotensin-converting enzyme inhibitors (e.g., enalapril or lisinopril). Malignant pulmonary effusions may be drained initially in the outpatient department. Hospital admission is necessary for patients with recurrent malignant effusions requiring chest tube placement and pleurodesis. Clinically evident tamponade requires immediate hospitalization for surgical creation of a pericardial window or pericardiocentesis followed by catheter drainage. SVC syndrome often requires admission for rapid diagnostic biopsy and initiation of therapy. If caused by lymphoma or small cell lung cancer, SVC syndrome is treated with chemotherapy alone. Other etiologies of SVC syndrome are treated with radiotherapy, which is delivered emergently if upper airway obstruction is present. Bronchoscopy-guided laser therapy can relieve selected cases of bronchial obstruction. Patients with neutropenia (absolute neutrophil count $< 1000/mm^3$) and fever (temperature $> 38.3°C$) should be admitted for empiric broad-spectrum antibiotics.

Cross-references: Death of Clinic Patients (Section 6), Dyspnea (Section 19), Pleural Effusion (Section 65), Lower Respiratory Infection (Section 67), Thoracentesis (Section 70), Arterial Blood Gas (Section 71), Congestive Heart Failure (Section 79), Radionuclide Assessment of Cardiac Function (Section 87), Echocardiography (Section 90), Anemia (Section 201).

REFERENCES

1. Helms SR, Carlson MD. Cardiovascular emergencies. Semin Oncol 1989;16(6):463–470.
    Especially useful for the discussion of malignant pericardial effusions.

2. Hughes WT, Armstrong D, Bodey GP, et al. Guidelines for the use of antimicrobial agents in neutropenic patients with unexplained fever. J Infect Dis 1990;161(3):381–396; published erratum appears in J Infect Dis 1990;161(6):1316.
    A comprehensive but pragmatic review; contains helpful algorithms for nearly every step in managing fever and neutropenia. This ought to be in the files of every house officer and practitioner caring for cancer patients.

3. Tattersall MH, Boyer MJ. Management of malignant pleural effusions. Thorax. 1990; 45(2):81–82.
    Best recent review.

4. Yellin A, Rosen A, Reichert N, et al. Superior vena cava syndrome. The myth—the facts. Am Rev Respir Dis 1990;141(5 Pt 1):1114–1118.
    Discusses why SVC syndrome is rarely a bona-fide emergency.

208 BACK PAIN IN THE CANCER PATIENT

Symptom

STEPHAN D. FIHN

EPIDEMIOLOGY/ETIOLOGY. Symptomatic metastases to the spine occur in 5% to 10% of all patients with carcinoma, affecting 20,000 persons a year. In males, the most common causative primary tumor is lung cancer (25%), followed by prostate (20%), carcinoma of unknown primary (15%), sarcoma (10%), myeloma, and gastrointestinal (each about 5%). In females, breast cancer is most common (≥50%). Less common tumors include hematologic malignancies, melanoma, and cancers of the head and neck, thyroid, and kidney. Spinal metastases occur most often in the fifth and sixth decades, involving the thoracic spine in 50% of cases, the lumbosacral spine in 30%, and cervical region in 15%.

Patients frequently report their first symptoms to their primary care provider. Early recognition of spinal involvement is critical, even in the terminally ill, in order to avoid paralysis and institutionalization during the patient's final weeks or months of life.

SYMPTOMS AND SIGNS. Pain is the initial symptom in 85% to 95% of patients. The pain is most commonly local but may be radicular, referred, or diffuse due to compression of the spinal tracts. The pain is often nonmechanical (i.e., unrelieved with bed rest), but this feature does not reliably differentiate malignant from benign processes. Spinal tenderness is present in about one-third of patients.

Cervical lesions are often slowly growing and produce bony pain as the first symptom. Root compression causes paresthesias and hyporeflexia in the arms. Leg weakness is more insidious and often preceded by spasticity, hyperreflexia, and the appearance of extensor plantar reflexes. **Thoracic lesions** usually cause local pain, followed by radicular pain and dysesthesia in a bandlike, dermatomal pattern. Paraplegia and bowel and bladder dysfunction are late signs. **Lesions of the conus medullaris** occur with involvement at the T-12/L-1 level and produce early bladder and bowel incontinence, along with saddle anesthesia. Cremasteric and bulbocavernosus reflexes are abnormal, and anal wink is absent. This syndrome occurs in less than 1% of cases of spinal epidural compression. The **cauda equina syndrome** occurs in 15% of spinal metastatic lesions, producing weakness, hypotonia, and hyporeflexia. Signs and symptoms may be patchy and asymmetric due to uneven compression of nerve roots.

CLINICAL APPROACH.   The neurologic examination should concentrate on autonomic, motor, and sensory function. Spinal tracts vary in susceptibility to injury by ischemia. The corticospinal tracts, posterior columns, and spinocerebellar tracts are most vulnerable, while the spinothalamic tracts and autonomic fibers are more resilient. As a result, weakness, spasticity, and hyperactive reflexes tend to be early manifestations followed shortly by loss of vibratory and position sense. Loss of pain and temperature and of bowel and bladder function tend to be late signs. Changes in reflexes and proprioception are absent in patients with underlying neuropathy, such as those who have received high doses of vincristine. In addition to metastatic disease, the differential diagnosis back pain with neurologic impairment includes disc herniation or spinal stenosis due to benign causes, carcinomatous meningitis, radiation myelitis, or bilateral compression of the lumbar plexus by enlarged lymph nodes or tumor, simulating a cauda equina syndrome.

Further diagnostic evaluation and treatment should be based on findings from the neurologic examination and radiographs of the spine. Patients with evidence of myelopathy should receive corticosteroids immediately and urgent myelography. Patients with radiculopathy should undergo myelography as soon as possible. Patients with back pain and no neurologic abnormality should have an erythrocyte sedimentation rate and spine films performed. If spine films are positive, myelography should be performed. If the clinician is suspicious of bony metastases but spine films are negative, radionuclide bone imaging may be helpful, especially if the sedimentation rate is greater than 20 mm/hr. If the sedimentation rate is less than 20 mm/hr and spine films are negative, careful follow-up without further diagnostic tests is in order.

Magnetic resonance imaging (MRI) may rival myelography in detecting extradural lesions compressing the cord and may be superior in detecting noncompressing lesions. It is less accurate in identifying subarachnoid lesions. Bone scanning is less specific than plain radiographs but is a sensitive method for detecting bony lesions that cause extradural compression. Routine use of bone scanning in suspected spinal metastasis is not warranted.

MANAGEMENT.   In terms of neurologic outcome, radiation alone appears equivalent to decompressive laminectomy plus radiation, although rigorous comparisons are lacking. Laminectomy is associated with greater short-term mortality (3–7%) and morbidity. Surgery is to be avoided except when a biopsy is required for diagnosis, the patient has received previous irradiation to the involved location, there is an unstable lesion requiring fixation, or the patient's symptoms progress during radiation.

Treatment with dexamethasone should begin immediately in all cases of suspected spinal compression, although the optimal dose is uncertain. Animal and uncontrolled human studies suggest that higher doses (e.g., 100 mg stat followed by 24 mg four times a day for 72 hours and then a 2-week taper) provide better results compared with standard doses of 4 mg four times a day.

FOLLOW-UP.   Recovery of function depends on several factors. The worse the initial function is, the worse is the outcome. On average, 18% of patients have improvement in ambulation following treatment with surgery or radiation. Complete paraplegia is rarely improved. Bowel and bladder dysfunction are poor prognostic signs. Radiosensitive tumors (seminoma, myeloma) have the best response irrespective of the method of treatment. Patients with breast and prostate cancer frequently demonstrate neurologic recovery and significant survival. Lung cancer, gastrointestinal cancers, and sarcomas respond poorly. Mean survival for patients with spinal cord compression due to lung cancer is 1 month. Mean survival for other types of cancer ranges from 6 months to 2 years. Patients with a slow onset of symptoms appear to have a better outlook, although this may be a function of tumor type.

Cross-references: Death of Clinic Patients (Section 6), Low Back Pain (Section 108), Hip Pain (Section 110), Muscular Weakness (Section 139), Peripheral Neuropathy (Section 149), Urinary Incontinence (Section 174), Prostate Cancer (Section 175), Management of Pain in the Patient with Cancer (Section 206).

REFERENCES

1. Deyo RA, Diehl AK. Cancer as a cause of back pain: Frequency, clinical presentation, and diagnostic strategies. J Gen Int Med 1988;3:230–238.

   Of 1975 patients presenting to a walk-in clinic with back pain, 13 (0.7%) had underlying cancer. Factors significantly associated with cancer were age 50 years or over, previous history of cancer, pain for more than 1 month, failure to improve with conservative therapy, and elevated sedimentation rate.

2. Gilbert RW, Kim J-H, Posner JB. Epidural spinal cord compression from metastatic tumor: Diagnosis and treatment. Ann Neurol 1978;3:40–45.

   An uncontrolled, retrospective review of 235 patients with spinal cord compression. Back pain was the presenting feature in 95%. Weakness on examination was present in 87%. Sensory complaints were never a presenting symptom but developed in 78%. Ambulation after treatment was as common following radiation alone as after surgery plus radiation.

3. Hollis PH, Malis LI, Zappulla RA. Neurological deterioration after lumbar puncture below complete spinal subarachnoid block. J Neurosurg 1986;64:253–256.

   In patients with complete spinal subarachnoid block, the incidence of neurologic deterioration after lumbar puncture was 14%.

4. Portenoy RK, Lipton RB, Foley KM. Back pain in the cancer patient: An algorithm for evaluation and management. Neurology 1987;37:134–138.

   A sensible approach that outlines important neurologic features.

5. Rodichok LD, Harper GR, Ruckdeschel JC, et al. Early diagnosis of spinal epidural metastases. Am J Med 1981;70:1181–1188.

   A study of 87 patients with back pain and known or suspected cancer. Thirty-six percent of patients with normal neurologic examinations had epidural metastases on myelography; all had abnormal plain radiographs.

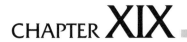
THE PREGNANT PATIENT

209 DIAGNOSIS OF PREGNANCY

Screening

DIANE L. ELLIOT

EPIDEMIOLOGY. The prevalence of unsuspected pregnancy is unknown, although one study reported that 2 of 110 women hospitalized for nonobstetric reasons were found to have unsuspected pregnancies.

RATIONALE. The patient interview (e.g., sexual activity, contraceptive practices, last menses) does not reliably exclude pregnancy. Because history and physical examination are neither sensitive nor specific for the early diagnosis of pregnancy, laboratory tests are needed.

The urine latex or hemagglutination tests detect only high levels of human chorionic gonadotropin (hCG) (500–3500 mIU/ml) and generally have been replaced by monoclonal antibody tests for the intact molecule or its beta subunit. Two weeks after conception, the hCG is approximately 80 mIU/ml and doubles each 2 days. The levels in serum and concentrated urine are comparable. Serum testing detects a lower hCG level and generally is slightly more expensive. Both the urine and monoclonal serum assays are more than 90% sensitive at the time of the first missed menses. Home urine tests use monoclonal antibodies and have 95% specificity but are less sensitive and are associated with a user error rate of up to 10%.

Transabdominal ultrasound can detect a gestational sac at 5 weeks to 6 weeks and a fetal heartbeat at 7 weeks to 8 weeks. Fetal heart tones are heard by Doppler at 10 weeks to 12 weeks and by fetoscope at 16 weeks to 20 weeks. Quickening occurs at 16 weeks to 20 weeks.

Although ectopic pregnancies result in lower hCG levels, more than 95% of women with proved ectopic pregnancy have a serum hCG in excess of 40 mIU/ml. Quantitative hCG levels may be needed to distinguish ectopic from intrauterine pregnancy prior to the sixth week because both groups may have pos-

652

itive qualitative pregnancy tests and negative ultrasonography. An intrauterine pregnancy should be associated with an hCG doubling at least every 2.2 days. In addition, an intrauterine pregnancy with a serum hCG exceeding 6500 mIU/ml usually is associated with a gestational sac by transabdominal ultrasound.

Not all hCG elevations indicate pregnancy. Over 20% of conceptions result in a subclinical abortion. Following a miscarriage, low and declining hCG levels may persist for 2 months. Detectable levels also can occur with choriocarcinoma and breast cancer.

STRATEGY. Laboratory tests are appropriate for women with amenorrhea, suspected pregnancy, pelvic pain, or scheduled radiographic studies. After the first missed menses, serum and urine monoclonal tests have comparable sensitivity; test choice depends on considerations of cost and convenience. Serum tests are preferred when evaluating a suspected ectopic pregnancy.

ACTION. A positive pregnancy test leads to review of the implications and limitations of the test. Ultrasound may be required when evaluating pelvic pain or a suspected ectopic pregnancy (see Section 163, Pelvic Pain in Women), as well as to date the pregnancy. In established intrauterine pregnancy, the clinician should discuss the woman's feelings about the pregnancy and emphasize the importance of early and continuous prenatal care. The clinician should assess the patient's diet, review her medications for contraindicated drugs, and emphasize discontinuation of smoking and alcohol. Laboratory tests (complete blood count, blood type, Rh antibody screen, rubella titer, urinalysis, VDRL, Pap smear, vaginal cultures) usually are deferred until the first prenatal visit with the health care provider who will care for the woman during pregnancy.

Cross-references: Abdominal Pain (Section 95), Pelvic Pain in Women (Section 163).

REFERENCES

1. Bluestern D. Should I trust office pregnancy tests? Postgrad Med 1990;87(6):57–68.
   Reviews test characteristics for urine, serum and home kits, and use with early and ectopic pregnancies.

2. Ramoska EA, Sacchetti AD, Nepp M. Reliability of patient history in determining the possibility of pregnancy. Ann Emerg Med 1986;18:48–50.
   Historical features could not be used to exclude pregnancy.

210 BACTERIURIA IN PREGNANCY

Screening

STEPHAN D. FIHN

EPIDEMIOLOGY. The prevalence of bacteriuria in pregnancy is 4% to 7%, which is similar to the rate among young, sexually active women in general. Bacteriuria is more common among women of low socioeconomic status and black women with sickle cell trait.

RATIONALE. Twenty percent to 40% of pregnant women with asymptomatic bacteriuria detected in the first trimester will develop acute pyelonephritis if left untreated, which results in a substantial risk of prematurity and possible perinatal morbidity. Placebo-controlled trials have shown that treatment of asymptomatic bacteriuria can substantially reduce the incidence of pyelonephritis.

STRATEGY. Screening all pregnant women for bacteriuria in early pregnancy will detect 40% to 70% of those who would otherwise develop symptomatic infections; the remainder develop bacteriuria later in pregnancy. For most patients, one screening culture should be obtained at the first prenatal visit. Cultures growing 10^5 bacteria/ml or more should be considered positive. Use of dip-slide cultures for screening in this setting is quite appropriate. All positive cultures should be confirmed with a quantitative, midstream culture. Women who test negative at the first screening but have a history of recurrent urinary tract infection (UTI) should be screened again at the beginning of the third trimester.

ACTION. The preferred oral drugs for treating asymptomatic bacteriuria or cystitis in pregnancy are amoxicillin, ampicillin and the oral cephalosporins. Infection due to Group B *Streptococcus* is readily treated with penicillin VK. Nitrofurantoin has been used, but its safety in pregnancy remains in question. Tetracycline, trimethoprim-sulfa, and the quinolones should be avoided.

Cross-references: Principles of Screening (Section 12), Urinary Tract Infections in Women (Section 177).

REFERENCES

1. Andriole VT, Patterson TF. Epidemiology, natural history, and management of urinary tract infections in pregnancy. Med Clin North Am 1991:75:359–373.
   A thoughtful review.

2. Stenqvist K, Dahlen-Nilsson I, Liden-Janson G, et al. Bacteruria in pregnancy. Am J Epidemiol 1989;129:372.

A recent study of over 3000 women that found a steady increase in the incidence of bacteriuria from 0.8% at the twelfth gestational week to 1.9% prior to delivery. The authors suggest that a single screening performed at 16 weeks might be the most efficient strategy.

211 ASTHMA IN PREGNANCY

Problem

DIANE L. ELLIOT

EPIDEMIOLOGY.   Asthma is the most common respiratory disease during pregnancy, with a prevalence of 0.4% to 1.3%.

SYMPTOMS AND SIGNS.   The course of asthma during pregnancy is variable and cannot be predicted from patient characteristics. In general, approximately half of women remain stable, 25% improve, and 25% worsen. Dyspnea is a nonspecific symptom during pregnancy and occurs in 60% of nonasthmatic women during the first and second trimesters. The signs and symptoms of an asthma exacerbation are not different during pregnancy.

CLINICAL APPROACH.   Because pregnancy results in only minor alternation in pulmonary function, changes in spirometry are reliable indicators of the patient's asthma. Chest radiography should be avoided; if it is absolutely indicated, special shielding is necessary.

MANAGEMENT.   Management is similar to that of nonpregnant individuals. Aminophylline crosses the placenta, but other than rare reports of newborn jitteriness, it is safe during pregnancy. Its clearance is reduced in the third trimester, and levels should be monitored. Inhaled and oral beta-2 agonists also can be used during pregnancy. They are tocolytic agents and rarely have been reported to inhibit labor. Because no data on inhaled ipratropium during pregnancy are available, this drug is best avoided.

Prednisone is metabolized by the placenta, which limits fetal exposure to the active drug. Corticosteroids, both inhaled and systemically administered, can be used during pregnancy. The risk of an asthma exacerbation compromising pregnancy far outweighs any potential corticosteroid risk.

Most exacerbations of asthma are associated with respiratory infections, which may require antibiotic treatment. Erythromycin (avoiding the estolate esters), penicillins, and first- and second-generation cephalosporins can be used during pregnancy; tetracycline and trimethoprim-sulfamethoxazole are contraindicated.

FOLLOW-UP.   Depending on severity, women are seen every 1 week to 4 weeks.

Cross-references: Upper Respiratory Infection (Section 66), Asthma and Chronic Obstructive Pulmonary Disease (Section 68), Pulmonary Function Testing (Section 69).

REFERENCES

1. D'Alonzo GE. The pregnant asthmatic patient. Sem Perinatol 1990;14:119–129.
    A review article that includes protocols for management and discusses treatment during labor and delivery and of nursing mothers.

2. Greenberger PA, Patterson R. Management of asthma during pregnancy. N Engl J Med 1985;312:897–902.
    A useful review article.

212 THYROID DISORDERS IN PREGNANCY

Problem

DIANE L. ELLIOT

EPIDEMIOLOGY.   Hyperthyroidism develops during 0.02% to 0.3% of pregnancies. Because hypothyroidism frequently is associated with anovulation, coexistent hypothyroidism and pregnancy are rare. Postpartum thyroid dysfunction has an incidence of approximately 5%. Risk factors include a family or personal history of postpartum thyroid dysfunction and the presence of antimicrosomal antibodies.

SYMPTOMS AND SIGNS.   Certain findings of hyperthyroidism (such as tachycardia, sensation of warmth, fatigue) are also features of a normal pregnancy. Hyperthyroidism during pregnancy may cause an inappropriately low weight gain rather than the traditional symptom of weight loss.

Although the presentation of postpartum thyroid dysfunction is variable, most individuals develop hyperthyroidism 4 weeks to 6 weeks postpartum, followed by hypothyroidism, with return of normal thyroid function by 6 months postpartum.

CLINICAL APPROACH.   Because treating hyperthyroidism improves the pregnancy's outcome, the clinician should have a low threshold for obtaining thyroid function tests. Thyroid binding globulin increases during pregnancy, leading to elevations of total thyroxine and a decreased T3 resin uptake. Free thyroxine and the calculated thyroid index accurately reflect thyroid function during pregnancy and are used for diagnosis. Thyroid-stimulating hormone (TSH) remains a useful screening test for hypothyroidism and for assessing the adequacy of thyroid hormone replacement.

Hyperthyroid pregnant women are presumed to have Graves' disease, and thyroid scanning is contraindicated during pregnancy. Molar pregnancies that produce large amounts of hCG, a hormone that weakly cross-reacts with TSH, rarely can cause hyperthyroidism.

MANAGEMENT.   The hyperthyroid pregnancy patient should be treated medically with propylthiouracil (PTU) 100 mg three times a day. Beta-blockers may be necessary transiently to control initial symptoms. Radioactive iodine is absolutely contraindicated during pregnancy. Surgery is reserved for the rare individual with complications from medical therapy. Hypothyroid pregnant women should begin full replacement doses of thyroxine.

FOLLOW-UP.   PTU treatment usually reduces the thyroid hormone level within 3 to 4 weeks, at which time the dose is tapered to 50 mg three times a day. Thyroid function is monitored each 3 to 4 weeks. Because PTU crosses the placenta, while thyroid hormones and TSH do not, the therapeutic goal is to minimize fetal exposure to PTU by using the lowest dose that maintains the woman's thyroid hormone in the high-normal range. Graves' disease may worsen postpartum, and because fetal exposure is no longer a consideration, many clinicians empirically increase the PTU dose following delivery.

For women on thyroid replacement, the physician should monitor TSH levels each trimester and adjust the replacement dose as appropriate.

Postpartum hyperthyroidism is transient and treated symptomatically with beta-blockers. Hypothyroidism also is usually transient and can be managed with several months of thyroid replacement, with a subsequent attempt to discontinue therapy slowly.

Cross-reference: Common Thyroid Disorders (Section 156).

REFERENCES

1. Burrow GN. Thyroid disease. In GN Burrow and TF Ferris, Eds. Medical Complications during Pregnancy. W.B. Saunders Co., Philadelphia, 1988, pp. 224–253.
    A thorough review from an extremely useful text.

2. Gerstein HC. How common is postpartum thyroiditis? Arch Intern Med 1990;150:1397–1400.
    Meta-analysis of postpartum thyroiditis, indicating that the incidence in unselected cohorts is 4.9%.

3. Mandel SJ, Larsen R, Seeley EW, et al. Increased need for thyroxine during pregnancy in women with primary hypothyroidism. N Engl J Med 1990;323:91–96.
    Nine of twelve women needed increased replacement dose, based on TSH elevation during pregnancy.

213 DIABETES MELLITUS IN PREGNANCY

Problem

DIANE L. ELLIOT

EPIDEMIOLOGY. Most women with type I diabetes do well during pregnancy, although perinatal mortality and congenital malformations are increased. Risk factors for maternal morbidity are established renal disease and atherosclerotic vascular disease.

MANAGEMENT. Organogenesis occurs early in the first trimester. Because tight blood glucose control during this interval appears to decrease congenital malformations, optimal control is appropriate when women are considering pregnancy and early in gestation. Management includes patient education, nutrition, and insulin therapy.

The recommended diet is 30 kcal/kg to 35 kcal/kg per day, and weight gain during pregnancy should be approximately 25 pounds. Calories are divided as three meals and two snacks a day: 20%, breakfast; 30%, lunch; 35%, dinner; 10%, evening snack; 5%, mid-morning snack.

Women must be able to monitor their blood glucose and obtain several values per day (fasting, following breakfast, late afternoon, and evenings). In addition, women should check morning ketones at least once a week, or more frequently if the blood glucose fluctuates unduly or remains over 150 mg/dl.

Insulin is administered in two or three injections per day, adjusted to maintain a fasting glucose of approximately 80 mg/dl and less than 130 mg/dl during the remainder of the day. Insulin requirements increase during pregnancy, but actual adjustments are variable. The physician should emphasize the need for early recognition of hypoglycemia, with management by oral glucose and, when needed, intramuscular (IM) glucogon.

Hospitalization for an intense interval of patient education and glucose control may be appropriate early in gestation. Additional indications for hospitalization include nausea and vomiting, poor glucose control that is unresponsive to insulin adjustments, and persistent ketonuria.

FOLLOW-UP. The obstetrician coordinates care with the internist and the pediatrician near delivery. Follow-up appointments are every 1 to 2 weeks and weekly after 30 weeks. Women with diabetes are at increased risk for urinary tract infections and preeclampsia. Renal function should be assessed each month. Because retinopathy can progress, patients should be examined by an ophthalmologist each trimester. Postpartum insulin requirements decrease and are reduced by one-half to two-thirds by 1 week after delivery.

Cross-references: Diabetic Retinopathy (Section 44), Diabetes Mellitus (Section 157), Bacteriuria in Pregnancy (Section 210), Pregnancy and Hypertension (Section 215).

REFERENCES

1. Hollingsworth DR. Pregnancy, Diabetes and Birth: A Management Guide. Williams and Wilkins, Baltimore, 1984.
   Detailed information on all aspects of care.
2. Kitzmiller JL, Gavin LA, Gin GD, et al. Preconception care of diabetes. Glycemic control prevents congenital anomalies. JAMA 1989;265:731–736.
   Animal studies and clinical reports support the importance of normalizing glycosylated hemoglobin prior to conception to reduce spontaneous abortions and congenital malformation.
3. Kitzmiller JK, Gunderson E, Gavin LA, et al. Managing diabetes and pregnancy. Curr Probl Obstet Gynecol Fertil 1988;11:105–167.
   Extensive review of the consequences of diabetes during pregnancy, with explicit management recommendations.

214 GESTATIONAL DIABETES MELLITUS

Problem

DIANE L. ELLIOT

EPIDEMIOLOGY.   Gestational diabetes develops in 1% to 6% of pregnant women. Risk factors include obesity, older age, family history of type II diabetes, and prior delivery of a large (>9 lb) infant.

SYMPTOMS AND SIGNS.   Gestational diabetes is asymptomatic when diagnosed.

CLINICAL APPROACH.   Because control of elevated blood glucose decreases newborn macrosomia, the Centers for Disease Control recommends screening all women at 24 weeks to 28 weeks with a glucose measurement obtained 1 hour after 50 g of oral glucose. A serum glucose higher than 140 mg/dl or whole blood glucose higher than 170 mg/dl is considered positive. This screen is 90% sensitive and 80% specific. A 100-g 3-hour glucose tolerance test confirms gestational diabetes.

MANAGEMENT.   Diet should include 30 kcal/kg to 35 kcal/kg per day (based on desirable body weight), with 50% carbohydrates, and 100 g protein per day. Women should avoid "concentrated" sweets and nonnutritive artificial sweeteners. Oral hypoglycemics are contraindicated during pregnancy.

Fifteen percent of women with gestational diabetes require insulin therapy, which is initiated when the fasting glucose exceeds 105 mg/dl or 2-hour postprandial glucose exceeds 120 mg/dl on two occasions within 2 weeks. The initial human insulin dose is 0.3 units/kg to 0.7 units/kg (based on prepregnancy weight). Management is the same as that for women with type I diabetes mellitus (see Section 213, Diabetes Mellitus in Pregnancy).

FOLLOW-UP.   The obstetrician coordinates care. Women are usually followed at 2-week intervals until 32 weeks, when visits are weekly. Fasting and 2-hour postprandial blood glucose levels are obtained at each visit.

Cross-references: Diabetes Mellitus (Section 157), Diabetes Mellitus in Pregnancy (Section 213).

REFERENCES

1. Hollingsworth DR. Pregnancy, Diabetes and Birth: A Management Guide. Williams and Wilkins, Baltimore, 1984.
    Detailed information on all aspects of care.

2. Kitzmiller JL, Gavin LA, Gin GD, et al. Preconception care of diabetes. Glycemic control prevents congenital anomalies. JAMA 1989;265:731–736.
    Animal studies and clinical reports support the importance of normalizing glycosylated hemoglobin prior to conception to reduce spontaneous abortions and congenital malformation.

3. Kitzmiller JK, Gunderson E, Gavin LA, et al. Managing diabetes and pregnancy. Curr Probl Obstet Gynecol Fertil 1988;11:105–107.
    Extensive review of the consequences of diabetes during pregnancy, with explicit management recommendations.

215 PREGNANCY AND HYPERTENSION

Problem

DIANE L. ELLIOT

EPIDEMIOLOGY. Hypertension during pregnancy is classified as preeclampsia, pregnancy-induced hypertension, or essential hypertension. The prevalence of hypertension during pregnancy is 10% to 20%; most cases are pregnancy-induced hypertension (hypertension without other features of preeclampsia). Because blood pressure normally decreases during the first trimester and increases during the third trimester, distinguishing essential from pregnancy-induced hypertension is difficult when blood pressure readings before pregnancy are not known. Risk factors for preeclampsia include the first pregnancy, underlying renal disease, previous hypertension, twin pregnancies, and a family history of preeclampsia.

SYMPTOMS AND SIGNS. Preeclampsia usually develops during the third trimester and produces rapid weight gain (>2 lb per week), proteinuria (>0.5 g/24hr), and hypertension (blood pressure > 140/90 mm Hg, systolic increase of 30 mm Hg or more, or diastolic increase of 15 mm Hg or more). Diastolic pressure increases more than systolic, with systolic levels often less than 160 mm Hg. Additional findings may include headache, epigastric pain, or diffuse edema. The spectrum of manifestations varies, and the presence of all features is not required for diagnosis.

CLINICAL APPROACH. Physicians should obtain a urinalysis from all women with rapid weight gain, edema, or elevated blood pressure. Although there are fewer than 200 reported cases, pheochromocytoma during pregnancy produces significant morbidity and mortality. Findings suggesting the diagnosis include newly diagnosed or fluctuating hypertension, headache, excessive perspiration, and palpitations. To screen for coarctation of the aorta, arm and leg blood pressures should be measured.

MANAGEMENT. Hypertension without proteinuria is usually treated with bed rest and medication. Exactly when to initiate blood pressure medications is controversial, but most authorities recommend medications when the diastolic blood pressure, monitored by the patient at home, persistently exceeds 90 mm Hg. The experience with antihypertension medication in pregnancy appears in Table 215–1.

In women who were hypertensive before pregnancy, the usual blood pressure decrease during the first and second trimesters may allow the gradual discon-

TABLE 215–1.   SAFETY OF ANTIHYPERTENSIVE DRUGS DURING PREGNANCY[1]

Drug	Comment
Safe	
Methyldopa	Extensive use; no adverse effects
Beta-blockers	Extensive use; rare anecdotal report of neonatal bradycardia and hypoglycemia
Hydralazine	Used in combination; extensive use; no adverse effects
Controversial[2]	
Calcium-channel blockers	No data as chronic treatment; tocolytic effects
Diuretics	Use is controversial; may be continued if used prior to pregnancy but should not be initiated for hypertension during pregnancy
Contraindicated	
Angiotensin-converting enzyme inhibitors	Reports of neonatal renal failure

[1]Drugs with limited use during pregnancy (clonidine, prazosin) should be switched to a drug with established safety.
[2]Should consult an expert before use.

tinuation of diuretics and other antihypertensive medications. Treatment then resumes during the third trimester, if indicated, with methyldopa or a beta-blocker.

Preeclampsia is a multisystem disorder usually managed by the obstetrician. Because the woman's condition may deteriorate rapidly, patients require immediate hospitalization, medical management, and delivery of the infant.

FOLLOW-UP.   The obstetrician usually closely follows women with hypertension, with consultation from the internist. Visits are scheduled every 2 weeks to 3 weeks until approximately week 32, when they occur weekly. During each encounter, the physician assesses symptoms, blood pressure, weight, edema, and proteinuria.

Cross-references: Essential Hypertension (Section 86), Proteinuria (Section 183).

REFERENCES

1. Ferris TF. Pregnancy complicated by hypertension and renal disease. Adv Intern Med 1990;35:269–288.
    Discusses drug therapy of hypertension during pregnancy, including those with underlying renal disease.

2. Liedheimer MD, Katz AI. Hypertension in pregnancy. N Engl J Med 1985;313:675–680.
    A brief review.

3. Sibai BM. Preeclampsia-eclampsia. Curr Prob Obstetr Gynecol Fertil 1990;13:1–45.
    Thorough discussion of pathophysiology, multisystem problems, and management.

XX CHAPTER

THE PREOPERATIVE PATIENT

216 GENERAL PRINCIPLES OF CONSULTATION

C. SCOTT SMITH

OBJECTIVES. When the generalist is asked to examine a patient preoperatively, there are three main goals of the evaluation: (1) to predict surgical risk and suggest modifications to improve that risk; (2) to identify current medical problems and assist in their perioperative management (e.g., hypertension, diabetes, anticoagulation); and (3) to suggest appropriate measures designed to prevent postoperative medical sequelae (e.g., deep venous thrombosis/pulmonary embolus, endocarditis).

PRINCIPLES. Effective consultation requires that the question being asked and the consultant's role in management be clearly identified and understood. The consultant must establish the urgency of the consult and communicate directly with the referring practitioner if possible.

When performing the consultation, it is important that the consultant gather firsthand data, including history, physical examination, and an independent review of the medical record, laboratory data, electrocardiograms, and radiographs.

One accepted format for the consultation note appears in Table 216–1. The

TABLE 216–1. THE CONSULTATION NOTE

1. Identify the patient and question(s) asked (or reason for consultation).
2. Record assessment and problem list.
3. Make recommendations as concise and explicit as possible. Attempt to list five or fewer in decreasing order of importance. Drug formulations, route of administration, and dosage should be specified. Contingency plans should also be included.
4. Record pertinent history and physical and laboratory data.
5. Discussion of clinical features, differential diagnosis, management options, and recent reports in the literature (optional).
6. References (optional).

importance of discussing the assessment and recommendations directly with the consulting practitioner cannot be overemphasized.

Frequent follow-up will keep the consultant abreast of changes and ensure optimal care for the patient.

REFERENCES

1. Carson JL, Elliot DL. Care of the pregnant patient with medical illness. J Gen Intern Med 1988;3:577–588.
    Reviews normal physiologic changes and special considerations when consulting on pregnant patients.

2. Goldman L, Lee T, Rudd P. Ten commandments for effective consultation. Arch Int Med 1983;143:1753–1755.
    Outlines not only the ethics and format of consultation but the possible political and educational goals of a consult service.

3. Keating HJ, Lubin MF. Perioperative responsibility of the physician/geriatrician. Clin Geriatric Med 1990;6(3):459–467.
    Reviews the features unique to consulting on older patients.

4. Marshall JB. How to make consultations work. Postgrad Med 1988;84(2):253–257.
    Pragmatic approach for getting the information clearly understood.

217 PREOPERATIVE CARDIOVASCULAR PROBLEMS

Problem

C. SCOTT SMITH

The medical management of patients undergoing general anesthesia and non-cardiac surgery depends on the length and physiologic stress of the procedure. The following recommendations are generalizations.

HYPERTENSION

EPIDEMIOLOGY.   Approximately 30% of surgical patients have hypertension, either long-standing or newly discovered. Only diastolic blood pressures greater than 110 mm Hg independently increase perioperative risk, unless the

TABLE 217–1.   DRUGS USED FOR RAPID CONTROL OF POSTOPERATIVE HYPERTENSION

Drug	Dose	Cost ($)[1]
Nitroglycerine ointment	1–2 in. q.4–6h.	0.01 (1 in.)
Nifedipine	10 mg PO q.3–4h.	0.38 (10 mg)
Labetalol	10–20 mg IV q.10min (maximum = 300 mg/24 h)	2.65 (10 mg)
Hydralazine	10–20 mg IM or IV; repeat PRN	2.55 (10 mg)
Nitroprusside	0.5–10 μg/kg/min IV drip	1.34 (10 mg)
Treatment of beta-blocker withdrawal		
Propranolol	1 mg/min until desired effect, appearance of toxicity, or maximum dose of 0.15 mg/kg is reached 1–2 mg IV q.1h. as needed	4.17 (1 mg)

[1]Average wholesale price, 1991 Drug Topics Red Book.

patient has an undiagnosed pheochromocytoma, in which case any hypertension is significant and associated with a mortality as high as 50%. Since perioperative ischemia is twice as likely to be caused by tachycardia than either hypo- or hypertension, it is usually more prudent to keep patients on their current antihypertensive drugs than to stop them abruptly, producing rebound tachycardia. Nonetheless, patients with long-standing hypertension often have generalized atherosclerosis and end-organ damage, making them more susceptible to the complication of intraoperative hypotension. Careful management is essential.

CLINICAL APPROACH.   Elective surgery should be postponed if the patient's recent diastolic blood pressure measurements exceed 110 mm Hg. When postoperative hypertension occurs, the physician should consider the following common causes: pain (35% of cases), hypercapnia (15%), postanesthetic effects (16%), volume overload, and bladder distension.

MANAGEMENT.   Patients with adequate preoperative blood pressure control should continue their regular medications until the morning of surgery. Table 217–1 lists potential drugs to use in the postoperative period until oral medications can be resumed. In those who take beta-blockers, intravenous propranolol is often necessary to prevent a withdrawal syndrome. A transdermal clonidine patch, placed 2 days to 3 days before surgery, is an effective substitute for those on oral clonidine.

ARRHYTHMIAS AND CONDUCTION ABNORMALITIES

EPIDEMIOLOGY.   Although almost 85% of patients develop perioperative arrhythmias, only 5% are hemodynamically significant. Risk factors for arrhythmias include hypokalemia, hypoxia, pain, hypo- or hypervolemia, anemia, myocardial infarction, pulmonary embolus, and pericarditis.

During insertion of a pulmonary artery catheter, right bundle branch block occurs in 5% of patients; in those with preexisting left bundle branch block, complete heart block may occur but is usually transient.

CLINICAL APPROACH.   The physician should avoid or correct any risk factors that may be present. Asymptomatic ventricular ectopy is a marker for organic heart disease but does not independently increase the risk of perioperative arrhythmia and, by itself, does not require prophylactic antiarrhythmic therapy.

MANAGEMENT.   Although controversial, preoperative digitalization is best reserved for high-risk patients such as those with moderate aortic or mitral stenosis (who do not tolerate rapid heart rate) or those with previous symptomatic supraventricular tachyarrhythmias.

Prophylactic lidocaine (1–2 mg/min by intravenous injection) is indicated in patients with myocardial ischemia during the previous 72 hours. A cardiologist should be asked to assist with the management of patients who have a history of sudden death or symptomatic ventricular arrhythmias.

The sensing and pacing function of permanent pacemakers should be checked preoperatively. Because cautery may inhibit demand pacemakers, cautery bursts should be few and short, with the ground placed as far as possible from the pacing unit. Alternatively, the pacemaker may be reprogrammed to fixed rate. A temporary pacemaker should be available to the operating room.

Indications for temporary pacemaker include new perioperative bifasicular block and symptomatic carotid hypersensitivity. It should also be considered in those with left bundle branch block prior to placement of a pulmonary artery catheter.

Automatic implantable cardiac defibrillators should be turned off prior to surgery.

VALVULAR DISEASE

MANAGEMENT.   Patients with valvular heart disease require antibiotic prophylaxis for endocarditis prior to surgery. (See Section 218, Preoperative Infectious Disease Problems.)

Aortic Stenosis.   Known aortic stenosis (AS) carries a likelihood ratio for operative mortality of approximately 4 (i.e., for any given risk, the presence of AS increases the risk of death fourfold).

Patients with critical AS (valve area < 0.4 cm^2/M^2 BSA) require valve replacement prior to elective surgery. Because patients with moderate AS have difficulty increasing cardiac output in response to stress, the clinician should treat perioperative volume depletion, fever, or rapid atrial fibrillation aggressively. Prophylactic digitalization, an arterial line, and a pulmonary artery catheter may be warranted in some patients.

Mitral Stenosis.   Patients with significant mitral stenosis (valve area < 1 cm^2/ M^2 BSA) should undergo valve replacement before elective surgery. Because of the stenotic valve and chronically elevated left atrial pressures, these patients are exquisitely sensitive to both volume overload and depletion. If not already prescribed, digoxin should be started. Perioperative monitoring with an arterial line and pulmonary artery catheter is usually warranted.

Aortic/Mitral Insufficiency.   The operative risk among patients with aortic insufficiency or mitral insufficiency depends mainly on their left ventricular function. These patients rarely require hemodynamic monitoring or further testing.

Bradycardia may be poorly tolerated in patients with aortic insufficiency (prolonged diastole leads to increased regurgitant fraction). In both disorders, hypovolemia should be avoided, and forward cardiac output may be augmented, if necessary, by increasing heart rate or decreasing afterload resistance (with vasodilators).

ISCHEMIC HEART DISEASE

EPIDEMIOLOGY.   Ischemic heart disease increases the risk of perioperative cardiovascular complications (Table 217–2). By age 80 years, 50% of asymptomatic patients have occult coronary disease and are at increased risk of postoperative cardiovascular mortality.

CLINICAL APPROACH.   When ischemic heart disease is suspected preoperatively, the patient should undergo exercise treadmill testing or, if unable to exercise sufficiently, a dipyridamole-thallium scan. The latter test is most useful in those who are over age 70 years, have Q waves on a resting electrocardiogram (ECG), are diabetic, have angina, or who have a history of ventricular ectopy. If over age 65, inability to exercise at least 2 minutes to achieve a pulse of at least 99 on an exercise treadmill is associated with a higher risk of perioperative cardiac complications.

MANAGEMENT.   Patients with known ischemic disease should continue their usual medications until surgery. Topical or intravenous nitrates and intravenous

TABLE 217–2.   RISK OF PERIOPERATIVE INFARCT OR SUDDEN CARDIAC DEATH

Prior myocardial infarction	
0–3 months:	25–40%
3–6 months:	10–15%
> 6 months:	4–6% (equal to baseline)
Congestive heart failure	
NYHA class I:	5%
NYHA class II:	10%
NYHA class III:	25%
NYHA class IV:	67%

beta-blockers are used until the patient is again able to take oral medications. Patients with severe disease should be evaluated for coronary artery bypass graft (CABG) or angioplasty. The indications for these procedures are no different than for patients not scheduled for surgery. The overall risk for those undergoing CABG prior to elective surgery (2.3%) is little different than for those simply going directly to surgery (2.4%), if carefully managed. (The 2.3% mortality includes that following CABG surgery [1.4%] plus the average mortality of elective surgery after CABG [0.9%].) Heart failure should be controlled prior to surgery.

Elective surgery should be postponed in patients with unstable angina, NYHA class III or IV heart failure, or myocardial infarction within the preceding 6 months. If delay is impossible, perioperative care includes an arterial line, pulmonary artery catheter, antianginal therapy, and consideration of an intra-aortic balloon pump.

PREDICTING CARDIAC RISK

Spinal anesthesia poses the same cardiac risk as general anesthesia. The risk of regional or local blocks is substantially lower. Although several standardized systems for calculating perioperative cardiac risk exist (see References), most predict higher-than-average risk for patients with "poor general medical status," age 70 years or more, arrhythmias, or remote congestive heart failure or myocardial infarction (i.e., greater than 6 months previously); intermediate risk (i.e., relatively contraindicating surgery), for patients with myocardial infarction within the past 3 months to 6 months, poorly controlled angina, or recent

TABLE 217–3.   LIKELIHOOD RATIOS FOR PERIOPERATIVE CARDIAC COMPLICATIONS IN VARIOUS CLINICAL SITUATIONS[1]

	Ratio
Remote MI, no history of CHF, age > 70,[2] normal sinus rhythm, good health	1
Remote MI, remote CHF, age <70 atrial fibrillation, good health	2
Aortic stenosis alone	4
Unstable angina alone	4
Remote MI, class III angina, remote CHF, and 8 premature ventricular beats on ECG	6
Age >70, MI in last 6 months, pulmonary edema in last week, atrial fibrillation	7.5

[1]Cardiac complications include perioperative myocardial infarction, sudden death, or congestive heart failure.

[2]i.e., Age > 70 per se, in an otherwise healthy patient, does not significantly increase the likelihood ratio.

congestive heart failure (CHF); and marked risk (i.e., elective surgery contraindicated) for unstable angina, myocardial infarction within 3 months, NYHA class IV congestive heart failure, or severe mitral or aortic stenosis.

Table 217–3 outlines likelihood ratios for perioperative cardiac complications of various clinical scenarios.

Cross-references: Angina (Section 78), Congestive Heart Failure (Section 79), Aortic Stenosis (Section 80), Other Valvular Disease (Section 82), Chronic Ventricular Arrhythmias (Section 84), Supraventricular Arrhythmias (Section 85), Essential Hypertension (Section 86), Radionuclide Assessment of Cardiac Function (Section 87), Exercise Tolerance Testing (Section 89), Echocardiography (Section 90), Peripheral Arterial Disease (Section 133).

REFERENCES

1. Detsky AS, Abrams HB, McLaughlin JR, et al. Predicting cardiac complications in patients undergoing non-cardiac surgery. J Gen Intern Med 1986;1:211–219.

   Modification of Goldman criteria that better estimates risk in the elderly and in vascular surgery. Uses likelihood ratios to generate a relative risk (based on pretest likelihood of cardiac problems).

2. Eagle KA, Coley CM, Newell JB, et al. Combining clinical and thallium data optimizes preoperative assessment of cardiac risk before major vascular surgery. Ann Intern Med 1989 Jun 1;110(11):859–866.

   Retrospective review of 200 vascular surgery patients that identifies clinical and thallium predictors of postoperative cardiac ischemic events.

3. Goldman L, Caldera DK, Southwick FS, et al. Multifactorial index of cardiac risk in non-cardiac surgical procedures. N Engl J Med 1977;297:845–850.

   The original gold standard of preoperative evaluation. Uses absolute risk. Tends to underestimate risk in the aged and in vascular surgery.

4. Goldman L, Lee TH. Noninvasive tests for diagnosing presence and extent of coronary artery disease. J Gen Int Med 1986;1:258–265.

   Excellent review of the efficacy of exercise testing with or without thallium as a predictor for cardiac complications.

5. Morise AP, McDowell DE, Savrin RA, et al. The prediction of cardiac risk in patients undergoing vascular surgery. Am J Med Sci 1987;293(3):150–158.

   Reviews risks in vascular surgery patients.

218 PREOPERATIVE INFECTIOUS DISEASE PROBLEMS

Problem

C. SCOTT SMITH

POSTOPERATIVE INFECTION PROPHYLAXIS

EPIDEMIOLOGY. The incidence of postoperative wound infection depends on the degree of contamination at the time of surgery (Table 218–1).

CLINICAL APPROACH. The principles of antibiotic prophylaxis before surgery are:

1. Target the most likely organisms (not all possible organisms).
2. Time the antibiotics to achieve maximal tissue levels at the time of surgery.
3. Discontinue antibiotics in a timely fashion. Antibiotics routinely administered longer than 24 hours promote antibiotic resistance with no further reduction in the incidence of infection.

Antibiotic prophylaxis is unnecessary in "clean" surgical procedures (e.g., soft tissue, orthopedic, cardiovascular procedures) unless the consequences of infection would be devastating (i.e., cardiac valve placement, orthopedic prosthetic devices, or vascular operations that involve placing a graft or making a groin incision).

In "clean contaminated" or "contaminated" surgery (entry into the respiratory or gastrointestinal tract, fresh trauma, or inflamed tissue), antibiotics decrease the incidence of postoperative wound infection by 5% to 15%.

"Dirty" surgery (abscess, purulent drainage, perforated abdominal viscus) requires broad-spectrum antibiotic coverage for longer periods of time (more appropriately considered treatment rather than prophylaxis).

MANAGEMENT. The first dose of prophylactic antibiotics should be given 1 to 2 hours prior to surgery (typically on call to the operating room). This en-

TABLE 218–1. INCIDENCE OF POSTOPERATIVE WOUND INFECTION

Type of Surgery	Percentage
Clean	< 5
Clean contaminated	10
Contaminated	20
Dirty	30–40

TABLE 218–2. GUIDELINES FOR PROPHYLACTIC ANTIBIOTIC USE

Wound	Drug	On Call Dose	Cost ($)[1]
Clean[2]	Cefazolin or	1g IV	3.52
	vancomycin[3]	1g IV	39.80
Contaminated (including clean contaminated)			
Colon or appendectomy[4]	Cefoxitin	1g IV	8.52
Other	Cefazolin	1g IV	3.52

[1]Average wholesale price, 1991 Drug Topics Red Book.
[2]Prophylactic antibiotics not required for all "clean" procedures. (see text.)
[3]Use in hospitals where infection with methicillin-resistant *S. aureus* or *S. epidermidis* is common.
[4]Many authorities recommend the addition of oral nonabsorbable antibiotics such as neomycin with or without erythromycin base. If surgery is elective, mechanical bowel preparation with nonabsorbable antibiotics is as efficacious as parenteral antibiotics.

sures maximal therapeutic tissue levels in the wound but does not allow time for the emergence of antibiotic-resistant bacteria. In general, a single preoperative dose of antibiotic is adequate unless surgery is prolonged, in which case a second dose may be advisable. Table 218–2 outlines some guidelines for prophylactic antibiotic use.

FOLLOW-UP. The patient's vital signs and wounds are monitored several times during the first 1 day to 2 days after the operation. Slight serosanguinous drainage and redness surrounding the incision and sutures are common and not necessarily signs of infection. Purulent or foul-smelling drainage requires culture, careful observation, and consideration of therapeutic antibiotics and surgical drainage.

PROPHYLAXIS OF BACTERIAL ENDOCARDITIS

EPIDEMIOLOGY/ETIOLOGY. Approximately 50% of the cases of native valve endocarditis are due to oral streptococci or enterococci. Of these cases, only 25% to 30% follow a procedure for which prophylaxis could have been given. There have been no controlled trials comparing prophylaxis with placebo in reducing the incidence of bacterial endocarditis. Nonetheless, it is empirically believed that patients with several types of cardiac lesions (Table 218–3) should receive prophylactic antibiotic therapy directed at these organisms.

The most common underlying cardiac lesions seen today in native valve endocarditis are: (1) mitral valve prolapse accompanied by regurgitation and thickened myxomatous valves (patients with simple clicks are not at heightened risk), (2) degenerative left-sided valvular lesions (usually associated with aging and a limited prognosis), and (3) congenital heart disease (bicuspid aortic valves, ventricular septal defects, pulmonary stenosis, etc.).

Of the bacteria that cause prosthetic valve endocarditis, 30% are oral streptococci and enterococci (more common in late infection), 30% are *Staphylo-*

TABLE 218–3.   BACTERIAL ENDOCARDITIS PROPHYLAXIS[1]

Cardiac conditions in which prophylaxis is indicated
Prosthetic valves (including bioprosthetic valves)
Mitral valve prolapse with regurgitation
Degenerative or rheumatic valvular lesions
Most left-sided congenital defects
Idiopathic hypertrophic subaortic stenosis
Prior endocarditis

Procedures in which prophylaxis is indicated
Any dental procedures or surgery/instrumentation of the respiratory tract likely to result in
   bleeding.
Any surgery/instrumentation of the genitourinary or gastrointestinal tract (except as noted
   under clinical approach)

[1]Specific guidelines appear in Dajani AS, Bisno AL, Chung KJ, et al. Prevention of bacterial
endocarditis. Recommendations by the American Heart Association. JAMA 1990;264(22):2919–2922.

coccus aureus and *S. epidermidis* (more common in early infection), and 30%
are miscellaneous organisms. The risk of endocarditis is 5% to 10% over the
life of the valve and is the same for mechanical and bioprosthetic valves.

CLINICAL APPROACH.   Table 218–3 outlines the lesions and procedures for
which endocarditis prophylaxis is recommended. In general, any cardiac lesion
resulting in a pressure gradient and turbulent flow poses a risk for endocarditis.
Thus, left-sided lesions (ventricular septal defect, aortic stenosis, mitral or aortic insufficiency, etc.) have the highest risk, and right-sided or low-flow lesions
(coronary artery bypass grafts or isolated secundum atrial septal defects with-

TABLE 218–4.   RECOMMENDED ENDOCARDITIS PROPHYLAXIS

Group	Drug	Cost ($)[1]
Respiratory Tract Procedures		
Low risk	Amoxicillin 3 g PO 1 hr before, 1.5 g PO 6 hr later	1.35
Penicillin-allergic	Erythromycin 1 g PO 1 hr before, 500 mg PO 6 hr later	1.20
High risk[2]	Ampicillin 2 g IM/IV ½ hr before, amoxicillin 1.5 g PO 6 hr later	5.95
Penicillin-allergic	Vancomycin 1 g IV over 1 hr starting 1 hr before; no second dose	39.80
Gastrointestinal or Genitourinary Procedures		
Low risk	Amoxicillin 3 g PO 1 hr before, 1.5 g PO 6 hr later[3]	1.35
High risk[2]	Ampicillin 2 g IM/IV 30 min before and gentamicin 1.5 mg/kg 30 min before (may repeat at 8 hr)	6.72
Any risk where *Penicillin-allergic*	Vancomycin 1 g over 1 hr starting 1 hr before and gentamicin 1.5 mg/kg 30 min before (may repeat at 8 hr)	41.02

[1]Average wholesale price, 1991 Drug Topics Red Book.
[2]Prosthetic valve, previous episode of endocarditis.
[3]Many authorities prefer parenteral drugs in this setting.

out patches) have low risk. Procedures that generally do not require prophylaxis include barium enema, upper gastrointestinal endoscopy or proctosigmoidoscopy without biopsy, liver biopsy, intrauterine device insertion and removal, and vaginal delivery. In high-risk patients (e.g., cardiac prosthesis, prior endocarditis), however, many physicians choose to administer antibiotics before even these low-risk procedures.

MANAGEMENT.   Specific recommendations are listed in Table 218–4.

FOLLOW-UP.   During the immediate postoperative period, intravenous devices and urinary catheters should be discontinued as soon as possible (especially with new prosthetic valves, because most early prosthetic valve endocarditis results from bacteremia from these sources).

Cross-references: Aortic Stenosis (Section 80), Mitral Valve Prolapse (Section 81), Other Valvular Disease (Section 82), Echocardiography (Section 90).

REFERENCES

1. Antibiotic prophylaxis for surgery. *Med Lett* 1992;34(862):5–8.
    Excellent concise review.

2. Dajani AS, Bisno AL, Chung KJ, et al. Prevention of bacterial endocarditis. Recommendations by the American Heart Association. JAMA 1990;264(22):2919–2922.
    Most recent recommendations on prophylaxis.

3. Guglielmo BJ, Hohn DC, Koo PJ, et al. Antibiotic prophylaxis in surgical procedures. A critical analysis of the literature. Arch Surg 1983;118:943–955.
    Comprehensive review of the studies to that date of surgical prophylaxis.

4. Kaiser AB. Antimicrobial prophylaxis in surgery. New Engl J Med 1986;315:1129–1138.
    Excellent overview.

5. Kaye D. Prophylaxis for infective endocarditis: An update. Ann Intern Med 1986;104:419–423.
    Good review of each of the categories of endocarditis.

219 PREOPERATIVE ENDOCRINE PROBLEMS

Problem

C. SCOTT SMITH

DIABETES MELLITUS

EPIDEMIOLOGY. Diabetes is present in 5% to 10% of all adults, with a higher prevalence among the elderly. Cardiovascular mortality is two to four times more common in diabetics. Clinically significant renal dysfunction, present in nearly half of patients with more than 10 years of diabetes, may complicate postoperative care. Autonomic neuropathy, also common, may be associated with respiratory depression or wide fluctuations of blood pressure intraoperatively. Moreover, diabetics have delayed wound healing and are more susceptible to wound infections, particularly when the blood glucose continuously exceeds 250 mg/dl in the weeks preceding surgery.

SYMPTOMS AND SIGNS. See Section 157 (Diabetes Mellitus).

CLINICAL APPROACH. Because myocardial infarctions may be asymptomatic in diabetics, an ECG should be obtained before and after major surgery. The clinician should carefully monitor the patient's electrolytes and renal function. Radiologic procedures involving intravenous contrast materials should be avoided if possible, but if the procedure is absolutely necessary, it should be performed only after adequate hydration.

Uncontrolled hyperglycemia (blood glucose > 350 mg/dl) or ketoacidosis should be reversed for at least 48 hours before any elective surgery.

MANAGEMENT. The stress of surgery causes an unpredictable release of counterregulatory hormones, including catecholamines, glucagon, cortisol, and growth hormone. In the perioperative period, most diabetics are relatively unstable and even those who do not normally use insulin may require it. During this time, the goal is to maintain the serum glucose between 150 mg/dl and 250 mg/dl, avoiding hypoglycemia while minimizing poor wound healing and any possible immunologic dysfunction. Specific recommendations appear in Table 219–1.

FOLLOW-UP. For 24 hours to 48 hours postoperatively, the patient should be followed closely, with finger-stick blood glucose determinations at least every 4 hours. Scrupulous care to avoid wound and urinary tract infections is required, and Foley catheters should be discontinued as soon as possible.

TABLE 219–1.   PERIOPERATIVE MANAGEMENT OF DIABETES

Patients controlled with oral agents
1. Stop agents prior to surgery.
   a. Short-acting (tolbutamide, tolazemide, acetohexamide, glyburide, glypizide) 1–2 days prior
   b. Long-acting (chlorpropamide) 3 days prior
2. Cover with q.i.d. finger-stick glucose determinations and sliding scale regular insulin while NPO.
3. Resume usual medication when tolerating oral intake.

Patients controlled with insulin
1. Previously well controlled, not seriously ill, minor procedure: "no insulin, no glucose."
2. Previously well controlled, major procedure:
   a. 5% dextrose in water (D5%) 1–2 ml/kg/hr and insulin drip 1–2 units/hr[1] *or*
   b. D5% 1–2 ml/kg/hr and ½ usual AM dose of insulin; sliding scale regular insulin while NPO.
   c. Finger-stick or serum glucose determinations q.1–2h for the first day.
3. Very ill or brittle
   a. D5% 1–2 ml/kg/hr and insulin drip 1–2 units/hr
   b. Finger-stick glucose determinations q.1–2h the first day.

[1]Some studies demonstrate reduced mortality and morbidity with this regimen.

THYROID DISEASE

EPIDEMIOLOGY.   Operating on thyrotoxic patients carries a 10% to 30% risk of thyroid storm, with an operative mortality of up to 60%.

Hypothyroid patients exhibit minimally increased perioperative mortality but have increased sensitivity to digitalis, anesthetics, and analgesics. In addition, hypothyroid patients are known to have decreased hypoxic ventilatory drive and impaired free water excretion, which may lead to carbon dioxide retention or hyponatremia.

CLINICAL APPROACH.   Elective surgery on hyperthyroid patients should be postponed until they are euthyroid (usually at least 1 month of treatment). Any patient with suspected hyperthyroidism should receive screening thyroid function tests (T_4 and a measure of free thyroxine index) prior to surgery. A thyroid-stimulating hormone level should be obtained in patients suspected of hypothyroidism.

Patients with autoimmune thyroid disorders (Graves' disease or Hashimoto's) should be screened for coexisting conditions, such as diabetes mellitus, Addison's disease, pernicious anemia, and myasthenia gravis.

MANAGEMENT.   The appropriate management of hyperthyroid patients during urgent or emergent surgery appears in Table 219–2. In patients with hyperthyroidism and atrial fibrillation, propranolol should be administered to control the heart rate if there are no contraindications (i.e., congestive heart failure, asthma).

When hypothyroidism is diagnosed, elective surgery is best postponed until a stable replacement dose is achieved (usually 2 months to 3 months). Replacement hormone is generally not started immediately before urgent surgery un-

TABLE 219–2.   MANAGEMENT OF HYPERTHYROIDISM IN EMERGENCY SURGERY

1. Propothiouracil (PTU) 200–400 mg PO/NG q.6 h.
2. Iodide
   a. Start 1–2 hr after propothiouracil
   b. Saturated solution of potassium iodide 5 drops PO/NG q.8h.
      or
      sodium iodide 1 g IV over 12 h q.12–24h.
3. Propranolol 20–120 mg PO/NG q.4–8h.
   or
   1–3 mg IV q.15min. as needed until desired effect, appearance of toxicity, or total dose of 0.15 mg/kg is reached; may repeat in 6–8hr.
4. Dexamethasone 2 mg PO/IV q.6h.

less the patient has myxedema coma, where delay in therapy leads to a poorer prognosis. In these patients, an initial dose of 300 μg to 500 μg of L-thyroxine should be administered slowly intravenously (IV), followed by 50 μg to 100 μg IV per day. Moreover, hypothyroid patients often lack adrenal reserve and, if surgery cannot be delayed, require treatment with hydrocortisone 100 mg IV every 8 hours starting the night before surgery and tapering rapidly the day following surgery (usually stopping within 72 hours).

FOLLOW-UP.   In the perioperative period, hyperthyroid patients should be monitored closely for fever, tachyarrhythmias, mental status changes, or dehydration, all signs that herald thyroid storm.

Hypothyroid patients should receive small doses of analgesics and be monitored closely for hyponatremia and, if they are not intubated, hypercapnia.

ADRENAL INSUFFICIENCY

ETIOLOGY.   The most common cause of adrenal insufficiency is suppression of the hypothalamic-pituitary-adrenal axis with exogenous glucocorticoids, followed by Addison's disease, pituitary dysfunction, and bilateral adrenalectomy.

SYMPTOMS AND SIGNS.   Signs of previous or current exogenous glucocorticoids are thinning of the skin, purple striae, truncal obesity, "moon" facies, plethoric cheeks, prominent fat pad of the posterior neck, and proximal muscle weakness. Symptoms of adrenal insufficiency include weakness, anorexia, weight loss, and postural lightheadedness. Signs include postural hypotension and, in Addison's disease, hyperpigmentation (especially of skin creases and pressure points).

CLINICAL APPROACH.   Patients who have received steroids in doses greater than 7.5 mg of prednisone or its equivalent per day for at least 4 weeks should be considered potentially adrenally suppressed. These patients, as well as those suspected of adrenal insufficiency from other causes, should receive empiric corticosteroids perioperatively or undergo a cosyntropin (ACTH) stimulation test of adrenal reserve.

MANAGEMENT.   The usual cosyntropin stimulation test involves at baseline and a 60-minute plasma cortisol sample after the intramuscular or IV administration of 0.25 mg of cosyntropin. A normal response is a 60-minute level of at least 18 µg/dl with an increment from baseline of at least 7 µg/dl.

Perioperative steroid coverage for adrenal insufficiency is the same as for hypothyroid patients.

FOLLOW-UP.   During withdrawal of steroid coverage, patients should be followed closely for findings that suggest too rapid a taper, such as hypotension, nausea, or anorexia.

Cross-references: Screening for Thyroid Disease (Section 153), Common Thyroid Disorders (Section 156), Diabetes Mellitus (Section 157).

REFERENCES

1. Gavin LA. Management of diabetes mellitus during surgery. West J Med 1989;151:525–529.
    Excellent review of continuous IV insulin approach.

2. Goldman DR, Brown FH, Levy WK, et al. Medical Care of the Surgical Patient: A Problem-Oriented Approach to Management. Philadelphia: JB Lippincott, 1982.
    One of the best reviews of the subject.

3. White VA, Kumagai LF. Preoperative endocrine and metabolic considerations. Med Clin North Am 1979;63(6):1321–1334.
    Good general review of perioperative endocrine problems.

220 PREOPERATIVE HEMATOLOGIC PROBLEMS

Problem

C. SCOTT SMITH

HEMATOLOGIC LABORATORY SCREENING

EPIDEMIOLOGY.   Over 50% of preoperative hematologic laboratory tests are ordered without recognizable indications. Less than 0.25% reveal abnormalities that might influence perioperative management.

CLINICAL APPROACH AND MANAGEMENT.   Table 220–1 lists the indications for various hematologic screening tests.

TABLE 220–1. INDICATIONS FOR HEMATOLOGIC SCREENING TESTS

Indication	Type/Screen	Hemoglobin	Prothrombin Time/Partial Thromboplastin Time	Platelets	White Blood Count
Major surgical procedure	+				
Malignancy		+[1]		+[1]	
Hepatobiliary disease		+	+	+	
Malnutrition/malabsorption		+	+		
Renal disease		+	+	+	
History of bleeding		+	+	+	
Anticoagulants			+		
Infection		+		+	+
History of chemotherapy/immunosuppression		+		+	+
Systemic lupus erythematosus		+	+	+	+

[1]Hematologic malignancy.

TABLE 220–2. PERIOPERATIVE MANAGEMENT OF PATIENTS ON CHRONIC ANTICOAGULATION

Thromboembolic Risk	Hemorrhagic Risk		
	Low (*Dental Extraction, Soft Tissue Biopsy, Arteriography*)	*Intermediate* (*Most Surgeries*)	*High* (*Ophthalmologic Surgery, Neurosurgery*)
High Caged ball or disk[1] mitral prosthetic valve; dialysis patient with previous shunt or graft thrombosis; previous multiple thromboemboli	No modification of anticoagulation	Tight control:[3] Heparin off 6 hr preoperatively; resume heparin 12–24 hr postoperatively	Tight control:[3] Heparin off 6–12 hr preoperatively; Resume heparin 24–48 hr postoperatively

Intermediate		
Other prosthetic valves (e.g., St. Jude, Medtronic, and other valves in aortic position)	No modification of anticoagulation	Intermediate control:[4] To OR when PT within 2–3 sec of control; start heparin 12–24 hr postoperatively	Intermediate control:[4] To OR when PT normal; start heparin 24–48 hr postoperatively
Low			
Previous deep venous thrombosis/pulmonary embolus; transient ischemic attack/cerebrovascular accident; myocardial infarction	Varies[2]	Loose control:[5] to OR when PT within 2–3 sec	Loose control:[5] To OR when PT normal

[1]Bjork Shiley, Lillehei-Kaster, and other tilting disk and caged ball protheses.

[2]Manage as intermediate hemorrhagic risk if thrombotic event occurred in previous month. If thrombotic event occurred more than 1 month prior, stop anticoagulants.

[3]**Tight control**
1. Admit 2–4 days preoperatively.
2. Start heparin and stop warfarin.
3. Stop heparin preoperatively; resume postoperatively.
4. Resume warfarin when tolerating oral medications.
5. After prothrombin time (PT) therapeutic, overlap heparin and warfarin for 24 hr.
6. If bleeding problems occur, use low-molecular-weight dextran for 2–3 days to minimize thrombosis.

[4]**Intermediate control**
1. Stop warfarin 2–4 days preoperatively.
2. Proceed to surgery when PT is at desired level.
3. Start heparin postoperatively.
4–6. As for "tight control."

[5]**Loose control**
1. Stop warfarin 3–4 days preoperatively.
2. Proceed to surgery when PT is at desired level.
3. Restart warfarin 1–2 days postoperatively or when tolerating oral medications.

DISCONTINUING CHRONIC ANTICOAGULATION THERAPY PERIOPERATIVELY

MANAGEMENT.   The risks of hemorrhage or thromboembolism vary according to the type of surgery and the underlying indication for anticoagulation. Table 220–2 outlines the management of perioperative anticoagulation.

PROPHYLAXIS FOR VENOUS THROMBOEMBOLISM

EPIDEMIOLOGY.   The incidence of venous thromboembolism is highest (>50%) in patients following hip fractures, hip or knee arthroplasty, and acute spinal cord injury. This incidence is reduced 50% by prophylaxis. The risk is intermediate (20–35%) in many gynecologic procedures (especially if for a gynecological malignancy) or abdominal urologic procedures, and prophylaxis is still warranted. The risk is estimated at 5% to 25% in other major surgical procedures, and prophylaxis is not indicated.

Stasis, endothelial abnormality or damage, and hypercoagulable states increase the likelihood of thrombosis.

MANAGEMENT.   Most surgeries require only low-dose heparin. Table 220–3 outlines the management of prophylaxis for venous thrombosis, including many procedures for which hemorrhagic complications would be catastrophic (e.g., intracranial neurologic and many ophthalmologic procedures) and procedures that produce a high risk of thrombotic complications.

Cross-references: Painful and Swollen Calf (Section 131), Bleeding (Section 197), Chronic Anticoagulation (Section 203), Transfusion Therapy (Section 204).

TABLE 220–3.   PROPHYLAXIS FOR VENOUS THROMBOEMBOLISM

Most surgeries	Heparin 5000 units SQ b.i.d.-t.i.d.
High hemorrhagic risk	Pneumatic compression device
High thrombotic risk	Two-step warfarin: Starting 10 days preoperatively, keep prothrombin time (PT) 2–3 sec prolonged. Postoperatively, give approximately twice the preoperative dose to increase PT ratio to 1.5.
	or
	Adjusted dose heparin: Start 2 days preoperatively with 3500 units SQ t.i.d. Check activated partial thromboplastin time (APTT) 6 hr after AM dose and adjust up or down by 500–1000 units to keep APTT at 30–40 sec.
	or
	Dextran-40: 10 ml/kg as 12-hr IV infusion on the day of surgery. Follow with 7 ml/kg/day as constant infusion for 5 days. May exacerbate heart failure.
	or
	Pneumatic compression device.

REFERENCES

1. Becker DM. Venous thromboembolism. J Gen Intern Med 1986;1:402–411.
   Excellent review.

2. Cygan R, Waitzkin H. Stopping and restarting medications in the perioperative period. J Gen Intern Med 1987;2:270–283.
   Very good reference for handling all kinds of medications during the perioperative period (including anticoagulation).

3. Fellin FM, Murphy S. Perioperative evaluation of patients with hematologic disorders. In Merli GJ and Weitz FH, Eds., Medical Management of the Surgical Patient. WB Saunders, Philadelphia, 1992, pp 84–115.
   A very thorough review.

4. Kaplan EB, Sheiner LB, Boeckmann AJ, et al. The usefulness of preoperative laboratory screening. JAMA 1985;253(24):3576–3581.
   Good review of the indications for many laboratory tests.

5. Merli GJ, Martinez J. Prophylaxis for deep vein thrombosis and pulmonary embolism in the surgical patient. In Merli GJ and Weitz FH, Eds., Medical Management of the Surgical Patient. WB Saunders, Philadelphia, 1992, pp 66–83.
   Up-to-date with practical guidance on specific regimens.

221 PREOPERATIVE PULMONARY PROBLEMS

Problem

C. SCOTT SMITH

EPIDEMIOLOGY. Although definitions vary, pulmonary complications develop in 10% to 20% of patients following general surgery. Independent risk factors include cigarette smoking, established obstructive lung disease, age, and site of operation. The incidence is greatest for thoracic operation (60%), followed by surgery of the upper abdomen, lower abdomen, and extremities (<1%). Patients with obstructive lung disease undergoing general surgery have a 3% to 7% mortality. Other risk factors appear in Table 221–1. Spinal anesthesia does not result in a better outcome compared with general anesthesia.

CLINICAL APPROACH. No delay in surgery is necessary for patients without risk factors (see Table 221–1) who are not undergoing a high-risk procedure (upper abdominal or thoracic surgery).

A baseline chest radiograph is recommended in all patients who are scheduled for a high-risk operation, who have an abnormal chest examination, or

TABLE 221–1.   RISK FACTORS FOR POSTOPERATIVE PULMONARY COMPLICATIONS

Risk Factor	Likelihood Ratio
Definite	
Obstructive lung disease	3–4
Age > 70	3
Smoker	2–6
Probable	
Anesthesia > 3 hr	2
Obesity	?
Respiratory infection	?

who have any pulmonary risk factors (see Table 221–1). Measurement of pulmonary function and arterial oxygen saturation are advisable when multiple risk factors are present or if the chest radiograph is abnormal. A maximal voluntary ventilation (MVV) less than 50% predicted or forced expiratory volume in one second (FEV_1) less than 2 liters has a positive predictive value for pulmonary complications of 40% to 45% in thoracic and upper abdominal operations. Arterial hypoxemia ($Pao_2 < 50$ mm Hg) or hypercapnia ($Paco_2 > 44$ mm Hg) are relative contraindications to surgery.

If pulmonary resection is contemplated, pulmonary function tests are quite helpful in predicting outcome. Patients with an FEV_1 of more than 2 liters and MVV more than 50% predicted may generally proceed to surgery. If the FEV_1 is less than 2 liters or the MVV is less than 50% predicted, a lung ventilation or perfusion scan is obtained to predict the postresection FEV_1 (postoperative FEV_1 = the preoperative FEV_1 multiplied by the percentage of perfusion or ventilation to the lung that will remain after surgery). If the predicted postresection FEV is greater than 800 cc, the surgery may proceed, although the risk of perioperative mortality is approximately 15%. Values below 800 cc are essentially an absolute contraindication to resection.

MANAGEMENT.   Measures that appear to prevent perioperative pulmonary complications include smoking cessation (for at least 8 weeks), intensive use of bronchodilators pre- and postoperatively, chest physiotherapy (including postural drainage), and incentive spirometry training. Patients with steroid-responsive obstructive lung disease may also benefit from corticosteroids, although the benefits must be balanced against the risk of impaired wound healing. Antibiotics are indicated only in those with an active infection. Elective surgery should be postponed until a full course of antibiotics is completed.

Measures of little or no benefit include intermittent positive pressure breathing, expiratory maneuvers, or carbon dioxide–induced hypercapnia (which attempts to stimulate deep breathing).

FOLLOW-UP.   The patient should be followed carefully several days postoperatively for respiratory symptoms, fever, tachypnea, or changes in the lung examination. Expected physiologic changes, which include decreased vital capacity and FEV_1 of up to 50% (peaking around 4 days), decreased tidal volume, and decreased sigh frequency, may promote atelectasis, hypoxemia, and infection.

Cross-references: Smoking Cessation (Section 11), Obesity (Section 15), Dyspnea (Section 19), Pleuritic Chest Pain (Section 61), Cough and Sputum (Section 63), Lower Respiratory Infection (Section 67), Asthma and Chronic Obstructive Pulmonary Disease (Section 68), Pulmonary Function Testing (Section 69), Arterial Blood Gas (Section 71).

REFERENCES

1. Bartlett RH, Gazzaniga AB, Geraghty TR. Respiratory maneuvers to prevent postoperative pulmonary complications. JAMA 1973;224(7):1017–1021.
   Reviews expiratory maneuvers, carbon dioxide–induced hyperventilation, intermittent positive-pressure breathing (IPPB), and inspiratory maneuvers. Inspiratory maneuvers are most effective.

2. Gracey DR, Divertie MB, Didier EP. Preoperative pulmonary preparation of patients with chronic obstructive pulmonary disease. A prospective study. Chest 1979;76(2):123–129.
   Uncontrolled study of the use of cigarette cessation, IPPB-delivered bronchodilators, chest physiotherapy, theophylline, and expectorants; showed a 50% reduction in pulmonary complications from historical controls.

3. Mohr DN, Jett JR. Preoperative evaluation of pulmonary risk factors. J Gen Intern Med 1988;3:277–287.
   Excellent scientific review of all the available data.

INDEX

Note: Page numbers in *italics* refer to illustrations; page numbers followed by t refer to tables.